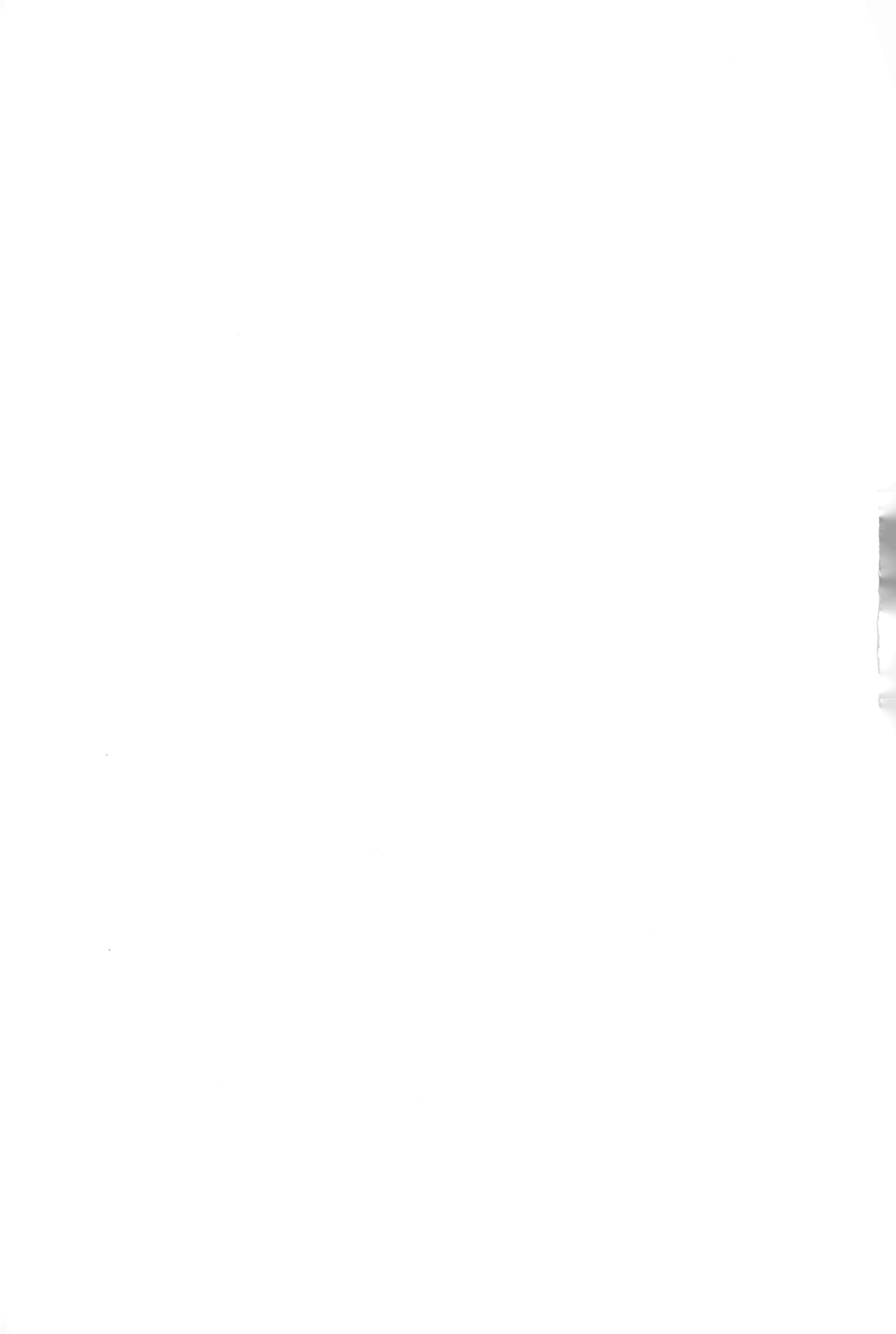

Genomics of Rare Hematologic Cancers

Genomics of Rare Hematologic Cancers

Editor

Francesc Solé

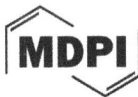

Basel • Beijing • Wuhan • Barcelona • Belgrade • Novi Sad • Cluj • Manchester

Editor
Francesc Solé
Institut de Recerca Contra la Leucèmia Josep Carreras
Barcelona
Spain

Editorial Office
MDPI
St. Alban-Anlage 66
4052 Basel, Switzerland

This is a reprint of articles from the Special Issue published online in the open access journal *Cancers* (ISSN 2072-6694) (available at: https://www.mdpi.com/journal/cancers/special_issues/rare_hematologic_cancers).

For citation purposes, cite each article independently as indicated on the article page online and as indicated below:

Lastname, A.A.; Lastname, B.B. Article Title. *Journal Name* **Year**, *Volume Number*, Page Range.

ISBN 978-3-0365-8956-5 (Hbk)
ISBN 978-3-0365-8957-2 (PDF)
doi.org/10.3390/books978-3-0365-8957-2

Cover image courtesy of Francesc Solé

© 2023 by the authors. Articles in this book are Open Access and distributed under the Creative Commons Attribution (CC BY) license. The book as a whole is distributed by MDPI under the terms and conditions of the Creative Commons Attribution-NonCommercial-NoDerivs (CC BY-NC-ND) license.

Contents

About the Editor vii

Preface ix

Silvia Ramos-Campoy, Anna Puiggros, Joanna Kamaso, Sílvia Beà, Sandrine Bougeon, María José Larráyoz, et al.
TP53 Abnormalities Are Underlying the Poor Outcome Associated with Chromothripsis in Chronic Lymphocytic Leukemia Patients with Complex Karyotype
Reprinted from: *Cancers* **2022**, *14*, 3715, doi:10.3390/cancers14153715 1

Marta Santiago, Alessandro Liquori, Esperanza Such, Ángel Zúñiga and José Cervera
The Clinical Spectrum, Diagnosis, and Management of GATA2 Deficiency
Reprinted from: *Cancers* **2023**, *15*, 1590, doi:10.3390/cancers15051590 19

Kunhwa Kim, Faustine Ong and Koji Sasaki
Current Understanding of DDX41 Mutations in Myeloid Neoplasms
Reprinted from: *Cancers* **2023**, *15*, 344, doi:10.3390/cancers15020344 35

Pamela Acha, Mar Mallo and Francesc Solé
Myelodysplastic Syndromes with Isolated del(5q): Value of Molecular Alterations for Diagnostic and Prognostic Assessment
Reprinted from: *Cancers* **2022**, *14*, 5531, doi:10.3390/cancers14225531 51

Ismail Elbaz Younes, Lubomir Sokol and Ling Zhang
Rosai–Dorfman Disease between Proliferation and Neoplasia
Reprinted from: *Cancers* **2022**, *14*, 5271, doi:10.3390/cancers14215271 65

Fernando Gallardo and Ramon M. Pujol
Genetics Abnormalities with Clinical Impact in Primary Cutaneous Lymphomas
Reprinted from: *Cancers* **2022**, *14*, 4972, doi:10.3390/cancers14204972 83

Alisa Förster, Melanie Decker, Brigitte Schlegelberger and Tim Ripperger
Beyond Pathogenic RUNX1 Germline Variants: The Spectrum of Somatic Alterations in RUNX1-Familial Platelet Disorder with Predisposition to Hematologic Malignancies
Reprinted from: *Cancers* **2022**, *14*, 3431, doi:10.3390/cancers14143431 99

Oscar González-López, Javier I. Muñoz-González, Alberto Orfao, IvánÁlvarez-Twose and Andrés C. García-Montero
Comprehensive Analysis of Acquired Genetic Variants and Their Prognostic Impact in Systemic Mastocytosis
Reprinted from: *Cancers* **2022**, *14*, 2487, doi:10.3390/cancers14102487 117

Eulàlia Genescà and Celia González-Gil
Latest Contributions of Genomics to T-Cell Acute Lymphoblastic Leukemia (T-ALL)
Reprinted from: *Cancers* **2022**, *14*, 2474, doi:10.3390/cancers14102474 143

Elizabeta A. Rojas and Norma C. Gutiérrez
Genomics of Plasma Cell Leukemia
Reprinted from: *Cancers* **2022**, *14*, 1594, doi:10.3390/cancers14061594 163

Claudia Fiñana, Noel Gómez-Molina, Sandra Alonso-Moreno and Laura Belver
Genomic and Epigenomic Landscape of Juvenile Myelomonocytic Leukemia
Reprinted from: *Cancers* **2022**, *14*, 1335, doi:10.3390/cancers14051335 177

David Oscier, Kostas Stamatopoulos, Amatta Mirandari and Jonathan Strefford
The Genomics of Hairy Cell Leukaemia and Splenic Diffuse Red Pulp Lymphoma
Reprinted from: *Cancers* **2022**, *14*, 697, doi:10.3390/cancers14030697 . . . . **197**

Juan José Rodríguez-Sevilla and Antonio Salar
Recent Advances in the Genetic of MALT Lymphomas
Reprinted from: *Cancers* **2022**, *14*, 176, doi:10.3390/cancers14010176 . . . . **221**

Oscar Molina, Alex Bataller, Namitha Thampi, Jordi Ribera, Isabel Granada, Pablo Velasco, et al.
Near-Haploidy and Low-Hypodiploidy in B-Cell Acute Lymphoblastic Leukemia: When Less Is Too Much
Reprinted from: *Cancers* **2022**, *14*, 32, doi:10.3390/cancers14010032 . . . . **245**

About the Editor

Francesc Solé

Dr. Francisco Solé is one of the world's leading authorities in Cytogenetics in Myelodysplastic Syndromes (MDS or MDS in English). He was involved in the recent IPSS-R and IPSS-M scoring systems at MDS. Dr. Solé is a reviewer for the following journals: American Journal of Hematology, Blood, The British Journal of Haematology, Cancers, Genes Chromosomes and Cancer, Haematologica, Leukemia, Leukemia Research, and Leukemia and Lymphoma. He is an associate professor at the Pompeu Fabra University (Barcelona, Spain), the University of Barcelona (UB) and the Autonomous University of Barcelona (Bellaterra, Spain). From 1996 to 2008, he was the coordinator of the Spanish Working Group on Cytogenetics in Hematology (GCECGH) of the SEHH (Spanish Society of Hematology and Hemotherapy). From 2004 to 2012, he was a member of the Eurogenest Hematology Quality Control Steering Committee. Since their creation, he has been a member of the Spanish Group of Myelodysplastic Syndromes (GESMD) and of the world MDS group, IWG-PM. In addition, since 2012, he has been a member of the ELN. Currently, he is the Scientific Coordinator of the Josep Carreras Leukemia Research Institute-ICO-GTiP Campus (Badalona), Coordinator of the Biological Sample Bank Unit for patients with hematological cancer, the Cytogenetics Unit and Microarray Unit, and Head of Group of the MDS Group. He is the author of more than 300 peer-reviewed publications and serves on multiple national committees and scientific advisory boards for numerous for-profit and non-profit organizations.

Preface

The aim of this Special Issue is to present the cytogenetic and genomic alterations that occur in the less prevalent hematologic cancers in order to determine their diagnostic and prognostic value. This Special Issue will present the main information to consider regarding the genetic diagnosis and prognosis of the rarest hematologic cancers.

Francesc Solé
Editor

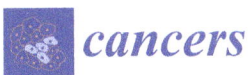

Article

TP53 Abnormalities Are Underlying the Poor Outcome Associated with Chromothripsis in Chronic Lymphocytic Leukemia Patients with Complex Karyotype

Silvia Ramos-Campoy [1,2,†], Anna Puiggros [1,2,*,†], Joanna Kamaso [1,2], Sílvia Beà [3,4], Sandrine Bougeon [5], María José Larráyoz [6], Dolors Costa [3,4], Helen Parker [7], Gian Matteo Rigolin [8], María Laura Blanco [9], Rosa Collado [10], Idoya Ancín [11], Rocío Salgado [12], Marco A. Moro-García [13], Tycho Baumann [3], Eva Gimeno [1,14], Carol Moreno [9], Marta Salido [1,2], Xavier Calvo [1,2], María José Calasanz [6], Antonio Cuneo [8], Florence Nguyen-Khac [15], David Oscier [16], Claudia Haferlach [17], Jonathan C. Strefford [7], Jacqueline Schoumans [5] and Blanca Espinet [1,2,*]

1. Molecular Cytogenetics and Hematological Cytology Laboratories, Pathology Department, Hospital del Mar, 08003 Barcelona, Spain; sramosca10@alumnes.ub.edu (S.R.-C.); jkamaso@imim.es (J.K.); egimenov@psmar.cat (E.G.); msalido@psmar.cat (M.S.); xcalvo@psmar.cat (X.C.)
2. Translational Research on Hematological Neoplasms Group, Cancer Research Program, Institut Hospital del Mar d'Investigacions Mèdiques (IMIM), 08003 Barcelona, Spain
3. Hematopathology Section, Department of Pathology, Hospital Clínic, Institut d'Investigacions Biomèdiques August Pi i Sunyer (IDIBAPS), University of Barcelona, 08036 Barcelona, Spain; sbea@clinic.cat (S.B.); dcosta@clinic.cat (D.C.); tychostephan.baumann@salud.madrid.org (T.B.)
4. Centro de Investigación Biomédica en Red de Cáncer (CIBERONC), 28029 Madrid, Spain
5. Oncogenomic Laboratory, Hematology Service, Lausanne University Hospital, 1011 Lausanne, Switzerland; sandrine.bougeon@chuv.ch (S.B.); jacqueline.schoumans@chuv.ch (J.S.)
6. Cytogenetics and Hematological Genetics Services, Department of Genetics, University of Navarra, 31008 Pamplona, Spain; mjlarra@unav.es (M.J.L.); mjcal@unav.es (M.J.C.)
7. Cancer Sciences, Faculty of Medicine, University of Southampton, Southampton SO16 6YD, UK; h.parker@soton.ac.uk (H.P.); jcs@soton.ac.uk (J.C.S.)
8. Hematology Section, St. Anna University Hospital, 44121 Ferrara, Italy; rglgmt@unife.it (G.M.R.); cut@unife.it (A.C.)
9. Department of Hematology, Hospital de la Santa Creu I Sant Pau, 08041 Barcelona, Spain; mlblanco@santpau.cat (M.L.B.); cmorenoa@santpau.cat (C.M.)
10. Department of Hematology, Consorcio Hospital General Universitario, 46014 Valencia, Spain; collado_ros@gva.es
11. Department of Hematology and Hemoterapia, Hospital Universitario Cruces, 48903 Bilbao, Spain; idoyamaria.ancinarteaga@osakidetza.eus
12. Cytogenetics Laboratory, Hematology Department, Fundación Jiménez Díaz, 28040 Madrid, Spain; rocio.salgado@quironsalud.es
13. Laboratory Medicine Department, Hospital Universitario Central de Asturias, 33011 Oviedo, Spain; marcoantonio.moro@sespa.es
14. Applied Clinical Research in Hematological Malignances, Cancer Research Program, Institut Hospital del Mar d'Investigacions Mèdiques (IMIM), 08003 Barcelona, Spain
15. Sorbonne University, Hematology Department, Hôpital Pitié-Salpêtrière, APHP, INSERM U1138, 75013 Paris, France; florence.nguyen-khac@aphp.fr
16. Department of Molecular Pathology, Royal Bournemouth Hospital, Bournemouth BH7 7DW, UK; david.oscier@sky.com
17. MLL Munich Leukemia Laboratory, 81377 Munich, Germany; claudia.haferlach@mll.com
* Correspondence: apuiggros@psmar.cat (A.P.); bespinet@psmar.cat (B.E.)
† These authors contributed equally to this work.

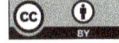

Simple Summary: Chromothripsis, a genomic event that generates massive chromosomal rearrangements, has been described in 1–3% of CLL patients and is associated with poor prognostic factors (e.g., *TP53* abnormalities and genomic complexity). However, previous studies have not assessed its role in CLL patients with complex karyotypes. Herein, we aimed to describe the genetic characteristics of 33 CLL patients with high genomic complexity and chromothripsis. Moreover, we analyzed the clinical impact of chromothripsis, comparing these patients against a cohort of 129 patients with complex karyotypes not presenting this catastrophic event. Nine cases were also assessed via the novel cytogenomic methodology known as optical genome mapping. We confirmed that this phenomenon is heterogeneous and associated with a shorter time to first treatment. Nonetheless, our findings suggested that *TP53* abnormalities, rather than chromothripsis itself, underlie the dismal outcome.

Abstract: Chromothripsis (cth) has been associated with a dismal outcome and poor prognosis factors in patients with chronic lymphocytic leukemia (CLL). Despite being correlated with high genome instability, previous studies have not assessed the role of cth in the context of genomic complexity. Herein, we analyzed a cohort of 33 CLL patients with cth and compared them against a cohort of 129 non-cth cases with complex karyotypes. Nine cth cases were analyzed using optical genome mapping (OGM). Patterns detected by genomic microarrays were compared and the prognostic value of cth was analyzed. Cth was distributed throughout the genome, with chromosomes 3, 6 and 13 being those most frequently affected. OGM detected 88.1% of the previously known copy number alterations and several additional cth-related rearrangements (median: 9, range: 3–26). Two patterns were identified: one with rearrangements clustered in the region with cth (3/9) and the other involving both chromothriptic and non-chromothriptic chromosomes (6/9). Cases with cth showed a shorter time to first treatment (TTFT) than non-cth patients (median TTFT: 2 m vs. 15 m; p = 0.013). However, when stratifying patients based on *TP53* status, cth did not affect TTFT. Only *TP53* maintained its significance in the multivariate analysis for TTFT, including cth and genome complexity defined by genomic microarrays (HR: 1.60; p = 0.029). Our findings suggest that *TP53* abnormalities, rather than cth itself, underlie the poor prognosis observed in this subset.

Keywords: chronic lymphocytic leukemia; genomic complexity; chromothripsis; *TP53*; genomic microarrays; optical genome mapping

1. Introduction

The therapeutic landscape for patients with chronic lymphocytic leukemia (CLL) has expanded with the emergence of new targeted agents. In this context, genomic complexity has become increasingly important due to its controversial role as a predictor of response to therapy. It has been associated with shorter survival and worse response rates in patients treated with standard chemoimmunotherapy [1–4], yet its role in patients receiving new treatment modalities is still not fully established. In the initial trials performed with BTK and BCL2 inhibitors (i.e., Ibrutinib, Acalabrutinib, Venetoclax), it appeared to be an independent prognostic factor [5–9]. However, this negative impact has been controversial in recent trials using different therapeutic combinations and in those previous studies after a longer follow-up [10–13]. Even though genomic complexity has been mainly defined by the detection of complex karyotypes (CK) by chromosome banding analysis (CBA), genomic microarrays (GM) are also a valuable tool to assess genomic complexity in CLL [14,15]. In addition, optical genome mapping (OGM) has arisen as a promising cytogenomic methodology for whole genome screening, able to detect all types of structural and copy number alterations (CNA) at a higher resolution than traditional cytogenetic methods. Recently, several groups have proven that OGM is a useful technique to detect a wide range of clinically significant cytogenomic abnormalities in different hematological neoplasms [16–19].

The emergence of GM and other high-resolution molecular techniques, such as next-generation sequencing, has allowed the identification of massive genomic alterations characterized by the occurrence of multiple genomic rearrangements, often generated in a single catastrophic event. These processes are globally referred to as chromoanagenesis and include chromothripsis, chromoanasynthesis and chromoplexy [20,21]. Chromothripsis (cth) (Greek, "chromo" for chromosome; "thripsis" for shattering into pieces) is a unique catastrophic event in which tens to hundreds of genomic fragments are shattered and randomly stitched together due to the subsequent erroneous repair mechanisms, producing highly derivative chromosomes. This process was initially described in a CLL patient as the presence of ≥10 oscillating switches between two or three copy number states in one or a few chromosomes [22]. Nonetheless, some authors also considered those with at least seven copy number switches to be cth events [23–25]. Several models have been proposed in order to explain its origin, including chromosome pulverization within a micronucleus, premature chromosome condensation or fragmentation of dicentric chromosomes during breakage–fusion–bridge cycles, among others [26–28]. However, the mechanisms underlying the formation of these complex patterns are still unknown. Its prevalence is highly variable and ranges between 2 to almost 100% among different tumors [29–31]. In CLL patients, cth prevalence is low (1–3% in unselected cohorts), and most studies are limited to a small number of cases [24,32]. Globally, reported cases present great heterogeneity in terms of the type and number of structural variants but also in the genomic regions and chromosomes affected. Nonetheless, this phenomenon preferentially occurs in certain chromosomes (2, 3, 6, 8, 9, 11, 13 and 17), and some authors have suggested a potential role of genes located in the recurrently abnormal regions in cth development [22–25,31–37]. In addition, no detailed comparison between patterns observed in chromothriptic chromosomes detected by GM or NGS and their corresponding karyotype has been performed to date. As for its clinical impact, it has been related to *TP53* abnormalities (found in approximately 70–80%) and a shorter time to first treatment and overall survival [23–25,32]. Nevertheless, the assessment of cth is not included in the International Workshop on CLL guidelines [38]. It is noteworthy that although it is known that cth is frequently found in the context of complex genomes, none of the aforementioned studies explored the impact of the overall genomic complexity on the evolution of these cases. In this regard, our group recently reported a strong association between cth and CK and the poor prognosis associated with cth, even within the CK subset [15]. However, the impact of *TP53* status and other clinico-biological characteristics in these patients with cth merits further exploration.

The aim of the present study was to describe the clinical and genomic characteristics of a cohort of 33 CLL patients with patterns of cth detected by GM, especially focusing on the relationship of cth with the overall genomic complexity. Furthermore, we compared cth cases with a cohort of non-chromothriptic CLL cases with CK to elucidate whether the presence of these highly complex patterns could have a negative effect on survival in this particular subgroup. Finally, we analyzed nine cases using OGM to determine the utility of this novel technique in the identification of cth.

2. Materials and Methods

2.1. Patient Cohort

A total of 162 CLL patients with genomic complexity detected by GM were selected. Among them, 33 showed patterns of cth by GM. The remaining 129 cases, which also showed CK by CBA (≥3 abnormalities in the same cell clone) but did not display cth, were considered as the control group for the comparison of clinical and biological characteristics [15]. All patients had CBA and GM results available at diagnosis or prior to treatment. Demographic, clinical and biological characteristics are summarized in Table 1. Thirty patients with cth and the control cohort were selected from a previous work from our group [15]. The three additional cases with chromothripsis were identified in another study from our group [39].

Table 1. Baseline characteristics of patients at diagnosis and last follow-up.

	Chromothripsis n = 33; n (%)	Control Group n = 129; n (%)	p-Value
Gender			
Men	23 (69.7%)	93 (72.1%)	0.785
Median age at diagnosis	66 years [33–91]	69 years [37–96]	0.177
Complex karyotype by CBA	30 (90.9%)	129 (100%)	0.008
3–4 abnormalities	7 (23.3%)	74 (57.4%)	
≥5 abnormalities	23 (76.7%)	55 (42.6%)	0.001
Stage at diagnosis			
MBL	1 (3.0%)	1 (0.8%)	0.367
CLL	32 (97.0%)	128 (99.2%)	
Binet A	16/30 (53.3%)	66/109 (60.6%)	0.532
Binet B/C	14/30 (46.7%)	43/109 (39.4%)	
Common CLL genomic aberrations *			
del(13)(q14)	19 (57.6%)	80 (62.0%)	0.641
Trisomy 12	1 (3.0%)	26 (20.2%)	0.018
del(11)(q22q23)	9 (27.3%)	42 (32.6%)	0.560
Aberrations in *TP53*	23 (69.7%)	49/127 (38.6%) **	0.001
del(17)(p13)	22 (66.7%)	45 (34.9%)	0.001
TP53 mutation	13/31 (41.9%)	32/119 (26.9%)	0.104
Unmutated IGHV	23/31 (74.2%)	71/110 (64.5%)	0.314
Median follow-up [range] ***	28 months [0–160]	33 months [1–160]	0.490
Time from diagnosis to cytogenetic study	1 month [0–298]	0 months [0–129]	0.163
Treatment ***			
Treated patients ^	29 (87.9%)	86 (66.7%)	0.017
Median time to first treatment [95% CI]	2 months [0–6]	15 months [9–21]	0.013
Survival ***			
Median overall survival [95% CI]	64 months [16–112]	90 months [59–121]	0.132

* Deletions and trisomy detected by FISH and/or genomic microarrays. ** Cases in which *TP53* mutation screening was not performed and FISH and/or genomic microarrays were negative for deletion were not considered. *** Data regarding treatment and follow-up from the control group were updated with respect to the previous publication. ^ Patients treated during the follow-up of the study. All samples used for the analysis, except one, were collected prior to treatment. Abbreviations: MBL = monoclonal B-cell lymphocytosis, CI = confidence interval.

2.2. Genomic Microarray Analyses

DNA was extracted from whole peripheral blood (PB) (n = 7; 21.2%), PB mononuclear cells (PBMCs) (n = 8; 24.2%), PB CD19+ purified cells (n = 13; 39.4%) or from bone marrow samples (n = 5; 15.2%) obtained no more than one year after CBA (median: 0 months; range: 0–12). Only DNA that fulfilled the required quality controls was amplified, labelled and hybridized using different genomic microarray platforms according to the manufacturers' protocols [ThermoFisher Scientific (n = 25; 75.8%), Agilent (n = 5; 15.2%) and Illumina (n = 3; 9.0%)] (Table S1). The number of abnormalities was recorded as previously described [15]. Chromothripsis was defined by the presence of ≥7 oscillating switches between two or three copy number states on an individual chromosome [23–25]. Coordinates were given according to the annotations of genome version GRCh37/hg19.

2.3. Optical Genome Mapping

For each sample, a minimum of 1.5 million PBMCs were used to extract ultra-high molecular weight (UHMW) DNA, following the manufacturer's instructions (Bionano Prep Frozen Cells DNA Isolation Protocol, Bionano Genomics, San Diego, CA, USA). Then,

UHMW DNA was enzymatically labeled in a sequence-specific manner using the Bionano Prep Direct Label and Stain (DLS) Protocol (Bionano Genomics). The molecules obtained, labeled around 15 times per 100 Kbp, were cleaned up and loaded onto a Saphyr chip and imaged via the Saphyr instrument (Bionano Genomics). In the chip, molecules were linearized in nanochannels by electrophoresis, and multiple cycles were run to reach an average genome coverage of $300\times$ (approximately 1300 Gb of data per sample). Imaged molecules $\geq$150 Kbp were analyzed using the rare variant pipeline (RVP) included in Bionano Solve software (v.3.5, Bionano Genomics, San Diego, CA, USA) and visualized in Bionano Access software (v1.6, Bionano Genomics, San Diego, CA, USA). The RVP included two algorithms: a structural variant (SV) analysis, based on the comparison of the labeling pattern against a reference assembly (hg19), and a tool to call large CNA inferred from the coverage of labels detected in each genomic interval. Default recommended confidence scores and an OGM control sample dataset provided by Bionano were used to pre-filter the abnormalities initially called by the software. The cut-off was set at 100 Kbp for SVs and 500 Kbp for CNA. Moreover, OGM results were manually reviewed to merge segmented CNA and discard variants found as benign polymorphisms in the Database of Genomic Variants (http://dgv.tcag.ca/dgv/app/home, accessed on 7 March 2022), SVs found to be duplicated in the results and low-quality translocation calls. Finally, the abnormalities detected by OGM in each patient were recorded and those involving chromothriptic regions were compared to the results previously obtained by GM and CBA techniques.

2.4. Whole Chromosome FISH Painting

Whole chromosome FISH painting (WCP) was performed in 6/9 cases analyzed by OGM to validate some selected cytogenomic abnormalities. Whole chromosome painting probes (MetaSystems, Altlussheim, Germany) for chromosomes 1, 2, 3, 6, 8, 9, 11, 13, 15, 17, 19 and Y were used. Chromosomes were counterstained with 4′,6′-diamidino-2-phenylindole (DAPI). FISH signals were observed under a fluorescence microscope in order to confirm or discard novel rearrangements revealed by OGM.

2.5. Statistical Analyses

Descriptive statistics were used to provide frequency distributions of discrete variables, while statistical measures were used to provide median values and ranges for quantitative variables. Groups were compared using Chi-square or Fisher exact tests for discrete variables and the Mann–Whitney U test for continuous variables. Time to first treatment (TTFT), the primary end-point of the study, was calculated from the date of cytogenetic study to the date of first treatment or last follow-up, whereas overall survival (OS) was defined from date of cytogenetic study to last follow-up or death. The Kaplan–Meier method was used to estimate the distribution of TTFT and OS. Comparisons among patient subgroups were performed via the Log-rank test. One patient with cth was excluded from survival analyses for having previously received treatment. A multivariate analysis using the Cox proportional hazards regression model was used to assess the independent prognostic impact on TTFT. Statistical analyses were performed using SPSS v.23 software (SPSS Inc., Chicago, IL, USA) and R v3.5.2. p-values < 0.05 were considered statistically significant.

3. Results

3.1. Identification of Chromothripsis Patterns by Genomic Microarrays

A total of 33 patients with cth detected by GM were included. Even though the majority of patients displayed cth in only one chromosome (25/33; 75.6%), eight patients showed complex patterns in several chromosomes (range: 2–4). Among the 46 chromothriptic events detected, 25 (54.3%) included changes that alternated between two copy number states, mostly between one and two copies, resulting in discontinuous deletions of several fragments. In 19/46 (41.3%) events, the oscillations involved both gains and losses, while in 2/46 (4.4%), the rearrangements implied only gains of chromosomal material. Furthermore, these oscillations in the copy number state were located either focally, involving only one chromosome arm, or throughout the whole chromosome (n = 17 and 29, respectively). Interestingly, no differences were observed between the patterns found in those chromothriptic events displaying 7–9 oscillating switches (n = 16) and those with ≥10 switches (n = 30) (Table S2). Cth was found in almost all chromosomes, with the most frequently involved chromosomes being 3, 6 and 13 (five cases each) (Figure S1). Of note, three of the five cases with cth in chromosome 3 carried a deletion of the 3p21.31 locus, which includes the *SETD2*, *CDC25A*, *MAP4*, *FBXW12* and *ATRIP* genes. As for cases with cth in chromosome 6, three of them displayed deletion of 6q21, which includes the *FOXO3a* gene. Regarding cth in chromosome 13, all had the 13q14 CLL common deleted region, which involved the *DLEU1* and *DLEU2* genes as well as the microRNAs miR-16-1 and miR-15a, with several additional deletions throughout the whole chromosome arm (Table S3).

In addition, cth patterns detected by GM were compared to the chromosomal aberrations found in the karyotype to assess whether CBA could suggest the presence of this phenomenon. In most of the chromothriptic events (15/46; 32.6%), the presence of multiple losses detected by GM was reported as monosomies by CBA. Notably, these were accompanied by chromosome markers or additional material of unknown origin, which could explain the apparent loss of the entire chromosome. Moreover, 24/46 (52.2%) of the chromosomes involved had different unbalanced structural aberrations, including unbalanced translocations (12/46; 26.1%), which might suggest the involvement of other chromosomes in the formation of cth, additional material of unknown origin (5/46; 10.9%) and single deletions (7/46; 15.2%). Unexpectedly, seven chromosomes with cth did not show any aberration by CBA. Nonetheless, in one of these cases, the karyotype was normal, suggesting non-division of the tumor clone, while in 6/7 cases, other abnormalities in different chromosomes were detected (Table S4 and Figure S2).

3.2. Detection of Different Chromothripsis Patterns by Optical Genome Mapping

Nine patients were analyzed using OGM. This methodology detected almost all the CNA related to cth previously visualized by GM (74/84; 88.1%), showing a high concordance in size and coordinates (Table S5). Remarkably, it also allowed the identification of several rearrangements involving chromothriptic regions (median: 9, range: 3–26), including intra-chromosomal (median: 6, range: 3–12) and inter-chromosomal translocations (median: 5, range: 0–14). Overall, two patterns of rearrangements could be observed. First, in 3/9 cases, the translocations identified by OGM only clustered in the cth region. These findings were in accordance with CBA and FISH results in two of the patients with an abnormal karyotype (cases #8 and #9 in Table S5). In particular, in one patient showing focal cth-related rearrangements on chromosome 6 (case #9), whole chromosome FISH painting (WCP) confirmed the presence of material from this chromosome only in the whole abnormal der(6) and in its normal counterpart (Figure 1A). In the second patient (case #8), OGM rearrangements were also limited to chromosome 6 but CBA identified an unbalanced t(6;19)(q12;p13) that was not detected by OGM, probably due to the limitations of this technique in the detection of abnormalities involving telomeric regions (Figure 1B). Further WCP analyses could not be performed on the third case (case #32), as cells from this patient did not yield abnormal metaphases for CBA. Notably, the three cases with clustered cth-related rearrangements displayed cth in chromosome 6. Notwithstanding, the abnormalities involved were very heterogeneous among these three cases and a commonly deleted region could not be identified. Only small deleted fragments (range: 0.64–2.83 Mb) were common between case #8 and the two remaining cases (cases #9 and #32), with no known gene included (Figure S3).

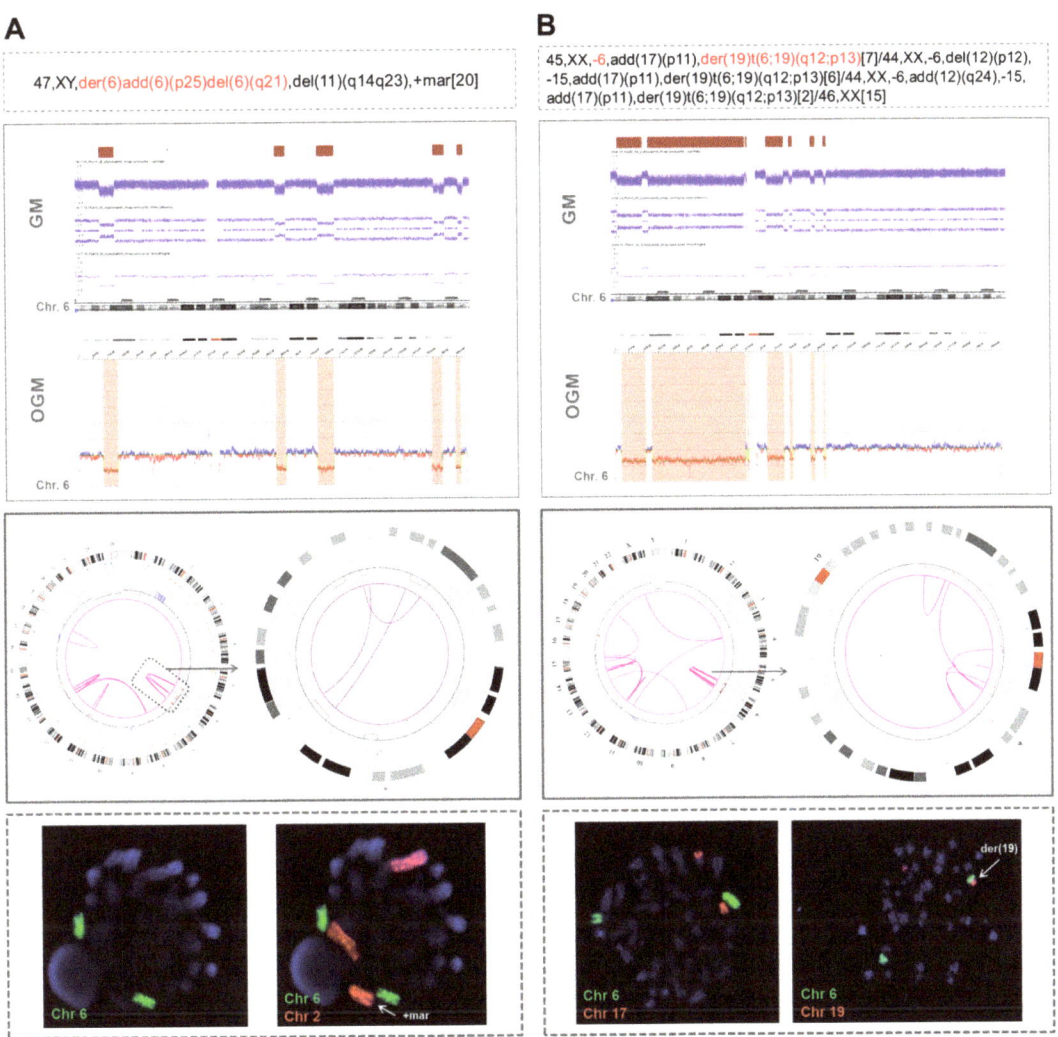

Figure 1. Two examples of cases analyzed by optical genome mapping showing only intra-chromosomal chromothripsis-related rearrangements. (**A**) A patient with chromothripsis in chromosome 6 in which OGM showed the presence of three intra-chromosomal translocations (case #9). When whole chromosome FISH painting (WCP) was performed, two green signals corresponding to chromosome 6 were observed, confirming the presence of material from this chromosome in the one initially reported as "der(6)add(6)(p25)del(6)(q21)" and in its normal counterpart. To ensure that this metaphase was abnormal, chromosome 2 was also stained, since both GM and OGM detected a duplication of 2p. WCP confirmed that the duplicated 2p was the marker chromosome found by CBA. (**B**) Patient with chromothripsis in chromosome 6 in which CBA identified a monosomy 6 and an unbalanced t(6;19)(q12;p13) (case #8). OGM revealed some rearrangements clustered in chromosome 6, but it did not detect this translocation. It was probably not called by OGM due to the involvement of the telomeric region of chromosome 19, a highly repetitive region in which the OGM detection of structural variants is known to be limited. The hybridization pattern obtained by WCP confirmed the presence of this translocation, since two different signals (orange and green), corresponding to both chromosomes, could be observed together but without showing a mixing of these signals, which

suggests that they rearranged after the process underlying chromothripsis. The abnormalities detected by CBA in chromosomes with chromothripsis are highlighted in red in the karyotype. Chromosome views show the comparison of the CNA profiles identified by GM and OGM in the chromothriptic chromosomes. The Circos plot represents the abnormalities identified by OGM for the whole genome (on the left) and the chromothriptic chromosome involved in this process (on the right). Different layers show, from outer to inner, cytobands of different chromosomes, structural variants (including deletions, duplications, inversions and insertions), copy number alterations and rearrangements, which are represented by lines joining the chromosomes involved.

Second, in 6/9 cases, OGM revealed the presence of rearrangements between the chromothriptic chromosome and other non-chromothriptic chromosomes (Figure 2).

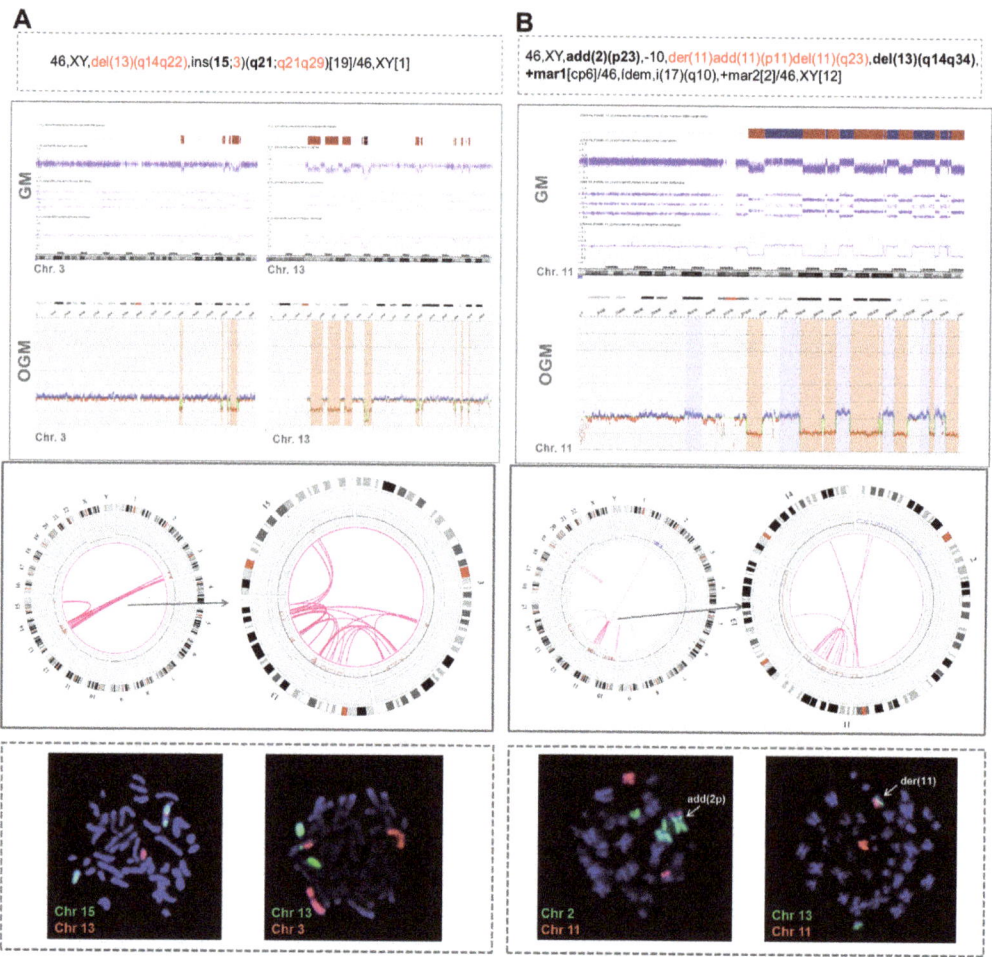

Figure 2. Two examples of cases with chromothripsis analyzed by optical genome mapping showing rearrangements between chromothriptic and non-chromothriptic chromosomes. (**A**) Patient with chromothripsis in chromosomes 3 and 13 (case #31). OGM detected 10 rearrangements between chromosomes 3 and 13 and four rearrangements between chromosomes 13 and 15. Whole chromosome FISH painting (WCP) revealed the presence of material from both chromosomes 3 and 13 inserted in chromosome 15. (**B**) Patient with chromothripsis in chromosome 11 (case #17). OGM revealed the presence of revealed the presence of

intra-chromosomal translocations and several additional rearrangements involving chromosomes 2, 13 and 14. Notably, t(2;11) and t(11;13) were validated by WCP. Conversely, despite showing only one line in the Circos plot, three parallel t(11;14) were identified by OGM and could not be validated by WCP. However, they could not be ruled out with certainty as true translocations since the rearranged fragment located between the breakpoints was very small and could be missed due to the low resolution of the technique. The abnormalities found by CBA in chromosomes with chromothripsis are highlighted in red in the karyotype. Additional chromosomes associated with chromothriptic events are highlighted in bold. Chromosome views show the comparison of the CNA profiles identified by GM and OGM in the chromothriptic chromosomes. The Circos plot represents the abnormalities identified by OGM for the whole genome (on the left) and for chromothriptic and non-chromothriptic chromosomes involved in this process (on the right). Different layers show, from outer to inner, cytobands of different chromosomes, structural variants (including deletions, duplications, inversions and insertions), copy number alterations and rearrangements, which are represented by lines joining the chromosomes involved.

These rearrangements involved 1 to 6 partners. In one case (case #16), 28 novel translocations were observed along the genome, leading to a very highly complex profile, which could suggest the presence of another catastrophic phenomenon known as chromoplexy (Figure 3). OGM results were compared with CBA data to see whether some of these rearrangements could also be detected in the karyotype. Interestingly, CBA could identify the translocations revealed by OGM in only two cases (cases #2 and #31 in Table S5). Nonetheless, most of the non-chromothriptic chromosomes with novel translocations revealed by OGM were altered, displaying either monosomies together with marker chromosomes or carrying deletions or additional material of unknown origin. Likewise, both GM and OGM also detected CNA in the breakpoints of these non-chromothriptic chromosomes related to chromothriptic events. Several genes were found in the breakpoints. However, none of the novel translocations or genes involved in the breakpoints were common among them (Table S5). Of note, WCP was carried out in six cases in order to validate the rearrangements found by OGM. Most of the novel translocations were confirmed, suggesting the involvement of other chromosomes in the development of cth. Only three new rearrangements could not be validated by WCP (t(11;14) in case #17 in Table S5). However, caution should be taken since the rearranged fragment could be missed due to the limited resolution of the WCP technique (Figure 2B).

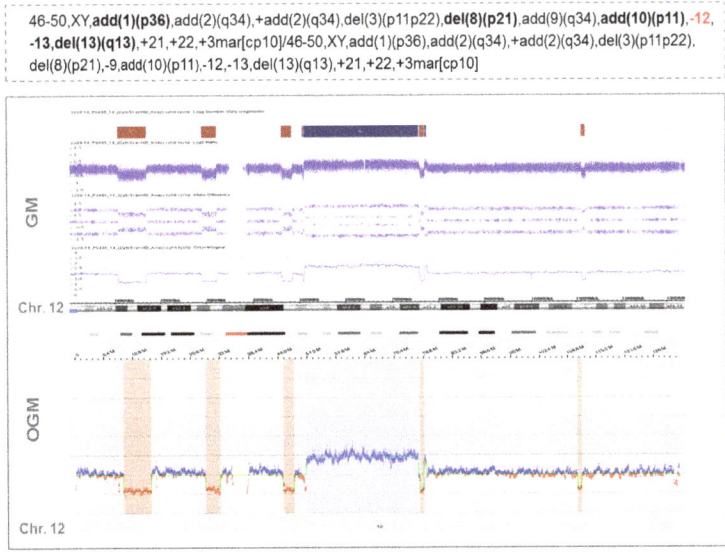

Figure 3. *Cont.*

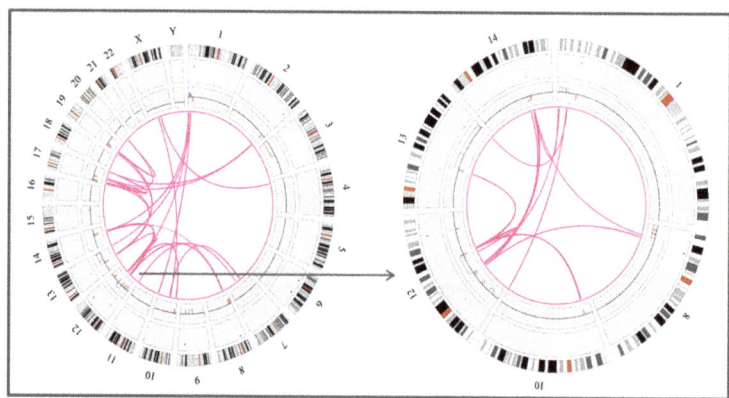

Figure 3. Example of a case with chromothripsis that shows multiple rearrangements with other chromosomes when analyzed by optical genome mapping. Overall, the karyotype of this patient presented a high complexity, with several bits of additional material found in different chromosomes and a few chromosome markers (case #16). Chromosome 12 displayed monosomy by CBA (highlighted in red in the karyotype) but when analyzed by GM and OGM, this chromosome showed an identical pattern of chromothripsis, with >10 switches between 2–3 copy number states. In addition, OGM identified several rearrangements among different chromosomes, as shown in the Circos plot depicted at the bottom of the figure. This highly complex profile could be associated with another catastrophic phenomenon known as chromoplexy, characterized by the presence of multiple chained translocations. Those additional chromosomes associated with chromothriptic events are highlighted in bold in the karyotype.

3.3. Association of Chromothripsis with Other Clinical Characteristics and Prognostic Impact

Clinical and biological features of patients with cth were compared between the different chromothriptic patterns observed. In the total cohort, 8/33 (24.2%) cases showed cth patterns in more than one chromosome. Among them, the majority (7/8; 87.5%) presented a high complexity, with ≥10 switches in at least one of the chromosomes involved, while only 1/8 (12.5%) displayed patterns with 7–9 switches. Conversely, patients with only one chromothriptic chromosome showed a similar frequency of patterns constituted by 7–9 (10/25; 40%) and ≥10 (15/25; 60%) switches. However, when comparing the abnormalities detected by CBA in both subgroups, no differences could be observed (median: 6 abn. [range: 0–16] in patients with one affected chromosome vs. 7.5 [range: 2–11] in those with >1 chromosome; $p = 0.481$). Likewise, no significant differences could be found among both subgroups in terms of gender, age, IGHV status or frequency of deletions and/or mutations in *TP53* (del/mut*TP53*) or del11q22q23 (*ATM*) (data not shown). Then, in the nine patients studied by OGM, clinical characteristics were compared between patients with only intra-chromosomal cth-related rearrangements and those with involvement of both chromothriptic and non-chromothriptic chromosomes. Overall, both subgroups were similar in gender (66.7% men in both groups), age (median: 67 vs. 66 years; $p = 0.362$), IGHV status (2/2, 100% vs. 5/6, 83.3%; $p = 1.000$) or frequency of del/mut*TP53* (66.7% vs. 50%; $p = 1.000$) or del(11q) (33.3% in both groups). However, the median number of abnormalities was higher in those patients with rearrangements involving non-chromothriptic chromosomes compared with those with clustered rearrangements. These differences were found when the number of abnormalities was recorded both by CBA (median: 8.5 [range: 2–16] vs. 0, 3 and 6 abnormalities, respectively) and GM (median: 19.5 [range: 11–30] vs. 15 [range: 10–15], respectively). Notwithstanding, it is important to note that statistical conclusions cannot be drawn from such a small subset of patients studied by OGM. Next, we aimed to determine whether the number of switches in the copy number state, 7–9 or ≥10, could have different impacts on the outcome of patients with cth. In this regard, patients having only 7–9 switches were compared to those with at least one cth event comprising ≥10. No significant differences were observed for TTFT between these two subgroups (median TTFT: 2 m vs. 2 m; p = 0.924) (Figure 4). Therefore, they were considered a unique group for subsequent analyses.

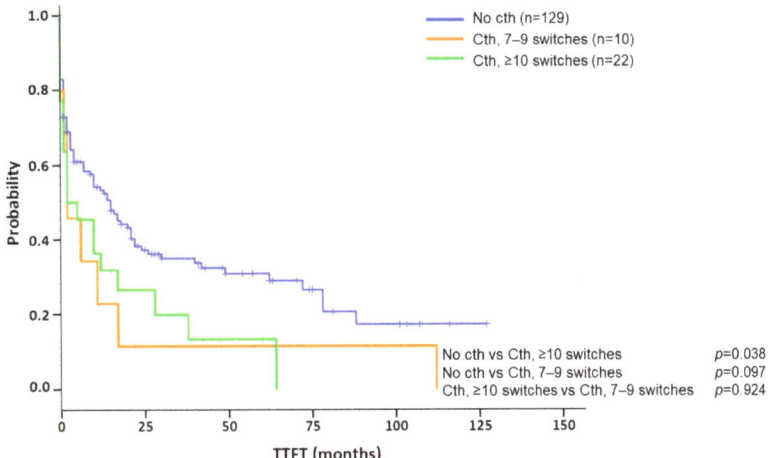

Figure 4. Kaplan–Meier plots for time to first treatment (TTFT) based on the presence of chromothripsis and the number of oscillating switches found in chromothripsis patterns. Kaplan–Meier estimation for TTFT in patients with 7–9 switches between 2–3 copy number states and ≥10 switches between 2–3 copy number states compared to a cohort of CLL cases carrying a complex karyotype (CK) without chromothripsis (cth). Of note, patients were classified into the "Cth ≥ 10 switches" group if they showed at least one chromothripsis event with these characteristics.

Concerning the prognostic impact of cth, patients included in the present series were compared to an aggressive cohort of CLL patients carrying CK without cth (Table 1) [15]. In this context, cth had a negative impact on TTFT compared with the control group (median TTFT: 2 m vs. 15 m; p = 0.013) (Figure 5A). Likewise, cases with cth showed a tendency towards a shorter OS (median OS: 64 m vs. 90 m; p = 0.205) (Figure 5B).

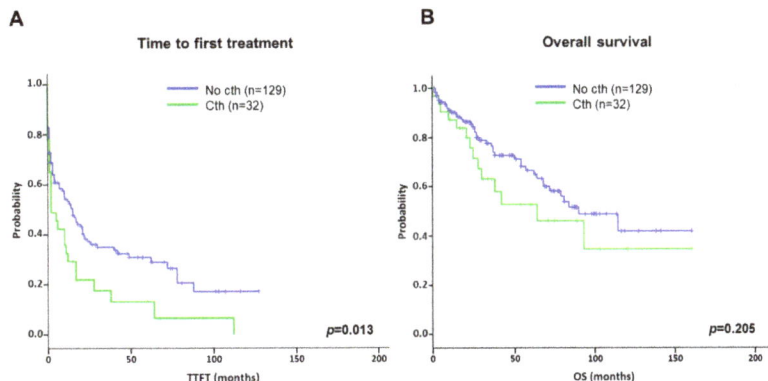

Figure 5. Kaplan–Meier plots for time to first treatment (TTFT) and overall survival (OS) based on the presence of chromothripsis. Kaplan–Meier estimation for TTFT (**A**) and OS (**B**) in patients with chromothripsis (Cth; including cases with 7–9 and ≥10 switches) compared to a cohort of CLL cases carrying complex karyotype (CK) without chromothripsis (No cth).

In addition, cth was associated with high genomic complexity and other genomic poor prognostic factors. Particularly, 30/33 patients carried a CK by CBA, with 23 (76.7%) cases having more than five abnormalities. The three non-CK cases by CBA showed genomic complexity as GM identified several abnormalities (median: 10; range: 10–24), with at least three of them ≥5 Mb (range: 3–6). In addition, unmutated IGHV (U-IGHV) and del(11q) were found at frequencies similar to the control group, which is known to be enriched in these poor prognostic markers (74.2% vs. 64.5%, p = 0.314, for U-IGHV; 27.3% vs. 32.6%, p = 0.560, for del(11q)). In contrast, patients with cth had a higher frequency of del/mut*TP53* than the control group (69.7% vs. 38.6%; p = 0.001). Of note, when patients were categorized according to their *TP53* status, cth did not significantly affect TTFT (del/mut*TP53* group, n = 72, median TTFT: 4 m vs. 2 m, p = 0.242, for non-cth and cth, respectively; WT *TP53* group, n = 87, median TTFT: 20 m vs. 17 m, p = 0.486, for non-cth and cth, respectively) (Figure 6).

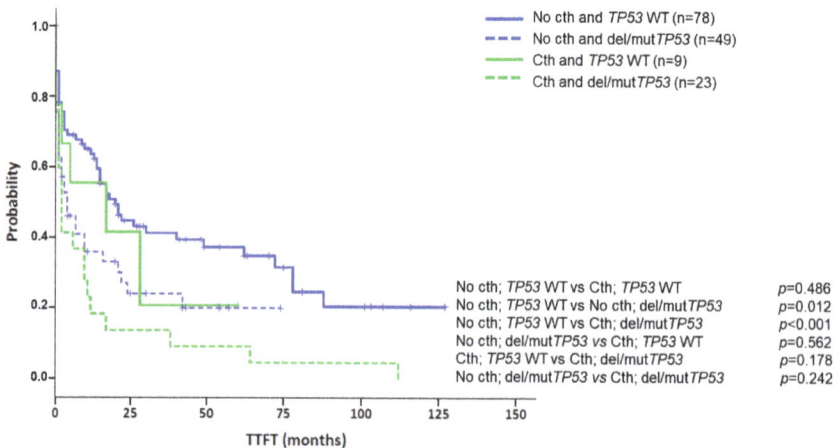

Figure 6. Kaplan–Meier plots for time to first treatment (TTFT) based on the presence of chromothripsis and abnormalities in *TP53* (deletions and/or mutations). Patients were classified according to the presence of chromothripsis (cth) and within each group (No cth vs. Cth), TTFT was assessed based on the presence of aberrations in *TP53* (deletions and/or mutations).

On the other hand, no significant differences were observed based on IGHV status or del(11q) for TTFT in the whole cohort (Table 2) and among patients with cth (Cth group, n = 30, median TTFT: 1 m vs. 6 m, p = 0.412, for mutated-IGHV and U-IGHV, respectively; Cth group, n = 32, median TTFT: 6 m vs. 2 m, p = 0.079, for non-del(11q) vs. del(11q), respectively). Notably, results from the mutated IGHV subset should be taken with caution since 6/8 cases also carried del/mut*TP53*. Therefore, the tendency towards a shorter TTFT could be attributed to the confounding effects of *TP53*. In the multivariate analysis for TTFT, including genome complexity defined by GM, *TP53* status and cth, only the presence of del/mut*TP53* retained significance (Table 2).

Table 2. Univariate and multivariate analysis for time to first treatment (TTFT).

Variable	Univariate Analysis *		Multivariate Analysis	
	Median TTFT in Months (95% CI)	p-Value	Hazard Ratio (95% CI)	p-Value
GM				
Intermediate-GC vs. low-GC	21 (4–38) vs. 17 (12–22)	0.941	0.91 (0.53–1.56)	0.719
High-GC vs. low-GC	3 (0–6) vs. 17 (12–22)	0.006	1.45 (0.82–2.57)	0.205
del/mutTP53	3 (1–5)	<0.001	1.60 (1.05–2.43)	0.029
U-IGHV	10 (3–17)	0.317	NA	NA
del(11)(q22q23)	14 (7–21)	0.614	NA	NA
Chromothripsis	2 (0–6)	0.013	1.21 (0.76–1.93)	0.422

* In comparison with the CK cohort extracted from Ramos-Campoy et al., 2022. Abbreviations: GM = genomic microarrays, GC = genomic complexity, low-GC = 0–2 copy number alterations (CNA) detected by genomic microarrays, intermediate-GC = 3–4 CNA, high-GC = ≥5 CNA, U-IGHV = CLL with unmutated IGHV, CI = confidence interval, NA = not assessed.

4. Discussion

Several works have focused on the study of cth in different types of hematological neoplasms and solid tumors due to its potential role in cancer onset and progression. In CLL, limited numbers of cases have been reported, and they were mainly associated with poor prognostic factors, such as abnormal *TP53* and genomic complexity and a dismal outcome (Table S6). Strikingly, none of the studies published explored the relationship between cth and overall genomic complexity. To the best of our knowledge, this is the largest cohort of CLL with cth assessed in the context of genomic complexity. Herein, an extensive study of the cytogenomic aberrations observed by genomic microarrays was performed, including a comparison with CBA results and an in-depth analysis with novel optical genome mapping technology.

Cth in CLL is highly heterogeneous in terms of the type and number of structural variants, but also in the genomic regions and chromosomes involved [22–25,31–37]. In this sense, chromothriptic events described in this cohort mostly involved losses of fragments or alternated losses and gains and were located indistinctly throughout whole chromosomes or focalized in one chromosome arm. The most recurrently involved regions in our series were located at 3p21, 6q21 and 13q14, which had been previously reported in CLL cases with cth [24,25,36]. Regarding the 3p21.31 locus, this region contains the *SETD2* gene, which encodes a histone methyltransferase involved not only in the regulation of gene transcription but also in maintenance of genomic stability, and whose inactivation was also found to be associated with genomic complexity, del/mut*TP53*, cth and aggressive disease [24,36]. Besides, the recurrent deletion affecting the 6q21 locus (containing the *FOXO3a* gene) has been described in 6% of CLL patients and associated with shorter progression-free survival [23,40]. In the context of cth, this region was also deleted in the patient studied by Bassaganyas et al. [34]. The deletion in 13q14, involving the *DLEU1* and *DLEU2* genes as well as the microRNAs miR-16-1 and miR-15a, is the most common cytogenetic lesion in patients with CLL, being present in more than 50% of cases at diagnosis and strongly associated with a favorable prognosis when found as the sole abnormality [41]. However, this good outcome vanishes when accompanied by many other anomalies constituting a pattern of cth [24]. On the other hand, we also found involvement of the previously reported 6p21.1 and 10q24 regions (including *NFKBIE* and *NFKB2*, respectively) in two patients, independently [34]. Likewise, our cohort included one previously reported case with a gain in 5p13.33, which had been suggested as a possible mechanism underlying the formation of these complex rearrangements through the increase in telomerase activity by the deregulation of the *TERT* gene [25]. However, no other case carrying this abnormality was found. Overall, our results confirm that no significant correlation could be established between any of these affected regions and cth onset, suggesting that it might not arise from deregulation of one potential driver gene; rather, it would be initiated by other mechanisms, as yet unknown, that could lead to the alteration of distinct genomic regions.

In the present study, we were able to compare the chromothriptic patterns detected by GM with the chromosomal abnormalities reported in the karyotype. As expected, due to its limited resolution, it was not possible to detect cth by CBA. However, our results confirmed that most of the chromothriptic chromosomes were already altered in the karyotype, carrying a monosomy, deletion or being involved in unbalanced rearrangements. Furthermore, although the chromothriptic chromosomes might display a simple aberration or even be normal, the presence of chromosome markers and additional material of unknown origin was a common feature in these cases, leading overall to more complex karyotypes than those without cth. This was reflected by the higher frequency of cases with ≥5 abnormalities compared with the control group. Thus, CBA can only suggest the presence of complex rearrangements through the detection of abnormalities involving material of unknown origin that might constitute patterns of cth. On the other hand, taking advantage of the structural information provided by the analysis of nine patients using OGM, we were able to reveal rearrangements associated with chromothriptic events, including intra-chromosomal and inter-chromosomal translocations. Even though some of the breakpoints directly overlapped or were close to coding genes, we did not find any common driver gene that could trigger the formation of cth. The novel rearrangements clustered in the chromothriptic chromosomes or involved different non-chromothriptic chromosomes. OGM also underscored a case with a higher complexity profile, comprising several chained translocations involving several chromosomes, which is characteristic of another catastrophic event called chromoplexy. This phenomenon was first identified in prostate cancer, with a prevalence of ~90%, and is also present in other solid tumors [42,43]. However, despite being described in some hematological neoplasms, such as multiple myeloma, mantle cell lymphoma or in previous reports on CLL [24,44–46], clinical and biological differences between both chromoplexy and cth and their impact on CLL have not been further explored. In this study, no differences in clinical characteristics could be identified among patients showing the aforementioned rearrangement patterns, although it should be noted that the cohort was too small to draw any conclusion. Even though it is still unknown whether the distinct patterns of rearrangements could affect the evolution of the disease, OGM is a novel technology that provides a more detailed description of these catastrophic events than GM and could shed light on the mechanisms involved in the development of cth. In addition, OGM data analysis is based on a user-friendly interface and could be potentially included in clinical practice. In contrast, even though whole genome sequencing methods have been extensively used for the characterization of cth [22,24,31,34,37], several issues, including high costs and the need for more harmonized analysis pipelines, preclude their incorporation in a routine setting.

Regarding clinical impact, we have shown that CLL patients with cth had a shorter TTFT compared with patients with genomic complexity lacking cth. These results are in accordance with prior studies performed in large CLL cohorts, which reported poor outcomes associated with cth in terms of progression-free survival, TTFT and OS [23–25,32]. However, it is noteworthy that the present study only comprised cases with CK and/or genomic complexity detected by GM. Thus, our results should not be extrapolated to a real-life CLL population, where complex cases account for around 10% of patients. Even though cth has been previously associated with genomic complexity, this is the first study focused on this high-risk group. Unfortunately, our series was based on a retrospective and multicenter cohort, including patients receiving different therapeutic agents, which hindered the assessment of overall survival or response to new targeted modalities. As expected, the cth group showed an enrichment of patients with high complexity (≥5 aberrations by CBA) and del/mut*TP53* (both being found in 70% of patients). These frequencies were similar to those defined in previous publications, which, despite not describing results from CBA data, reported high complexity in these cases and a significant association of cth with *TP53* abnormalities (up to 81%) [23–25,32]. Notwithstanding, these known independent poor prognostic markers were significantly increased, even when cth patients were compared with the control group with CK, also known to be related to these features. It is therefore conceivable that the poorer evolution observed in cases with cth might be related not only to the chromothriptic event itself but also to the presence of high complexity by CBA or *TP53* abnormalities. In this regard, cth did not affect TTFT when cases were categorized according to *TP53* status. Indeed, in the multivariate analysis, *TP53* was the only parameter maintaining its prognostic significance, reinforcing this hypothesis. Therefore, cth does not represent an independent prognostic factor for CLL patients with genomic complexity, and its identification is not essential in the clinical setting. In summary, a strong connection between *TP53* and cth has been demonstrated. Nonetheless, it would be very interesting to better explore the characteristics and the clinical evolution of cth in cases with wild-type *TP53*, in which other mechanisms would promote the survival of the clones with cth and the confounding effects of *TP53* dysfunction on survival would be avoided.

5. Conclusions

In conclusion, chromothripsis is a recurrent event in CLL patients with genomic complexity and is strongly associated with an increased frequency of *TP53* abnormalities. In this sense, the short survival observed in CK cases with cth might actually be due to the increased prevalence of del/mut*TP53*. In addition, OGM has proven to be a valuable cytogenomic tool, capable of detecting previously known abnormalities and identifying new rearrangements, affording an improved view of the highly complex genomic landscape of these patients. However, important questions remain regarding the mechanisms underlying cth and the impact of these patterns on the onset and evolution of CLL. Therefore, further studies with larger cohorts, including more cases with cth and preserved *TP53*, are needed to better understand the role of this phenomenon in CLL pathogenesis and prognosis, particularly in patients treated with new therapeutic agents, to better elucidate the potential of cth as a predictive marker.

Supplementary Materials: The following supporting information can be downloaded at: https://www.mdpi.com/article/10.3390/cancers14153715/s1, Figure S1. Number of cases showing chromothripsis for each chromosome. Chromosomes are represented on the X-axis and the total number of cases showing chromothripsis for each chromosome is represented on the Y-axis. The chromosomes involved most in the cohort (3, 6 and 13) are highlighted in blue. Figure S2. Copy number profiles of some of the chromothriptic chromosomes. Copy number profiles derived from genomic microarray analyses were available for 18 cases. Figure S3. Chromothripsis detected in chromosome 6 in those cases in which optical genome mapping only revealed intra-chromosomal chromothripsis-related rearrangements. Whole chromosome 6 view of genomic microarray results from cases #8, #9 and #32, which carried intra-chromosomal rearrangements when analyzed by OGM, are represented. Only small deleted fragments were common between case #8 and the other two remaining cases. Specifically, three fragments of 2.83 Mb (10,743,398–13,571,692), 1.20 Mb (16,137,146–17,257,084) and 1.17 Mb (86,948,132–88,115,441) were shared between cases #8 and #9 (highlighted in green), and three fragments of 1.79 Mb (7,651,724–9,438,895), 0.64 Mb (19,953,714–20,591,009) and 1.28 Mb (36,084,473–37,366,801) were common between cases #8 and #32 (highlighted in red). Table S1. Genomic microarray platforms used in this study. Table S2. Patterns of chromothripsis found in cases with 7–9 switches and those with ≥10 switches between 2–3 copy number states. Table S3. Detailed information of the chromothriptic events detected by GM, including the genes involved in the rearrangements (*shown in the excel file attached*). Table S4. Detailed information of the chromothriptic events detected by GM and karyotypes obtained by CBA (*shown in the excel file attached*). Table S5. Results obtained by optical genome mapping in those chromosomes with chromothripsis (*shown in the excel file attached*). Table S6. Review of the literature published about chromothripsis in CLL (*shown in the excel file attached*).

Author Contributions: Conceptualization, A.P. and B.E.; Methodology, S.R.-C., A.P. and B.E.; Formal Analysis, S.R.-C. and A.P.; Investigation, S.R.-C., A.P., S.B. (Sandrine Bougeon), J.S., S.B. (Sílvia Beà), J.K. and B.E.; Resources, S.R.-C., A.P., J.K., S.B. (Sílvia Beà), M.J.L., D.C., H.P., G.M.R., M.L.B., R.C., I.A., R.S., M.A.M.-G., T.B., E.G., C.M., M.S., X.C., M.J.C., A.C., F.N.-K., D.O., C.H., J.C.S. and B.E.; Data Curation, S.R.-C.; Writing-Original Draft Preparation, S.R.-C., A.P. and B.E.; Writing—Review and Editing, S.R.-C., A.P., J.K., S.B. (Sílvia Beà), S.B. (Sandrine Bougeon), M.J.L., D.C., H.P., G.M.R., M.L.B., R.C., I.A., R.S., M.A.M.-G., T.B., E.G., C.M., M.S., X.C., M.J.C., A.C., F.N.-K., D.O., C.H., J.C.S., J.S. and B.E.; Supervision, Project Administration and Funding Acquisition, B.E. All authors have read and agreed to the published version of the manuscript.

Funding: This work was partly supported by grants from Generalitat de Catalunya (17SGR437), Gilead Sciences Fellowship (GLD17/00282), Ministerio de Universidades of Spain (FPU17/00361), Fundación Española de Hematología y Hemoterapia (FEHH-Janssen), Instituto de Salud Carlos III/FEDER (PT17/0015/0011) and the "Xarxa de Bancs de tumors", sponsored by Pla Director d'Oncologia de Catalunya (XBTC).

Institutional Review Board Statement: The study was conducted in accordance with national and international guidelines (Professional Code of Conduct, Declaration of Helsinki) and approved by the Drug Research Ethical Committee (CEIm) of the Hospital del Mar, Barcelona (2017/7565/I).

Informed Consent Statement: Informed consent was obtained from all patients involved in the study.

Data Availability Statement: Detailed chromosome banding analyses, genomic microarrays and optical genome mapping profiles for selected cases are provided in Supplementary Tables. Please contact either bespinet@psmar.cat or apuiggros@psmar.cat for additional data.

Acknowledgments: The authors would like to thank Gonzalo Blanco, Ferran Nadeu and Julio Delgado for their contribution to the study, providing patients samples and data; the MARGenomics Platform from Institut Hospital del Mar d'Investigacions Mèdiques (Barcelona) for performing part of the genomic microarrays and Alexander Hoischen and Tuomo Mantere from the Radboud University Medical Center and scientists and staff at Bionano Genomics, including Yannick Delpu, Chloe Tessereau, Michaela West, Rachel Fourdin and Karl Hong, for their support with the OGM analyses.

Conflicts of Interest: The authors declare no conflict of interest.

References

1. Herling, C.D.; Klaumünzer, M.; Rocha, C.K.; Altmüller, J.; Thiele, H.; Bahlo, J.; Kluth, S.; Crispatzu, G.; Herling, M.; Schiller, J.; et al. Complex karyotypes and KRAS and POT1 mutations impact outcome in CLL after chlorambucil-based chemotherapy or chemoimmunotherapy. *Blood* **2016**, *128*, 395–404. [CrossRef] [PubMed]
2. Puiggros, A.; Collado, R.; Calasanz, M.J.; Ortega, M.; Ruiz-Xivillé, N.; Rivas-Delgado, A.; Luño, E.; González, T.; Navarro, B.; García-Malo, M.D.; et al. Patients with chronic lymphocytic leukemia and complex karyotype show an adverse outcome even in absence of TP53/ATM FISH deletions. *Oncotarget* **2017**, *8*, 54297–54303. [CrossRef] [PubMed]
3. Rigolin, G.M.; Cavallari, M.; Quaglia, F.M.; Formigaro, L.; Lista, E.; Urso, A.; Guardalben, E.; Liberatore, C.; Faraci, D.; Saccenti, E.; et al. In CLL, comorbidities and the complex karyotype are associated with an inferior outcome independently of CLL-IPI. *Blood* **2017**, *129*, 3495–3498. [CrossRef] [PubMed]
4. Baliakas, P.; Jeromin, S.; Iskas, M.; Puiggros, A.; Plevova, K.; Nguyen-Khac, F.; Davis, Z.; Rigolin, G.M.; Visentin, A.; Xochelli, A.; et al. Cytogenetic complexity in chronic lymphocytic leukemia: Definitions, associations, and clinical impact. *Blood* **2019**, *133*, 1205–1216. [CrossRef] [PubMed]
5. Thompson, P.A.; O'Brien, S.M.; Wierda, W.G.; Ferrajoli, A.; Stingo, F.; Smith, S.C.; Burger, J.A.; Estroy, Z.; Jain, N.; Kantarjian, H.M.; et al. Complex karyotype is a stronger predictor than del(17p) for an inferior outcome in relapsed or refractory chronic lymphocytic leukemia patients treated with ibrutinib-based regimens. *Cancer* **2015**, *121*, 3612–3621. [CrossRef]
6. Byrd, J.C.; Harrington, B.; O'Brien, S.; Jones, J.A.; Schuh, A.; Devereux, S.; Chaves, J.; Wierda, W.G.; Awan, F.T.; Brown, J.R.; et al. Acalabrutinib (ACP-196) in Relapsed Chronic Lymphocytic Leukemia. *N. Engl. J. Med.* **2016**, *374*, 323–332. [CrossRef]
7. Chanan-Khan, A.; Cramer, P.; Demirkan, F.; Fraser, G.; Silva, R.S.; Grosicki, S.; Pristupa, A.; Janssens, A.; Mayer, J.; Bartlett, N.L.; et al. Ibrutinib combined with bendamustine and rituximab compared with placebo, bendamustine, and rituximab for previously treated chronic lymphocytic leukaemia or small lymphocytic lymphoma (HELIOS): A randomised, double-blind, phase 3 study. *Lancet Oncol.* **2016**, *17*, 200–211. [CrossRef]
8. Anderson, M.A.; Tam, C.; Lew, T.E.; Juneja, S.; Juneja, M.; Westerman, D.; Wall, M.; Lade, S.; Gorelik, A.; Huang, D.C.S.; et al. Clinicopathological features and outcomes of progression of CLL on the BCL2 inhibitor venetoclax. *Blood* **2017**, *129*, 3362–3370. [CrossRef]

9. O'Brien, S.; Furman, R.R.; Coutre, S.; Flinn, I.W.; Burger, J.A.; Blum, K.; Sharman, J.; Wierda, W.; Jones, J.; Zhao, W.; et al. Single agent ibrutinib in treatment-naïve and relapsed/refractory chronic lymphocytic leukemia: A 5-year experience. *Blood* **2018**, *131*, 1910–1919. [CrossRef]

10. Brown, J.R.; Hillmen, P.; O'Brien, S.; Barrientos, J.C.; Reddy, N.M.; Coutre, S.E.; Tam, C.S.; Mulligan, S.P.; Jaeger, U.; Barr, P.M.; et al. Extended follow-up and impact of high-risk prognostic factors from the phase 3 RESONATE study in patients with previously treated CLL/SLL. *Leukemia* **2018**, *32*, 83–91. [CrossRef]

11. Mato, A.R.; Thompson, M.; Allan, J.N.; Brander, D.M.; Pagel, J.M.; Ujjani, C.S.; Hill, B.T.; Lamanna, N.; Lansigan, F.; Jacobs, R.; et al. Real-world outcomes and management strategies for venetoclax-treated chronic lymphocytic leukemia patients in the United States. *Haematologica* **2018**, *103*, 1511–1517. [CrossRef]

12. Al-Sawaf, O.; Lilienweiss, E.; Bahlo, J.; Robrecht, S.; Fink, A.M.; Patz, M.; Tandon, M.; Jiang, Y.; Schary, W.; Ritgen, M.; et al. High efficacy of venetoclax plus obinutuzumab in patients with complex karyotype and chronic lymphocytic leukemia. *Blood* **2020**, *135*, 866–870. [CrossRef]

13. Kater, A.P.; Wu, J.Q.; Kipps, T.; Eichhorst, B.; Hillmen, P.; D'Rozario, J.; Assouline, S.; Owen, C.; Robak, T.; de la Serna, J.; et al. Venetoclax Plus Rituximab in Relapsed Chronic Lymphocytic Leukemia: 4-Year Results and Evaluation of Impact of Genomic Complexity and Gene Mutations from the MURANO Phase III Study. *J. Clin. Oncol.* **2020**, *38*, 4042–4054. [CrossRef] [PubMed]

14. Chun, K.; Wenger, G.D.; Chaubey, A.; Dash, D.P.; Kanagal-Shamanna, R.; Kantarci, S.; Kolhe, R.; Van Dyke, D.L.; Wang, L.; Wolff, D.J.; et al. Assessing copy number aberrations and copy-neutral loss-of-heterozygosity across the genome as best practice: An evidence-based review from the Cancer Genomics Consortium (CGC) working group for chronic lymphocytic leukemia. *Cancer Genet.* **2018**, *228–229*, 236–250. [CrossRef] [PubMed]

15. Ramos-Campoy, S.; Puiggros, A.; Beà, S.; Bougeon, S.; Larráyoz, M.J.; Costa, D.; Parker, H.; Rigolin, G.M.; Ortega, M.; Blanco, M.L.; et al. Chromosome banding analysis and genomic microarrays are both useful but not equivalent methods for genomic complexity risk stratification in chronic lymphocytic leukemia patients. *Haematologica* **2022**, *107*, 593–603. [CrossRef]

16. Levy, B.; Baughn, L.B.; Chartrand, S.; LaBarge, B.; Claxton, D.; Lennon, A.; Akkari, Y.; Cujar, C.; Kolhe, R.; Kroeger, K.; et al. A National Multicenter Evaluation of the Clinical Utility of Optical Genome Mapping for Assessment of Genomic Aberrations in Acute Myeloid Leukemia. *medRxiv* **2020**. [CrossRef]

17. Neveling, K.; Mantere, T.; Vermeulen, S.; Oorsprong, M.; van Beek, R.; Kater-Baats, E.; Pauper, M.; van der Zande, G.; Smeets, D.; Weghuis, D.O.; et al. Next-generation cytogenetics: Comprehensive assessment of 52 hematological malignancy genomes by optical genome mapping. *Am. J. Hum. Genet.* **2021**, *108*, 1423–1435. [CrossRef]

18. Yang, H.; García-Manero, G.; Rush, D.; Montalban-Bravo, G.; Mallampati, S.; Medeiros, L.J.; Levy, B.; Luthra, R.; Kanagal-Shamanna, R. Application of Optical Genome Mapping for Comprehensive Assessment of Chromosomal Structural Variants for Clinical Evaluation of Myelodysplastic Syndromes. *medRxiv* **2021**. [CrossRef]

19. Rack, K.; De Bie, J.; Ameye, G.; Gielen, O.; Demeyer, S.; Cools, J.; De Keersmaecker, K.; Vermeesch, J.R.; Maertens, J.; Segers, H.; et al. Optimizing the diagnostic workflow for acute lymphoblastic leukemia by optical genome mapping. *Am. J. Hematol.* **2022**, *in press*. [CrossRef]

20. Holland, A.J.; Cleveland, D.W. Chromoanagenesis and cancer: Mechanisms and consequences of localized, complex chromosomal rearrangements. *Nat. Med.* **2012**, *18*, 1630–1638. [CrossRef]

21. Pellestor, F. Chromoanagenesis: Cataclysms behind complex chromosomal rearrangements. *Mol. Cytogenet.* **2019**, *12*, 6. [CrossRef] [PubMed]

22. Stephens, P.J.; Greenman, C.D.; Fu, B.; Yang, F.; Bignell, G.R.; Mudie, L.J.; Pleasance, E.D.; Lau, K.W.; Beare, D.; Stebbings, L.A.; et al. Massive genomic rearrangement acquired in a single catastrophic event during cancer development. *Cell* **2011**, *144*, 27–40. [CrossRef] [PubMed]

23. Edelmann, J.; Holzmann, K.; Miller, F.; Winkler, D.; Bühler, A.; Zenz, T.; Bullinger, L.; Kühn, M.W.; Gerhardinger, A.; Bloehdorn, J.; et al. High-resolution genomic profiling of chronic lymphocytic leukemia reveals new recurrent genomic alterations. *Blood* **2012**, *120*, 4783–4794. [CrossRef] [PubMed]

24. Puente, X.S.; Beà, S.; Valdés-Mas, R.; Villamor, N.; Gutiérrez-Abril, J.; Martín-Subero, J.I.; Munar, M.; Rubio-Pérez, C.; Jares, P.; Aymerich, M.; et al. Non-coding recurrent mutations in chronic lymphocytic leukaemia. *Nature* **2015**, *526*, 519–524. [CrossRef] [PubMed]

25. Salaverria, I.; Martín-Garcia, D.; López, C.; Clot, G.; García-Aragonés, M.; Navarro, A.; Delgado, J.; Baumann, T.; Pinyol, M.; Martin-Guerrero, I.; et al. Detection of chromothripsis-like patterns with a custom array platform for chronic lymphocytic leukemia. *Genes Chromosomes Cancer* **2015**, *54*, 668–680. [CrossRef] [PubMed]

26. Crasta, K.; Ganem, N.J.; Dagher, R.; Lantermann, A.B.; Ivanova, E.V.; Pan, Y.; Nezi, L.; Protopopov, A.; Chowdhury, D.; Pellman, D. DNA breaks and chromosome pulverization from errors in mitosis. *Nature* **2012**, *482*, 53–58. [CrossRef] [PubMed]

27. Maciejowski, J.; Li, Y.; Bosco, N.; Campbell, P.J.; de Lange, T. Chromothripsis and kataegis induced by telomere crisis. *Cell* **2015**, *163*, 1641–1654. [CrossRef] [PubMed]

28. Zhang, C.Z.; Spektor, A.; Cornils, H.; Francis, J.M.; Jackson, E.K.; Liu, S.; Meyerson, M.; Pellman, D. Chromothripsis from DNA damage in micronuclei. *Nature* **2015**, *522*, 179–184. [CrossRef]

29. Kim, T.M.; Xi, R.; Luquette, L.J.; Johnson, M.D.; Park, P.J. Functional genomic analysis of chromosomal aberrations in a compendium of 8000 cancer genomes. *Genome Res.* **2013**, *23*, 217–227. [CrossRef]

30. Cai, H.; Kumar, N.; Bagheri, H.C.; von Mering, C.; Robinson, M.D.; Baudis, M. Chromothripsis-like patterns are recurring but heterogeneously distributed features in a survey of 22,347 cancer genome screens. *BMC Genom.* **2014**, *15*, 82. [CrossRef]
31. Cortés-Ciriano, I.; Lee, J.J.; Xi, R.; Jain, D.; Jung, Y.L.; Yang, L.; Gordenin, D.; Klimczak, L.J.; Zhang, C.Z.; Pellman, D.S.; et al. Comprehensive analysis of chromothripsis in 2658 human cancers using whole-genome sequencing. *Nat. Genet.* **2020**, *52*, 331–341. [CrossRef] [PubMed]
32. Leeksma, A.C.; Baliakas, P.; Moysiadis, T.; Puiggros, A.; Plevova, K.; Van der Kevie-Kersemaekers, A.M.; Posthuma, H.; Rodriguez-Vicente, A.E.; Tran, A.N.; Barbany, G.; et al. Genomic arrays identify high-risk chronic lymphocytic leukemia with genomic complexity: A multi-center study. *Haematologica* **2021**, *106*, 87–97. [CrossRef] [PubMed]
33. Pei, J.; Jhanwar, S.C.; Testa, J.R. Chromothripsis in a Case of TP53-Deficient Chronic Lymphocytic Leukemia. *Leuk. Res. Rep.* **2012**, *1*, 4–6. [CrossRef]
34. Bassaganyas, L.; Beà, S.; Escaramís, G.; Tornador, C.; Salaverria, I.; Zapata, L.; Drechsel, O.; Ferreira, P.G.; Rodríguez-Santiago, B.; Tubio, J.M.; et al. Sporadic and reversible chromothripsis in chronic lymphocytic leukemia revealed by longitudinal genomic analysis. *Leukemia* **2013**, *27*, 2376–3379. [CrossRef] [PubMed]
35. Tan, L.; Xu, L.H.; Liu, H.B.; Yang, S.J. Small lymphocytic lymphoma/chronic lymphocytic leukemia with chromothripsis in an old woman. *Chin. Med. J.* **2015**, *128*, 985–987. [CrossRef]
36. Parker, H.; Rose-Zerilli, M.J.; Larráyoz, M.; Clifford, R.; Edelmann, J.; Blakemore, S.; Gibson, J.; Wang, J.; Ljungström, V.; Wojdacz, T.K.; et al. Genomic disruption of the histone methyltransferase SETD2 in chronic lymphocytic leukaemia. *Leukemia* **2016**, *30*, 2179–2186. [CrossRef]
37. Burns, A.; Alsolami, R.; Becq, J.; Stamatopoulos, B.; Timbs, A.; Bruce, D.; Robbe, P.; Vavoulis, D.; Clifford, R.; Cabes, M.; et al. Whole-genome sequencing of chronic lymphocytic leukaemia reveals distinct differences in the mutational landscape between IgHVmut and IgHVunmut subgroups. *Leukemia* **2018**, *32*, 332–342. [CrossRef]
38. Hallek, M.; Cheson, B.D.; Catovsky, D.; Caligaris-Cappio, F.; Dighiero, G.; Döhner, H.; Hillmen, P.; Keating, M.; Montserrat, E.; Chiorazzi, N.; et al. iwCLL guidelines for diagnosis, indications for treatment, response assessment, and supportive management of CLL. *Blood* **2018**, *131*, 2745–2760. [CrossRef]
39. Puiggros, A.; Ramos-Campoy, S.; Kamaso, J.; de la Rosa, M.; Salido, M.; Melero, C.; Rodríguez-Rivera, M.; Bougeon, S.; Collado, R.; Gimeno, E.; et al. Optical Genome Mapping: A promising new tool to assess genomic complexity in chronic lymphocytic leukemia (CLL). *Cancers* **2022**, *14*, 3376. [CrossRef]
40. Jarosova, M.; Hruba, M.; Oltova, A.; Plevova, K.; Kruzova, L.; Kriegova, E.; Fillerova, R.; Koritakova, E.; Doubek, M.; Lysak, D.; et al. Chromosome 6q deletion correlates with poor prognosis and low relative expression of FOXO3 in chronic lymphocytic leukemia patients. *Am. J. Hematol.* **2017**, *92*, E604–E607. [CrossRef]
41. Döhner, H.; Stilgenbauer, S.; Benner, A.; Leupolt, E.; Kröber, A.; Bullinger, L.; Döhner, K.; Bentz, M.; Lichter, P. Genomic aberrations and survival in chronic lymphocytic leukemia. *N. Engl. J. Med.* **2000**, *343*, 1910–1916. [CrossRef] [PubMed]
42. Baca, S.C.; Prandi, D.; Lawrence, M.S.; Mosquera, J.M.; Romanel, A.; Drier, Y.; Park, K.; Kitabayashi, N.; MacDonald, T.Y.; Ghandi, M.; et al. Punctuated evolution of prostate cancer genomes. *Cell* **2013**, *153*, 666–677. [CrossRef] [PubMed]
43. Shen, M.M. Chromoplexy: A new category of complex rearrangements in the cancer genome. *Cancer Cell* **2013**, *23*, 567–569. [CrossRef] [PubMed]
44. Costa, D.; Granada, I.; Espinet, B.; Collado, R.; Ruiz-Xivillé, N.; Puiggros, A.; Uribe, M.; Arias, A.; Gómez, C.; Delgado, J.; et al. Balanced and unbalanced translocations in a multicentric series of 2843 patients with chronic lymphocytic leukemia. *Genes Chromosomes Cancer* **2022**, *61*, 37–43. [CrossRef]
45. Nadeu, F.; Martin-Garcia, D.; Clot, G.; Díaz-Navarro, A.; Duran-Ferrer, M.; Navarro, A.; Vilarrasa-Blasi, R.; Kulis, M.; Royo, R.; Gutiérrez-Abril, J.; et al. Genomic and epigenomic insights into the origin, pathogenesis, and clinical behavior of mantle cell lymphoma subtypes. *Blood* **2020**, *136*, 1419–1432. [CrossRef]
46. Neuse, C.J.; Lomas, O.C.; Schliemann, C.; Shen, Y.J.; Manier, S.; Bustoros, M.; Ghobrial, I.M. Genome instability in multiple myeloma. *Leukemia* **2020**, *34*, 2887–2897. [CrossRef]

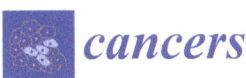

Review

The Clinical Spectrum, Diagnosis, and Management of GATA2 Deficiency

Marta Santiago [1,2], Alessandro Liquori [2,3,*], Esperanza Such [1,2,3], Ángel Zúñiga [4] and José Cervera [1,2,3,4]

1. Hematology Department, Hospital La Fe, 46026 Valencia, Spain
2. Hematology Research Group, Instituto de Investigación Sanitaria La Fe, 46026 Valencia, Spain
3. Centro de Investigación Biomédica en Red de Cáncer (CIBERONC), 28029 Madrid, Spain
4. Genetics Unit, Hospital La Fe, 46026 Valencia, Spain
* Correspondence: liquorialessandro@gmail.com

Simple Summary: A predisposition to myeloid neoplasms has recently been recognized as a defined clinical entity by the World Health Organization. One of the most well-known syndromes within this group is GATA2 deficiency, which is a highly heterogeneous disorder that can include pulmonary and vascular involvement, immunodeficiency, and myeloid neoplasms. The only curative treatment for this syndrome is allogeneic hematopoietic stem cell transplantation (HSCT), which should be performed in patients with GATA2 deficiency before irreversible organ damage. These patients should be referred to a multidisciplinary team to assess all potential and specific organ-system manifestations that could impact the patient's treatment, and consultations with appropriate subspecialists should be facilitated. Additionally, genetic testing should be offered to first-degree relatives, particularly those considered for donation when an HSCT with a sibling donor is feasible.

Abstract: Hereditary myeloid malignancy syndromes (HMMSs) are rare but are becoming increasingly significant in clinical practice. One of the most well-known syndromes within this group is GATA2 deficiency. The *GATA2* gene encodes a zinc finger transcription factor essential for normal hematopoiesis. Insufficient expression and function of this gene as a result of germinal mutations underlie distinct clinical presentations, including childhood myelodysplastic syndrome and acute myeloid leukemia, in which the acquisition of additional molecular somatic abnormalities can lead to variable outcomes. The only curative treatment for this syndrome is allogeneic hematopoietic stem cell transplantation, which should be performed before irreversible organ damage happens. In this review, we will examine the structural characteristics of the *GATA2* gene, its physiological and pathological functions, how *GATA2* genetic mutations contribute to myeloid neoplasms, and other potential clinical manifestations. Finally, we will provide an overview of current therapeutic options, including recent transplantation strategies.

Keywords: GATA2 deficiency; GATA2 haploinsufficiency; germline mutation; predisposition to myeloid neoplasms

1. Background

Familial myelodysplastic syndromes (MDSs) and acute myeloid leukemia (AML), also known as hereditary myeloid malignancy syndromes (HMMSs), have been recognized phenotypically for more than a century, with the first molecular basis discovered in 1999 through the identification of germline *RUNX1* mutations [1]. Since then, and recently accelerated by the advent of next-generation sequencing (NGS), a growing number of genes have been associated with germline predisposition to myeloid malignancies, including the *ANKRD26* [2–4], *ETV6* [5–7], *CEBPA* [8], *DDX41* [9], *GATA2* [10], *RBBP6* [11], *TERT*, *TERC* [12], and, most recently, the *SAMD9* [13] and *SAMD9L* genes [14,15]. Although they are traditionally considered very rare entities, it is now known that 4–13% of pediatric and 5–15% of adult MDS/AML cases are caused by germline predisposition [16–21].

Although most of these entities have only recently been described, the World Health Organization (WHO) incorporated some of them as provisional categories in its fourth revised classification [22]. In recognition of the robustness of data, HMMSs have also been integrated into other guidelines and expert recommendations, such as the Nordic Guidelines and the European Leukemia Network [23,24], highlighting the need to identify, diagnose, and correctly manage patients with hereditary syndromes. Finally, the growing recognition and molecular identification of this subset of myeloid malignancies have led to their being formalized in the most recent revisions by the WHO and the International Consensus Classification (ICC) of myeloid neoplasms [25,26]. The WHO 2022 update reinforces this category and includes it within the group of secondary myeloid neoplasms [25]. On the other hand, the 2022 ICC proposes to place these entities within the category of pediatric and/or germline mutation-associated disorders due to their overlap with other childhood disorders [26].

This review focuses on one of these entities, specifically the phenotypic spectrum of patients diagnosed with GATA2 deficiency, recognized as a major myeloid neoplasia predisposition syndrome with pleiotropic manifestations. We discuss the structural characteristics of the *GATA2* gene and describe how its genetic alterations might contribute to the onset of myeloid neoplasms as a result of aberrant induced hematopoiesis [27]. In addition, we will summarize diagnostic clues for proper identification and management of this syndrome.

2. *GATA2* Molecular Insights

The *GATA binding protein 2* (*GATA2*) gene is located on the long arm of human chromosome 3 at cytoband 21.3 (i.e., 3q21.3) and encodes two main isoforms (NM_032638 and NM_001145661) identical in their coding regions, but differing in the 5' untranslated region [28,29]. The GATA2 protein belongs to the GATA binding factors family, which modulates the expression of several genes by binding to the DNA motif GATA and other transcription factors [30]. This is managed by two highly conserved zinc finger domains (ZF1 and ZF2), which are responsible for the DNA-binding ability of GATA2. In addition, the GATA2 protein contains two transactivation domains, a nuclear localization signal, and a negative regulatory domain [29].

The precise role of *GATA2* in hematopoiesis is still not entirely understood. Hematopoietic stem cells (HSCs) found in the bone marrow of $GATA2^{+/-}$ mice were found to be impaired in terms of both number and functionality, as evidenced by serial transplantation assays [31]. *GATA2* heterozygosity is associated with decreased proliferation ability and increased quiescence and apoptosis in HSCs [31]. Moreover, *GATA2* haploinsufficiency impairs the function of granulocyte-macrophage progenitors but not that of other committed myeloid progenitors [32]. Despite this, $GATA2^{+/-}$ mice do not develop MDS/AML, which makes it challenging to study the impact of *GATA2* haploinsufficiency on leukemic progression in these models.

On the other hand, the overexpression of *GATA2* results in the self-renewal of myeloid progenitors and hampers lymphoid differentiation in mouse bone marrow [33]. Additionally, the overexpression of *GATA2* promotes proliferation in human embryonic stem cells (hESCs) but quiescence in hESC-derived HSCs [34]. Elevated levels of *GATA2* have been observed in AML patients, both adults and children, who have poor prognoses [35]. These findings indicate that, in addition to its function as a tumor suppressor, *GATA2* may also act as an oncogene when overexpressed.

In line with these data, and focusing on adult hematopoiesis, the GATA2 protein, together with several transcription factors (e.g., FLI1, LMO2, and RUNX1), is involved in HSC survival and self-renewal, thus participating in early lineage commitment. Meanwhile, during hematopoietic differentiation, GATA2 modulates downstream fate decisions by interacting with CEBPA, GATA1, and SPI1 [36,37].

To date, roughly 500 GATA2-deficient patients have been reported, and the syndrome was confirmed to be inherited according to an autosomal dominant pattern in 50% of cases, de novo in 5% of cases, and uncertain in the rest of the cases [38]. This is unexpectedly different from previous studies, in which de novo occurrence was estimated in two thirds of all cases [39,40]. However, there is a lack of a well-characterized series in which segregation studies have been carried out systematically or in which penetrance or expressivity were considered. Therefore, these data should be viewed with caution.

In addition, almost 200 unique (likely) pathogenic variants have been described that can be classified into four groups: truncating mutations (splice site, nonsense, frameshift, and whole-gene deletions) proximal to or within the ZF2 domain; missense mutations within the ZF2 domain; mutations resulting in aberrant mRNA splicing (e.g., synonymous changes) (Figure 1) [38,41,42]; and other regulatory variants, such as those located in the *GATA2* intronic +9.5 kb enhancer site (e.g., c.1017+572C>T, the c.1017+532A>T, and the c.1017+513_1017+540del [c.1017+512del28]), which is essential for hematopoiesis [42–46]. Overall, germline *GATA2* (likely) pathogenic variants are hypothesized to result in haploinsufficiency because truncated alleles lead to clinical phenotypes similar to missense variants [31,45]. Strikingly, some variants have been associated with only partial loss-of-function (p.T354M) or even gain-of-function (p.L359V) mechanisms, suggesting more complex pathways [47,48].

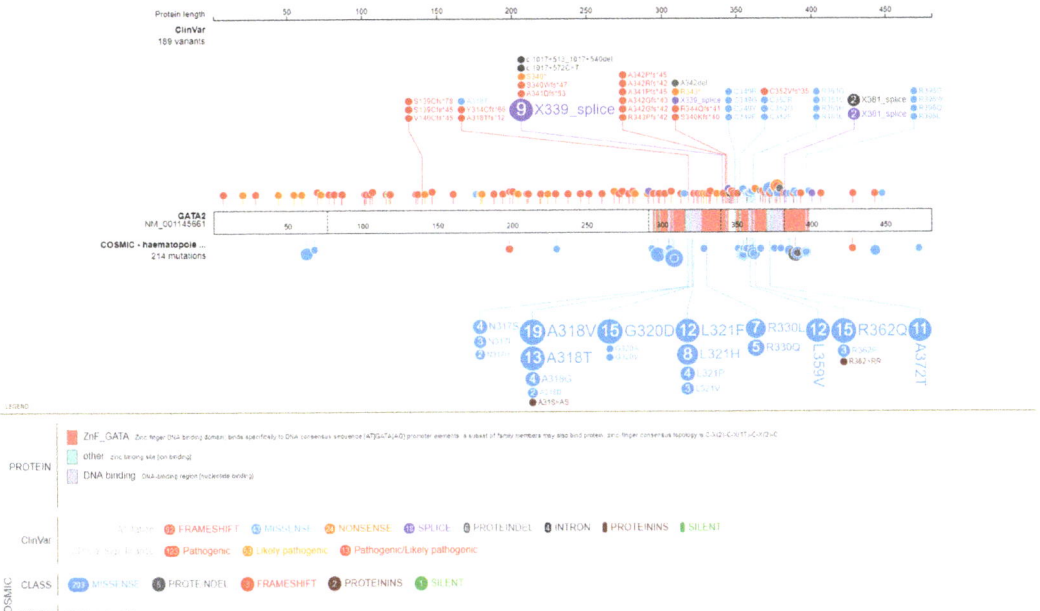

Figure 1. Germline and somatic *GATA2* (likely) pathogenic variants obtained from ClinVar and COSMIC databases, respectively. Somatic variants are restricted to those found in hematopoietic malignancies. Variants were visualized using the ProteinPaint web application (https://pecan.stjude.cloud/home, accessed on 27 January 2023) and colored based on their functional type (e.g., frameshift and missense). Since the effect of splice variants is often undetermined, these were annotated on the position of the closest amino acid that would be involved (e.g., the NM_001145661:c.1018-1G>T variant is annotated as X339_splice). Numbers in circles indicate the number of entries and/or reported cases. All variants are annotated to NM_001145661.

Although most deleterious changes are private, it is possible to recognize some mutational hotspots. Recurrent variants in the extended ZF2 domain have been identified, including p.T354M and p.R396W/Q/W, found in roughly one fifth of the reported cases, as well as the c.1017+572C>T intronic variant, found in 20 patients [38].

Germline *GATA2* mutations are usually necessary but not sufficient for myeloid disease development. It has been proposed that different environmental stressors may modify the expression of these germline variants during embryogenesis or after birth, inducing disorder in tissues where limited GATA2 expression is inadequate for their normal cellular function [38]. Particularly in bone marrow (BM), such stressors can lead to certain cytogenetic and molecular alterations that accumulate over time, selecting clonality and triggering myeloid transformation. Indeed, the germline variant can also modify the BM microenvironment, contributing to clonal selection [38].

In patients with progression to a malignant neoplasm, certain cytogenetic and molecular alterations appear recurrently. The most frequent cytogenetic alterations in patients with germline *GATA2*-mutated myeloid neoplasms involve chromosome 7, including its monosomy, partial deletion of 7q and der(1;7)(q10;p10), and trisomy of chromosome 8 [27,40,49]. These neoplasms tend to show fewer somatic mutations and a different molecular landscape compared to non-*GATA2* MDS/AML. The most frequent recurrent somatic mutations identified in *GATA2*-MDS/AML patients are in the *SETBP1*, *ASXL1*, and *STAG2* genes, and the RAS pathway. By contrast, deleterious *SF3B1*, *U2AF1*, *NPM1*, and *FLT3* changes are infrequent in *GATA2*-mutated myeloid neoplasms [21,50–60].

Interestingly, *GATA2* can also be mutated in somatic cells of sporadic MDS/AML. Different from germline *GATA2* mutations, which mainly include truncated and ZF2 missense changes, somatic *GATA2* mutations are usually missense variants located in the ZF1 domain (e.g., p.N317-L321 hotspot) or in-frame indels in the C-terminus (Figure 1) [38]. This suggests a likely difference in GATA2 function during the leukemogenic process between germline and somatic cases [61]. Of note, somatic *GATA2* mutations are often associated with both monoallelic and biallelic *CEBPA* somatic mutations [62–64]. Additionally, somatic mutations in *GATA2*, although rare, have also been linked to milder forms of the immunodeficiency phenotype observed in patients with germline mutant *GATA2* [65,66].

3. *GATA2* Phenotypic Spectrum

Heterozygous pathogenic variants in the *GATA2* gene cause a highly heterogeneous disorder with incomplete penetrance [67]. This may present with immunodeficiency (including monocytopenia with *Mycobacterium avium* complex (MonoMAC) infection and dendritic cell (DC), monocyte, B, and natural killer (NK) lymphoid (DCML) deficiency syndromes); syndromic features, such as congenital deafness and lymphedema (originally defining Emberger syndrome), or pulmonary and vascular involvement [49], and there is a high probability of evolving to MDS and/or AML. In 2011, these diverse clinical syndromes were linked to define a common genetic diagnosis of the GATA2 deficiency syndrome [10,45,68,69].

Except for a few cases, the relationship between genotype and phenotype in these patients is poorly understood due to significant variations in clinical presentation, even among individuals within the same family [41,49]. Therefore, determining the true clinical penetrance of this disorder would require a comprehensive examination of the genotypes of a large number of first-degree relatives of patients. It is worth noting some of the reported phenotype/genotype correlations: (1) patients with noncoding variants (which can account for up to 10% of cases) have been observed to exhibit reduced disease penetrance [41,49,70,71]; (2) the p.T354M variant seemed to be associated with a predominance of myeloid malignancies (83% of cases; 44/53), while p.R398W/Q variants were more commonly associated with immunodeficiency (88% of cases; 23/26) in a relatively large series [38]; (3) there have been indications that complete haploinsufficiency or loss of GATA2 function, rather than missense mutations, may be required for the development of lymphedema [72].

These complex and variable presentations pose a significant challenge for clinicians when diagnosing and managing patients with *GATA2* mutations.

4. Hematological Presentation

The first hematoimmunologic manifestation typically occurs between the second and third decade of life, with a median age that varies in different studies (ranging from 12 to 19 years) [38,39,41,49,71]. While some patients present with cytopenias, immunodeficiency, or BM failure during childhood, others can develop MDS without preexisting clinical features during young adulthood (Figure 2) [27].

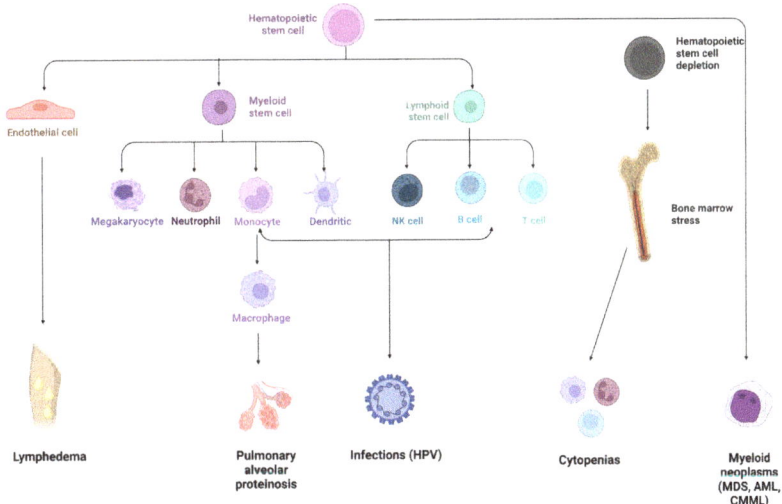

Figure 2. GATA2 deficiency clinical spectrum. HPV, human papilloma virus; MDS, myelodysplastic syndromes; AML, acute myeloid leukemia; CMML, chronic myelomonocytic leukemia. Figure made using https://www.biorender.com/, accessed on 27 January 2023.

4.1. Bone Marrow Failure

Unlike other germline alterations predisposing to HMMSs that preferentially lead to thrombocytopenia (e.g., *ANKRD26, RUNX1, ETV6*) [73–75], neutropenia may be the first and leading form of cytopenia in these patients. Although a decreased white blood cells (WBC) count can lead to a complex differential diagnosis, neutropenia with profound monocytopenia should prompt consideration of GATA2 deficiency [67]. Paradoxically, monocytosis can be the initial presenting sign in patients who develop *GATA2*-related MDS [27].

Bone marrow morphology can reveal altered cellularity (hypo- and normal or hypercellular marrow in patients with cytopenia or MDS, respectively), pronounced erythropoiesis, multilineage dysplasia, and fibrosis [40,67].

4.2. Myeloid Neoplasms

GATA2 haploinsufficiency is a major contributor to MDS/AML in adolescents and young adults. While some patients who develop MDS have a high risk of progressing to AML or chronic myelomonocytic leukemia (CMML), a small subset presents directly with AML [27]. Other reported hematological disorders include acute lymphoblastic leukemia (ALL), juvenile myelomonocytic leukemia (JMML), and myelofibrosis [71,76,77].

The prevalence of GATA2 deficiency is currently unknown, but given the significant disease penetrance and low tolerance to pathogenic mutations in the *GATA2* gene, it is likely that most carriers of the mutation will develop hematologic or immunologic complications over the course of their lifetime. In one study that reviewed 18 published series (>350 individuals), the penetrance of myeloid neoplasms was estimated to reach 75% in *GATA2*-mutated carriers [27], with an increased risk of developing MDS/AML as they aged. The risk of developing MDS/AML was calculated to be 6% at 10 years, 39% at 20 years, and 81% at 40 years in a series of 79 patients [39,71,76].

While MDS/AML is the most common neoplasm in GATA2 deficiency, the EWOG-MDS study [49], which included 426 patients, found that *GATA2* germline mutations were present in up to 7% of all pediatric cases with primary MDS and 15% of advanced MDS in examined series [49,78,79]. Monosomy 7 is the most frequent cytogenetic alteration, being present in 37–57% of all patients with *GATA2* MDS and 48–72% of adolescents (>12 years old) with *GATA2* MDS [22,49,76]. Since MDS is very uncommon during childhood, it would seem mandatory to screen all children with this diagnosis for *GATA2* germline mutations [22,49,76].

5. Immunodeficiency Disorder

GATA2 deficiency is a unique primary immune deficiency that is also known as immunodeficiency 21, DCML, or MonoMAC (OMIM #614172). The immune defect may appear in adult life, as the number of hematopoietic stem and progenitor cells (HSPCs) decreases with age, which makes GATA2 deficiency a unique primary immune deficiency [80]. It is characterized by immunophenotype features resembling those seen in chronic infection or age-related immunosenescence. The spectrum of alterations can include dendritic cell deficiency, monocytopenia, loss of transitional B cells, the absence of CD56 bright NK cells (which presents an altered *CXCL12/CXCR4*-dependent chemotaxis [76,81–84]), reversed CD4:CD8 ratio, an excess of CD45RA+ CD8+ T cells, and poor-quality humoral response [27,85] despite normal levels of immunoglobulins and an adequate presence of bone marrow plasma cells in most patients [40,86,87].

As a result of immune deficiency, GATA2 carriers have an increased frequency of infections, with significant differences in the severity between patients [80]. Due to the deficit and dysfunction of dendritic cells, NK cells, and monocytes/macrophages, the identification of viruses and intracellular pathogens is compromised, leading to the severe spread of viral infections and mycobacterial susceptibility [40,41]. Donadieu and colleagues described severe bacterial infections as the most frequent pathogenic occurrences in *GATA2* carriers, with a cumulative rate of 33% at 20 years and 64% at 40 years [71]. On the other hand, Spinner et al. reported that severe viral infections were the most common ones in their series (70%), in particular those related to the human papilloma virus (HPV), which occurred in about two thirds of carriers [41]. The most important complication derived from underlying HPV infection is the development of recurrent warts or condyloma that can lead to dysplasia and/or squamous carcinoma [88]. Infections with other disseminated pathogens are frequently observed in GATA2-deficient patients, including non-tuberculous mycobacteria, herpes virus (varicella zoster virus, Epstein–Barr virus, and cytomegalovirus), and fungi (invasive aspergillosis, disseminated histoplasmosis, and candidiasis) [41].

Therefore, various immunological factors are highly suggestive of GATA2 deficiency and should make the clinician think of this disorder. These include prior immunodeficiency in a patient with MDS, atypical mycobacterial infections in patients with monocytopenia, persistent warts or severe herpes virus infections in cytopenic patients, and loss of B cells and their precursors, especially in patients who develop MDS [27,41,84,85].

Eventually, as in other immunodeficiencies, these patients can also present with autoimmune manifestations, described in 11–30% of cases [41,71,89], which may overshadow typical features of GATA2 deficiency and delay the diagnosis. Amarnani et al. reported rheumatological findings in 18% of their GATA2 deficiency cohort, with notable manifestations, including early onset osteoarthritis, piezogenic pedal papules, ankylosing spondylitis, and seronegative erosive rheumatoid arthritis [89].

6. Non-Hemato-/Immunologic Manifestations

6.1. Pulmonary Involvement

Pulmonary dysfunction is a common finding in up to 50% of patients with GATA2 deficiency [90], even in the absence of hematopoietic disease, leading to progressive compromised pulmonary function with diffusion defects, ventilatory defects, or a mixed pattern, along with significant clinical and radiographic disease [41,71,76,91].

In addition to recurrent infections, pulmonary alveolar proteinosis (PAP) is one of the most distinctive lung features. This rare disorder is characterized by the lack of anti-GM-CSF autoantibodies and the accumulation of surfactant proteins and subsequent impaired gas exchange [40]. It results from impaired function of the alveolar macrophages in GATA2-deficiency patients, which are responsible for inadequate clearance, and is associated with increased restrictive ventilatory defects and pulmonary arterial hypertension (PAH) [40,90]. Depending on the studied cohort, PAP and PAH may be present in 4–20% of patients [41,71,90].

Therefore, it is recommended to screen patients with PAP and/or immunodeficiency and/or myeloid malignancies without anti-GM-CSF antibodies for *GATA2* alterations. It is important to note that clinical variability within families, including asymptomatic relatives identified through family screening, has also been reported in the case of pulmonary dysfunction [41,90].

Radiographic findings might be unspecific and will depend on the underlying disorder. Several structural abnormalities have been identified on chest computed tomography, including nodular and reticular opacities, ground-glass opacities, consolidations, a "crazy-paving" pattern, subpleural blebbing, and paraseptal emphysema [41,76,90].

Although some of the lung manifestations, including PAP, PAH, and underlying infections, can be reversed as a result of an allogeneic hematopoietic stem cell transplantation (allo-HSCT) [41,92,93], it should be noted that HSCT toxicity related to the conditioning regimen and pulmonary graft-versus-host disease (GvHD) can also harm lung function [41,90].

Therefore, individuals with GATA2 deficiency should undergo regular, ongoing monitoring of their lung function throughout their lifetime. Although there are no guidelines for the pulmonary follow-up of these patients, it should be individualized and tailored to each patient's needs. This may involve regular visits to a pulmonologist for symptom monitoring and pulmonary function testing to assess respiratory capacity. Imaging tests, such as chest X-rays or computerized tomography (CT) scans, may also be used to evaluate lung changes. Additionally, if there is suspicion of alveolar proteinosis, a diagnosis confirmation can be made through bronchoscopy with bronchoalveolar lavage (BAL) and/or parenchymal biopsy.

6.2. Emberger Syndrome: Dysmorphic Features

Emberger syndrome (OMIM #614038) is characterized by the association of primary lymphedema (a common feature found in 11–20% of *GATA2* carriers, typically affecting one or both lower limbs, frequently involving the genitals in the form of a hydrocele), with AML (often preceded by pancytopenia or MDS), with or without congenital sensorineural hearing loss [38,40,41,68,71,76,94–97].

6.3. Other Dysmorphic Features

Additional dysmorphic features that have been described, include hypothyroidism, bilateral syndactyly of the toes, hypotelorism, and epicanthal folds, behavioral disorder, and urogenital malformations, among others [27,41].

7. Management and Surveillance

7.1. Allogeneic-HSCT

Although allo-HSCT is the only curative therapy for the impaired hematopoietic and lymphoid systems of patients with GATA2 deficiency [93,98–100], it represents a therapeutic challenge due to disease-associated comorbidities and clinical heterogeneity. Meanwhile, determining who should be candidates for allo-HSCT and when it should be performed (so that the benefits outweigh the risks) are questions that remain under debate [93,100]. Moreover, due to the low prevalence and relatively recent description of GATA2 deficiency syndrome, most outcomes and complications following allo-HSCT have been described in case reports or small series [93,98,100–104]. While some studies have reported an overall survival (OS) rate in 5-year posttransplant patients with clonal events at a rate of 55–60% [41,71,101], other reports have shown superior outcomes after the procedure [98–100,103]. Notably, Nichol-Vinueza et al. showed a 4-year posttransplant OS rate of 85.1% [100]. However, these cohorts are not necessarily comparable due to the heterogeneity of conditioning regimens and GvHD prophylaxis, donor type source, HSCT-related risk factors, duration of follow-up, and the clinical status or comorbidities of the GATA2 patient population [98,99,101].

7.1.1. Indications for and Timing of allo-HSCT

While hematologic malignancy development may be the most dangerous complication and a primary indication for transplant, it is not the only one. Restoring normal immunity and lung function is also important in the decision to proceed with SCT [93].

The lack of a genotype-phenotype correlation makes the natural history of GATA2 deficiency unpredictable, to the point that there are patients who become symptomatic after many decades. However, once symptoms appear, survival declines, with a probability of survival by 40 years of 60–80% according to different series [41,71]. In this regard, the ideal time for allo-HSCT should be after the onset of symptoms but before irreversible organ damage occurs [93,98,99], although more specific criteria for the timing need to be defined [105]. While some authors report better outcomes when HSCT is performed earlier after diagnosis and when there are fewer comorbidities [71,100,101], the EWOG-MDS 2017 guidelines on childhood MDS recommend watchful waiting if blood cells are stable and high-risk genetic aberrations are absent [49]. By contrast, other authors go as far as to propose that preemptive allo-HSCT could improve overall outcomes before malignancy develops [106–108]. More specific treatment strategies have yet to be fully elucidated.

There are three major indications for HSCT. Firstly, diagnosis of MDS/AML, however, it is not clear if better timing for HSCT is during the hypocellular MDS phase or when the patients develop cytogenetics abnormalities/excess of blasts [40,41,49,71,98,99,102,103,105]. Secondly, history of severe, recurrent, or treatment-refractory infections, particularly aggressive HPV infection. Relapsed/refractory precancerous or malignant disease due to HPV should be an indication for allo-HSCT. In this sense, considering the iatrogenic immunosuppression after HSCT, rigorous evaluation for HPV must take place before and after transplantation so that surgical and other therapeutic measures can be undertaken in cases with new or persistent disease [93,99,102–105]. Thirdly, progressive lung injury from infection and PAP, which leads to deteriorated lung function [93,99,102,103,105].

7.1.2. Conditioning, Graft Source, and Donors

Transplanting GATA2-deficient patients is a controversial topic due to the variable disease progression and the timing of HSCT [100,109]. Although nonmyeloablative HSCT can reverse clinical manifestations and was the strategy used in the earlier years, relapse rates, engraftment failure, and late graft rejections led to the consideration of more intensive conditioning regimens [93,102]. In this regard, several reports have demonstrated similar outcomes when using myeloablative regimens in patients with mutated and wild-type (wt) GATA2 [49,98,101]. However, in patients with low-stage and hypocellular MDS, myeloablation may not be necessary due to low rates of relapse [98], and the intensity can be reduced by using a controlled approach [110]. Therefore, some authors propose that the choice of conditioning scheme choice for GATA2-deficient patients should be based on the patient's MDS phenotype and cytogenetics [101,103,105,110].

The donor source constitutes a critical variable in the outcome of HSCT. Although it is still unclear which donor source will yield better outcomes for GATA2-deficient patients [102], it has been suggested that bone marrow should be preferred over peripheral blood, while umbilical cord blood should be avoided [102,103]. Matched related donors remain the best choice, although haploidentical HSCT could be an appropriate alternative [103,110].

7.1.3. HSCT-Derived Complications

Bortnick et al. conducted a study of 65 cases and found that pediatric patients with GATA2 deficiency had a similar risk of transplant-related toxicity (TRT) or transplant-related mortality (TRM) as compared to those with wt *GATA2* [98]. However, they also reported that three patients developed transplant-associated microangiopathy, which might indicate a distinct endothelial vulnerability in GATA2 patients, consistent with the known role of *GATA2* in the perturbation of normal vascular development [41,111,112]. Simonis et al. conducted a systematic review of 183 patients (median age 23 years) from January 2010 until March 2018 and reported that the risk of TRT was not higher in patients with GATA2 deficiency compared to those without it [93]. Similarly, Hofmann et al. reported no differences in TRM and overall organ toxicity between a pediatric cohort with GATA2 deficiency and controls [101]. However, they did observe a small number of serious and unusual infectious/immunologic complications and neurologic toxicities in the GATA2 population, as well as a higher rate of thrombotic events in GATA2 patients, with complete resolution after transplantation [101].

Although information about GvHD is often not available in these series, it seems that the proportion of patients with acute or chronic GvHD is similar to that of other transplant cohorts [93,100,101]. Reducing the severity of both acute and chronic GvHD is being evaluated in GATA2 deficiency patients with promising outcomes by administering post-cyclophosphamide (PTCy) after HSCT, as seen in wt GATA2 patients [100,103,105]. However, when HSCT is indicated but no preexisting malignancies are present, strategies to prevent GvHD are of the greatest importance, as there is no advantage to this complication [110].

In summary, considering that there are no formal recommendations on the indications for allo-HSCT, conditioning regimen, GvHD prophylaxis, donor source, and antibiotic prophylaxis in GATA2-deficiency patients, the decision to perform an allo-HSCT requires careful and individualized management [99]. Although treatment-related morbidity is manageable in these patients, an individualized approach should be taken into consideration for optimal outcomes.

7.2. Antibiotic Prophylaxis, Immunoglobulins, and Vaccination

Prior to performing allo-HSCT, it is crucial to effectively treat any severe infections to create a favorable environment for the transplanted donor stem cells to thrive [105]. Although opportunistic infections that manifest before transplantation do not seem to pose a major issue in terms of overall outcomes, patients are typically kept on antibiotic prophylaxis to prevent such infections. While most case reports of allo-HSCT do not provide details on the antibiotic prophylaxis regimen, in a study by Simonis et al., patients treated for non-tuberculous mycobacterium before HSCT took prophylactic azithromycin until the time of transplant and for about one year afterward [93]. For patients still receiving treatment for active infection at the time of HSCT, antimycobacterial drugs were administered for 6–12 months after the transplant [93]. Spinner et al. also recommend azithromycin for all patients with GATA2 deficiency even before HSCT is indicated [41].

Although rare, GATA2 patients may experience humoral deficiency [87,113]. In such cases, immunoglobulin replacement may be necessary [40].

Due to the high susceptibility of patients to HPV and the potential for recurrent and life-threatening oncogenic HPV lesions, early vaccination is likely to be beneficial [40,41,71].

7.3. Surveillance

Given the complexity of information available on GATA2 deficiency syndrome and other HMMSs, patients should be referred to multidisciplinary teams that include physicians who are well-versed in these conditions. This would facilitate the assessment of potential organ-system manifestations that could impact the patient's treatment, and promote consultation with appropriate subspecialists.

Since most patients with symptomatic GATA2 deficiency will eventually require an allo-HSCT, close monitoring is crucial in order to perform the procedure before organ damage occurs [93,98]. Therefore, a donor search should be conducted as soon as the deficiency is diagnosed, with systematic testing of potential relatives considered for donation [71,99].

Allo-HSCT can eradicate clonal malignancy, restore normal hematopoiesis, clear underlying infections, and improve pulmonary symptoms and function in patients with PAP [93,98,103]. However, it cannot reverse extra-hematopoietic manifestations of GATA2 deficiency, so patients remain at risk for non-hematopoietic issues and will require lifelong follow-up [101,105]. It is worth mentioning that HPV can persist after allo-HSCT, so gynecologists play an important role in guiding the management and surveillance of these patients [104,114], especially during the period of immunosuppression following the procedure.

7.4. Family Monitoring

Genetic testing should be offered to first-degree relatives, particularly to potential donors of HSC progenitors, to identify asymptomatic carriers with GATA2 deficiency. According to some authors, hematological surveillance of carriers should include annual bone marrow analysis with morphological, cytogenetic, and molecular evaluation to prevent the appearance of new driver acquisitions [99]. Moreover, some researchers recommend avoiding exposure to corticosteroids and immunosuppressive drugs and monitoring pulmonary function regularly to prevent complications [27].

7.5. Genetic Counseling

It is important to note that genetic counseling should be offered to family members who test positive for *GATA2* mutations to help them understand the implications of the diagnosis and the potential risks of passing the condition on to their own children, and they should receive proper information about the different reproductive or prenatal diagnostic options.

8. Conclusions

Recognizing GATA2 deficiency in clinical care is crucial for several reasons [115]. Firstly, an accurate diagnosis can help patients understand their specific disorder and avoid inappropriate treatments. Secondly, a genetic diagnosis can aid in selecting the most suitable HSCs donor for an allo-HSCT. TShirdly, identifying GATA2 syndrome can impact treatment recommendations and disease management for patients and their families. As patients with this condition face various complications affecting many systems, HSCT is often an attractive therapeutic option. The choice of therapy largely depends on the patient´s age, the availability of a compatible donor, and any co-existing medical conditions. Thus, early and accurate diagnosis of these patients allows for tailored therapy.

9. Future Directions

As awareness of GATA2 deficiency grows within the scientific community, early diagnosis will help in avoiding unnecessary diagnostic procedures and enable tailored strategies, for both treatment and surveillance [49].

Moreover, we may be able to identify patients who are at high risk of transforming to myeloid malignancies based on factors such as molecular alterations, cytogenetic evolution, or severity of cytopenias. By managing these patients early, we can aim for better outcomes before organ dysfunction occurs.

Author Contributions: M.S.; writing—original draft preparation, M.S., A.L., E.S., Á.Z. and J.C.; writing—review and editing, J.C.; supervision. All authors have read and agreed to the published version of the manuscript.

Funding: This study was supported by research funding from FEDER funds (CIBERONC [CB16/12/00284]), Instituto de Salud Carlos III (ISCIII) grants PI18/1472, PI19/00812, and PI22/01633, Fundació La Marató de TV3 grant 228/C/2020, as well as from the Conselleria de Educación, Cultura y Deporte CIGE/2021/015. M.S. is the recipient of the "Clinico Junior 2019" (CLJUN19005SANT) and Rio Hortega (CM22/00191) fellowships granted by the Asociación Española contra el Cáncer (AECC) and the ISCIII, respectively. A.L. is the recipient of the APOSTD/2021/212 Generalitat Valenciana post-doctoral fellowship.

Institutional Review Board Statement: Not applicable.

Informed Consent Statement: Not applicable.

Data Availability Statement: Not applicable.

Conflicts of Interest: The authors declare no conflict of interest.

References

1. Song, W.J.; Sullivan, M.G.; Legare, R.D.; Hutchings, S.; Tan, X.; Kufrin, D.; Ratajczak, J.; Resende, I.C.; Haworth, C.; Hock, R.; et al. Haploinsufficiency of CBFA2 Causes Familial Thrombocytopenia with Propensity to Develop Acute Myelogenous Leukaemia. *Nat. Genet.* **1999**, *23*, 166–175. [CrossRef] [PubMed]
2. Pippucci, T.; Savoia, A.; Perrotta, S.; Pujol-Moix, N.; Noris, P.; Castegnaro, G.; Pecci, A.; Gnan, C.; Punzo, F.; Marconi, C.; et al. Mutations in the 5′ UTR of ANKRD26, the Ankirin Repeat Domain 26 Gene, Cause an Autosomal-Dominant Form of Inherited Thrombocytopenia, THC2. *Am. J. Hum. Genet.* **2011**, *88*, 115–120. [CrossRef] [PubMed]
3. Noris, P.; Perrotta, S.; Seri, M.; Pecci, A.; Gnan, C.; Loffredo, G.; Pujol-Moix, N.; Zecca, M.; Scognamiglio, F.; de Rocco, D.; et al. Mutations in ANKRD26 Are Responsible for a Frequent Form of Inherited Thrombocytopenia: Analysis of 78 Patients from 21 Families. *Blood* **2011**, *117*, 6673–6680. [CrossRef] [PubMed]
4. Noris, P.; Favier, R.; Alessi, M.C.; Geddis, A.E.; Kunishima, S.; Heller, P.G.; Giordano, P.; Niederhoffer, K.Y.; Bussel, J.B.; Podda, G.M.; et al. ANKRD26-Related Thrombocytopenia and Myeloid Malignancies. *Blood* **2013**, *122*, 1987–1989. [CrossRef]
5. Zhang, M.Y.; Churpek, J.E.; Keel, S.B.; Walsh, T.; Lee, M.K.; Loeb, K.R.; Gulsuner, S.; Pritchard, C.C.; Sanchez-Bonilla, M.; Delrow, J.J.; et al. Germline ETV6 Mutations in Familial Thrombocytopenia and Hematologic Malignancy. *Nat. Genet.* **2015**, *47*, 180. [CrossRef]
6. Noetzli, L.; Lo, R.W.; Lee-Sherick, A.B.; Callaghan, M.; Noris, P.; Savoia, A.; Rajpurkar, M.; Jones, K.; Gowan, K.; Balduini, C.L.; et al. Germline Mutations in ETV6 Are Associated with Thrombocytopenia, Red Cell Macrocytosis and Predisposition to Lymphoblastic Leukemia. *Nat. Genet.* **2015**, *47*, 535–538. [CrossRef]
7. Topka, S.; Vijai, J.; Walsh, M.F.; Jacobs, L.; Maria, A.; Villano, D.; Gaddam, P.; Wu, G.; McGee, R.B.; Quinn, E.; et al. Germline ETV6 Mutations Confer Susceptibility to Acute Lymphoblastic Leukemia and Thrombocytopenia. *PLoS Genet.* **2015**, *11*, e1005262. [CrossRef]
8. Smith, M.L.; Cavenagh, J.D.; Lister, T.A.; Fitzgibbon, J. Mutation of CEBPA in Familial Acute Myeloid Leukemia. *N. Engl. J. Med.* **2004**, *351*, 2403–2407. [CrossRef]
9. Polprasert, C.; Schulze, I.; Sekeres, M.A.; Makishima, H.; Przychodzen, B.; Hosono, N.; Singh, J.; Padgett, R.A.; Gu, X.; Phillips, J.G.; et al. Inherited and Somatic Defects in DDX41 in Myeloid Neoplasms. *Cancer Cell* **2015**, *27*, 658–670. [CrossRef]
10. Hahn, C.N.; Chong, C.E.; Carmichael, C.L.; Wilkins, E.J.; Brautigan, P.J.; Li, X.C.; Babic, M.; Lin, M.; Carmagnac, A.; Lee, Y.K.; et al. Heritable GATA2 Mutations Associated with Familial Myelodysplastic Syndrome and Acute Myeloid Leukemia. *Nat. Genet.* **2011**, *43*, 1012. [CrossRef]
11. Harutyunyan, A.S.; Giambruno, R.; Krendl, C.; Stukalov, A.; Klampfl, T.; Berg, T.; Chen, D.; Feenstra, J.D.M.; Jäger, R.; Gisslinger, B.; et al. Germline RBBP6 Mutations in Familial Myeloproliferative Neoplasms. *Blood* **2016**, *127*, 362–365. [CrossRef]
12. Kirwan, M.; Vulliamy, T.; Marrone, A.; Walne, A.J.; Beswick, R.; Hillmen, P.; Kelly, R.; Stewart, A.; Bowen, D.; Schonland, S.O.; et al. Defining the Pathogenic Role of Telomerase Mutations in Myelodysplastic Syndrome and Acute Myeloid Leukemia. *Hum. Mutat.* **2009**, *30*, 1567–1573. [CrossRef]
13. Narumi, S.; Amano, N.; Ishii, T.; Katsumata, N.; Muroya, K.; Adachi, M.; Toyoshima, K.; Tanaka, Y.; Fukuzawa, R.; Miyako, K.; et al. SAMD9 Mutations Cause a Novel Multisystem Disorder, MIRAGE Syndrome, and Are Associated with Loss of Chromosome 7. *Nat. Genet.* **2016**, *48*, 792–797. [CrossRef]
14. Chen, D.H.; Below, J.E.; Shimamura, A.; Keel, S.B.; Matsushita, M.; Wolff, J.; Sul, Y.; Bonkowski, E.; Castella, M.; Taniguchi, T.; et al. Ataxia-Pancytopenia Syndrome Is Caused by Missense Mutations in SAMD9L. *Am. J. Hum. Genet.* **2016**, *98*, 1146–1158. [CrossRef]
15. Tesi, B.; Davidsson, J.; Voss, M.; Rahikkala, E.; Holmes, T.D.; Chiang, S.C.C.; Komulainen-Ebrahim, J.; Gorcenco, S.; Nilsson, A.R.; Ripperger, T.; et al. Gain-of-Function SAMD9L Mutations Cause a Syndrome of Cytopenia, Immunodeficiency, MDS, and Neurological Symptoms. *Blood* **2017**, *129*, 2266–2279. [CrossRef]

16. Akpan, I.J.; Osman, A.E.G.; Drazer, M.W.; Godley, L.A. Hereditary Myelodysplastic Syndrome and Acute Myeloid Leukemia: Diagnosis, Questions, and Controversies. *Curr. Hematol. Malig. Rep.* **2018**, *13*, 426–434. [CrossRef]
17. Huang, K.L.; Mashl, R.J.; Wu, Y.; Ritter, D.I.; Wang, J.; Oh, C.; Paczkowska, M.; Reynolds, S.; Wyczalkowski, M.A.; Oak, N.; et al. Pathogenic Germline Variants in 10,389 Adult Cancers. *Cell* **2018**, *173*, 355–370.e14. [CrossRef]
18. Lu, C.; Xie, M.; Wendl, M.C.; Wang, J.; McLellan, M.D.; Leiserson, M.D.M.; Huang, K.L.; Wyczalkowski, M.A.; Jayasinghe, R.; Banerjee, T.; et al. Patterns and Functional Implications of Rare Germline Variants across 12 Cancer Types. *Nat. Commun.* **2015**, *6*, 10086. [CrossRef]
19. Wartiovaara-Kautto, U.; Hirvonen, E.A.M.; Pitkänen, E.; Heckman, C.; Saarela, J.; Kettunen, K.; Porkka, K.; Kilpivaara, O. Germline Alterations in a Consecutive Series of Acute Myeloid Leukemia. *Leukemia* **2018**, *32*, 2282–2285. [CrossRef]
20. Yang, F.; Long, N.; Anekpuritanang, T.; Bottomly, D.; Savage, J.C.; Lee, T.; Solis-Ruiz, J.; Borate, U.; Wilmot, B.; Tognon, C.; et al. Identification and Prioritization of Myeloid Malignancy Germline Variants in a Large Cohort of Adult Patients with AML. *Blood* **2022**, *139*, 1208–1221. [CrossRef]
21. Drazer, M.W.; Kadri, S.; Sukhanova, M.; Patil, S.A.; West, A.H.; Feurstein, S.; Calderon, D.A.; Jones, M.F.; Weipert, C.M.; Daugherty, C.K.; et al. Prognostic Tumor Sequencing Panels Frequently Identify Germ Line Variants Associated with Hereditary Hematopoietic Malignancies. *Blood Adv.* **2018**, *2*, 146–150. [CrossRef] [PubMed]
22. Arber, D.A.; Orazi, A.; Hasserjian, R.; Thiele, J.; Borowitz, M.J.; le Beau, M.M.; Bloomfield, C.D.; Cazzola, M.; Vardiman, J.W. The 2016 Revision to the World Health Organization Classification of Myeloid Neoplasms and Acute Leukemia. *Blood*. **2016**, *127*, 2391–2405, Erratum in *Blood* **2016**, *128*, 462–463. [CrossRef]
23. Baliakas, P.; Tesi, B.; Wartiovaara-Kautto, U.; Stray-Pedersen, A.; Friis, L.S.; Dybedal, I.; Hovland, R.; Jahnukainen, K.; Raaschou-Jensen, K.; Ljungman, P.; et al. Nordic Guidelines for Germline Predisposition to Myeloid Neoplasms in Adults: Recommendations for Genetic Diagnosis, Clinical Management and Follow-Up. *Hemasphere* **2019**, *3*, e321. [CrossRef] [PubMed]
24. Döhner, H.; Wei, A.H.; Appelbaum, F.R.; Craddock, C.; DiNardo, C.D.; Dombret, H.; Ebert, B.L.; Fenaux, P.; Godley, L.A.; Hasserjian, R.P.; et al. Diagnosis and Management of AML in Adults: 2022 Recommendations from an International Expert Panel on Behalf of the ELN. *Blood* **2022**, *140*, 1345–1377. [CrossRef] [PubMed]
25. Khoury, J.D.; Solary, E.; Abla, O.; Akkari, Y.; Alaggio, R.; Apperley, J.F.; Bejar, R.; Berti, E.; Busque, L.; Chan, J.K.C.; et al. The 5th Edition of the World Health Organization Classification of Haematolymphoid Tumours: Myeloid and Histiocytic/Dendritic Neoplasms. *Leukemia* **2022**, *36*, 1703–1719. [CrossRef]
26. Arber, D.A.; Orazi, A.; Hasserjian, R.P.; Borowitz, M.J.; Calvo, K.R.; Kvasnicka, H.M.; Wang, S.A.; Bagg, A.; Barbui, T.; Branford, S.; et al. International Consensus Classification of Myeloid Neoplasms and Acute Leukemias: Integrating Morphologic, Clinical, and Genomic Data. *Blood* **2022**, *140*, 1200–1228. [CrossRef]
27. Wlodarski, M.W.; Collin, M.; Horwitz, M.S. GATA2 Deficiency and Related Myeloid Neoplasms. *Semin Hematol.* **2017**, *54*, 81–86. [CrossRef]
28. McGowan-Jordan, J.; Simon, A.; Schmid, M. *An International System for Human Cytogenetic Nomenclature*; Karger: Basel, Switzerland; New York, NY, USA, 2016.
29. Hsu, A.P.; Sampaio, E.P.; Khan, J.; Calvo, K.R.; Lemieux, J.E.; Patel, S.Y.; Frucht, D.M.; Vinh, D.C.; Auth, R.D.; Freeman, A.F.; et al. Mutations in GATA2 Are Associated with the Autosomal Dominant and Sporadic Monocytopenia and Mycobacterial Infection (MonoMAC) Syndrome. *Blood* **2011**, *118*, 2653–2655. [CrossRef]
30. Rodrigues, N.P.; Tipping, A.J.; Wang, Z.; Enver, T. GATA-2 Mediated Regulation of Normal Hematopoietic Stem/Progenitor Cell Function, Myelodysplasia and Myeloid Leukemia. *Int. J. Biochem. Cell Biol.* **2012**, *44*, 457–460. [CrossRef]
31. Rodrigues, N.P.; Janzen, V.; Forkert, R.; Dombkowski, D.M.; Boyd, A.S.; Orkin, S.H.; Enver, T.; Vyas, P.; Scadden, D.T. Haploinsufficiency of GATA-2 Perturbs Adult Hematopoietic Stem-Cell Homeostasis. *Blood* **2005**, *106*, 477–484. [CrossRef]
32. Rodrigues, N.P.; Boyd, A.S.; Fugazza, C.; May, G.E.; Guo, Y.P.; Tipping, A.J.; Scadden, D.T.; Vyas, P.; Enver, T. GATA-2 Regulates Granulocyte-Macrophage Progenitor Cell Function. *Blood* **2008**, *112*, 4862–4873. [CrossRef]
33. Nandakumar, S.K.; Johnson, K.; Throm, S.L.; Pestina, T.I.; Neale, G.; Persons, D.A. Low-Level GATA2 Overexpression Promotes Myeloid Progenitor Self-Renewal and Blocks Lymphoid Differentiation in Mice. *Exp. Hematol.* **2015**, *43*, 565–577. [CrossRef]
34. Zhou, Y.; Zhang, Y.; Chen, B.; Dong, Y.; Zhang, Y.; Mao, B.; Pan, X.; Lai, M.; Chen, Y.; Bian, G.; et al. Overexpression of GATA2 Enhances Development and Maintenance of Human Embryonic Stem Cell-Derived Hematopoietic Stem Cell-like Progenitors. *Stem Cell Rep.* **2019**, *13*, 31–47. [CrossRef]
35. Menendez-Gonzalez, J.B.; Vukovic, M.; Abdelfattah, A.; Saleh, L.; Almotiri, A.; Thomas, L.A.; Agirre-Lizaso, A.; Azevedo, A.; Menezes, A.C.; Tornillo, G.; et al. Gata2 as a Crucial Regulator of Stem Cells in Adult Hematopoiesis and Acute Myeloid Leukemia. *Stem Cell Rep.* **2019**, *13*, 291–306. [CrossRef]
36. Beck, D.; Thoms, J.A.I.; Perera, D.; Schütte, J.; Unnikrishnan, A.; Knezevic, K.; Kinston, S.J.; Wilson, N.K.; O'Brien, T.A.; Göttgens, B.; et al. Genome-Wide Analysis of Transcriptional Regulators in Human HSPCs Reveals a Densely Interconnected Network of Coding and Noncoding Genes. *Blood* **2013**, *122*, e12–e22. [CrossRef]
37. May, G.; Soneji, S.; Tipping, A.J.; Teles, J.; McGowan, S.J.; Wu, M.; Guo, Y.; Fugazza, C.; Brown, J.; Karlsson, G.; et al. Dynamic Analysis of Gene Expression and Genome-Wide Transcription Factor Binding during Lineage Specification of Multipotent Progenitors. *Cell Stem Cell* **2013**, *13*, 754–768. [CrossRef]
38. Homan, C.C.; Venugopal, P.; Arts, P.; Shahrin, N.H.; Feurstein, S.; Rawlings, L.; Lawrence, D.M.; Andrews, J.; King-Smith, S.L.; Harvey, N.L.; et al. GATA2 Deficiency Syndrome: A Decade of Discovery. *Hum. Mutat.* **2021**, *42*, 1399–1421. [CrossRef]

39. Bruzzese, A.; Leardini, D.; Masetti, R.; Strocchio, L.; Girardi, K.; Algeri, M.; del Baldo, G.; Locatelli, F.; Mastronuzzi, A. GATA2 Related Conditions and Predisposition to Pediatric Myelodysplastic Syndromes. *Cancers* **2020**, *12*, 2962. [CrossRef] [PubMed]
40. Collin, M.; Dickinson, R.; Bigley, V. Haematopoietic and Immune Defects Associated with GATA2 Mutation. *Br. J. Haematol.* **2015**, *169*, 173–187. [CrossRef]
41. Spinner, M.A.; Sanchez, L.A.; Hsu, A.P.; Shaw, P.A.; Zerbe, C.S.; Calvo, K.R.; Arthur, D.C.; Gu, W.; Gould, C.M.; Brewer, C.C.; et al. GATA2 Deficiency: A Protean Disorder of Hematopoiesis, Lymphatics, and Immunity. *Blood* **2014**, *123*, 809–821. [CrossRef]
42. Kozyra, E.J.; Pastor, V.B.; Lefkopoulos, S.; Sahoo, S.S.; Busch, H.; Voss, R.K.; Erlacher, M.; Lebrecht, D.; Szvetnik, E.A.; Hirabayashi, S.; et al. Synonymous GATA2 Mutations Result in Selective Loss of Mutated RNA and Are Common in Patients with GATA2 Deficiency. *Leukemia* **2020**, *34*, 2673–2687. [CrossRef] [PubMed]
43. Wehr, C.; Grotius, K.; Casadei, S.; Bleckmann, D.; Bode, S.F.N.; Frye, B.C.; Seidl, M.; Gulsuner, S.; King, M.C.; Percival, M.B.; et al. A Novel Disease-Causing Synonymous Exonic Mutation in GATA2 Affecting RNA Splicing. *Blood* **2018**, *132*, 1211–1215. [CrossRef] [PubMed]
44. Bresnick, E.H.; Jung, M.M.; Katsumura, K.R. Human GATA2 Mutations and Hematologic Disease: How Many Paths to Pathogenesis? *Blood Adv.* **2020**, *4*, 4584–4592. [CrossRef] [PubMed]
45. Hsu, A.P.; Johnson, K.D.; Falcone, E.L.; Sanalkumar, R.; Sanchez, L.; Hickstein, D.D.; Cuellar-Rodriguez, J.; Lemieux, J.E.; Zerbe, C.S.; Bresnick, E.H.; et al. GATA2 Haploinsufficiency Caused by Mutations in a Conserved Intronic Element Leads to MonoMAC Syndrome. *Blood* **2013**, *121*, 3830–3837. [CrossRef] [PubMed]
46. You, X.; Zhou, Y.; Chang, Y.I.; Kong, G.; Ranheim, E.A.; Johnson, K.D.; Soukup, A.A.; Bresnick, E.H.; Zhang, J. Gata2 +9.5 Enhancer Regulates Adult Hematopoietic Stem Cell Self-Renewal and T-Cell Development. *Blood Adv.* **2022**, *6*, 1095–1099. [CrossRef]
47. al Seraihi, A.F.; Rio-Machin, A.; Tawana, K.; Bödör, C.; Wang, J.; Nagano, A.; Heward, J.A.; Iqbal, S.; Best, S.; Lea, N.; et al. GATA2 Monoallelic Expression Underlies Reduced Penetrance in Inherited GATA2-Mutated MDS/AML. *Leukemia* **2018**, *32*, 2502–2507. [CrossRef]
48. Zhang, S.J.; Ma, L.Y.; Huang, Q.H.; Li, G.; Gu, B.W.; Gao, X.D.; Shi, J.Y.; Wang, Y.Y.; Gao, L.; Cai, X.; et al. Gain-of-Function Mutation of GATA-2 in Acute Myeloid Transformation of Chronic Myeloid Leukemia. *Proc. Natl. Acad. Sci. USA* **2008**, *105*, 2076–2081. [CrossRef]
49. Wlodarski, M.W.; Hirabayashi, S.; Pastor, V.; Starý, J.; Hasle, H.; Masetti, R.; Dworzak, M.; Schmugge, M.; van den Heuvel-Eibrink, M.; Ussowicz, M.; et al. Prevalence, Clinical Characteristics, and Prognosis of GATA2-Related Myelodysplastic Syndromes in Children and Adolescents. *Blood* **2016**, *127*, 1387–1397. [CrossRef]
50. West, R.R.; Calvo, K.R.; Embree, L.J.; Wang, W.; Tuschong, L.M.; Bauer, T.R.; Tillo, D.; Lack, J.; Droll, S.; Hsu, A.P.; et al. ASXL1 and STAG2 Are Common Mutations in GATA2 Deficiency Patients with Bone Marrow Disease and Myelodysplastic Syndrome. *Blood Adv.* **2022**, *6*, 793–807. [CrossRef]
51. McReynolds, L.J.; Calvo, K.R.; Holland, S.M. Germline GATA2 Mutation and Bone Marrow Failure. *Hematol. Oncol. Clin. N. Am.* **2018**, *32*, 713–728. [CrossRef]
52. Bödör, C.; Renneville, A.; Smith, M.; Charazac, A.; Iqbal, S.; Étancelin, P.; Cavenagh, J.; Barnett, M.J.; Kramarzová, K.; Krishnan, B.; et al. Germ-Line GATA2 p.THR354MET Mutation in Familial Myelodysplastic Syndrome with Acquired Monosomy 7 and ASXL1 Mutation Demonstrating Rapid Onset and Poor Survival. *Haematologica* **2012**, *97*, 890–894. [CrossRef]
53. McReynolds, L.J.; Zhang, Y.; Yang, Y.; Tang, J.; Mulé, M.; Hsu, A.P.; Townsley, D.M.; West, R.R.; Zhu, J.; Hickstein, D.D.; et al. Rapid Progression to AML in a Patient with Germline GATA2 Mutation and Acquired NRAS Q61K Mutation. *Leuk Res. Rep.* **2019**, *12*, 100176. [CrossRef]
54. Fisher, K.E.; Hsu, A.P.; Williams, C.L.; Sayeed, H.; Merritt, B.Y.; Tarek Elghetany, M.; Holland, S.M.; Bertuch, A.A.; Gramatges, M.M. Somatic Mutations in Children with GATA2-Associated Myelodysplastic Syndrome Who Lack Other Features of GATA2 Deficiency. *Blood Adv.* **2017**, *1*, 443–448. [CrossRef] [PubMed]
55. Pastor Loyola, V.B.; Hirabayashi, S.; Pohl, S.; Kozyra, E.J.; Catala, A.; de Moerloose, B.; Dworzak, M.; Hasle, H.; Masetti, R.; Schmugge, M.; et al. Somatic Genetic and Epigenetic Architecture of Myelodysplastic Syndromes Arising from GATA2 Deficiency. *Blood* **2015**, *126*, 299. [CrossRef]
56. Churpek, J.E.; Pyrtel, K.; Kanchi, K.L.; Shao, J.; Koboldt, D.; Miller, C.A.; Shen, D.; Fulton, R.; O'Laughlin, M.; Fronick, C.; et al. Genomic Analysis of Germ Line and Somatic Variants in Familial Myelodysplasia/Acute Myeloid Leukemia. *Blood* **2015**, *126*, 2484–2490. [CrossRef]
57. Zhang, M.Y.; Keel, S.B.; Walsh, T.; Lee, M.K.; Gulsuner, S.; Watts, A.C.; Pritchard, C.C.; Salipante, S.J.; Jeng, M.R.; Hofmann, I.; et al. Genomic Analysis of Bone Marrow Failure and Myelodysplastic Syndromes Reveals Phenotypic and Diagnostic Complexity. *Haematologica* **2015**, *100*, 42–48. [CrossRef]
58. Keel, S.B.; Scott, A.; Bonilla, M.S.; Ho, P.A.; Gulsuner, S.; Pritchard, C.C.; Abkowitz, J.L.; King, M.C.; Walsh, T.; Shimamura, A. Genetic Features of Myelodysplastic Syndrome and Aplastic Anemia in Pediatric and Young Adult Patients. *Haematologica* **2016**, *101*, 1343–1350. [CrossRef]
59. Wang, X.; Muramatsu, H.; Okuno, Y.; Sakaguchi, H.; Yoshida, K.; Kawashima, N.; Xu, Y.; Shiraishi, Y.; Chiba, K.; Tanaka, H.; et al. GATA2 and Secondary Mutations in Familial Myelodysplastic Syndromes and Pediatric Myeloid Malignancies. *Haematologica* **2015**, *100*, e398–e401. [CrossRef]

60. Kotmayer, L.; Romero-Moya, D.; Marin-Bejar, O.; Kozyra, E.; Català, A.; Bigas, A.; Wlodarski, M.W.; Bödör, C.; Giorgetti, A. GATA2 Deficiency and MDS/AML: Experimental Strategies for Disease Modelling and Future Therapeutic Prospects. *Br. J. Haematol.* **2022**, *199*, 482–495. [CrossRef]
61. Martignoles, J.A.; Delhommeau, F.; Hirsch, P. Genetic Hierarchy of Acute Myeloid Leukemia: From Clonal Hematopoiesis to Molecular Residual Disease. *Int. J. Mol. Sci.* **2018**, *19*, 3850. [CrossRef]
62. Fasan, A.; Eder, C.; Haferlach, C.; Grossmann, V.; Kohlmann, A.; Dicker, F.; Kern, W.; Haferlach, T.; Schnittger, S. GATA2 Mutations Are Frequent in Intermediate-Risk Karyotype AML with Biallelic CEBPA Mutations and Are Associated with Favorable Prognosis. *Leukemia* **2013**, *27*, 482–485. [CrossRef] [PubMed]
63. Greif, P.A.; Dufour, A.; Konstandin, N.P.; Ksienzyk, B.; Zellmeier, E.; Tizazu, B.; Sturm, J.; Benthaus, T.; Herold, T.; Yaghmaie, M.; et al. GATA2 Zinc Finger 1 Mutations Associated with Biallelic CEBPA Mutations Define a Unique Genetic Entity of Acute Myeloid Leukemia. *Blood* **2012**, *120*, 395–403. [CrossRef]
64. Theis, F.; Corbacioglu, A.; Gaidzik, V.I.; Paschka, P.; Weber, D.; Bullinger, L.; Heuser, M.; Ganser, A.; Thol, F.; Schlegelberger, B.; et al. Clinical Impact of GATA2 Mutations in Acute Myeloid Leukemia Patients Harboring CEBPA Mutations: A Study of the AML Study Group. *Leukemia* **2016**, *30*, 2248–2250. [CrossRef]
65. Alfayez, M.; Wang, S.A.; Bannon, S.A.; Kontoyiannis, D.P.; Kornblau, S.M.; Orange, J.S.; Mace, E.M.; DiNardo, C.D. Myeloid Malignancies with Somatic GATA2 Mutations Can Be Associated with an Immunodeficiency Phenotype. *Leuk Lymphoma* **2019**, *60*, 2025–2033. [CrossRef] [PubMed]
66. Sekhar, M.; Pocock, R.; Lowe, D.; Mitchell, C.; Marafioti, T.; Dickinson, R.; Collin, M.; Lipman, M. Can Somatic GATA2 Mutation Mimic Germ Line GATA2 Mutation? *Blood Adv.* **2018**, *2*, 904. [CrossRef]
67. Saettini, F.; Coliva, T.; Vendemini, F.; Moratto, D.; Savoldi, G.; Borlenghi, E.; Masetti, R.; Niemeyer, C.M.; Biondi, A.; Balduzzi, A.; et al. When to Suspect GATA2 Deficiency in Pediatric Patients: From Complete Blood Count to Diagnosis. *Pediatr. Hematol. Oncol.* **2021**, *38*, 510–514. [CrossRef]
68. Ostergaard, P.; Simpson, M.A.; Connell, F.C.; Steward, C.G.; Brice, G.; Woollard, W.J.; Dafou, D.; Kilo, T.; Smithson, S.; Lunt, P.; et al. Mutations in GATA2 Cause Primary Lymphedema Associated with a Predisposition to Acute Myeloid Leukemia (Emberger Syndrome). *Nat. Genet.* **2011**, *43*, 929–931. [CrossRef]
69. Dickinson, R.E.; Griffin, H.; Bigley, V.; Reynard, L.N.; Hussain, R.; Haniffa, M.; Lakey, J.H.; Rahman, T.; Wang, X.N.; McGovern, N.; et al. Exome Sequencing Identifies GATA-2 Mutation as the Cause of Dendritic Cell, Monocyte, B and NK Lymphoid Deficiency. *Blood* **2011**, *118*, 2656–2658. [CrossRef]
70. Oleaga-Quintas, C.; de Oliveira-Júnior, E.B.; Rosain, J.; Rapaport, F.; Deswarte, C.; Guérin, A.; Sajjath, S.M.; Zhou, Y.J.; Marot, S.; Lozano, C.; et al. Inherited GATA2 Deficiency Is Dominant by Haploinsufficiency and Displays Incomplete Clinical Penetrance. *J. Clin. Immunol.* **2021**, *41*, 639–657. [CrossRef]
71. Donadieu, J.; Lamant, M.; Fieschi, C.; de Fontbrune, F.S.; Caye, A.; Ouachee, M.; Beaupain, B.; Bustamante, J.; Poirel, H.A.; Isidor, B.; et al. Natural History of GATA2 Deficiency in a Survey of 79 French and Belgian Patients. *Haematologica* **2018**, *103*, 1278–1287. [CrossRef]
72. Kazenwadel, J.; Secker, G.A.; Liu, Y.J.; Rosenfeld, J.A.; Wildin, R.S.; Cuellar-Rodriguez, J.; Hsu, A.P.; Dyack, S.; Fernandez, C.V.; Chong, C.E.; et al. Loss-of-Function Germline GATA2 Mutations in Patients with MDS/AML or MonoMAC Syndrome and Primary Lymphedema Reveal a Key Role for GATA2 in the Lymphatic Vasculature. *Blood* **2012**, *119*, 1283–1291. [CrossRef] [PubMed]
73. Hayashi, Y.; Harada, Y.; Huang, G.; Harada, H. Myeloid Neoplasms with Germ Line RUNX1 Mutation. *Int. J. Hematol.* **2017**, *106*, 183–188. [CrossRef] [PubMed]
74. Marconi, C.; Canobbio, I.; Bozzi, V.; Pippucci, T.; Simonetti, G.; Melazzini, F.; Angori, S.; Martinelli, G.; Saglio, G.; Torti, M.; et al. 5′UTR Point Substitutions and N-Terminal Truncating Mutations of ANKRD26 in Acute Myeloid Leukemia. *J. Hematol. Oncol.* **2017**, *10*, 18. [CrossRef]
75. Feurstein, S.; Godley, L.A. Germline ETV6 Mutations and Predisposition to Hematological Malignancies. *Int. J. Hematol.* **2017**, *106*, 189–195. [CrossRef]
76. Fabozzi, F.; Strocchio, L.; Mastronuzzi, A.; Merli, P. GATA2 and Marrow Failure. *Best Pract. Res. Clin. Haematol.* **2021**, *34*, 101278. [CrossRef]
77. Rütsche, C.V.; Haralambieva, E.; Lysenko, V.; Balabanov, S.; Theocharides, A.P.A. A Patient with a Germline GATA2 Mutation and Primary Myelofibrosis. *Blood Adv.* **2021**, *5*, 791–795. [CrossRef]
78. Sahoo, S.S.; Pastor, V.B.; Goodings, C.; Voss, R.K.; Kozyra, E.J.; Szvetnik, A.; Noellke, P.; Dworzak, M.; Starý, J.; Locatelli, F.; et al. Clinical Evolution, Genetic Landscape and Trajectories of Clonal Hematopoiesis in SAMD9/SAMD9L Syndromes. *Nat. Med.* **2021**, *27*, 1806–1817. [CrossRef]
79. Sahoo, S.S.; Kozyra, E.J.; Wlodarski, M.W. Germline Predisposition in Myeloid Neoplasms: Unique Genetic and Clinical Features of GATA2 Deficiency and SAMD9/SAMD9L Syndromes. *Best Pract. Res. Clin. Haematol.* **2020**, *33*, 101197. [CrossRef]
80. Shamriz, O.; Zahalka, N.; Simon, A.J.; Lev, A.; Barel, O.; Mor, N.; Tal, Y.; Segel, M.J.; Somech, R.; Yonath, H.; et al. GATA2 Deficiency in Adult Life Is Characterized by Phenotypic Diversity and Delayed Diagnosis. *Front. Immunol.* **2022**, *13*, 886117. [CrossRef]

81. Mace, E.M.; Hsu, A.P.; Monaco-Shawver, L.; Makedonas, G.; Rosen, J.B.; Dropulic, L.; Cohen, J.I.; Frenkel, E.P.; Bagwell, J.C.; Sullivan, J.L.; et al. Mutations in GATA2 Cause Human NK Cell Deficiency with Specific Loss of the CD56(Bright) Subset. *Blood* **2013**, *121*, 2669–2677. [CrossRef]
82. Maciejewski-Duval, A.; Meuris, F.; Bignon, A.; Aknin, M.-L.; Balabanian, K.; Faivre, L.; Pasquet, M.; Barlogis, V.; Fieschi, C.; Bellanné-Chantelot, C.; et al. Altered Chemotactic Response to CXCL12 in Patients Carrying GATA2 Mutations. *J. Leukoc Biol.* **2016**, *99*, 1065–1076. [CrossRef] [PubMed]
83. Ganapathi, K.A.; Townsley, D.M.; Hsu, A.P.; Arthur, D.C.; Zerbe, C.S.; Cuellar-Rodriguez, J.; Hickstein, D.D.; Rosenzweig, S.D.; Braylan, R.C.; Young, N.S.; et al. GATA2 Deficiency-Associated Bone Marrow Disorder Differs from Idiopathic Aplastic Anemia. *Blood* **2015**, *125*, 56–70. [CrossRef] [PubMed]
84. Nováková, M.; Žaliová, M.; Suková, M.; Wlodarski, M.; Janda, A.; Froňková, E.; Campr, V.; Lejhancová, K.; Zapletal, O.; Pospíšilová, D.; et al. Loss of B Cells and Their Precursors Is the Most Constant Feature of GATA-2 Deficiency in Childhood Myelodysplastic Syndrome. *Haematologica* **2016**, *101*, 707–716. [CrossRef] [PubMed]
85. Dickinson, R.E.; Milne, P.; Jardine, L.; Zandi, S.; Swierczek, S.I.; McGovern, N.; Cookson, S.; Ferozepurwalla, Z.; Langridge, A.; Pagan, S.; et al. The Evolution of Cellular Deficiency in GATA2 Mutation. *Blood* **2014**, *123*, 863–874. [CrossRef] [PubMed]
86. Vinh, D.C.; Patel, S.Y.; Uzel, G.; Anderson, V.L.; Freeman, A.F.; Olivier, K.N.; Spalding, C.; Hughes, S.; Pittaluga, S.; Raffeld, M.; et al. Autosomal Dominant and Sporadic Monocytopenia with Susceptibility to Mycobacteria, Fungi, Papillomaviruses, and Myelodysplasia. *Blood* **2010**, *115*, 1519–1529. [CrossRef]
87. Chou, J.; Lutskiy, M.; Tsitsikov, E.; Notarangelo, L.D.; Geha, R.S.; Dioun, A. Presence of Hypogammaglobulinemia and Abnormal Antibody Responses in GATA2 Deficiency. *J. Allergy Clin. Immunol.* **2014**, *134*, 223–226. [CrossRef]
88. Toboni, M.D.; Bevis, K.S. Vulvar Cancer as a Result of GATA2 Deficiency, a Rare Genetic Immunodeficiency Syndrome. *Obstet. Gynecol.* **2018**, *132*, 1112–1115. [CrossRef]
89. Amarnani, A.A.; Poladian, K.R.; Marciano, B.E.; Daub, J.R.; Williams, S.G.; Livinski, A.A.; Hsu, A.P.; Palmer, C.L.; Kenney, C.M.; Avila, D.N.; et al. A Panoply of Rheumatological Manifestations in Patients with GATA2 Deficiency. *Sci. Rep.* **2020**, *10*, 8305. [CrossRef]
90. Marciano, B.E.; Olivier, K.N.; Folio, L.R.; Zerbe, C.S.; Hsu, A.P.; Freeman, A.F.; Filie, A.C.; Spinner, M.A.; Sanchez, L.A.; Lovell, J.P.; et al. Pulmonary Manifestations of GATA2 Deficiency. *Chest* **2021**, *160*, 1350–1359. [CrossRef]
91. Raffáč, Š.; Aljubouri, M.A.S.; Gabzdilová, J. Alveolar Proteinosis, Infectious Complications and Monocytopenia Associated with GATA2 Deficiency. *Neuro Endocrinol. Lett.* **2021**, *41*, 290–295.
92. Cuellar-Rodriguez, J.; Gea-Banacloche, J.; Freeman, A.F.; Hsu, A.P.; Zerbe, C.S.; Calvo, K.R.; Wilder, J.; Kurlander, R.; Olivier, K.N.; Holland, S.M.; et al. Successful Allogeneic Hematopoietic Stem Cell Transplantation for GATA2 Deficiency. *Blood* **2011**, *118*, 3715–3720. [CrossRef] [PubMed]
93. Simonis, A.; Fux, M.; Nair, G.; Mueller, N.J.; Haralambieva, E.; Pabst, T.; Pachlopnik Schmid, J.; Schmidt, A.; Schanz, U.; Manz, M.G.; et al. Allogeneic Hematopoietic Cell Transplantation in Patients with GATA2 Deficiency-a Case Report and Comprehensive Review of the Literature. *Ann. Hematol.* **2018**, *97*, 1961–1973. [CrossRef] [PubMed]
94. Kazenwadel, J.; Betterman, K.L.; Chong, C.E.; Stokes, P.H.; Lee, Y.K.; Secker, G.A.; Agalarov, Y.; Demir, C.S.; Lawrence, D.M.; Sutton, D.L.; et al. GATA2 Is Required for Lymphatic Vessel Valve Development and Maintenance. *J. Clin. Investig.* **2015**, *125*, 2879–2994. [CrossRef] [PubMed]
95. Nakazawa, H.; Yamaguchi, T.; Sakai, H.; Maruyama, M.; Kawakami, T.; Kawakami, F.; Nishina, S.; Ishikawa, M.; Kosho, T.; Ishida, F. A Novel Germline GATA2 Frameshift Mutation with a Premature Stop Codon in a Family with Congenital Sensory Hearing Loss and Myelodysplastic Syndrome. *Int. J. Hematol.* **2021**, *114*, 286–291. [CrossRef]
96. Saida, S.; Umeda, K.; Yasumi, T.; Matsumoto, A.; Kato, I.; Hiramatsu, H.; Ohara, O.; Heike, T.; Adachi, S. Successful Reduced-Intensity Stem Cell Transplantation for GATA2 Deficiency before Progression of Advanced MDS. *Pediatr Transplant.* **2016**, *20*, 333–336. [CrossRef]
97. Rio-Machin, A.; Vulliamy, T.; Hug, N.; Walne, A.; Tawana, K.; Cardoso, S.; Ellison, A.; Pontikos, N.; Wang, J.; Tummala, H.; et al. The Complex Genetic Landscape of Familial MDS and AML Reveals Pathogenic Germline Variants. *Nat. Commun.* **2020**, *11*, 1044. [CrossRef]
98. Bortnick, R.; Wlodarski, M.; de Haas, V.; de Moerloose, B.; Dworzak, M.; Hasle, H.; Masetti, R.; Starý, J.; Turkiewicz, D.; Ussowicz, M.; et al. Hematopoietic Stem Cell Transplantation in Children and Adolescents with GATA2-Related Myelodysplastic Syndrome. *Bone Marrow Transplant.* **2021**, *56*, 2732–2741. [CrossRef]
99. Jørgensen, S.F.; Buechner, J.; Myhre, A.E.; Galteland, E.; Spetalen, S.; Kulseth, M.A.; Sorte, H.S.; Holla, Ø.L.; Lundman, E.; Alme, C.; et al. A Nationwide Study of GATA2 Deficiency in Norway-the Majority of Patients Have Undergone Allo-HSCT. *J. Clin. Immunol.* **2022**, *42*, 404–420. [CrossRef]
100. Nichols-Vinueza, D.X.; Parta, M.; Shah, N.N.; Cuellar-Rodriguez, J.M.; Bauer, T.R.; West, R.R.; Hsu, A.P.; Calvo, K.R.; Steinberg, S.M.; Notarangelo, L.D.; et al. Donor Source and Post-Transplantation Cyclophosphamide Influence Outcome in Allogeneic Stem Cell Transplantation for GATA2 Deficiency. *Br. J. Haematol.* **2022**, *196*, 169–178. [CrossRef]
101. Hofmann, I.; Avagyan, S.; Stetson, A.; Guo, D.; Al-Sayegh, H.; London, W.B.; Lehmann, L. Comparison of Outcomes of Myeloablative Allogeneic Stem Cell Transplantation for Pediatric Patients with Bone Marrow Failure, Myelodysplastic Syndrome and Acute Myeloid Leukemia with and without Germline GATA2 Mutations. *Biol. Blood Marrow Transplant.* **2020**, *26*, 1124–1130. [CrossRef]

102. Grossman, J.; Cuellar-Rodriguez, J.; Gea-Banacloche, J.; Zerbe, C.; Calvo, K.; Hughes, T.; Hakim, F.; Cole, K.; Parta, M.; Freeman, A.; et al. Nonmyeloablative Allogeneic Hematopoietic Stem Cell Transplantation for GATA2 Deficiency. *Biol. Blood Marrow Transplant.* **2014**, *20*, 1940–1948. [CrossRef]
103. Parta, M.; Shah, N.N.; Baird, K.; Rafei, H.; Calvo, K.R.; Hughes, T.; Cole, K.; Kenyon, M.; Schuver, B.B.; Cuellar-Rodriguez, J.; et al. Allogeneic Hematopoietic Stem Cell Transplantation for GATA2 Deficiency Using a Busulfan-Based Regimen. *Biol Blood Marrow Transplant.* **2018**, *24*, 1250–1259. [CrossRef]
104. Parta, M.; Cole, K.; Avila, D.; Duncan, L.; Baird, K.; Schuver, B.B.; Wilder, J.; Palmer, C.; Daub, J.; Hsu, A.P.; et al. Hematopoietic Cell Transplantation and Outcomes Related to Human Papillomavirus Disease in GATA2 Deficiency. *Transplant. Cell Ther.* **2021**, *27*, 435.e1–435.e11. [CrossRef]
105. Bogaert, D.J.; Laureys, G.; Naesens, L.; Mazure, D.; de Bruyne, M.; Hsu, A.P.; Bordon, V.; Wouters, E.; Tavernier, S.J.; Lambrecht, B.N.; et al. GATA2 Deficiency and Haematopoietic Stem Cell Transplantation: Challenges for the Clinical Practitioner. *Br. J. Haematol.* **2020**, *188*, 768–773. [CrossRef]
106. Khan, N.E.; Rosenberg, P.S.; Alter, B.P. Preemptive Bone Marrow Transplantation and Event-Free Survival in Fanconi Anemia. *Biol. Blood Marrow Transplant.* **2016**, *22*, 1888–1892. [CrossRef]
107. Godley, L.A.; Shimamura, A. Genetic Predisposition to Hematologic Malignancies: Management and Surveillance. *Blood* **2017**, *130*, 424–432. [CrossRef]
108. Hamilton, K.V.; Maese, L.; Marron, J.M.; Pulsipher, M.A.; Porter, C.C.; Nichols, K.E. Stopping Leukemia in Its Tracks: Should Preemptive Hematopoietic Stem-Cell Transplantation Be Offered to Patients at Increased Genetic Risk for Acute Myeloid Leukemia? *J. Clin. Oncol.* **2019**, *37*, 2098–2104. [CrossRef]
109. Connelly, J.A.; Savani, B.N. Finding the Best Haematopoietic Stem Cell Transplant Regimen for GATA2 Haploinsufficiency: How Close Are We? *Br. J. Haematol.* **2022**, *196*, 13–14. [CrossRef]
110. Hickstein, D. HSCT for GATA2 Deficiency across the Pond. *Blood* **2018**, *131*, 1272–1274. [CrossRef]
111. Linnemann, A.K.; O'Geen, H.; Keles, S.; Farnham, P.J.; Bresnick, E.H. Genetic Framework for GATA Factor Function in Vascular Biology. *Proc. Natl. Acad. Sci. USA* **2011**, *108*, 13641–13646. [CrossRef]
112. Johnson, K.D.; Hsu, A.P.; Ryu, M.J.; Wang, J.; Gao, X.; Boyer, M.E.; Liu, Y.; Lee, Y.; Calvo, K.R.; Keles, S.; et al. Cis-Element Mutated in GATA2-Dependent Immunodeficiency Governs Hematopoiesis and Vascular Integrity. *J. Clin. Investig.* **2012**, *122*, 3692–3704. [CrossRef] [PubMed]
113. Portich, J.P.; Condino Neto, A.; Faulhaber, G.A.M. Humoral Deficiency in a Novel GATA2 Mutation: A New Clinical Presentation Successfully Treated with Hematopoietic Stem Cell Transplantation. *Pediatr. Blood Cancer* **2020**, *67*, e28374. [CrossRef] [PubMed]
114. Yüksel, H.; Zafer, E. Gynecologic Manifestations in Emberger Syndrome. *Turk. J. Obstet Gynecol.* **2021**, *18*, 65–67. [CrossRef] [PubMed]
115. Feurstein, S.; Drazer, M.W.; Godley, L.A. Genetic Predisposition to Leukemia and Other Hematologic Malignancies. *Semin Oncol.* **2016**, *43*, 598–608. [CrossRef]

Disclaimer/Publisher's Note: The statements, opinions and data contained in all publications are solely those of the individual author(s) and contributor(s) and not of MDPI and/or the editor(s). MDPI and/or the editor(s) disclaim responsibility for any injury to people or property resulting from any ideas, methods, instructions or products referred to in the content.

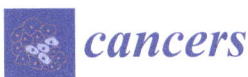

Review

Current Understanding of *DDX41* Mutations in Myeloid Neoplasms

Kunhwa Kim, Faustine Ong and Koji Sasaki *

Department of Leukemia, The University of Texas MD Anderson Cancer Center, Houston, TX 77030, USA
* Correspondence: ksasaki1@mdanderson.org

Simple Summary: The DEAD-box RNA helicase 41, *DDX41*, is one of the most frequently identified mutations in myeloid neoplasms with germline predispositions, which represents 2% of the entire MDS/AML population. *DDX41* is located at 5q35.3, and its mutation has unique features of male predominance and long-term cytopenia before the development of myeloid neoplasms. So far, mechanism studies revealed that *DDX41* mutations, affected by both germline and somatic mutations, can be pathogenic by impairments in the normal function of genes involving RNA splicing and processing, ribosomal biogenesis, metabolism, cycle progression, and innate immunity. We are gaining a better understanding of disease from more studies coming out with larger cohorts. The survival impact of the mutation remains unclear, although recent larger studies suggest a better treatment response and survival in higher risk MDS/AML. Several studies showed a good response to lenalidomide in certain patients with MDS with *DDX41* mutations. Early identification of stem-cell transplant donors in the family for patients with *DDX41* mutations is crucial to avoid donor-derived leukemia from germline carriers. In this article, we reviewed the current understanding of DDX41 mutations in AML/MDS, including its pathogenesis and clinical characteristics, outcome, and treatment.

Abstract: The DEAD-box RNA helicase 41 gene, *DDX41*, is frequently mutated in hereditary myeloid neoplasms, identified in 2% of entire patients with AML/MDS. The pathogenesis of *DDX41* mutation is related to the defect in the gene's normal functions of RNA and innate immunity. About 80% of patients with germline *DDX41* mutations have somatic mutations in another allele, resulting in the biallelic *DDX41* mutation. Patients with the disease with *DDX41* mutations reportedly often present with the higher-grade disease, but there are conflicting reports about its impact on survival outcomes. Recent studies using larger cohorts reported a favorable outcome with a better response to standard therapies in patients with *DDX41* mutations to patients without *DDX41* mutations. For stem-cell transplantation, it is important for patients with *DDX41* germline mutations to identify family donors early to improve outcomes. Still, there is a gap in knowledge on whether germline DDX41 mutations and its pathology features can be targetable for treatment, and what constitutes an appropriate screening/surveillance strategy for identified carriers. This article reviews our current understanding of *DDX41* mutations in myeloid neoplasms in pathologic and clinical features and their clinical implications.

Keywords: *DDX41* mutations; myelodysplastic syndrome; acute myeloid leukemia; hereditary myeloid neoplasms

Citation: Kim, K.; Ong, F.; Sasaki, K. Current Understanding of *DDX41* Mutations in Myeloid Neoplasms. *Cancers* 2023, *15*, 344. https://doi.org/10.3390/cancers15020344

Academic Editors: Francesc Solé and Eishi Ashihara

Received: 19 August 2022
Revised: 22 December 2022
Accepted: 23 December 2022
Published: 5 January 2023

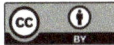

Copyright: © 2023 by the authors. Licensee MDPI, Basel, Switzerland. This article is an open access article distributed under the terms and conditions of the Creative Commons Attribution (CC BY) license (https://creativecommons.org/licenses/by/4.0/).

1. Introduction

The assessment of next-generation sequencing in the study of myelodysplastic syndromes (MDS) and acute myeloid leukemia (AML) is now guiding treatment decisions and predicting survival along with age and comorbidity considerations at the time of diagnosis [1–19]. The application of targeted therapies with *FLT3* inhibitors, *IDH* inhibitors, and venetoclax has further improved outcomes in patients with MDS and AML in newly diagnosed and relapsed settings [20–31].

In recent years, the accumulation of genetic data in myeloid neoplasms from next-generation sequencing has resulted in a rapid gain in understanding of hereditary myeloid neoplasms and identification of their related pathogenic germline mutations [32]. Patients with myeloid neoplasms with germline predisposition represent approximately 5–15% of all adult MDS and AML cases. The World Health Organization designated a new category of myeloid neoplasms with germline predisposition in 2016 [33].

The DEAD-box RNA helicase-1 gene (*DDX41*) is one of the most frequently identified mutations in myeloid neoplasms with a genetic predisposition. The *DDX41* gene is located at chromosome 5q35.3, and the gene can be affected by germline and somatic mutations [34]. Large cohort studies have shown that 1.5–3.8% of patients with myeloid neoplasms have *DDX41* mutations [35–37]. First identified in 2015 as predisposing mutations for myeloid neoplasms by a study of an index family with a strong history of MDS/AML, a significant proportion of hereditary myeloid neoplasms were associated with the *DDX41* mutations by affecting RNA biology and innate immunity [34]. Many studies have come out in recent years, which provide a better understanding of pathogenesis and clinical implications of *DDX41* mutations. In particular, as a common mutation in the association of hereditary myeloid neoplasms, understanding *DDX41* mutations can help establish the strategy for surveillance and management of germline mutation carriers, and screening and early identification for stem-cell transplant donors for the patients with MDS/AML with germline *DDX41* mutations.

This article reviews our current understanding of *DDX41* mutations in MDS/AML, focusing on pathogenic mechanisms, and pathologic and clinical data.

2. DDX41 Mutations and Their Role in MDS/AML Pathogenesis

The pathology of *DDX41* mutations in myeloid neoplasms may be related to a disruption of the gene's normal functions involving multiple functions in RNA biology [34]. *DDX41* encodes a member of the DEAD-box ATP-dependent RNA helicases, which are involved in pre-mRNA splicing, RNA processing, ribosome biogenesis, and small nucleolar RNA processing [34,38,39]. In addition, *DDX41* interacts with intracellular DNA in dendritic cells and macrophages, and activates innate immunity through the stimulator of interferon genes (STING)-interferon pathway [40,41]. More studies have come out in past years describing and identifying the pathomechanism of *DDX41* mutations.

Changes in *DDX41* expression have demonstrated variable effects in vitro and in vivo. For example, the knockdown of *DDX41* in K562 cells was shown to increase their proliferation in vitro and accelerate their tumor growth in a xenograft model [34]. Conversely, the knockout of *DDX41* in a mouse model impaired the differentiation and development of hematopoietic cells, particularly myeloid lineage cells, and decreased their proliferation capacity both in vivo and ex vivo [42].

A recent mouse model study demonstrated that monoallelic germline mutations of *DDX41* cause age-dependent myelodysplastic changes, whereas biallelic mutations resulting from the acquisition of somatic mutations on the other allele cause hematopoietic defects at a young age, likely by dysregulating small nucleolar RNA processing and ribosomal function [39]. *DDX41* mutations may also have an oncogenic effect by dysregulating the STING-interferon pathway, thereby impairing innate immunity [40,43].

Additionally, Mosler et al. proposed that an increased level of R-loop, RNA-DNA hybrids and displaced strand of DNA can be caused by dysregulation from loss of *DDX41*, as outlined in a recent study using quantitative mass spectrometry-based proteomics using human cells [44]. The study showed pathogenic variants of *DDX41* mutations resulted in the accumulation of double-strand breaks in human hematopoietic stem cells causing inflammatory responses. These enhanced inflammatory responses from R-loop accumulation and the dysregulation of hematopoietic stem cell production were also shown in a study using zebra fish by Weinreb et al. [45]. These studies propose the role of *DDX41* in genomic stability against R-loop generations.

DDX41 mutations are clinically associated with an increased lifetime risk of myeloid neoplasms, including the early presentation of idiopathic cytopenia of undetermined significance (ICUS) [46]. Diseases reported to be associated with *DDX41* mutations include myeloproliferative neoplasms, chronic lymphocytic leukemia, chronic myeloid leukemia, multiple myeloma, and Hodgkin and non-Hodgkin lymphomas other than myeloid neoplasms [35,47–49]. *DDX41* mutations are also associated with blood disorders, including macrocytosis [47]. Some studies found *DDX41* mutations to be associated with an increased risk of autoimmune disorders or solid cancers, but these findings require further investigation [35,47]. The specific risk for hematologic malignancies including MDS/AML conveyed by *DDX41* mutations remains unclear.

3. Pathologic Features of Myeloid Neoplasms with *DDX41* Mutations

In common practice, next-generation sequencing panels at diagnosis of myeloid neoplasms or follow-up can detect *DDX41* mutations [47]. Comprehensive genomic testing with exome or genome sequencing can be used to identify variants that gene-targeted sequencing might miss [47]. The results of germline pathogenic variant testing can be confirmed by specimen without blood contamination obtained from skin fibroblasts [47].

In a recently published study using a multi-national cohort, *DDX41* germline mutations account for about 80% of patients with myeloid neoplasms with germline predisposition [37]. The study further showed that pathologic or likely pathogenic germline mutations of DDX41 were identified 10 times more frequently in patients with myeloid neoplasms than the general population [37]. Germline *DDX41* mutations are passed from parent to child through autosomal dominant inheritance, but the penetrance of *DDX41* mutations remains unclear. Only about 30% of patients with germline *DDX41* mutations have a family history of hematologic malignancy, but a familial series study showed high penetrant patterns in some families [35,49]. Interestingly, the *DDX41*-mutant MDS/AML has a male predominance, with a male-to-female ratio of 3:1 [35,50]. The etiology of male predominance remains unknown.

Up to 80% of carriers of germline *DDX41* mutations who develop MDS/AML have additional somatic mutations on the other *DDX41* allele, which has been reported by multiple studies [34,49,50]. The pattern of biallelic mutations from secondary somatic mutations in *DDX41* mutations also can be seen in somatic mutations in the CCAAT enhancer binding protein alpha gene, *CEBPA*, in AML [34]. The role of additional somatic mutation and biallelic mutation as pathogenesis of *DDX41* mutations were described by Chlon et al. as mentioned above.

Notably, germline and somatic *DDX41* mutations tend to have different patterns and locations of mutations on the gene.

Most patients with germline mutations have pathogenic variants with either nonsense, frameshift, or splicing site mutations [49,51]. One of the most frequently identified germline mutations, p.D140fs, causes protein truncation [52]. Other germline mutations are associated with loss of function and derangements in splicing [49]. A study of 346 patients with germline *DDX41* mutations reported that MDS patients with truncating variants of *DDX41* germline mutations were observed to have shorter duration to AML transformation, about 2.5 times faster, compared to patients with non-truncating variants [37]. However, there was no difference in overall survival between the two groups [37]. The most frequent somatic mutation is the p.R525H missense mutation [36,51]. The mutation is located at the C-terminus of the helicase domain at the site of ATP interaction and hydrolyzation, which can cause deranged interactions with ATP in the helicase domain without directly changing the main domain [38]. One study showed that cord blood cells and leukemia cells harboring the p.R525H mutation had deranged pre-mRNA processing and ribosomal biogenesis from mutation-related change, resulting in impaired E2 factor activity and, thus, defective cell cycle progression [38].

In a next-generation sequencing study of patients with *DDX41*-mutant disease, most germline mutations (93%) were upstream of the helicase 2 domain or involved loss of the start codon (30%). In contrast, most somatic mutations (78%) were within the helicase 2 domain [36].

Ethnicity-based differences in the frequencies of *DDX41* mutations have been noted. Several studies from cohorts of Asian patients showed a distinct mutations profile. In a study of 28 Korean patients, the most common germline mutation was p.V152G, which was detected in 10 patients, followed by p.Y259C, p.A500fs, and p.E7* [46]. Similarly, in a Japanese population, p.A500fs and p.E7* were the most frequent germline mutations, and p.R525H was the most common somatic mutation [53]. In a study of Chinese patients, the most common mutations were c.935 + 4A>T and p.T360Ifs*33, which were detected in three patients each [54]. This ethnic difference in mutations was shown in a recent study by Li et al. with large data including 176 patients with germline mutations [50]. In the study, p.A500fs was only identified in Asian patients, and 92% of patients with Y295C (n = 12) were Asian patients. The majority, over 90%, of patients with p.M1I or p.D140fs were Caucasians. Interestingly, the study also showed a more frequent loss of function in germline mutations (85% vs. 51%) in Caucasians than in Asians.

Prior reports of mutation-related protein changes are summarized in Table 1. The study by Makishima et al., was published upon acceptance of our manuscript, and was not included in the table [37].

Table 1. Summary of *DDX41* studies and identified germline mutations.

Study Characteristics (Author, Year, Cohort, Database)	Total Number of Data	Nucleotide Change	Amino Acid Change	Number of Patients or Families (% of Studied Patients or Families)	No. of Patients with Concomitant Somatic *DDX41* Mutations	No. of Patients with Hematologic Malignancies
Polprasert et al., 2015 [34]; a cohort of MDS/secondary AML, multicenter (US/Germany), and TCGA database	27/1034 patients and 7 index families (19 patients with germline mutation)	c.419insGATG (c.415_418dupGATG)	p.D140fs	14 (74%)	5/14	8 AML 6 MDS/CMML
		c.T1187C	p.I396T	2 (10%)	2/2	2 MDS
		c.156_157insA	p.Q52fs	1 (5%)	1/1	1 AML
		c.G465A	p.M155I	1 (5%)	0/1	1 MDS
		Not mentioned	p.F183I	1 (5%)	1/1	1 MDS
Lewinsohn et al., 2016 [49]; a cohort of families with suspected inherited hematologic malignancies, multicenter (Australian/US) familial hematologic malignancies registry	9/289 families	c.415_418dupGATG	p.D140Gfs	3 families	Not reported	3 AMLs
		c.3G>A	p.M1I	2 families	Not reported	3 AML (1 with NHL involvement), 1 MDS, 1 CML
		c.435-2_435-1delAGinsCA	(predicted to produce p.W146Hfsand p.S145Rfs)	1 family	Not reported	1 MDS
		c.490C>T	p.R164W	1 family	Not reported	3 NHL
		c.1574G>A	p.R525H (suspected germline)	1 family	Not reported	2 MDS, 1 AML
		c.1589G>A	p.G530D	1 family	Not reported	3 AML
Cardoso et al., 2016 [55]; a cohort of families with at least two cases of bone marrow failure and at least one of whom having MDS or AML (no detailed description of the study cohort)	4/78 families	c.3G>A	p.M1I	1 family	Not reported	2 MDS
		c.155dupA	p. R53Afs	1 family	Not reported	3 MDS, 1 carrier (1 CML family history with unchecked mutation)
		c.719delTinsCG	p.I240Tfs	1 family	Not reported	1 AML (1 AML family history with unchecked mutation)
		c.1586-1587delCA	p.T529Rfs	1 family	Not reported	1 MDS, 1 carrier (1 AML family history with unchecked mutation)

Table 1. Cont.

Study Characteristics (Author, Year, Cohort, Database)	Total Number of Data	Nucleotide Change	Amino Acid Change	Number of Patients or Families (% of Studied Patients or Families)	No. of Patients with Concomitant Somatic DDX41 Mutations	No. of Patients with Hematologic Malignancies
Sebert et al., 2019 [35]; a cohort of families with a family history of MDS, AML, AA, single-center (France) data	43/1385 patients (33 patients with causal germline variants)	c.G517A	p.G173R	6 (18%)	6/6	3 MDS, 1 AML, 2 AA
		c.G3A	p.M1I	3 (9%)	3/3	2 AML, 1 MDS
		c.992_994del	p.K331del	3 (9%)	2/3	1 MDS/MPN, 1 MDS, 1 AML
		c.C121T	p.Q41*	2 (6%)	1/2	2 MDS
		c.418_419insGATG	p.D140fs	2 (6%)	1/2	1 AML, 1 MDS/MPN
		c.C1015T	p.R339C	2 (6%)	1/2	1 AA, 1 MDS
		c.A1C	p.M1L	1 (3%)	1/1	1 MDS
		c.69delC	p.S23fs	1 (3%)	1/1	1 MDS
		c.A316T	p.K106*	1 (3%)	0/1	1 CMML
		c.342_346del	p.E114fs	1 (3%)	1/1	1 MDS
		c.542+2A>G	-	1 (3%)	0/1	1 MDS
		c.644+1G>A	-	1 (3%)	1/1	1 MDS
		c.T649C	p.S217P	1 (3%)	1/1	1 MDS
		c.A734G	p.E245G	1 (3%)	1/1	1 MDS
		c.799-2T>A	-	1 (3%)	1/1	1 AML
		c.945delC	p.H315fs	1 (3%)	1/1	1 AML
		c.A1031G	p.D344G	1 (3%)	1/1	neutropenia only
		c.1088_1090del	p.S363del	1 (3%)	1/1	1 AML
		c.C1108T	p.Q370*	1 (3%)	1/1	1 AML
		c.1298dupC	p.P433fs	1 (3%)	0/1	1 AML
		c.1791_1792del	p.K597fs	1 (3%)	1/1	1 AML
Quesada et al., 2019 [36]; a cohort of known/suspected myeloid neoplasms, single-center (US) data	34/1002 patients (32 patients with germline mutations)	c.3G>A	p.M1I	9 (28%)	9/9	1 AML, 4 MDS->AML, 4 MDS
		c.415_418dupGATG	p.D140Gfs	4 (13%)	4/4	2 AML, 1 MDS->AML, 1 MDS
		c.121C>T	p.Q41*	2 (6%)	2/2	2 MDS
		c.25A>G	p.K9E	1 (3%)	0/1	1 MDS/CMML->AML
		c.38C>T	p.T13I	1 (3%)	0/1	1 Post PV-MF
		c.59G>A	p.G20E	1 (3%)	0/1	1 MDS
		c.62_63del	p.S21Tfs	1 (3%)	1/1	1 AML
		c.142C>T	p.Q48*	1 (3%)	1/1	1 MDS->AML
		c.298+2_298+4delTGG	Splice	1 (3%)	1/1	1 MDS->AML
		c.475C>T	p.R159*	1 (3%)	1/1	1 MDS->AML
		c.476G>A	p.R159Q	1 (3%)	0/1	MPN
		c.572-1G>A	Splice	1 (3%)	1/1	1 AML
		c.608A>G	p.H203R	1 (3%)	0/1	1 MDS->AML
		c.649T>C	p.S217P	1 (3%)	1/1	1 AML
		c.821A>G	p.H274R	1 (3%)	0/1	1 MPN
		c.1046T>A	p.M349K	1 (3%)	1/1	1 suspected MDS
		c.1105C>T	p.R369*	1 (3%)	1/1	1 MDS->AML
		c.1105C>G	p.R369G	1 (3%)	1/1	1 MDS
		c.1771C>T	p.R591W	1 (3%)	0/1	1 MDS->AML
		c.1766G>A	p.G589D	1 (3%)	0/1	1 CMML

Table 1. Cont.

Study Characteristics (Author, Year, Cohort, Database)	Total Number of Data	Nucleotide Change	Amino Acid Change	Number of Patients or Families (% of Studied Patients or Families)	No. of Patients with Concomitant Somatic DDX41 Mutations	No. of Patients with Hematologic Malignancies
Choi et al., 2021 [46]; a cohort of patients with ICUS/MDS/AML, single-center (Korea) data	39/457 patients (34 patients with germline mutations)	c.455T>G	p.V152G	10 (29%)	10/10	2 ICUS, 8 MDS
		c.776A>G	p.Y259C	9 (26%)	8/9	2 ICUS, 7 MDS
		c.1496dupC	p.A500fs	6 (18%)	6/6	1 ICUS, 2 MDS, 3 AML
		c.19G>T	p.E7*	3 (9%)	2/3	2 MDS, 1 AML
			p.D139G	2 (6%)	0/2	1 MDS, 1 AML
			p.E3K	1 (3%)	0/1	1 AML
			p.Y33C	1 (3%)	0/1	1 AML
			p.K187R	1 (3%)	0/1	1 AML
		c.983T>G	p.L328R	1 (3%)	1/1	1 MDS
Bannon et al., 2021 [51]; a cohort of patients who were referred to genetic counseling and testing for hematologic malignancies with DDX41 mutations, single-center (US) data	33 (38 referred)/90 DDX41 germline mutations (out of 5801 heme malignancies patients)	c.415_418dupGATG	p.D140fs	10 (30%)	7/10	5 AML, 4 MDS (1 carrier)
		c.3A>G	p.M1I	8 (24%)	2/8	4 AML, 1 MDS->AML, 2 MDS, 1 CLL
		c.121C>T	p.Q41*	3 (9%)	2/3	2 AML, 1 MDS
		c.337del	p.E113fs	1 (3%)	1/1	1 MDS->AML
		c.434+1G>A	-	1 (3%)	0/1	1 MDS
		c.475C>T	p.R159*	1 (3%)	0/1	1 MDS/MPN
		c.547T>G	p.F183V (VUS)	1 (3%)	1/1	1 MDS
		c.572-1G>A	-	1 (3%)	1/1	1 AML
		c.653G>A	p.G218D (VUS)	1 (3%)	0/1	1 MDS->AML
		c.847del	p.L283fs	1 (3%)	0/1	1 MDS
		c.946_947del	p.M316fs	1 (3%)	1/1	1 MDS
		c.1004dupT	p.D336fs	1 (3%)	1/1	1 MDS
		c.1105C>G	p.R369G (VUS)	1 (3%)	1/1	1 MDS
		c.1187T>C	p.I396T	1 (3%)	1/1	1 MDS
		c.1273_1276dupCTCG	p.E426fs	1 (3%)	1/1	1 AML
Qu et al., 2021 [54]; a cohort of myeloid neoplasms, single-center (China) data	47/1529 patients (25 patients with germline mutation)	c.1077_1078dupTA	p.T360Ifs	3 (12%)	3/3	3 MDS
		c.935+4A>T	-	3 (12%)	2/3	1 AML, 1 MDS, 1 Post-ET MF
		c. C1105T	p.R369*	2 (8%)	2/2	1 AML, 1 MDS
		c. T455G	p.V152G	2 (8%)	2/2	2 MDS
		c.647dupT	p.S217Ifs	2 (8%)	1/2	1 MDS, 1 Post-ET MF
		c. C931T	p.R311*	2 (8%)	2/2	2 MDS
		c. G3T	p.M1I	1 (4%)	1/1	1 MDS
		c. G391T	p.E131*	1 (4%)	1/1	1 MDS
		c. G553T	p.E185*	1 (4%)	1/1	1 AML
		c.572-1G>C	-	1 (4%)	1/1	1 MDS
		c. C773T	p.P258L	1 (4%)	1/1	1 MDS
		c.865delT	p.S289Hfs	1 (4%)	0/1	1 MDS
		c.1213_1216del	p.S405Wfs	1 (4%)	1/1	1 MDS
		c.1296_1298dup	p.P434dup	1 (4%)	1/1	1 MDS
		c. G1531T	p.E511*	1 (4%)	1/1	1 MDS
		c. A776G	p.Y259C	1 (4%)	1/1	1 MDS
		c.T983G	p.L328R	1 (4%)	1/1	1 MDS

Table 1. Cont.

Study Characteristics (Author, Year, Cohort, Database)	Total Number of Data	Nucleotide Change	Amino Acid Change	Number of Patients or Families (% of Studied Patients or Families)	No. of Patients with Concomitant Somatic DDX41 Mutations	No. of Patients with Hematologic Malignancies
Alkhateeb et al., 2022 [56]; a cohort of myeloid neoplasm patients, single-center (US) data	33/4524 patients (likely 25 germline patients)	c.3G>A	p.M1I	10 (40%)	1/10	4 AML, 5 MDS (1 carrier)
		c.415_418dup	p.D140Gfs	5 (20%)	0/5	4 MDS, 1 AML
		c.1589G>A	p.G530D	2 (8%)	0/2	1 MDS, 1 AML
		c.121C>T	p.Q41*	1 (4%)	0/1	1 AML
		c.305_306del	p.K102Rfs	1 (4%)	1/1	1 AML
		c.337del	p.E113Kfs	1 (4%)	0/1	1 MPN
		c.434+1G>A	-	1 (4%)	0/1	1 MDS
		c.776A>G	p.Y259C	1 (4%)	1/1	1 MDS
		c.931C>T	p.R311*	1 (4%)	1/1	1 AML
		c.946_947del	p.M316D	1 (4%)	0/1	1 MDS
		c.1102C>T	p.Q368*	1 (4%)	0/1	1 MDS
Li et al., 2022 [50]; a cohort of patients with hematologic malignancies, multi-center (US) data **	176/9821 patients, 116 patients with causal variants	c.3G>A	p.M1I	42 (36%)	35/42	24 AML, 13 MDS, 5 CCUS
		c.415_418dup	p.D140fs	23 (20%)	15/23	18 AML, 2 MDS, 1 MPN, 2 CCUS
		c.475C>T	p.R159*	3 (3%)	3/3	1 AML, 1 MDS, 1 CCUS
		c.931C>T	p.R311*	3 (3%)	3/3	1 AML, 2 MDS
		c.946_947del	p.M316fs	3 (3%)	2/3	1 AML, 1 MPN, 1 CCUS
		c.992_994del	p.K331del	3 (3%)	2/3	1 AML, 2 MDS
		c.1105C>T	p.R369*	3 (3%)	3/3	2 AML, 1 CCUS
		c.121C>T	p.Q41*	2 (2%)	1/2	2 AML
		c.773C>T	p.P258L	2 (2%)	2/2	1 AML, 1 CCUS
		c.1046T>A	p.M349K	2 (2%)	0/2	2 AML
		c.1105C>G	p.R369G	2 (2%)	2/2	1 AML, 1 MDS
		c.130C>T	p.Q44*	1 (1%)	1/1	1 MDS
		c.323del	p.K108fs	1 (1%)	1/1	1 AML
		c.430del	p.T144fs	1 (1%)	1/1	1 CCUS
		c.566C>T	p.P189L	1 (1%)	1/1	1 MDS
		c.645-1G>T	-	1 (1%)	1/1	1 AML
		c.646C>G	p.L216V	1 (1%)	1/1	1 AML
		c.649T>C	p.S217P	1 (1%)	1/1	1 CCUS
		c.653G>A	p.G218D	1 (1%)	1/1	1 AML
		c.668dup	p.I224fs	1 (1%)	1/1	1 AML
		c.710T>G	p.L237W	1 (1%)	1/1	1 MDS
		c.776A>G	p.Y259C	1 (1%)	1/1	1 CCUS
		c.847del	p.L283fs	1 (1%)	1/1	1 AML
		c.916C>T	p.Q306*	1 (1%)	0/1	1 MPN
		c.967C>T	p.R323C	1 (1%)	1/1	1 AML
		c.1015C>T	p.R339C	1 (1%)	1/1	1 MDS
		c.1016G>A	p.R339H	1 (1%)	0/1	1 MDS
		c.1016G>T	p.R339L	1 (1%)	1/1	1 CCUS
		c.1018T>A	p.Y340N	1 (1%)	1/1	1 MDS
		c.1108C>T	p.Q370*	1 (1%)	1/1	1 AML
		c.1141A>T	p.K381*	1 (1%)	1/1	1 MPN

Table 1. *Cont.*

Study Characteristics (Author, Year, Cohort, Database)	Total Number of Data	Nucleotide Change	Amino Acid Change	Number of Patients or Families (% of Studied Patients or Families)	No. of Patients with Concomitant Somatic *DDX41* Mutations	No. of Patients with Hematologic Malignancies
		c.1354del	p.L452fs	1 (1%)	1/1	1 CCUS
		c.1394del	p.G465fs	1 (1%)	1/1	1 AML
		c.1399G>T	p.D467Y	1 (1%)	1/1	1 AML
		c.1496dup	p.A500fs	1 (1%)	1/1	1 MDS
		c.1504C>T	p.Q502*	1 (1%)	1/1	MDS
		c.1574G>A	p.R525H	1 (1%)	0/1	1 AML
		c.1586_1587delCA	p.T529fs	1 (1%)	0/1	1 CCUS
		c.1628C>G	p.S543*	1 (1%)	1/1	1 CCUS
Duployez et al, 2022 [57]; a cohort of 5 prospective trials and additional diagnostic samples, multi-center (France) data	191 AML patients with germline mutations	c.415_418dup	p.D140fs	32 (17%)	27/32	All AML patients
		c.3G>A	p.M1?	19 (10%)	15/19	
		c.517G>A	p.G173R	10 (5%)	8/10	
		c.847del	p.L283fs	9 (5%)	7/9	
		c.1088_1090del	p.S363del	9 (%)	8/9	
		c.138+1G>C		6	5/6	
		c.653G>A	p.G218D	5	5/5	
		c.992_994del	p.K331del	5	4/5	
		c.268C>T	p.Q90*	4	4/4	
		c.305_306del	p.K102fs	4	4/4	
		c.804del	p.E268fs	4	4/4	
		c.55G>T	p.G19*	3	2/3	
		c.121C>T	p.Q41*	3	3/3	
		c.936-1G>A	-	3	2/3	
		c.1212_1226delinsAG	p.S405fs	3	3/3	
		c.1334_1336del	p.V445del	3	2/3	
		c.1496del	p.P499fs	3	3/3	
		c.1A>C	p.M1?	2	2/2	
		c.316A>T	p.K106*	2	2/2	
		c.571G>A	p.A191T	2	2/2	
		c.656G>A	p.R219H	2	0/2	
		c.935+2T>C	-	2	1/2	
		c.945del	p.H315fs	2	1/2	
		c.1031A>G	p.D344G	2	2/2	
		c.1098+1G>A	-	2	2/2	
		c.1105C>T	p.R369*	2	1/2	
		c.1298del	p.P433fs	2	2/2	
		c.1504C>T	p.Q502*	2	1/2	
		c.1585dup	p.T529fs	2	1/2	
		c.2T>C	p.M1?	1	1/1	
		c.69del	p.S23fs	1	1/1	
		c.130C>T	p.Q44*	1	0/1	
		c.142C>T	p.Q48*	1	1/1	
		c.156_157delinsTT	p.Q52_R53delinsH	1	1/1	
		c.325C>T	p.Q109*	1	1/1	
		c.342_346del	p.E114fs	1	1/1	

Table 1. Cont.

Study Characteristics (Author, Year, Cohort, Database)	Total Number of Data	Nucleotide Change	Amino Acid Change	Number of Patients or Families (% of Studied Patients or Families)	No. of Patients with Concomitant Somatic DDX41 Mutations	No. of Patients with Hematologic Malignancies
		c.364G>T	p.E122*	1	1/1	
		c.373+1G>A	-	1	0/1	
		c.434+1G>T	-	1	1/1	
		c.436T>C	p.W146R	1	1/1	
		c.475C>T	p.R159*	1	1/1	
		c.622C>G	p.Q208E	1	1/1	
		c.643A>C	p.I215L	1	0/1	
		c.644T>C	p.I215T	1	0/1	
		c.649T>C	p.S217P	1	1/1	
		c.668G>A	p.G223D	1	1/1	
		c.758C>G	p.S252*	1	1/1	
		c.791G>A	p.C264Y	1	1/1	
		c.799-2A>T	-	1	1/1	
		c.805dup	p.L269fs	1	0/1	
		c.931C>T	p.R311*	1	0/1	
		c.958A>T	p.T320S	1	0/1	
		c.959C>T	p.T320I	1	1/1	
		c.967C>A	p.R323S	1	1/1	
		c.967C>T	p.R323C	1	0/1	
		c.968G>A	p.R323H	1	1/1	
		c.998T>A	p.V333D	1	1/1	
		c.1033G>A	p.E345K	1	1/1	
		c.1037C>A	p.A346D	1	1/1	
		c.1105C>G	p.R369G	1	1/1	
		c.1108C>T	p.Q370*	1	1/1	
		c.1118_1127del	p.L373fs	1	1/1	
		c.1212_1224del	p.L406fs	1	1/1	
		c.1252G>T	p.E418*	1	1/1	
		c.1298dup	p.P433fs	1	1/1	
		c.1463C>A	p.A488D	1	1/1	
		c.1514T>A	p.I505N	1	1/1	
		c.1615del	p.A539fs	1	1/1	
		c.1628C>G	p.S543*	1	1/1	
		c.1732+1del	-	1	1/1	
		c.1791_1792del	p.K597fs	1	1/1	

Abbreviation: AML: acute myeloid leukemia, ICUS: idiopathic cytopenia of undetermined significance, CML: chronic myeloid leukemia, CMML: chronic myelomonocytic leukemia, MDS: myeloid dysplastic syndrome, MPN: myeloproliferative neoplasm, NHL: non-Hodgkin's lymphoma, post-PV MF: post-polycythemia vera myelofibrosis, post-ET MF: post-essential thrombocythemia myelofibrosis, VUS: variant of uncertain significance. ** Only included causal variants in the table (excluded VUS).

Bone marrow examination often shows hypocellularity and erythroid dysplasia [46,52]. 70–80% of patients with germline *DDX41* mutations have a normal karyotype [34–36]. In addition, 3–30% of patients have concomitant *TP53* mutations [35,36,56]. A systematic review study of pooled studies of *DDX41* mutations showed 47% of patients have concomitant other somatic mutations, most frequently *ASXL1*(26%), *TP53* (23%), followed by *TET2*, *EZH2*, *SRSF2*, and *DNMT3A* [48]. Interestingly, the recent study by Makishima et al. including 346 patients with pathogenic or likely pathogenic germline *DDX41* mutations showed that co-mutations, including TP53, did not affect outcomes [37].

4. Clinical Presentation and Outcomes

The age at diagnosis of MDS/AML patients with germline *DDX41* mutations has been reported within a wide range from 57 to 70 years, but most studies reported that it is comparable to patients with general MDS/AML [34–36,50,58].

Some studies showed that MDS/AML patients with germline *DDX41* mutations often have a higher-grade disease than those with wildtype *DDX41* [34,36,51]. However, the survival effect of germline *DDX41* mutations was reported to vary.

Several studies have assessed outcomes in MDS/AML patients with *DDX41* mutations. Polprasert et al. showed that MDS/AML patients with *DDX41* mutations had worse survival than patients with wildtype *DDX41* in a large cohort of MDS and secondary AML patients of 1034 patients (hazard ratio, 3.5; $p < 0.0001$) [34]. In a smaller study that included 28 patients with ICUS, MDS, or AML having *DDX41* germline mutations, Choi et al. found no difference in survival by *DDX41* mutation status [46].

Sebert et al. showed that the median survival duration of patients with germline *DDX41* mutations (5.2 years) was longer than that of patients with wildtype *DDX41* (2.7 years) in a propensity score-matched study with 18 matched patients with *DDX41* mutations, but this difference was not statistically significant. They also found that patients with germline mutations had a good overall response to intensive chemotherapy (response rate at 100%, $n = 9$) and hypomethylating agent (response rate at 73%, $n = 11$), and a median response duration of 2.5 years [35].

Li et al. showed that 81 patients with *DDX41* germline causal variants had superior overall survival compared to age-matched or general MDS or AML cases with wild-type *DDX41* or a variant of unknown significance (median OS: not reached) [50].

A recent study by Duployez et al. showed prolonged survival in *DDX41* germline mutant AML patients, with a good response to intensive chemotherapy in intermediate or high-risk patients with AML, in a large cohort study using five prospective clinical trials of 191 newly diagnosed *DDX41* mutant AML patients [57]. The median overall survival of AML patients with *DDX41* germline mutations of all variants was 28.1 months (Interquartile range, IQR, at 10.7–82.7 months) when censored at stem-cell transplant, and median relapse-free survival at 18.7 months (IQR 8.3–80.9 months).

These conflicting results are likely due to different study populations, heterogeneity of MDS/AML clinical course and treatments, and a limited number of study patients from a low prevalence of mutations. While Sebert et al. studied patients with germline *DDX41* mutations and analyzed the survival of only those patients who were treated for high-risk MDS and AML, Polprasert et al. included all patients with either germline or somatic mutations in the survival analyses. Choi et al. included patients with either germline or somatic mutations, but analyzed survival by diagnosis. Li et al. studied patients with germline pathogenic variants. Duployez et al. studied AML patients only.

As the prevalence of *DDX41*-associated MDS/AML is relatively low, further accumulation of clinical data may help clarify the prognostic role of *DDX41* mutations.

5. Treatment—General Approaches

So far, there are no randomized studies focusing on patients with *DDX41* mutations for specific therapeutic approaches. The treatment approaches of *DDX41*-mutant myeloid neoplasms generally follow standard care for general MDS/AML treatments. Two recent studies reported treatment responses in *DDX41* mutant patients. Li et al. reported a higher response rate at 78%, and superior survival (not reached) in a matched case-control study including 28 patients with AML having *DDX41* germline mutations. In the study, most (about 80%) patients were treated with hypomethylating agents with or without venetoclax [59]. Duployez et al., as mentioned above, also reported a better response to intensive chemotherapy in patients with intermediate or adverse *DDX41* germline-mutant patients in AML.

Interestingly, a few studies showed a good response to lenalidomide in MDS patients with *DDX41* mutations [34]. Lenalidomide is a well-established standard therapy for the low-risk MDS with a 5q deletion [60]. Lenalidomide has demonstrated its efficacy in MDS/AML patients with *DDX41* mutations, even in the absence of a full 5q deletion [34]. Only 26% of patients with MDS with 5q deletion have the deletion at 5q35, where *DDX41* is located at [34].

In a study of 111 patients treated with lenalidomide, Polprasert et al. reported that the response rate among patients with *DDX41* mutations (100% (8/8 patients)) was significantly higher than that among patients with wildtype *DDX41* (53% (55/103 patients); $p = 0.01$). In another prediction model study using 137 patients with MDS or other myeloid neoplasms, the mutation of any DEAD-box RNA helicase gene, including *DDX41*, was associated with higher response to lenalidomide (odds ratio 3.4, $p = 0.04$). Among seven patients with heterozygous *DDX41* mutations or deletions, the lenalidomide response rate was 57%. For the three patients who had *DDX41* mutations only, the response rate was 100% [61].

In addition, there is a case report about single-agent lenalidomide with the successful treatment of one patient with high-risk MDS (i.e., MDS with excess blasts type 2) [62]. The patient, who had a germline mutation (p.D140fs) and a low burden of *DDX41* p.R525H mutation, had a good response and had improved blood counts and rare dysplasia after 4 months of lenalidomide monotherapy. The blast percentage had decreased from 16% before treatment to 3% [62].

6. Treatment—Special Considerations: SCT

SCT is an essential part of treatment in hereditary myeloid neoplasms, especially in fit, younger patients. Donor cell leukemia is a particular concern in *DDX41* germline mutant myeloid neoplasms with its severity and fatality.

Berger et al. were the first to report a case of a *DDX41* mutation giving rise to donor cell leukemia. They described a patient who received an allogeneic SCT from an HLA-matched related donor carrying a germline *DDX41* mutation (c.3G>A; p.(MET1?)) and other somatic mutations [63]. The patient's family had a strong history of leukemia; the patient's father died of leukemia, and one of the patient's two brothers (not the donor) developed AML. The donor remained free of disease, but the patient developed high-risk MDS that might have been associated with stress from post-transplant changes [63].

Kobayashi et al. similarly reported a case of donor cell leukemia in a patient who received stem cells from a donor with a germline *DDX41* mutation (p.F498fs). There was also a significant increase in the variant allele frequency (7.9% vs 0.4%) of a somatic *DDX41* mutation (p.R525H) in a carrier after transplant [64]. Larger studies have since investigated the effects of donor clonal hematopoiesis in SCT. In a recent study of 1727 patients who received stem cells from donors with clonal hematopoiesis, only eight cases of donor cell leukemia were identified; in two of these cases, germline *DDX41* mutations were present [65].

Therefore, the early identification of the related donors' germline *DDX41* mutation carrier status is one strategy to avoid SCT delay in MDS/AML patients with germline *DDX41* mutations. In a report on the experience of a single tertiary cancer center, Bannon et al. reported that such identification of optimal related donors was effective [51].

7. Family Screening and Surveillance

There are no specific guidelines for family screening, or the surveillance of germline carriers identified from family screening. Family screening might be considered only for patients with germline mutations because somatic *DDX41* mutations are not heritable, and *DDX41* mutations are rare among the general population [52]. However, the risk of malignancy and penetrance of disease in germline carriers remains unclear, and methods for detecting or preventing myeloid neoplasms and other cancers in these individuals have not been established [66].

As a first step, surveillance methods and the timing for the family members identified as germline *DDX41* need to be established. Lewinsohn et al. reported that germline *DDX41* mutation carriers had cytopenia and other complete blood count (CBC) abnormalities at the time of MDS/AML diagnosis, but mostly lacked these abnormalities before diagnosis [49]. Further studies showed earlier CBC changes in carriers; Polprasert et al. reported macrocytosis and monocytosis in carriers, and Bannon et al. and Sebert et al. reported that 50–60% of carriers who were later diagnosed with hematologic malignancies had antecedent cytopenia [34,35,51]. In a study by Choi et al., five of 28 patients with germline *DDX41* mutations had ICUS [46]. Therefore, CBCs can be helpful in the screening or surveillance of carriers identified from family screening, but specific recommendations are not yet available. Makishima et al., reported an increasing risk of developing myeloid neoplasms by age in germline carriers [37]. The risk for myeloid neoplasms in patients with three major pathogenic variants under the age of 40 were negligible, but it increases rapidly after the age of 40 [37]. Age 40 could be a cut-off for a surveillance in germline carriers based on study results, although further accumulation of data would be helpful.

Several papers have described the experiences of patients with germline *DDX41* mutations in genetics clinics. One review, which detailed multiple cases from MD Anderson's genetics clinic, described the experience of a patient who had a biallelic *DDX41* mutation with a hotspot germline *DDX41* mutation and the screening of the patient's adult children [66]. Bannon et al. described how *DDX41* mutation carriers were offered education and follow-up; all unaffected family members, including potential stem cell transplant (SCT) donors, were offered genetic testing and counseling [51]. This enabled the prompt transition to stem-cell donor identification within 15 days after family screening [51].

Other considerations for the screening and surveillance of patients and their families should include the early detection of secondary hematologic malignancies, both myeloid and lymphoid malignancies, including follicular lymphoma and Hodgkin's lymphoma. It should also include autoimmune diseases in MDS/AML patients who have had disease remission, and the early detection of primary hematologic malignancies or autoimmune diseases in germline mutation carriers.

8. Conclusions

We are rapidly gaining knowledge about hereditary MDS/AML through recent clinical and translational research endeavors, particularly of *DDX41*-associated hereditary myeloid neoplasms. MDS/AML with *DDX41* mutations has become a study of interest with its unique features of pathophysiology, genetic and clinical characteristics. There is the potential therapeutic implication of an expected good treatment response to standard therapies, and the need for early donor identifications for SCT.

Despite the rapid advancements in this field, there still is a gap in knowledge that future studies need to address for patients with *DDX41*-associated myeloid neoplasms. Further understanding of the clinical impact of the *DDX41* mutations, including learning further prognostic or clinical information of *DDX41* mutant AML/MDS patients, and studying whether *DDX41* mutations can be targetable for therapeutic or preventive applications would be essential. Additionally, establishing standardized approaches for cancer and other medical surveillance/screening in family members (i.e., germline-carriers) is essential.

Author Contributions: Conceptualization, K.K. and K.S.; Data Curation, K.K., F.O. and K.S.; Writing—Original Draft Preparation, K.K.; Writing—Review & Editing, F.O. and K.S.; Supervision, K.S.; Project Administration, K.S. All authors have read and agreed to the published version of the manuscript.

Funding: This review was supported by the MD Anderson Cancer Center Support Grant CA016672 from the National Cancer Institute.

Acknowledgments: We thank Joseph Munch (senior scientific editor, Research Medical Library at the University of Texas MD Anderson Cancer Center) for editing this review.

Conflicts of Interest: K.K.: none. F.O.: none. K.S.: Daiichi Sankyo: Consultancy; Novartis: Consultancy, Research Funding; Pfizer Japan: Consultancy; Otsuka: Honoraria.

References

1. Montalban-Bravo, G.; Kanagal-Shamanna, R.; Class, C.A.; Sasaki, K.; Ravandi, F.; Cortes, J.E.; Daver, N.; Takahashi, K.; Short, N.J.; DiNardo, C.D.; et al. Outcomes of acute myeloid leukemia with myelodysplasia related changes depend on diagnostic criteria and therapy. *Am. J. Hematol.* **2020**, *95*, 612–622. [CrossRef] [PubMed]
2. Sasaki, K.; Kanagal-Shamanna, R.; Montalban-Bravo, G.; Assi, R.; Jabbour, E.; Ravandi, F.; Kadia, T.; Pierce, S.; Takahashi, K.; Nogueras Gonzalez, G.; et al. Impact of the variant allele frequency of ASXL1, DNMT3A, JAK2, TET2, TP53, and NPM1 on the outcomes of patients with newly diagnosed acute myeloid leukemia. *Cancer* **2020**, *126*, 765–774. [CrossRef] [PubMed]
3. Morita, K.; Kantarjian, H.M.; Wang, F.; Yan, Y.; Bueso-Ramos, C.; Sasaki, K.; Issa, G.C.; Wang, S.; Jorgensen, J.; Song, X.; et al. Clearance of Somatic Mutations at Remission and the Risk of Relapse in Acute Myeloid Leukemia. *J. Clin. Oncol.* **2018**, *36*, 1788–1797. [CrossRef] [PubMed]
4. Chien, K.S.; Class, C.A.; Montalban-Bravo, G.; Wei, Y.; Sasaki, K.; Naqvi, K.; Ganan-Gomez, I.; Yang, H.; Soltysiak, K.A.; Kanagal-Shamanna, R.; et al. LILRB4 expression in chronic myelomonocytic leukemia and myelodysplastic syndrome based on response to hypomethylating agents. *Leuk. Lymphoma* **2020**, *61*, 1493–1499. [CrossRef] [PubMed]
5. Quesada, A.E.; Montalban-Bravo, G.; Luthra, R.; Patel, K.P.; Sasaki, K.; Bueso-Ramos, C.E.; Khoury, J.D.; Routbort, M.J.; Bassett, R.; Hidalgo-Lopez, J.E.; et al. Clinico-pathologic characteristics and outcomes of the World Health Organization (WHO) provisional entity de novo acute myeloid leukemia with mutated RUNX1. *Mod. Pathol.* **2020**, *33*, 1678–1689. [CrossRef]
6. Lachowiez, C.A.; Loghavi, S.; Furudate, K.; Montalban-Bravo, G.; Maiti, A.; Kadia, T.; Daver, N.; Borthakur, G.; Pemmaraju, N.; Sasaki, K.; et al. Impact of splicing mutations in acute myeloid leukemia treated with hypomethylating agents combined with venetoclax. *Blood Adv.* **2021**, *5*, 2173–2183. [CrossRef]
7. Venugopal, S.; Shoukier, M.; Konopleva, M.; Dinardo, C.D.; Ravandi, F.; Short, N.J.; Andreeff, M.; Borthakur, G.; Daver, N.; Pemmaraju, N.; et al. Outcomes in patients with newly diagnosed TP53-mutated acute myeloid leukemia with or without venetoclax-based therapy. *Cancer* **2021**, *127*, 3541–3551. [CrossRef]
8. Kim, K.; Maiti, A.; Loghavi, S.; Pourebrahim, R.; Kadia, T.M.; Rausch, C.R.; Furudate, K.; Daver, N.G.; Alvarado, Y.; Ohanian, M.; et al. Outcomes of TP53-mutant acute myeloid leukemia with decitabine and venetoclax. *Cancer* **2021**, *127*, 3772–3781. [CrossRef]
9. Issa, G.C.; Zarka, J.; Sasaki, K.; Qiao, W.; Pak, D.; Ning, J.; Short, N.J.; Haddad, F.; Tang, Z.; Patel, K.P.; et al. Predictors of outcomes in adults with acute myeloid leukemia and KMT2A rearrangements. *Blood Cancer J.* **2021**, *11*, 162. [CrossRef]
10. Sasaki, K.; Kadia, T.; Begna, K.; DiNardo, C.D.; Borthakur, G.; Short, N.J.; Jain, N.; Daver, N.; Jabbour, E.; Garcia-Manero, G.; et al. Prediction of early (4-week) mortality in acute myeloid leukemia with intensive chemotherapy. *Am. J. Hematol.* **2022**, *97*, 68–78. [CrossRef]
11. Fiskus, W.; Boettcher, S.; Daver, N.; Mill, C.P.; Sasaki, K.; Birdwell, C.E.; Davis, J.A.; Takahashi, K.; Kadia, T.M.; DiNardo, C.D.; et al. Effective Menin inhibitor-based combinations against AML with MLL rearrangement or NPM1 mutation (NPM1c). *Blood Cancer J.* **2022**, *12*, 5. [CrossRef] [PubMed]
12. Sasaki, K.; Ravandi, F.; Kadia, T.; DiNardo, C.; Borthakur, G.; Short, N.; Jain, N.; Daver, N.; Jabbour, E.; Garcia-Manero, G.; et al. Prediction of survival with intensive chemotherapy in acute myeloid leukemia. *Am. J. Hematol.* **2022**, *97*, 865–876. [CrossRef]
13. Jabbour, E.; Faderl, S.; Sasaki, K.; Kadia, T.; Daver, N.; Pemmaraju, N.; Patel, K.; Khoury, J.D.; Bueso-Ramos, C.; Bohannan, Z.; et al. Phase 2 study of low-dose clofarabine plus cytarabine for patients with higher-risk myelodysplastic syndrome who have relapsed or are refractory to hypomethylating agents. *Cancer* **2017**, *123*, 629–637. [CrossRef] [PubMed]
14. Jabbour, E.; Short, N.J.; Montalban-Bravo, G.; Huang, X.; Bueso-Ramos, C.; Qiao, W.; Yang, H.; Zhao, C.; Kadia, T.; Borthakur, G.; et al. Randomized phase 2 study of low-dose decitabine vs low-dose azacitidine in lower-risk MDS and MDS/MPN. *Blood* **2017**, *130*, 1514–1522. [CrossRef] [PubMed]
15. Short, N.J.; Jabbour, E.; Naqvi, K.; Patel, A.; Ning, J.; Sasaki, K.; Nogueras-Gonzalez, G.M.; Bose, P.; Kornblau, S.M.; Takahashi, K.; et al. A phase II study of omacetaxine mepesuccinate for patients with higher-risk myelodysplastic syndrome and chronic myelomonocytic leukemia after failure of hypomethylating agents. *Am. J. Hematol.* **2019**, *94*, 74–79. [CrossRef]
16. Montalban-Bravo, G.; Kanagal-Shamanna, R.; Sasaki, K.; Patel, K.; Ganan-Gomez, I.; Jabbour, E.; Kadia, T.; Ravandi, F.; DiNardo, C.; Borthakur, G.; et al. NPM1 mutations define a specific subgroup of MDS and MDS/MPN patients with favorable outcomes with intensive chemotherapy. *Blood Adv.* **2019**, *3*, 922–933. [CrossRef] [PubMed]
17. Montalban-Bravo, G.; Class, C.A.; Ganan-Gomez, I.; Kanagal-Shamanna, R.; Sasaki, K.; Richard-Carpentier, G.; Naqvi, K.; Wei, Y.; Yang, H.; Soltysiak, K.A.; et al. Transcriptomic analysis implicates necroptosis in disease progression and prognosis in myelodysplastic syndromes. *Leukemia* **2020**, *34*, 872–881. [CrossRef] [PubMed]
18. Montalban-Bravo, G.; Kanagal-Shamanna, R.; Benton, C.B.; Class, C.A.; Chien, K.S.; Sasaki, K.; Naqvi, K.; Alvarado, Y.; Kadia, T.M.; Ravandi, F.; et al. Genomic context and TP53 allele frequency define clinical outcomes in TP53-mutated myelodysplastic syndromes. *Blood Adv.* **2020**, *4*, 482–495. [CrossRef]
19. Sasaki, K.; Ravandi, F.; Kadia, T.M.; DiNardo, C.D.; Short, N.J.; Borthakur, G.; Jabbour, E.; Kantarjian, H.M. De novo acute myeloid leukemia: A population-based study of outcome in the United States based on the Surveillance, Epidemiology, and End Results (SEER) database, 1980 to 2017. *Cancer* **2021**, *127*, 2049–2061. [CrossRef]
20. DiNardo, C.D.; Lachowiez, C.A.; Takahashi, K.; Loghavi, S.; Kadia, T.; Daver, N.; Xiao, L.; Adeoti, M.; Short, N.J.; Sasaki, K.; et al. Venetoclax combined with FLAG-IDA induction and consolidation in newly diagnosed acute myeloid leukemia. *Am. J. Hematol.* **2022**, *97*, 1035–1043. [CrossRef]

21. Perl, A.E.; Martinelli, G.; Cortes, J.E.; Neubauer, A.; Berman, E.; Paolini, S.; Montesinos, P.; Baer, M.R.; Larson, R.A.; Ustun, C.; et al. Gilteritinib or Chemotherapy for Relapsed or Refractory FLT3-Mutated AML. *N. Engl. J. Med.* **2019**, *381*, 1728–1740. [CrossRef] [PubMed]
22. DiNardo, C.D.; Stein, E.M.; de Botton, S.; Roboz, G.J.; Altman, J.K.; Mims, A.S.; Swords, R.; Collins, R.H.; Mannis, G.N.; Pollyea, D.A.; et al. Durable Remissions with Ivosidenib in IDH1-Mutated Relapsed or Refractory AML. *N. Engl. J. Med.* **2018**, *378*, 2386–2398. [CrossRef] [PubMed]
23. Kadia, T.M.; Reville, P.K.; Wang, X.; Rausch, C.R.; Borthakur, G.; Pemmaraju, N.; Daver, N.G.; DiNardo, C.D.; Sasaki, K.; Issa, G.C.; et al. Phase II Study of Venetoclax Added to Cladribine Plus Low-Dose Cytarabine Alternating With 5-Azacitidine in Older Patients With Newly Diagnosed Acute Myeloid Leukemia. *J. Clin. Oncol.* **2022**, *40*, 3848–3857. [CrossRef] [PubMed]
24. Yalniz, F.; Abou Dalle, I.; Kantarjian, H.; Borthakur, G.; Kadia, T.; Patel, K.; Loghavi, S.; Garcia-Manero, G.; Sasaki, K.; Daver, N.; et al. Prognostic significance of baseline FLT3-ITD mutant allele level in acute myeloid leukemia treated with intensive chemotherapy with/without sorafenib. *Am. J. Hematol.* **2019**, *94*, 984–991. [CrossRef]
25. Sasaki, K.; Kantarjian, H.M.; Kadia, T.; Patel, K.; Loghavi, S.; Garcia-Manero, G.; Jabbour, E.J.; DiNardo, C.; Pemmaraju, N.; Daver, N.; et al. Sorafenib plus intensive chemotherapy improves survival in patients with newly diagnosed, FLT3-internal tandem duplication mutation-positive acute myeloid leukemia. *Cancer* **2019**, *125*, 3755–3766. [CrossRef]
26. Maiti, A.; Franquiz, M.J.; Ravandi, F.; Cortes, J.E.; Jabbour, E.J.; Sasaki, K.; Marx, K.; Daver, N.G.; Kadia, T.M.; Konopleva, M.Y.; et al. Venetoclax and BCR-ABL Tyrosine Kinase Inhibitor Combinations: Outcome in Patients with Philadelphia Chromosome-Positive Advanced Myeloid Leukemias. *Acta Haematol.* **2020**, *143*, 567–573. [CrossRef]
27. Abou Dalle, I.; Ghorab, A.; Patel, K.; Wang, X.; Hwang, H.; Cortes, J.; Issa, G.C.; Yalniz, F.; Sasaki, K.; Chihara, D.; et al. Impact of numerical variation, allele burden, mutation length and co-occurring mutations on the efficacy of tyrosine kinase inhibitors in newly diagnosed FLT3- mutant acute myeloid leukemia. *Blood Cancer J.* **2020**, *10*, 48. [CrossRef]
28. DiNardo, C.D.; Maiti, A.; Rausch, C.R.; Pemmaraju, N.; Naqvi, K.; Daver, N.G.; Kadia, T.M.; Borthakur, G.; Ohanian, M.; Alvarado, Y.; et al. 10-day decitabine with venetoclax for newly diagnosed intensive chemotherapy ineligible, and relapsed or refractory acute myeloid leukaemia: A single-centre, phase 2 trial. *Lancet Haematol.* **2020**, *7*, e724–e736. [CrossRef]
29. Shoukier, M.; Kadia, T.; Konopleva, M.; Alotaibi, A.S.; Alfayez, M.; Loghavi, S.; Patel, K.P.; Kanagal-Shamanna, R.; Cortes, J.; Samra, B.; et al. Clinical characteristics and outcomes in patients with acute myeloid leukemia with concurrent FLT3-ITD and IDH mutations. *Cancer* **2021**, *127*, 381–390. [CrossRef]
30. Maiti, A.; Qiao, W.; Sasaki, K.; Ravandi, F.; Kadia, T.M.; Jabbour, E.J.; Daver, N.G.; Borthakur, G.; Garcia-Manero, G.; Pierce, S.A.; et al. Venetoclax with decitabine vs. intensive chemotherapy in acute myeloid leukemia: A propensity score matched analysis stratified by risk of treatment-related mortality. *Am. J. Hematol.* **2021**, *96*, 282–291. [CrossRef]
31. Yilmaz, M.; Kantarjian, H.; Short, N.J.; Reville, P.; Konopleva, M.; Kadia, T.; DiNardo, C.; Borthakur, G.; Pemmaraju, N.; Maiti, A.; et al. Hypomethylating agent and venetoclax with FLT3 inhibitor "triplet" therapy in older/unfit patients with FLT3 mutated AML. *Blood Cancer J.* **2022**, *12*, 77. [CrossRef] [PubMed]
32. Huang, K.L.; Mashl, R.J.; Wu, Y.; Ritter, D.I.; Wang, J.; Oh, C.; Paczkowska, M.; Reynolds, S.; Wyczalkowski, M.A.; Oak, N.; et al. Pathogenic Germline Variants in 10,389 Adult Cancers. *Cell* **2018**, *173*, 355–370.e314. [CrossRef]
33. Arber, D.A.; Orazi, A.; Hasserjian, R.; Thiele, J.; Borowitz, M.J.; Le Beau, M.M.; Bloomfield, C.D.; Cazzola, M.; Vardiman, J.W. The 2016 revision to the World Health Organization classification of myeloid neoplasms and acute leukemia. *Blood* **2016**, *127*, 2391–2405. [CrossRef] [PubMed]
34. Polprasert, C.; Schulze, I.; Sekeres, M.A.; Makishima, H.; Przychodzen, B.; Hosono, N.; Singh, J.; Padgett, R.A.; Gu, X.; Phillips, J.G.; et al. Inherited and Somatic Defects in DDX41 in Myeloid Neoplasms. *Cancer Cell* **2015**, *27*, 658–670. [CrossRef] [PubMed]
35. Sebert, M.; Passet, M.; Raimbault, A.; Rahme, R.; Raffoux, E.; Sicre de Fontbrune, F.; Cerrano, M.; Quentin, S.; Vasquez, N.; Da Costa, M.; et al. Germline DDX41 mutations define a significant entity within adult MDS/AML patients. *Blood* **2019**, *134*, 1441–1444. [CrossRef] [PubMed]
36. Quesada, A.E.; Routbort, M.J.; DiNardo, C.D.; Bueso-Ramos, C.E.; Kanagal-Shamanna, R.; Khoury, J.D.; Thakral, B.; Zuo, Z.; Yin, C.C.; Loghavi, S.; et al. DDX41 mutations in myeloid neoplasms are associated with male gender, TP53 mutations and high-risk disease. *Am. J. Hematol.* **2019**, *94*, 757–766. [CrossRef]
37. Makishima, H.; Saiki, R.; Nannya, Y.; Korotev, S.C.; Gurnari, C.; Takeda, J.; Momozawa, Y.; Best, S.; Krishnamurthy, P.; Yoshizato, T.; et al. Germline DDX41 mutations define a unique subtype of myeloid neoplasms. *Blood* **2022**. [CrossRef]
38. Kadono, M.; Kanai, A.; Nagamachi, A.; Shinriki, S.; Kawata, J.; Iwato, K.; Kyo, T.; Oshima, K.; Yokoyama, A.; Kawamura, T.; et al. Biological implications of somatic DDX41 p.R525H mutation in acute myeloid leukemia. *Exp. Hematol.* **2016**, *44*, 745–754.e744. [CrossRef]
39. Chlon, T.M.; Stepanchick, E.; Hershberger, C.E.; Daniels, N.J.; Hueneman, K.M.; Kuenzi Davis, A.; Choi, K.; Zheng, Y.; Gurnari, C.; Haferlach, T.; et al. Germline DDX41 mutations cause ineffective hematopoiesis and myelodysplasia. *Cell Stem Cell* **2021**, *28*, 1966–1981.e1966. [CrossRef]
40. Lee, K.G.; Kim, S.S.; Kui, L.; Voon, D.C.; Mauduit, M.; Bist, P.; Bi, X.; Pereira, N.A.; Liu, C.; Sukumaran, B.; et al. Bruton's tyrosine kinase phosphorylates DDX41 and activates its binding of dsDNA and STING to initiate type 1 interferon response. *Cell Rep.* **2015**, *10*, 1055–1065. [CrossRef]
41. Zhang, Z.; Yuan, B.; Bao, M.; Lu, N.; Kim, T.; Liu, Y.J. The helicase DDX41 senses intracellular DNA mediated by the adaptor STING in dendritic cells. *Nat. Immunol.* **2011**, *12*, 959–965. [CrossRef] [PubMed]

42. Ma, J.; Mahmud, N.; Bosland, M.C.; Ross, S.R. DDX41 is needed for pre- and postnatal hematopoietic stem cell differentiation in mice. *Stem Cell Rep.* **2022**, *17*, 879–893. [CrossRef] [PubMed]
43. Jiang, Y.; Zhu, Y.; Liu, Z.J.; Ouyang, S. The emerging roles of the DDX41 protein in immunity and diseases. *Protein Cell* **2017**, *8*, 83–89. [CrossRef] [PubMed]
44. Mosler, T.; Conte, F.; Longo, G.M.C.; Mikicic, I.; Kreim, N.; Mockel, M.M.; Petrosino, G.; Flach, J.; Barau, J.; Luke, B.; et al. R-loop proximity proteomics identifies a role of DDX41 in transcription-associated genomic instability. *Nat. Commun.* **2021**, *12*, 7314. [CrossRef] [PubMed]
45. Weinreb, J.T.; Ghazale, N.; Pradhan, K.; Gupta, V.; Potts, K.S.; Tricomi, B.; Daniels, N.J.; Padgett, R.A.; De Oliveira, S.; Verma, A.; et al. Excessive R-loops trigger an inflammatory cascade leading to increased HSPC production. *Dev. Cell* **2021**, *56*, 627–640.e625. [CrossRef] [PubMed]
46. Choi, E.J.; Cho, Y.U.; Hur, E.H.; Jang, S.; Kim, N.; Park, H.S.; Lee, J.H.; Lee, K.H.; Kim, S.H.; Hwang, S.H.; et al. Unique ethnic features of DDX41 mutations in patients with idiopathic cytopenia of undetermined significance, myelodysplastic syndrome, or acute myeloid leukemia. *Haematologica* **2022**, *107*, 510–518. [CrossRef] [PubMed]
47. Churpek, J.E.; Smith-Simmer, K. DDX41-Associated Familial Myelodysplastic Syndrome and Acute Myeloid Leukemia. Available online: https://www.ncbi.nlm.nih.gov/books/NBK574843/ (accessed on 15 August 2022).
48. Wan, Z.; Han, B. Clinical features of DDX41 mutation-related diseases: A systematic review with individual patient data. *Ther. Adv. Hematol.* **2021**, *12*, 20406207211032433. [CrossRef]
49. Lewinsohn, M.; Brown, A.L.; Weinel, L.M.; Phung, C.; Rafidi, G.; Lee, M.K.; Schreiber, A.W.; Feng, J.; Babic, M.; Chong, C.E.; et al. Novel germ line DDX41 mutations define families with a lower age of MDS/AML onset and lymphoid malignancies. *Blood* **2016**, *127*, 1017–1023. [CrossRef]
50. Li, P.; Brown, S.; Williams, M.; White, T.; Xie, W.; Cui, W.; Peker, D.; Lei, L.; Kunder, C.A.; Wang, H.Y.; et al. The genetic landscape of germline DDX41 variants predisposing to myeloid neoplasms. *Blood* **2022**, *140*, 716–755. [CrossRef]
51. Bannon, S.A.; Routbort, M.J.; Montalban-Bravo, G.; Mehta, R.S.; Jelloul, F.Z.; Takahashi, K.; Daver, N.; Oran, B.; Pemmaraju, N.; Borthakur, G.; et al. Next-Generation Sequencing of DDX41 in Myeloid Neoplasms Leads to Increased Detection of Germline Alterations. *Front. Oncol.* **2020**, *10*, 582213. [CrossRef]
52. Cheah, J.J.C.; Hahn, C.N.; Hiwase, D.K.; Scott, H.S.; Brown, A.L. Myeloid neoplasms with germline DDX41 mutation. *Int. J. Hematol.* **2017**, *106*, 163–174. [CrossRef] [PubMed]
53. Makishima, H.; Nannya, Y.; Takeda, J.; Momozawa, Y.; Saiki, R.; Yoshizato, T.; Atsuta, Y.; Iijima-Yamashita, Y.; Yoshida, K.; Shiraishi, Y.; et al. Clinical Impacts of Germline DDX41 Mutations on Myeloid Neoplasms. *Blood* **2020**, *136*, 38–40. [CrossRef]
54. Qu, S.; Li, B.; Qin, T.; Xu, Z.; Pan, L.; Hu, N.; Huang, G.; Peter Gale, R.; Xiao, Z. Molecular and clinical features of myeloid neoplasms with somatic DDX41 mutations. *Br. J. Haematol.* **2021**, *192*, 1006–1010. [CrossRef] [PubMed]
55. Cardoso, S.R.; Ryan, G.; Walne, A.J.; Ellison, A.; Lowe, R.; Tummala, H.; Rio-Machin, A.; Collopy, L.; Al Seraihi, A.; Wallis, Y.; et al. Germline heterozygous DDX41 variants in a subset of familial myelodysplasia and acute myeloid leukemia. *Leukemia* **2016**, *30*, 2083–2086. [CrossRef] [PubMed]
56. Alkhateeb, H.B.; Nanaa, A.; Viswanatha, D.; Foran, J.M.; Badar, T.; Sproat, L.; He, R.; Nguyen, P.; Jevremovic, D.; Salama, M.E.; et al. Genetic features and clinical outcomes of patients with isolated and comutated DDX41-mutated myeloid neoplasms. *Blood Adv.* **2022**, *6*, 528–532. [CrossRef]
57. Duployez, N.; Largeaud, L.; Duchmann, M.; Kim, R.; Rieunier, J.; Lambert, J.; Bidet, A.; Larcher, L.; Lemoine, J.; Delhommeau, F.; et al. Prognostic impact of DDX41 germline mutations in intensively treated acute myeloid leukemia patients: An ALFA-FILO study. *Blood* **2022**, *140*, 756–768. [CrossRef]
58. Kennedy, A.L.; Shimamura, A. Genetic predisposition to MDS: Clinical features and clonal evolution. *Blood* **2019**, *133*, 1071–1085. [CrossRef]
59. Li, P.; White, T.; Xie, W.; Cui, W.; Peker, D.; Zeng, G.; Wang, H.Y.; Vagher, J.; Brown, S.; Williams, M.; et al. AML with germline DDX41 variants is a clinicopathologically distinct entity with an indolent clinical course and favorable outcome. *Leukemia* **2022**, *36*, 664–674. [CrossRef]
60. List, A.; Dewald, G.; Bennett, J.; Giagounidis, A.; Raza, A.; Feldman, E.; Powell, B.; Greenberg, P.; Thomas, D.; Stone, R.; et al. Lenalidomide in the myelodysplastic syndrome with chromosome 5q deletion. *N. Engl. J. Med.* **2006**, *355*, 1456–1465. [CrossRef]
61. Negoro, E.; Radivoyevitch, T.; Polprasert, C.; Adema, V.; Hosono, N.; Makishima, H.; Przychodzen, B.; Hirsch, C.; Clemente, M.J.; Nazha, A.; et al. Molecular predictors of response in patients with myeloid neoplasms treated with lenalidomide. *Leukemia* **2016**, *30*, 2405–2409. [CrossRef]
62. Abou Dalle, I.; Kantarjian, H.; Bannon, S.A.; Kanagal-Shamanna, R.; Routbort, M.; Patel, K.P.; Hu, S.; Bhalla, K.; Garcia-Manero, G.; DiNardo, C.D. Successful lenalidomide treatment in high risk myelodysplastic syndrome with germline DDX41 mutation. *Am. J. Hematol.* **2020**, *95*, 227–229. [CrossRef] [PubMed]
63. Berger, G.; van den Berg, E.; Sikkema-Raddatz, B.; Abbott, K.M.; Sinke, R.J.; Bungener, L.B.; Mulder, A.B.; Vellenga, E. Re-emergence of acute myeloid leukemia in donor cells following allogeneic transplantation in a family with a germline DDX41 mutation. *Leukemia* **2017**, *31*, 520–522. [CrossRef] [PubMed]
64. Kobayashi, S.; Kobayashi, A.; Osawa, Y.; Nagao, S.; Takano, K.; Okada, Y.; Tachi, N.; Teramoto, M.; Kawamura, T.; Horiuchi, T.; et al. Donor cell leukemia arising from preleukemic clones with a novel germline DDX41 mutation after allogenic hematopoietic stem cell transplantation. *Leukemia* **2017**, *31*, 1020–1022. [CrossRef] [PubMed]

65. Gibson, C.J.; Kim, H.T.; Zhao, L.; Murdock, H.M.; Hambley, B.; Ogata, A.; Madero-Marroquin, R.; Wang, S.; Green, L.; Fleharty, M.; et al. Donor Clonal Hematopoiesis and Recipient Outcomes After Transplantation. *J. Clin. Oncol.* **2022**, *40*, 189–201. [CrossRef] [PubMed]
66. DiNardo, C.D.; Routbort, M.J.; Bannon, S.A.; Benton, C.B.; Takahashi, K.; Kornblau, S.M.; Luthra, R.; Kanagal-Shamanna, R.; Medeiros, L.J.; Garcia-Manero, G.; et al. Improving the detection of patients with inherited predispositions to hematologic malignancies using next-generation sequencing-based leukemia prognostication panels. *Cancer* **2018**, *124*, 2704–2713. [CrossRef]

Disclaimer/Publisher's Note: The statements, opinions and data contained in all publications are solely those of the individual author(s) and contributor(s) and not of MDPI and/or the editor(s). MDPI and/or the editor(s) disclaim responsibility for any injury to people or property resulting from any ideas, methods, instructions or products referred to in the content.

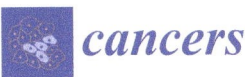

Review

Myelodysplastic Syndromes with Isolated del(5q): Value of Molecular Alterations for Diagnostic and Prognostic Assessment

Pamela Acha [1], Mar Mallo [1,2] and Francesc Solé [1,2,*]

1. MDS Group, Institut de Recerca Contra la Leucèmia Josep Carreras, ICO-Hospital Germans Trias i Pujol, Universitat Autònoma de Barcelona, 08916 Badalona, Spain
2. Microarrays Unit, Institut de Recerca Contra la Leucèmia Josep Carreras, ICO-Hospital Germans Trias i Pujol, Universitat Autònoma de Barcelona, 08916 Badalona, Spain
* Correspondence: fsole@carrerasresearch.org; Tel.: +34-93-557-2806

Simple Summary: Myelodysplastic syndromes with isolated del(5q) constitute the only MDS subtype defined by a cytogenetic alteration. The results of several clinical studies and the advances in new technologies have provided a better understanding of the biological basis of this disease. Specific genetic alterations have been found to be associated with prognosis and response to treatments. This review intends to summarize the current knowledge of the molecular background of MDS with isolated del(5q), focusing on the clinical and prognostic relevance of cytogenetic alterations and somatic mutations.

Abstract: Myelodysplastic syndromes (MDS) are a group of clonal hematological neoplasms characterized by ineffective hematopoiesis in one or more bone marrow cell lineages. Consequently, patients present with variable degrees of cytopenia and dysplasia. These characteristics constitute the basis for the World Health Organization (WHO) classification criteria of MDS, among other parameters, for the current prognostic scoring system. Although nearly half of newly diagnosed patients present a cytogenetic alteration, and almost 90% of them harbor at least one somatic mutation, MDS with isolated del(5q) constitutes the only subtype clearly defined by a cytogenetic alteration. The results of several clinical studies and the advances of new technologies have allowed a better understanding of the biological basis of this disease. Therefore, since the first report of the "5q- syndrome" in 1974, changes and refinements have been made in the definition and the characteristics of the patients with MDS and del(5q). Moreover, specific genetic alterations have been found to be associated with the prognosis and response to treatments. The aim of this review is to summarize the current knowledge of the molecular background of MDS with isolated del(5q), focusing on the clinical and prognostic relevance of cytogenetic alterations and somatic mutations.

Keywords: myelodysplastic syndromes; chromosome 5q deletion; somatic mutations; cytogenetic alterations

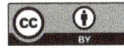

1. Introduction

Myelodysplastic syndromes (MDS) are a group of clonal hematological neoplasms characterized by ineffective hematopoiesis in one or more bone marrow (BM) cell lineages. Consequently, patients present with variable degrees of cytopenia and dysplasia, which are essential features for establishing a diagnosis according to the World Health Organization (WHO) classification [1,2].

Although nearly half of newly diagnosed patients present a cytogenetic alteration and almost 90% of them harbor at least one somatic mutation, MDS with isolated chromosome 5q deletion (MDS-5q) constitutes the only subtype clearly defined by a cytogenetic alteration [3–6]. The results of several clinical studies and advances in new technologies have allowed better characterization of this entity. As a consequence, since the first report of the 5q- syndrome, changes and refinements have been made in the definition and characteristics of the patients that pertain to this subtype [7]. Moreover, specific genetic alterations have been found to be associated with prognosis and response to treatments [1,2,8,9].

While preparing this review, the overview of the next WHO classification and the proposal of the International Consensus Classification (ICC) of myeloid neoplasms and acute leukemias were published [2,8]. Consequently, MDS-5q will be renamed and the inclusion criteria will be slightly modified, as will be explained in the subsequent section.

In the present review, we aimed to summarize the current knowledge of the molecular background of MDS-5q, focusing on the clinical and prognostic relevance of cytogenetic alterations and somatic mutations.

2. From "5q- Syndrome" to MDS-5q

In 1974, Van den Berghe et al. reported a group of three patients with refractory anemia and interstitial deletion of the long arm of chromosome 5. Such cases were later recognized as the "5q- syndrome". Features of the syndrome included macrocytic anemia, low-normal leukocyte counts, and normal to elevated platelet counts. The BM showed erythroid hypoplasia, hypolobulated megakaryocytes, and a blast count <15% [7]. According to the French–American–British (FAB) cooperative group classification criteria, most of the patients with these characteristics pertain to the group of patients with refractory anemia [10].

It was not until the 2001 edition of the WHO classification that the 5q- syndrome was recognized as a unique and well-defined MDS subtype [11]. In addition to previously described characteristics of this syndrome, in this classification, the blast count threshold was redefined to <5%, and the absence of Auer roads was considered to define 5q- syndrome patients. In 2008, the subtype "MDS with isolated del(5q)" was introduced and the term 5q-syndrome remained restricted to a subset of cases within this category that presented with macrocytic anemia, normal or elevated platelet count, BM erythroid hypoplasia, and a blast count <5% in BM and <1% in peripheral blood (PB) [12]. In the 2017 WHO classification, these cases remained within the MDS with isolated del(5q) subtype. Additionally, the diagnosis of this subtype can be established even if there is one additional cytogenetic abnormality besides the del(5q), unless this abnormality is monosomy 7 or del(7q) [1,13]. This is based on data showing that there is no adverse effect of one chromosomal abnormality in addition to the del(5q) in such patients [14].

As mentioned previously, the overview of the next WHO classification has recently been published [2]. In this new proposal, MDS with isolated del(5q) has been renamed as "myelodysplastic neoplasm with low blast and isolated del(5q)" (abbreviated MDS-5q). The diagnostic criteria have not changed, and it is stated that although an *SF3B1* or *TP53* mutation (not multi-hit) may potentially alter the biology and/or prognosis of the disease, the presence of such mutations does not per se override the diagnosis of this entity. Regarding the ICC proposal for the classification of MDS, MDS with isolated del(5q) has been retained with no changes from the revised fourth edition of the WHO classification, although the name has been simplified to "MDS with del(5q)". Similarly to the new WHO proposal, the ICC also specifies that *TP53* mutations are admitted in this MDS subtype unless a multi-hit state is detected [8].

It is important to remark that although del(5q) is the most frequent cytogenetic alteration in MDS and is present in roughly 20% of cytogenetic abnormal cases, only about 5% are classified in the MDS-5q category. Features such as higher blast count, alterations in chromosome 7, or a multi-hit *TP53* state impact disease prognosis and would reclassify these remaining patients into other, more aggressive, disease subtypes [2,8,15].

The changes in terms and inclusion criteria over time are produced as a consequence of the advances in technology and discoveries, which directly impact our knowledge and the management of this disease (Figure 1).

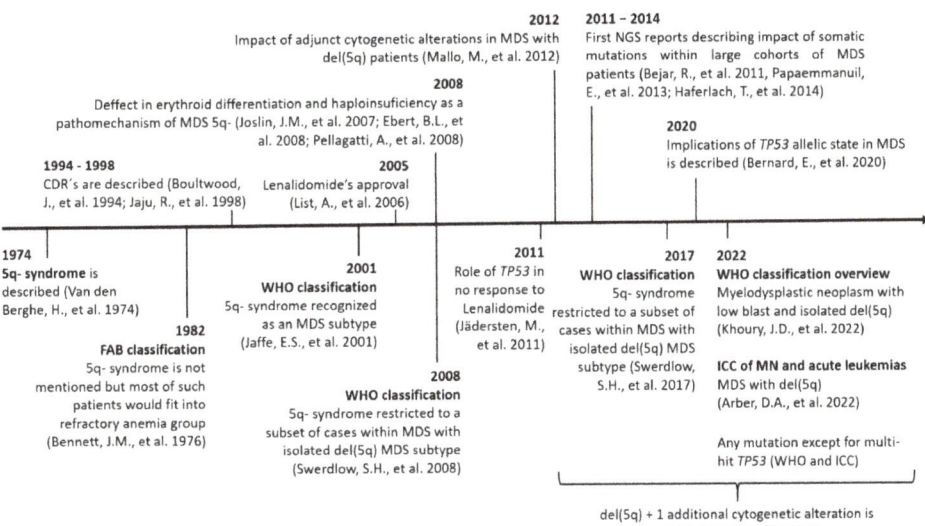

Figure 1. Timeline showing the main discoveries involving MDS-5q and the changes in nomenclature and inclusion criteria. Abbreviations: CDR, commonly deleted region; chr, chromosome; ICC: International Consensus Classification; MN, myeloid neoplasms; NGS, next-generation sequencing.

3. Role of Conventional Cytogenetics in MDS-5q

Conventional cytogenetics (CC) constitutes the gold standard for the genetic diagnosis and prognosis of MDS. However, fluorescence in situ hybridization (FISH) of 5q31 could be useful in cases without evidence of del(5q) by CC. When the presence of MDS-5q is suspected and/or if the cytogenetic study shows no metaphases or an aberrant karyotype with chromosome 5 is involved (no 5q deletion), it is recommended to perform FISH analysis [16,17]. Figure 2 shows the genetic studies available for the diagnosis and characterization of MDS-5q. During follow-up, genetics studies will be adapted to each patient, considering their comorbidities. A new BM aspiration, and the corresponding genetic study, will be performed on suspicion of disease evolution and no response to treatment. In the case of clonal evolution, the approach can be decided according to the general patient status.

The karyotype is a prognostic variable included in the International Prognostic Scoring System (IPSS) and the revised edition of the IPSS (IPSS-R) [18,19]. Del(5q) alone has always been considered a good prognostic variable and, in the IPSS-R, a concomitant cytogenetic alteration has been included. This change was based on a scoring system proposed by Schanz et al. based on an international data collection of 2902 patients [15]. Deletion 5q is a classical alteration detected in around 15–20% of MDS patients, with half being isolated, around 17% having an additional alteration, and 36% being part of a complex karyotype [3]. The prognostic impact of the accompanying abnormalities in del(5q) is difficult to determine because double abnormalities are highly variable. In 2011, Mallo et al. published an international collaborative study including a large series of del(5q) patients to determine the prognostic impact of adjunct prognostic abnormalities. The multivariate analysis showed that karyotype complexity was one of the main prognostic factors together with platelet count and BM blasts [14]. The good prognosis of del(5q) with one accompanying alteration was included in the MDS with the del(5q) category of the 2017 WHO classification, excluding cases harboring a chromosome 7 alteration [1].

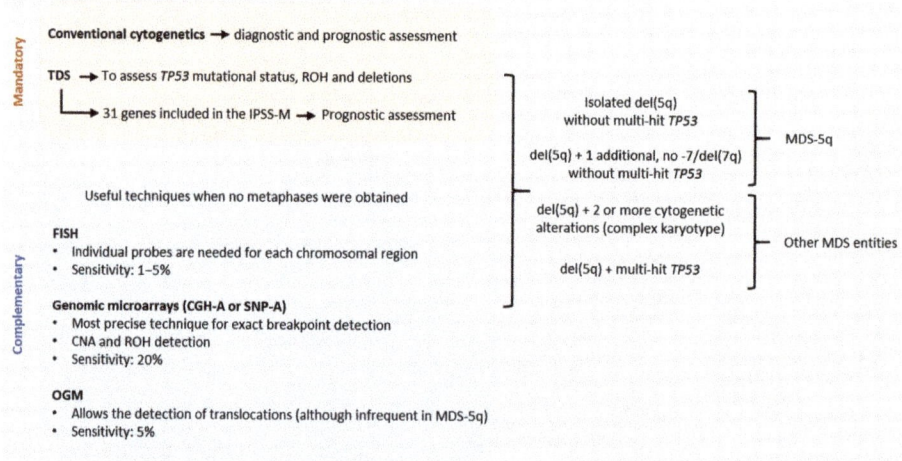

Figure 2. Genetic studies of MDS-5q according to the new diagnostic and prognostic guidelines: techniques available for correct diagnostic and prognostic assessment of MDS-5q according to the criteria of the next World Health Organization (WHO) classification, the proposal of the International Consensus Classification (ICC) and the Molecular International Prognosis Scoring System (IPSS-M). Abbreviations: CGH-A, comparative genomic hybridization; CNA, copy number alteration; FISH, fluorescence in situ hybridization; OGM, optical genome mapping; ROH, region of homozygosity; SNP-A, single nucleotide polymorphism array; TDS, targeted gene sequencing (assuming the use of probes that allow the detection of small CNA and ROH. Otherwise, SNP-A would be recommended to assess CNA and ROH in *TP53* for accurate diagnostic and prognostic assessment).

3.1. Commonly Deleted Regions in Chromosome 5q

Two "commonly deleted regions" (CDR) were originally described by Boultwood and colleagues: a 1.5 Mb deletion encompassing 5q32–5q33, which was originally associated with the 5q- syndrome and better prognosis, and a more proximal CDR at 5q31. The latter was associated with other MDS subtypes and cases of acute myeloid leukemia (AML) cases, with complex karyotypes and a worse prognosis [20–23]. High-resolution techniques, such as genomic microarrays and optical genome mapping (OGM), can detect cryptic alterations accompanying the del(5q) and can help define the breakpoint. However, since high-density genomic microarrays work with DNA probes, this approach has become the most suitable technique to obtain precise del(5q) breakpoint genomic coordinates.

Most patients have large deletions that encompass both CDRs. This was corroborated by subsequent studies combining conventional cytogenetics and single nucleotide polymorphism arrays, with Mallo et al., describing a wider CDR that extended from q22.3 to q31.3. This region encompasses 14.6 Mb, while the median size of the total deletion detected in most cases is around 70 Mb [17].

Several studies have focused on the study of the 5q CDR, but in 2012, Jerez et al., published an article emphasizing the importance of the common retained region (CRR) [24]. Their work reinforces the idea that in the 5q- syndrome, the proximal and terminal regions are always retained. Thus, two CRRs were described: CRR1 for the proximal region (spanning 81.7 Mb and ending at band 5q14.2) and CRR2 for the distal region (5q34), with both being associated with disease subtypes. No CRR could be identified in other forms of MDS and AML with del(5q). As was previously described, patients with CRR had a lower number of genomic lesions and correlate with better prognosis. Additionally, this study supports the idea that genomic microarrays can add prognostic information to prognostic scoring systems as was reported by Arenillas et al., in 2013 [25]. Figure 3 shows the CDR and CRR identified for chromosome 5q.

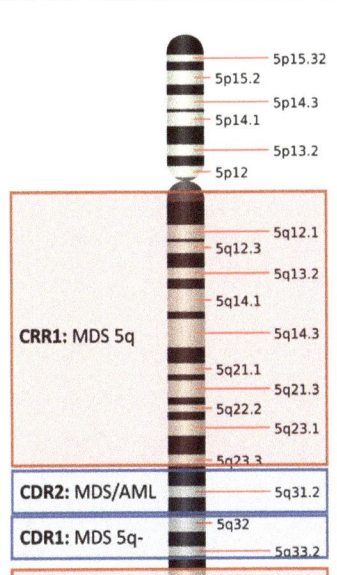

Figure 3. Commonly deleted regions (CDR) and commonly retained regions (CRR) in chromosome 5q.

It is widely known that additional techniques can help to describe the karyotype. Most of the complex cases carrying an apparent monosomy 5 have shown that, following studies with additional techniques such as FISH or genomic arrays, this apparent monosomy presents a partially retained 5q. As previously mentioned, genomic microarrays can help to accurately define the breakpoints [24,26].

Molecular studies revealed that haploinsufficiency of several genes (particularly *RPS14*, *CSNK1A1*, *EGR1*, *miR-145*, and *miR-14a*) located in 5q CDR contribute to the pathogenesis and hematological phenotype associated with MDS-5q [27–29]. For example, miR-145 and miR-14a are micro RNAs that have been found to be responsible for the negative regulation of effector molecules that regulate megakaryocytic differentiation. Thus, a deficiency of these micro RNAs is responsible for the thrombosis and megakaryocytic dysplasia (hypolobulated megakaryocytes) which characterize MDS-5q [30,31].

3.2. Karyotyping: Present and Future Directions

Point mutations have been described as a frequent event in MDS patients. In 2011, Bejar et al. described the clinical effects of these mutations and stated that the prognosis of these patients may be driven by the association of prognostic variables. Specific genes were found to be associated with specific risk groups such as *TET2* in cases with a normal karyotype and *TP53* in cases with a complex karyotype [32]. In 2022, the IPSS-M, a prognostic scoring system based on molecular data was published. This scoring system takes into account the mutational status of 31 genes; however, it still retains the karyotype as a prognostic parameter [9].

OGM has emerged as a promising non-sequencing-based technique for high resolution genome-wide structural variant profiling. It can simplify lab workflow by reducing multiple tests. Parallel studies with standard-of-care tests have been performed in hematological neoplasms and have shown high concordance [33]. A recent study published by Yang et al. showed that OGM results changed the comprehensive cytogenetic scoring system and the

IPSS-R risk groups in 21% and 17%, respectively, of their MDS patient's cohort with an improved prediction of prognosis. Although more studies especially focused on MDS-5q are needed, the combination of OGM and next-generation sequencing (NGS) seems to be a promising approach for the evaluation of prognosis [34].

4. Prognostic Impact of Somatic Mutations in MDS-5q

It has been described that one-third of MDS-5q patients present with no somatic alterations, while nearly half of patients (43%) can present with an isolated mutation [35,36]. The pattern of recurrently mutated genes is similar to other MDS subtypes, except for *TP53* mutations that were found to be enriched in this subtype of patients [35,37,38]. In the subsequent section, the genes most frequently mutated in MDS-5q are described and Table 1 summarizes their biological and clinical associations and main characteristics and frequencies.

Table 1. Recurrently mutated genes in MDS-5q: clinical and biological correlations.

Gene	Pathway/Function	Frequency	Clinical and Biological Correlations
SF3B1	Splicing factor	19–20%	• Associated with RS • Controvert data regarding outcome of concomitant *SF3B1* mutation and del(5q)
DNMT3A	DNA methylation	18%	• Recurrent founder lesion (DTA mutations)
TP53	Checkpoint/cell cycle	18%	• Aggressive disease course • Higher risk of transformation to AML • Shorter OS • Resistance to lenalidomide treatment
TET2	DNA methylation	12%	• Recurrent founder lesion (DTA mutations)
CSNK1A1	Proliferation, apoptosis, DNA damage response	7–10%	• Associated with older age
ASXL1	Chromatin modification	6%	• Recurrent founder lesion (DTA mutations)
JAK2	Tyrosine kinase	6%	• Associated with elevated platelet counts

Abbreviations: AML, acute myeloid leukemia; DTA, *DNMT3A*, *TET2*, and *ASXL1*; OS, overall survival; RS, ring sideroblasts.

Based on data from Meggendorfer et al. [35], Malcovati et al. [39], Heuser et al. [40], and Mossner et al. [41].

4.1. SF3B1 Mutation

The *SF3B1* gene encodes subunit 1 of the splicing factor 3b protein complex, which is a core component of the RNA splicing machinery. Mutations in *SF3B1* have been reported in around 20% of MDS-5q cases and have been associated with a variable proportion of ring sideroblasts [5,6,39,42]. Evidence provided by several reports suggests that, in some cases of MDS-5q, the *SF3B1* mutation might precede the cytogenetic alteration [41,43–45]. Despite the order of acquisition of such genetic events, cases with concomitant *SF3B1* and del(5q) would still be classified within the category of MDS-5q in the WHO classification system, as well as in the ICC system [2,8].

Controversial data have been published regarding the prognosis of *SF3B1* mutations in MDS-5q patients. On one hand, a study published by Meggendorfer et al., demonstrated a significantly shorter overall survival (OS) in patients harboring both alterations compared with MDS-5q patients without *SF3B1* mutation [35]. On the other hand, no significant difference in OS was reported by Malcovati et al. when analyzing the same in their respective cohort [39].

4.2. DNMT3A, TET2 and ASXL1 Mutations

Mutations affecting the genes *DNMT3A*, *TET2*, and *ASXL1* genes—commonly known as DTA mutations—are frequently found in clonal hematopoiesis of indeterminate potential (CHIP), which is a non-malignant condition associated with increased risk of progression to hematologic neoplasia compared with individuals without detectable mutations [46,47]. In line with this, in mutational hierarchy studies performed by Mossner et al., DTA mutations were found to be recurrent "founder" lesions in MDS patients, including the MDS-5q cases analyzed [36,41].

DNMT3A codifies for DNA methyltransferase 3 alpha, which is required for genome-wide de novo methylation and is essential for the establishment of DNA methylation patterns during development [48]. On the contrary, *TET2* codifies for tet methylcytosine dioxygenase 2, which catalyzes the conversion of the modified genomic base 5-methylcytosine (5mC) into 5-hydroxymethylcytosine (5hmC) and plays a key role in active DNA demethylation. As mentioned previously, both genes are recurrently mutated in MDS. Specifically, in MDS-5q, *DNMT3A* mutations were found in roughly 18% of cases while *TET2* mutations were described in nearly 12% of patients [35].

Some studies have reported that in MDS patients, *DNMT3A* mutations were associated with a higher risk of leukemia transformation and shorter OS, but no specific study describing either phenotypic or survival associations was exclusively performed in MDS-5q patients [49,50].

A report by Scharenberg et al. described that progression in patients with low- and intermediate-1-risk del(5q) MDS is predicted by mutations in a limited number of genes, among which *TET2* is included. Specifically, 6/13 patients with evidence of disease progression presented mutations in the *TET2* gene [51]. In MDS patient cohorts including all disease subtypes, *TET2* mutations were found to be associated with shorter OS after hematopoietic stem cell transplantation and lower response rate to hypomethylating agents [9,52,53].

Located in chromosome 20q, additional sex combs 1 (*ASXL1*) codifies for a protein involved in transcriptional regulation. Mutations of mostly the frameshift type have been described in MDS patients in variable frequencies ranging from 14–24% in different cohorts [5,6,9,32,53,54]. Concretely in MDS-5q, they are less abundant and most studies describe frequencies of around 6% [35,53–55]. While it is a common event in early disease, Fernandez-Mercado et al. reported higher frequencies of this mutation of up to 25% among advanced cases of the disease, suggesting a role in disease progression in MDS-5q [36]. Similarly to *DNMT3A* and *TET2*, *ASXL1* mutations were mostly studied among MDS patient cohorts, including all subtypes, finding an association with worse prognosis and a shorter OS, but no specific associations were mentioned between *ASXL1* mutations and outcomes in MDS-5q cases have been described.

4.3. TP53 Mutations

The tumor-suppressor p53 gene (*TP53*) is located in chromosome band 17p13 and is essential for genome integrity. *TP53* encodes for the p53 protein, which is a transcription factor involved in essential cell functions, such as DNA repair, cell cycle control, apoptosis, aging, and stemness [56,57].

TP53 gene mutations are detected in approximately 18% of MDS-5q [58,59]. It is the only mutation that was found to be significantly enriched in this MDS subtype compared with the other subtypes (18% vs. 6%) [35]. Data regarding the time of acquisition of this mutation are controversial. While it seems that there was a group of patients in which the mutation is already present in the early phases of the disease, there was another in which the *TP53* mutation arises during disease evolution, especially after treatment with lenalidomide [43,51,59].

Mutations in the *TP53* gene in MDS patients are associated with generally unfavorable outcomes, aggressive disease course, higher risk of transformation to AML, shorter overall survival (OS), and resistance to lenalidomide treatment [17,37,51,59].

Double or even triple hits in the *TP53* gene locus were already reported in 2013 by Kulasekararaj et al. [37]. A more recent study published by Bernard et al., provides new insights regarding the importance of the *TP53* allelic state (multi-hit). After studying 3324 patients, four main *TP53* mutational profiles were identified: (1) monoallelic mutations; (2) multiple mutations; (3) mutation and concomitant deletion affecting 17p; and (4) mutation and concomitant loss of heterozygosity of the 17p region. They found that two-thirds of patients with a *TP53* mutation present with multiple hits, while only one-third present with monoallelic mutations. Associations with high-risk presentation and poor outcomes were only specific to multi-hit patients, while surprisingly, monoallelic patients did not differ from *TP53* wild-type patients in outcome and response to therapy. The authors described that the *TP53* allelic state segregates patient outcomes across WHO subtypes, despite monoallelic *TP53* being enriched by MDS-5q. Moreover, they found that patients with monoallelic *TP53* mutations had longer survival compared with multi-hit patients [58].

In the 2017 edition, the WHO recommended assessing *TP53* mutational status in MDS-5q to identify high-risk cases [1]. However, the upcoming edition of the WHO classification takes into consideration new insights regarding the allelic state of this gene to redefine a specific subtype of MDS associated with the presence of multiple alterations affecting the *TP53* locus (Figure 2). This subtype is called MDS with biallelic *TP53* inactivation (MDS-bi*TP53*). However, the presence of a single *TP53* mutation (unless it is multi-hit) does not per se exclude the diagnosis of MDS-5q [2]. Similarly, the ICC proposal takes into account the *TP53* allelic state to define a new disease category called "myeloid neoplasms with mutated *TP53*". In the case of MDS-5q, only single-hit *TP53* mutations are admitted, otherwise, the diagnosis would change to the newly mentioned category [8].

4.4. CSNK1A1 Mutations

Located in the CDR 5q32, *CSNK1A1* encodes for casein kinase 1A1 (CK1 α), a serine/threonine kinase that participates in many cellular processes, including growth and proliferation via the β catenin and Wnt signaling pathway, apoptosis, and response to DNA damage [60–62]. In 2015, a study by Kronke et al., identified CK1α as a lenalidomide target in myeloid cells and found that heterozygous deletion of *CSNK1A1* in del(5q) MDS provides a therapeutic window for selective targeting of the malignant cells [63].

Missense mutations have been reported in exons 3 and 4 in 7–10% of MDS-5q patients [35,40,44,64,65]. Detected variant allele frequency values range from 3–78% and mimic a homozygous mutation status, which is consistent with the location of the *CSNK1A1* gene and the CDR [35,40].

CSNK1A1 mutations were found to be associated with older age and some reports show a trend towards decreased response to lenalidomide, but no independent prognostic impact on OS has been described to date [40,60]. In a study performed by Meggendorfer et al., *CSNK1A1* mutations were found to co-occur with *SF3B1* mutations in 42% of the cases [35].

4.5. JAK2 Mutations

Janus kinase 2 (*JAK2*) encodes a non-receptor tyrosine kinase that plays a central role in cytokine and growth factor signaling. Somatic mutations in *JAK2* constitute a major diagnostic criterion for myeloproliferative neoplasms (MPN) and are found in approximately 95% of polycythemia vera cases and 50% of essential thrombocythemia and primary myelofibrosis [2,9,66,67].

Mutations in this gene, specifically the V617F hotspot, were reported in approximately 6% of patients with MDS-5q and were found to correlate with higher platelet counts when compared with *JAK2* wild-type patients [35,55,68]. Sangiorgio et al., performed a detailed microscopic analysis of BM aspirates of MDS-5q cases with concomitant *JAK2* mutations and found greater reticulin fibrosis in mutated cases. Additionally, they found a combination of hypolobulated megakaryocytes (typically found in MDS-5q) and large forms with hyperlobulated nuclei, which are commonly seen in MPN [69].

Although the phenotypic characteristics have been described, no significant differences in OS or disease progression were found in such MDS-5q *JAK2* mutated cases when compared with *JAK2* wild-type cases [55,69].

5. Clonal Evolution

As mentioned previously, several authors have described the commonly mutated genes and concomitant copy number alterations in MDS-5q, but few studies have explored clonal evolution in this specific subtype of MDS.

The first systematic study providing molecular monitoring of long-term serial follow-up samples in a significant cohort of patients was by Mossner et al. [41]. As in most of the subsequent publications, such clonal evolution studies are based on bulk sequencing (exome or gene panel), in which clonal composition and evolutionary patterns are reconstructed based on variant allele frequency values of the detected mutations. The authors described that MDS "founder" lesions recurrently affected genes involved in the regulation of DNA methylation (e.g., *TET2*, *DNMT3A*), chromatin remodeling (e.g., *ASXL1*), or RNA splicing (e.g., *SF3B1*), and that del(5q) was acquired as a secondary lesion or constituted a minor independent clone in 62% of patients classified as MDS-5q. This is in contrast to previous studies proposing del(5q) as the initiating lesion in such patients [44]. In line with this, single-cell studies performed by our group demonstrated that in some MDS-5q cases, del(5q) can appear as the initiating lesion, while it can appear as a secondary hit in other cases [43].

As expected, the emergence and disappearance of specific clones in the BM are frequently correlated with changes in the clinical features in PB, such as hemoglobin and platelet levels. Moreover, it has been described that, in almost all cases, treatment with lenalidomide induced an effective reduction of cells carrying del(5q), however, it did not induce complete molecular remission of all clones carrying typical MDS mutations [41]. Furthermore, loss of response to lenalidomide is correlated with the gradual growth of a non-related clonal population already detectable at low levels before treatment or the expansion of a descendent from the original clone of the diagnosis [70].

In another longitudinal study, Scharenberg et al. described that 37% of their MDS-5q cohort progressed to either higher-risk MDS or transformed into AML in a median of 85 months after diagnosis. Interestingly, they found that all the cases harbored recurrent mutations in *TP53*, *TET2*, or *RUNX1* in addition to del(5q) [51]. Thus, several patients showed an increased allele burden and gains of new mutations during the course of the disease and treatment. Particularly, the acquisition of *TP53* mutations was relatively common in the progression of patients treated with lenalidomide, with some of them exhibiting more than one *TP53* mutation.

In general, all the above-mentioned studies agreed that both linear and branched evolutionary patterns occur with and without disease-modifying treatments, and subclones that acquire additional mutations associated with treatment resistance or disease progression can be detected months before clinical changes become apparent [41,43,51,70].

6. Conclusions

Based on our understanding of MDS-5q, together with the changes in the inclusion criteria, the evaluation of prognosis evaluation and the management of the disease are clearly in line with the progress of molecular genetics, which at the same time are linked to the advances in technology and scientific discoveries.

With the arrival of the IPSS-M and the newly proposed classifications for MDS, NGS techniques are mandatory for correct disease classification and assessment of prognosis. However, the approaches to financing health care are extremely diverse and are country-specific, and therefore, there may still be situations in which NGS remains restricted to potentially guiding therapeutic decisions, such as treatment intensity or hematopoietic stem cell transplantation.

Although many advances have been achieved, especially in the last decade, unanswered questions remain. Techniques such as OGM and new single-cell techniques together with new clinical trials are just some future steps to better understanding this disease and ultimately improving patient care.

Author Contributions: P.A., M.M. and F.S. wrote, reviewed, and edited the manuscript. All authors have read and agreed to the published version of the manuscript.

Funding: This research received no external funding.

Institutional Review Board Statement: Not applicable.

Informed Consent Statement: Not applicable.

Data Availability Statement: Not applicable.

Conflicts of Interest: The authors declare no conflict of interest.

References

1. Swerdlow, S.H.; Campo, E.; Harris, N.L.; Jaffe, E.S.; Pileri, S.A.; Stein, H.; Thiele, J. (Eds.) *WHO Classification of Tumours of Hematopoietic and Lymphoid Tissues*, 4th ed.; IARC: Lyon, France, 2017.
2. Khoury, J.D.; Solary, E.; Abla, O.; Akkari, Y.; Alaggio, R.; Apperley, J.F.; Bejar, R.; Berti, E.; Busque, L.; Chan, J.K.C.; et al. The 5th Edition of the World Health Organization Classification of Haematolymphoid Tumours: Myeloid and Histiocytic/Dendritic Neoplasms. *Leukemia* **2022**, *36*, 1703–1719. [CrossRef] [PubMed]
3. Haase, D. Cytogenetic Features in Myelodysplastic Syndromes. *Ann. Hematol.* **2008**, *87*, 515–526. [CrossRef] [PubMed]
4. Haase, D.; Germing, U.; Schanz, J.; Pfeilstocker, M.; Nosslinger, T.; Hildebrandt, B.; Kundgen, A.; Lubbert, M.; Kunzmann, R.; Giagounidis, A.A.N.; et al. New Insights into the Prognostic Impact of the Karyotype in MDS and Correlation with Subtypes: Evidence from a Core Dataset of 2124 Patients. *Blood* **2007**, *110*, 4385–4395. [CrossRef]
5. Papaemmanuil, E.; Gerstung, M.; Malcovati, L.; Tauro, S.; Gundem, G.; Van Loo, P.; Yoon, C.J.; Ellis, P.; Wedge, D.C.; Pellagatti, A.; et al. Clinical and Biological Implications of Driver Mutations in Myelodysplastic Syndromes. *Blood* **2013**, *122*, 3616–3627. [CrossRef] [PubMed]
6. Haferlach, T.; Nagata, Y.; Grossmann, V.; Okuno, Y.; Bacher, U.; Nagae, G.; Schnittger, S.; Sanada, M.; Kon, A.; Alpermann, T.; et al. Landscape of Genetic Lesions in 944 Patients with Myelodysplastic Syndromes. *Leukemia* **2014**, *28*, 241–247. [CrossRef] [PubMed]
7. Van Den Berghe, H.; Cassiman, J.-J.; David, G.; Fryns, J.-P.; Michaux, J.-L.; Sokal, G. Distinct Haematological Disorder with Deletion of Long Arm of No. 5 Chromosome. *Nature* **1974**, *251*, 437–438. [CrossRef] [PubMed]
8. Arber, D.A.; Orazi, A.; Hasserjian, R.P.; Borowitz, M.J.; Calvo, K.R.; Kvasnicka, H.-M.; Wang, S.A.; Bagg, A.; Barbui, T.; Branford, S.; et al. International Consensus Classification of Myeloid Neoplasms and Acute Leukemias: Integrating Morphologic, Clinical, and Genomic Data. *Blood* **2022**, *140*, 1200–1228. [CrossRef]
9. Bernard, E.; Tuechler, H.; Greenberg, P.L.; Hasserjian, R.P.; Arango Ossa, J.E.; Nannya, Y.; Devlin, S.M.; Creignou, M.; Pinel, P.; Monnier, L.; et al. Molecular International Prognostic Scoring System for Myelodysplastic Syndromes. *NEJM Evid.* **2022**, *1*. [CrossRef]
10. Bennett, J.M.; Catovsky, D.; Daniel, M.T.; Flandrin, G.; Galton, D.A.; Gralnick, H.R.; Sultan, C. Proposals for the Classification of the Acute Leukaemias. French-American-British (FAB) Co-Operative Group. *Br. J. Haematol.* **1976**, *33*, 451–458. [CrossRef]
11. Jaffe, E.S.; Harris, N.L.; Stein, H.; Vardiman, J.W. (Eds.) *World Health Organization Classification of Tumours, Pathology and Genetics of Tumours of Haematopoietic and Lymphoid Tissues*; IARC Press: Lyon, France, 2001.
12. Swerdlow, S.H.; Campo, E.; Harris, N.L.; Jaffe, E.S.; Pileri, S.A.; Stein, H.; Thiele, J. (Eds.) *WHO Classification of Tumours of Hematopoietic and Lymphoid Tissues*; IARC: Lyon, France, 2008.
13. Arber, D.A.; Orazi, A.; Hasserjian, R.; Thiele, J.; Borowitz, M.J.; Le Beau, M.M.; Bloomfield, C.D.; Cazzola, M.; Vardiman, J.W. The 2016 Revision to the World Health Organization Classification of Myeloid Neoplasms and Acute Leukemia. *Blood* **2016**, *127*, 2391–2405. [CrossRef]
14. Mallo, M.; Cervera, J.; Schanz, J.; Such, E.; García-Manero, G.; Luño, E.; Steidl, C.; Espinet, B.; Vallespí, T.; Germing, U.; et al. Impact of Adjunct Cytogenetic Abnormalities for Prognostic Stratification in Patients with Myelodysplastic Syndrome and Deletion 5q. *Leukemia* **2011**, *25*, 110–120. [CrossRef] [PubMed]

15. Schanz, J.; Tüchler, H.; Solé, F.; Mallo, M.; Luño, E.; Cervera, J.; Granada, I.; Hildebrandt, B.; Slovak, M.L.; Ohyashiki, K.; et al. New Comprehensive Cytogenetic Scoring System for Primary Myelodysplastic Syndromes (MDS) and Oligoblastic Acute Myeloid Leukemia After MDS Derived From an International Database Merge. *JCO* **2012**, *30*, 820–829. [CrossRef] [PubMed]
16. Mallo, M.; Arenillas, L.; Espinet, B.; Salido, M.; Hernandez, J.M.; Lumbreras, E.; del Rey, M.; Arranz, E.; Ramiro, S.; Font, P.; et al. Fluorescence in Situ Hybridization Improves the Detection of 5q31 Deletion in Myelodysplastic Syndromes without Cytogenetic Evidence of 5q-. *Haematologica* **2008**, *93*, 1001–1008. [CrossRef] [PubMed]
17. Mallo, M.; Del Rey, M.; Ibáñez, M.; Calasanz, M.J.; Arenillas, L.; Larráyoz, M.J.; Pedro, C.; Jerez, A.; Maciejewski, J.; Costa, D.; et al. Response to Lenalidomide in Myelodysplastic Syndromes with Del(5q): Influence of Cytogenetics and Mutations. *Br. J. Haematol.* **2013**, *162*, 74–86. [CrossRef] [PubMed]
18. Greenberg, P.; Cox, C.; LeBeau, M.M.; Fenaux, P.; Morel, P.; Sanz, G.; Sanz, M.; Vallespi, T.; Hamblin, T.; Oscier, D.; et al. International Scoring System for Evaluating Prognosis in Myelodysplastic Syndromes. *Blood* **1997**, *89*, 2079–2088. [CrossRef]
19. Greenberg, P.L.; Tuechler, H.; Schanz, J.; Sanz, G.; Garcia-Manero, G.; Sole, F.; Bennett, J.M.; Bowen, D.; Fenaux, P.; Dreyfus, F.; et al. Revised International Prognostic Scoring System for Myelodysplastic Syndromes. *Blood* **2012**, *120*, 2454–2465. [CrossRef]
20. Boultwood, J.; Fidler, C.; Lewis, S.; Kelly, S.; Sheridan, H.; Littlewood, T.; Buckle, V.; Wainscoat, J. Molecular Mapping of Uncharacteristically Small 5q Deletions in Two Patients with the 5q- Syndrome: Delineation of the Critical Region on 5q and Identification of a 5q- Breakpoint. *Genomics* **1994**, *19*, 425–432. [CrossRef]
21. Boultwood, J.; Fidler, C.; Strickson, A.J.; Watkins, F.; Gama, S.; Kearney, L.; Tosi, S.; Kasprzyk, A.; Cheng, J.-F.; Jaju, R.J.; et al. Narrowing and Genomic Annotation of the Commonly Deleted Region of the 5q- Syndrome. *Blood* **2002**, *99*, 4638–4641. [CrossRef]
22. Jaju, R.; Boultwood, J.; Oliver, F.; Kostrzewa, M.; Fidler, C.; Parker, N.; McPherson, J.; Morris, S.; Müller, U.; Wainscoat, J.; et al. Molecular Cytogenetic Delineation of the Critical Deleted Region in the 5q- Syndrome. *Genes Chromosom. Cancer* **1998**, *22*, 251–256. [CrossRef]
23. Nybakken, G.E.; Bagg, A. The Genetic Basis and Expanding Role of Molecular Analysis in the Diagnosis, Prognosis, and Therapeutic Design for Myelodysplastic Syndromes. *J. Mol. Diagn.* **2014**, *16*, 145–158. [CrossRef]
24. Jerez, A.; Gondek, L.P.; Jankowska, A.M.; Makishima, H.; Przychodzen, B.; Tiu, R.V.; O'Keefe, C.L.; Mohamedali, A.M.; Batista, D.; Sekeres, M.A.; et al. Topography, Clinical, and Genomic Correlates of 5q Myeloid Malignancies Revisited. *JCO* **2012**, *30*, 1343–1349. [CrossRef] [PubMed]
25. Arenillas, L.; Mallo, M.; Ramos, F.; Guinta, K.; Barragán, E.; Lumbreras, E.; Larráyoz, M.-J.; De Paz, R.; Tormo, M.; Abáigar, M.; et al. Single Nucleotide Polymorphism Array Karyotyping: A Diagnostic and Prognostic Tool in Myelodysplastic Syndromes with Unsuccessful Conventional Cytogenetic Testing: Snp Array In Myelodysplastic Syndromes. *Genes Chromosom. Cancer* **2013**, *52*, 1167–1177. [CrossRef] [PubMed]
26. Galván, A.B.; Mallo, M.; Arenillas, L.; Salido, M.; Espinet, B.; Pedro, C.; Florensa, L.; Serrano, S.; Solé, F. Does Monosomy 5 Really Exist in Myelodysplastic Syndromes and Acute Myeloid Leukemia? *Leuk. Res.* **2010**, *34*, 1242–1245. [CrossRef]
27. Ebert, B.L.; Galili, N.; Tamayo, P.; Bosco, J.; Mak, R.; Pretz, J.; Tanguturi, S.; Ladd-Acosta, C.; Stone, R.; Golub, T.R.; et al. An Erythroid Differentiation Signature Predicts Response to Lenalidomide in Myelodysplastic Syndrome. *PLoS Med.* **2008**, *5*, e35. [CrossRef]
28. Pellagatti, A.; Hellström-Lindberg, E.; Giagounidis, A.; Perry, J.; Malcovati, L.; Della Porta, M.G.; Jädersten, M.; Killick, S.; Fidler, C.; Cazzola, M.; et al. Haploinsufficiency of RPS14 in 5q- Syndrome Is Associated with Deregulation of Ribosomal- and Translation-Related Genes. *Br. J. Haematol.* **2008**, *142*, 57–64. [CrossRef] [PubMed]
29. Joslin, J.M.; Fernald, A.A.; Tennant, T.R.; Davis, E.M.; Kogan, S.C.; Anastasi, J.; Crispino, J.D.; Le Beau, M.M. Haploinsufficiency of EGR1, a Candidate Gene in the Del(5q), Leads to the Development of Myeloid Disorders. *Blood* **2007**, *110*, 719–726. [CrossRef]
30. Kumar, M.S.; Narla, A.; Nonami, A.; Mullally, A.; Dimitrova, N.; Ball, B.; McAuley, J.R.; Poveromo, L.; Kutok, J.L.; Galili, N.; et al. Coordinate Loss of a MicroRNA and Protein-Coding Gene Cooperate in the Pathogenesis of 5q- Syndrome. *Blood* **2011**, *118*, 8. [CrossRef]
31. Starczynowski, D.T.; Kuchenbauer, F.; Argiropoulos, B.; Sung, S.; Morin, R.; Muranyi, A.; Hirst, M.; Hogge, D.; Marra, M.; Wells, R.A.; et al. Identification of MiR-145 and MiR-146a as Mediators of the 5q– Syndrome Phenotype. *Nat. Med.* **2010**, *16*, 49–58. [CrossRef]
32. Bejar, R.; Stevenson, K.; Abdel-Wahab, O.; Galili, N.; Nilsson, B.; Garcia-Manero, G.; Kantarjian, H.; Raza, A.; Levine, R.L.; Neuberg, D.; et al. Clinical Effect of Point Mutations in Myelodysplastic Syndromes. *N. Engl. J. Med.* **2011**, *364*, 2496–2506. [CrossRef]
33. Smith, A.C.; Neveling, K.; Kanagal-Shamanna, R. Optical Genome Mapping for Structural Variation Analysis in Hematologic Malignancies. *Am. J. Hematol.* **2022**, *97*, 975–982. [CrossRef]
34. Yang, H.; Garcia-Manero, G.; Sasaki, K.; Montalban-Bravo, G.; Tang, Z.; Wei, Y.; Kadia, T.; Chien, K.; Rush, D.; Nguyen, H.; et al. High-Resolution Structural Variant Profiling of Myelodysplastic Syndromes by Optical Genome Mapping Uncovers Cryptic Aberrations of Prognostic and Therapeutic Significance. *Leukemia* **2022**, *36*, 2306–2316. [CrossRef] [PubMed]
35. Meggendorfer, M.; Haferlach, C.; Kern, W.; Haferlach, T. Molecular Analysis of Myelodysplastic Syndrome with Isolated Deletion of the Long Arm of Chromosome 5 Reveals a Specific Spectrum of Molecular Mutations with Prognostic Impact: A Study on 123 Patients and 27 Genes. *Haematologica* **2017**, *102*, 1502–1510. [CrossRef] [PubMed]

36. Fernandez-Mercado, M.; Burns, A.; Pellagatti, A.; Giagounidis, A.; Germing, U.; Agirre, X.; Prosper, F.; Aul, C.; Killick, S.; Wainscoat, J.S.; et al. Targeted Re-Sequencing Analysis of 25 Genes Commonly Mutated in Myeloid Disorders in Del(5q) Myelodysplastic Syndromes. *Haematologica* **2013**, *98*, 1856–1864. [CrossRef] [PubMed]
37. Kulasekararaj, A.G.; Smith, A.E.; Mian, S.A.; Mohamedali, A.M.; Krishnamurthy, P.; Lea, N.C.; Gäken, J.; Pennaneach, C.; Ireland, R.; Czepulkowski, B.; et al. TP53 Mutations in Myelodysplastic Syndrome Are Strongly Correlated with Aberrations of Chromosome 5, and Correlate with Adverse Prognosis. *Br. J. Haematol.* **2013**, *160*, 660–672. [CrossRef]
38. Hosono, N.; Makishima, H.; Mahfouz, R.; Przychodzen, B.; Yoshida, K.; Jerez, A.; LaFramboise, T.; Polprasert, C.; Clemente, M.J.; Shiraishi, Y.; et al. Recurrent Genetic Defects on Chromosome 5q in Myeloid Neoplasms. *Oncotarget* **2017**, *8*, 6483–6495. [CrossRef]
39. Malcovati, L.; Stevenson, K.; Papaemmanuil, E.; Neuberg, D.; Bejar, R.; Boultwood, J.; Bowen, D.T.; Campbell, P.J.; Ebert, B.L.; Fenaux, P.; et al. SF3B1-Mutant Myelodysplastic Syndrome as a Distinct Disease Subtype—A Proposal of the International Working Group for the Prognosis of Myelodysplastic Syndromes (IWG-PM). *Blood* **2020**, *136*, 157–170. [CrossRef]
40. Heuser, M.; Meggendorfer, M.; Cruz, M.M.A.; Fabisch, J.; Klesse, S.; Köhler, L.; Göhring, G.; Ganster, C.; Shirneshan, K.; Gutermuth, A.; et al. Frequency and Prognostic Impact of Casein Kinase 1A1 Mutations in MDS Patients with Deletion of Chromosome 5q. *Leukemia* **2015**, *29*, 1942–1945. [CrossRef]
41. Mossner, M.; Jann, J.-C.; Wittig, J.; Nolte, F.; Fey, S.; Nowak, V.; Obländer, J.; Pressler, J.; Palme, I.; Xanthopoulos, C.; et al. Mutational Hierarchies in Myelodysplastic Syndromes Dynamically Adapt and Evolve upon Therapy Response and Failure. *Blood* **2016**, *128*, 1246–1259. [CrossRef]
42. Malcovati, L.; Karimi, M.; Papaemmanuil, E.; Ambaglio, I.; Jädersten, M.; Jansson, M.; Elena, C.; Gallì, A.; Walldin, G.; Della Porta, M.G.; et al. SF3B1 Mutation Identifies a Distinct Subset of Myelodysplastic Syndrome with Ring Sideroblasts. *Blood* **2015**, *126*, 233–241. [CrossRef]
43. Acha, P.; Palomo, L.; Fuster-Tormo, F.; Xicoy, B.; Mallo, M.; Manzanares, A.; Grau, J.; Marcé, S.; Granada, I.; Rodríguez-Luaces, M.; et al. Analysis of Intratumoral Heterogeneity in Myelodysplastic Syndromes with Isolated Del(5q) Using a Single Cell Approach. *Cancers* **2021**, *13*, 841. [CrossRef]
44. Woll, P.S.; Kjällquist, U.; Chowdhury, O.; Doolittle, H.; Wedge, D.C.; Thongjuea, S.; Erlandsson, R.; Ngara, M.; Anderson, K.; Deng, Q.; et al. Myelodysplastic Syndromes Are Propagated by Rare and Distinct Human Cancer Stem Cells In Vivo. *Cancer Cell* **2014**, *25*, 794–808. [CrossRef] [PubMed]
45. Mian, S.A.; Rouault-Pierre, K.; Smith, A.E.; Seidl, T.; Pizzitola, I.; Kizilors, A.; Kulasekararaj, A.G.; Bonnet, D.; Mufti, G.J. SF3B1 Mutant MDS-Initiating Cells May Arise from the Haematopoietic Stem Cell Compartment. *Nat. Commun.* **2015**, *6*, 10004. [CrossRef] [PubMed]
46. Steensma, D.P.; Bejar, R.; Jaiswal, S.; Lindsley, R.C.; Sekeres, M.A.; Hasserjian, R.P.; Ebert, B.L. Clonal Hematopoiesis of Indeterminate Potential and Its Distinction from Myelodysplastic Syndromes. *Blood* **2015**, *126*, 9–16. [CrossRef]
47. Jaiswal, S.; Fontanillas, P.; Flannick, J.; Manning, A.; Grauman, P.V.; Mar, B.G.; Lindsley, R.C.; Mermel, C.H.; Burtt, N.; Chavez, A.; et al. Age-Related Clonal Hematopoiesis Associated with Adverse Outcomes. *N. Engl. J. Med.* **2014**, *371*, 2488–2498. [CrossRef] [PubMed]
48. Chen, T.; Ueda, Y.; Xie, S.; Li, E. A Novel Dnmt3a Isoform Produced from an Alternative Promoter Localizes to Euchromatin and Its Expression Correlates with Activede Novo Methylation. *J. Biol. Chem.* **2002**, *277*, 38746–38754. [CrossRef] [PubMed]
49. Lin, M.-E.; Hou, H.-A.; Tsai, C.-H.; Wu, S.-J.; Kuo, Y.-Y.; Tseng, M.-H.; Liu, M.-C.; Liu, C.-W.; Chou, W.-C.; Chen, C.-Y.; et al. Dynamics of DNMT3A Mutation and Prognostic Relevance in Patients with Primary Myelodysplastic Syndrome. *Clin. Epigenet.* **2018**, *10*, 42. [CrossRef] [PubMed]
50. Thol, F.; Winschel, C.; Ludeking, A.; Yun, H.; Friesen, I.; Damm, F.; Wagner, K.; Krauter, J.; Heuser, M.; Ganser, A. Rare Occurrence of DNMT3A Mutations in Myelodysplastic Syndromes. *Haematologica* **2011**, *96*, 1870–1873. [CrossRef]
51. Scharenberg, C.; Giai, V.; Pellagatti, A.; Saft, L.; Dimitriou, M.; Jansson, M.; Jädersten, M.; Grandien, A.; Douagi, I.; Neuberg, D.S.; et al. Progression in Patients with Low- and Intermediate-1-Risk Del(5q) Myelodysplastic Syndromes Is Predicted by a Limited Subset of Mutations. *Haematologica* **2017**, *102*, 498–508. [CrossRef]
52. Itzykson, R.; Kosmider, O.; Cluzeau, T.; Mansat-De Mas, V.; Dreyfus, F.; Beyne-Rauzy, O.; Quesnel, B.; Vey, N.; Gelsi-Boyer, V.; Raynaud, S.; et al. Impact of TET2 Mutations on Response Rate to Azacitidine in Myelodysplastic Syndromes and Low Blast Count Acute Myeloid Leukemias. *Leukemia* **2011**, *25*, 1147–1152. [CrossRef]
53. Bejar, R.; Stevenson, K.E.; Caughey, B.; Lindsley, R.C.; Mar, B.G.; Stojanov, P.; Getz, G.; Steensma, D.P.; Ritz, J.; Soiffer, R.; et al. Somatic Mutations Predict Poor Outcome in Patients with Myelodysplastic Syndrome After Hematopoietic Stem-Cell Transplantation. *JCO* **2014**, *32*, 2691–2698. [CrossRef]
54. Thol, F.; Friesen, I.; Damm, F.; Yun, H.; Weissinger, E.M.; Krauter, J.; Wagner, K.; Chaturvedi, A.; Sharma, A.; Wichmann, M.; et al. Prognostic Significance of *ASXL1* Mutations in Patients With Myelodysplastic Syndromes. *JCO* **2011**, *29*, 2499–2506. [CrossRef] [PubMed]
55. Patnaik, M.M.; Lasho, T.L.; Finke, C.M.; Gangat, N.; Caramazza, D.; Holtan, S.G.; Pardanani, A.; Knudson, R.A.; Ketterling, R.P.; Chen, D.; et al. WHO-Defined 'Myelodysplastic Syndrome with Isolated Del(5q)' in 88 Consecutive Patients: Survival Data, Leukemic Transformation Rates and Prevalence of JAK2, MPL and IDH Mutations. *Leukemia* **2010**, *24*, 1283–1289. [CrossRef] [PubMed]

56. Lu, W.-J.; Amatruda, J.F.; Abrams, J.M. P53 Ancestry: Gazing through an Evolutionary Lens. *Nat. Rev. Cancer* **2009**, *9*, 758–762. [CrossRef] [PubMed]
57. Junttila, M.R.; Evan, G.I. P53—A Jack of All Trades but Master of None. *Nat. Rev. Cancer* **2009**, *9*, 821–829. [CrossRef]
58. Bernard, E.; Nannya, Y.; Hasserjian, R.P.; Devlin, S.M.; Tuechler, H.; Medina-Martinez, J.S.; Yoshizato, T.; Shiozawa, Y.; Saiki, R.; Malcovati, L.; et al. Implications of TP53 Allelic State for Genome Stability, Clinical Presentation and Outcomes in Myelodysplastic Syndromes. *Nat. Med.* **2020**, *26*, 1549–1556. [CrossRef]
59. Jädersten, M.; Saft, L.; Smith, A.; Kulasekararaj, A.; Pomplun, S.; Göhring, G.; Hedlund, A.; Hast, R.; Schlegelberger, B.; Porwit, A.; et al. TP53 Mutations in Low-Risk Myelodysplastic Syndromes with Del(5q) Predict Disease Progression. *J. Clin. Oncol.* **2011**, *29*, 1971–1979. [CrossRef]
60. Smith, A.; Jiang, J.; Kulasekararaj, A.G.; Mian, S.; Mohamedali, A.; Gaken, J.; Ireland, R.; Czepulkowski, B.; Best, S.; Mufti, G.J. CSNK1A1 Mutations and Isolated Del(5q) Abnormality in Myelodysplastic Syndrome: A Retrospective Mutational Analysis. *Lancet Haematol.* **2015**, *2*, e212–e221. [CrossRef]
61. Knippschild, U.; Gocht, A.; Wolff, S.; Huber, N.; Löhler, J.; Stöter, M. The Casein Kinase 1 Family: Participation in Multiple Cellular Processes in Eukaryotes. *Cell Signal.* **2005**, *17*, 675–689. [CrossRef]
62. Schittek, B.; Sinnberg, T. Biological Functions of Casein Kinase 1 Isoforms and Putative Roles in Tumorigenesis. *Mol. Cancer* **2014**, *13*, 231. [CrossRef]
63. Krönke, J.; Fink, E.C.; Hollenbach, P.W.; MacBeth, K.J.; Hurst, S.N.; Udeshi, N.D.; Chamberlain, P.P.; Mani, D.R.; Man, H.W.; Gandhi, A.K.; et al. Lenalidomide Induces Ubiquitination and Degradation of CK1α in Del(5q) MDS. *Nature* **2015**, *523*, 183–188. [CrossRef]
64. Schneider, R.K.; Ademà, V.; Heckl, D.; Järås, M.; Mallo, M.; Lord, A.M.; Chu, L.P.; McConkey, M.E.; Kramann, R.; Mullally, A.; et al. Role of Casein Kinase 1A1 in the Biology and Targeted Therapy of Del(5q) MDS. *Cancer Cell* **2014**, *26*, 509–520. [CrossRef] [PubMed]
65. Bello, E.; Pellagatti, A.; Shaw, J.; Mecucci, C.; Kušec, R.; Killick, S.; Giagounidis, A.; Raynaud, S.; Calasanz, M.J.; Fenaux, P.; et al. *CSNK1A1* Mutations and Gene Expression Analysis in Myelodysplastic Syndromes with Del(5q). *Br. J. Haematol.* **2015**, *171*, 210–214. [CrossRef] [PubMed]
66. Greenfield, G.; McMullin, M.F.; Mills, K. Molecular Pathogenesis of the Myeloproliferative Neoplasms. *J. Hematol. Oncol.* **2021**, *14*, 103. [CrossRef] [PubMed]
67. Nangalia, J.; Green, A.R. Myeloproliferative Neoplasms: From Origins to Outcomes. *Blood* **2017**, *130*, 2475–2483. [CrossRef]
68. Ingram, W.; Lea, N.C.; Cervera, J.; Germing, U.; Fenaux, P.; Cassinat, B.; Kiladjian, J.J.; Varkonyi, J.; Antunovic, P.; Westwood, N.B.; et al. The JAK2 V617F Mutation Identifies a Subgroup of MDS Patients with Isolated Deletion 5q and a Proliferative Bone Marrow. *Leukemia* **2006**, *20*, 1319–1321. [CrossRef]
69. Sangiorgio, V.F.I.; Geyer, J.T.; Margolskee, E.; Al-Kawaaz, M.; Mathew, S.; Tam, W.; Orazi, A. Myeloid Neoplasms with Isolated Del(5q) and *JAK2* V617F Mutation: A "Grey Zone" Combination of Myelodysplastic and Myeloproliferative Features? *Haematologica* **2020**, *105*, e276–e279. [CrossRef]
70. da Silva-Coelho, P.; Kroeze, L.I.; Yoshida, K.; Koorenhof-Scheele, T.N.; Knops, R.; van de Locht, L.T.; de Graaf, A.O.; Massop, M.; Sandmann, S.; Dugas, M.; et al. Clonal Evolution in Myelodysplastic Syndromes. *Nat. Commun.* **2017**, *8*, 15099. [CrossRef]

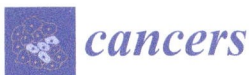

Review

Rosai–Dorfman Disease between Proliferation and Neoplasia

Ismail Elbaz Younes [1], Lubomir Sokol [2] and Ling Zhang [3,*]

[1] Department of Pathology, Cleveland Clinic, Cleveland, OH 44195, USA
[2] Department of Hematology and Oncology, Moffitt Cancer Center, Tampa, FL 33612, USA
[3] Department of Pathology, Moffitt Cancer Center, Tampa, FL 33612, USA
* Correspondence: ling.zhang@moffitt.org

Simple Summary: Rosai–Dorfman disease (RDD) was a benign histiocytic proliferative disorder rather than a neoplastic process. Emergent molecular studies have shown recurrent somatic gain-of-function mutations in genes of the MAPK pathway (e.g., *NRAS*, *KRAS*, *MAP2K1*, and *ARAF*) in a subset of RDD, suggesting a clonal histiocytic proliferative process. This review encompasses clinical characteristics, updated subclassification, diagnostic approaches, and treatment strategies, with an emphasis on the molecular profiles of RDD. This study includes the latest international consensus on diagnosing and managing this disease. This review will provide novel insights on the latest discoveries in RDD.

Abstract: Rosai–Dorfman disease (RDD) is a rare myeloproliferative disorder of histiocytes with a broad spectrum of clinical manifestations and peculiar morphologic features (accumulation of histiocytes with emperipolesis). Typically, the patient with RDD shows bilateral painless, massive cervical lymphadenopathy associated with B symptoms. Approximately 43% of patients presented with extranodal involvement. According to the 2016 revised histiocytosis classification, RDD belongs to the R group, including familial and sporadic form (classical nodal, extranodal, unclassified, or RDD associated with neoplasia or immune disease). Sporadic RDD is often self-limited. Most RDD needs only local therapies. Nevertheless, a small subpopulation of patients may be refractory to conventional therapy and die of the disease. Recent studies consider RDD a clonal neoplastic process, as approximately 1/3 of these patients harbor gene mutations involving the MAPK/ERK pathway, e.g., *NRAS*, *KRAS*, *MAP2K1*, and, rarely, the *BRAF* mutation. In addition to typical histiocytic markers (S100/fascin/CD68/CD163, etc.), recent studies show that the histiocytes in RDD also express BCL-1 and OCT2, which might be important in pathogenesis. Additionally, the heterozygous germline mutation involving the FAS gene *TNFRSF6* is identified in some RDD patients with an autoimmune lymphoproliferative syndrome type Ia. *SLC29A3* germline mutation is associated with familial or Faisalabad histiocytosis and H syndrome.

Keywords: Rosai–Dorfman disease; sinus histiocytosis; MAPK pathway; gene mutation; histiocytic disorder

1. Introduction

Rosai–Dorfman disease (RDD) was initially described by Pierre-Paul Destombes, who reported four cases in 1965 [1]; afterward, Reed and Azoury outlined and reported a classic case of RDD [2]. Later, Rosai and Dorfman described 34 cases and coined the name sinus histiocytosis with massive lymphadenopathy, which was later changed to RDD [3–5]. The largest cohort collected 423 cases from an international registry in 1990 where both nodal and extranodal RDD were documented [5].

RDD predominantly occurs in young black children and clinically manifests with massive bilateral cervical lymphadenopathy. Extranodal and cutaneous forms are present. Clinical course is variable, ranging from self-limited process to disseminated refractory disease with increased associated mortality. Given the disease heterogeneity, treatment options are different for RDD, including local or systemic approaches. Histologically, a biopsy of the lesion reveals characteristic features of abnormal S100$^+$, CD68$^+$, and CD1a$^-$ histiocytes with infrequent to overt emperipolesis. RDD can be an isolated or combined disorder. Increased polyclonal plasma cells and fibrosis in the background are often associated with IgG4 lymphoproliferative disorder. It is also not uncommon for RDD to be associated with autoimmune diseases, malignant tumors, and rare hereditary disorders [6].

The etiology of RDD is unclear. It has been postulated that an infectious agent is the etiologic cause of RDD; nonetheless, no microorganism has been detected. Epstein–Barr virus (EBV) was thought to play a role in RDD because many patients with RDD were positive for EBV; however, in situ hybridizations for EBV were negative [7]. Other virus candidates (e.g., HHV-6, HIV, and cytomegalovirus) were also proposed but never approved.

Recent studies showed that approximately 1/3 of RDD these patients harbor gene mutations involving the MAPK/ERK pathway, e.g., *NRAS*, *KRAS*, *MAP2K1*, and, rarely, *BRAF*, indicating a neoplastic process rather than a reactive disorder.

Genetic predisposition or hereditary forms of RDD has been hypothesized, as cases have been described in twins or family members, which supports this hypothesis [8]. Germline mutations in *SLC29A3* (at 10q23), which is associated with H syndrome (histiocytosis-lymphadenopathy plus syndrome), Faisalabad histiocytosis, and pigmented hypertrichotic dermatosis with insulin-dependent diabetes, have been found in cases of familial RDD. Another germline mutation (*TNFRSF*) that is found in autoimmune lymphoproliferative syndrome (ALPS) type I is also found in RDD.

This review outlines clinicopathologic features; updates the subclassification and treatment of RDD; emphasizes the novel molecular findings behind this entity; and aims to guide clinicians and pathologists on how to appropriately reach the diagnosis and proceed with targeted therapy.

2. Discussion

RDD is an abnormal proliferation of histiocytes with varieties of clinical pictures, either isolated or with other diseases, which requires an integrated clinical, radiological, pathological, and molecular diagnostic approach. According to the Society of Histiocytes expert consensus in 2016, histiocytosis and neoplasms of the macrophage-dendritic cell lineage are reclassified into five groups: (1) Langerhans-related (L group); (2) cutaneous and mucocutaneous (C group); (3) malignant histiocytosis (M group); (4) RDD (R group); and (5) hemophagocytic lymphohistiocytosis and macrophage-activation syndrome (H group) [9]. Despite RDD being considered an independent entity distinguished from other histiocytoses, the nature of RDD still needs further exploration, in particular, following the laboratory implications of the novel next generation sequencing (NGS) technique. The emergence of novel molecular data indicates that RDD is a neoplastic process. RDD was recently listed in the 5th Edition of the World Health Organization (WHO) Classification of Myeloid and Histiocytic/Dendritic Neoplasms [10].

3. Epidemiology

RDD is a relatively rare entity, with an incidence of 1:200,000, with around 100 new cases diagnosed annually in the United States [6]. RDD usually affects African American children and young adults, with a slight male predominance. The mean age at diagnosis of RDD is approximately 20.6 years with a male-to-female ratio of 3:2 [5]. In contrast to classic or nodal RDD, cutaneous RDD on the other hand is a different entity, with a mean age of 45 years and more common incidence in Caucasians and Asians [11].

4. Subclassification

Under the R group of non-Langerhans cell histiocytosis (LCH), RDD can be further classified into five subgroups: classical (nodal), familial, extranodal, neoplasia associated, and immune disease-associated RDD [9].

The classical RDD subgroup includes IgG4 lymphoproliferative disorder or those without IgG4 syndrome. Upon involved sites, extranodal RDD is further subgrouped into bone RDD, central nervous system (CNS) RDD (with or without IgG4 syndrome), single-organ, or disseminated RDD. The single-organ RDD does not include lymph nodes or CNS RDD and is further divided into two subtypes: with or without IgG4 syndrome. Of note, cutaneous RDD has been reclassified to be included in the C group under the nonxanthogranuloma family [9].

Certain hereditary conditions predispose to RDD. Familial RDD is unique, which can be linked with H syndrome or ALPS [9], and is considered in a separate category that will be discussed under the session of molecular mechanisms.

RDD has been associated with variable kinds of neoplasia or immune diseases. Approximately 10% of RDD coexists with immunologic diseases: Systemic lupus erythematosus (SLE) has been reported with RDD in many case reports. They are different from the pathogenesis perspective; however, some emerging case reports show that some mutations may lead to a newly discovered disease entity called RAS-associated autoimmune leukoproliferative disease, which is caused by gain-of-function mutations in the RAS-family (*NRAS* and *KRAS*). A case report shows the p.G13C mutation in the *KRAS* gene in a patient presenting with SLE and RDD, rendering the diagnosis of RAS-associated autoimmune leukoproliferative disease [12]. Idiopathic juvenile arthritis and autoimmune hemolytic anemia have been reported in association with RDD [13].

RDD can occur in patients with a history of lymphomas. However, composite lymphomas and RDD rarely occur. Many types of lymphomas can co-occur with RDD, including classic Hodgkin lymphoma and non-Hodgkin lymphoma. The two most common types of lymphomas associated with RDD are follicular lymphoma and nodular lymphocyte-predominant Hodgkin lymphoma. The latter was changed to nodular lymphocyte-predominant B-cell lymphoma, according to the most recent International Consensus Classification of Mature Lymphoid Neoplasms [14]. Additionally, RDD can co-occur with other lymphomas (marginal-zone lymphoma, peripheral T-cell lymphoma), cutaneous clear-cell sarcoma, myelodysplastic syndromes (MDS), allogeneic stem transplant for precursor B-cell acute lymphoblastic leukemia, and concurrent with or following L-group histiocytosis, e.g., LCH, Erdheim Chester disease (ECD), or malignant histiocytosis [6,15,16].

5. Clinical Presentation

RDD usually presents with bilateral cervical lymphadenopathy. Mediastinal, groin, and, rarely, or retroperitoneal cavity can be involved. Patients with RDD are often accompanied with B symptoms (fever, night sweat, and weight loss). Around 43% of patients develop extranodal disease [13], most commonly involving skin, nasal cavity, and orbit. Salivary, spleen, and testes can be involved [8]. Bone RDD manifested with solitary or multifocal lytic lesions, involving in long bones, vertebrae, and sacrum. [16,17]. The organ specific clinical presentation and imaging findings are summarized in Table 1.

Table 1. Clinical Symptoms and Signs of Nodal and Extranodal RDD—Organ and Tissue Specified [6,15,16,18–22].

Site	Incidence	Symptoms/Signs	Radiologic Findings
Nodal			
Lymph node	57% of cases	Bilateral cervical lymphadenopathy or other LN sites, manifested with palpable masses	Enlarged LNs
Extranodal			
Skin	10% of cases	Painless, macular, slow-growing papules, subcutaneous nodules. Any skin site can be affected.	Nodule(s) or mass(es)

Table 1. Cont.

Site	Incidence	Symptoms/Signs	Radiologic Findings
CNS	<5% of cases (75% intracranial and 25% spinal lesions), more than 300 cases have been reported. Cervical and thoracic regions are the most common areas affected in spinal-dural or epidural lesion	Headaches, seizures, gait difficulty. In familial cases, there is an association with damage to the auditory nerve pathway and deafness.	Dural lesion, extra-axial, homogeneously enhancing, mimicking nodular meningioma; or parenchymal (infratentorial) involvement
Orbit	11% of cases	Presents as a mass in different part of the orbit, e.g., conjunctiva, lacrimal glands, and cornea. It can also present as uveitis.	Orbital mass
Head and neck	11% of cases involving nasal cavity, more common among Asians	Nasal obstruction, epistaxis, and nasal dorsum deformity	Nodules, swelling, mass(es)
Intrathoracic	2% of patients, with pulmonary disease concurrent lymphadenopathy or systemic disease. Cardiac involvement is extremely rare ~0.1–0.2% of cases.	Chronic dry cough, progressive dyspnea, or acute respiratory failure. RDD affecting lower respiratory tract have a high mortality rate, reaching 45%.	Pulmonary nodular consolidation in all lobes of the lungs; pleural effusion with fibrosis or nodules
Retroperitoneal /genitourinary tract	Kidneys are affected in approximately 4% of cases.	Abdominal or flank pain, fullness, hematuria, renal failure, hypercalcemia, and/or nephrotic syndrome	Mass(es), hydronephrosis, urethral obstruction
Gastrointestinal tract	<1% of cases, commonly in middle-aged women with concurrent nodal or extranodal affection	Abdominal pain, constipation, hematochezia, and intestinal obstruction	Mass(es)
Bone	5% to 10% of cases, usually with concurrent nodal affection	Bone pain and, rarely, pathologic fractures	Cortex-based osteolytic lesion, commonly long bones, vertebrae, and sacrum

Abbreviations: CNS, central nervous system; RDD, Rosai–Dorfman disease. LN: lymph node

Laboratory evaluation of RDD patients shows approximately 2/3 of patients present with normochromic normocytic anemia, leukocytosis (neutrophilia most commonly). Polyclonal hypergammaglobulinemia was reported in approximately 90% of patients; increased erythrocyte sedimentation rate in approximately 90%; and hypoalbuminemia in approximately 60%. The CD4:CD8 ratio was found to be decreased. Other laboratory findings are present, such as elevated ferritin level and autoimmune hemolytic anemia.

According to the international expert consensus at the 32nd Histiocyte Society Meeting in 2018 and National Comprehensive Cancer Network (NCCN) Guidelines for Histiocytic Neoplasms (2020), comprehensive systemic physical examination should be conducted, including head and neck, intrathoracic/pulmonary/cardiovascular, gastrointestinal (GI), renal, genitourinary (GU) system, neuroendocrine, CNS, and cutaneous symptoms. The following recommendations are used for baseline evaluation of new/suspected cases of RDD [6,23].

1. Medical history
    a. Constitutional symptoms;
    b. Organ affection (head, eyes, ears, nose, and throat; cardiovascular; pulmonary; GI; GU; skin; CNS; and endocrine);
    c. History of autoimmune disease, LCH, or other histiocytic lesions, as well as hematologic malignancies;
    d. Family history for children.
2. Physical examination

a. Lymphadenopathy;
b. Organomegaly;
c. Cutaneous and extranodal lesions;
d. Neurologic changes.
3. Radiological evaluation
    a. All patients should have whole-body positron emission tomography (PET)/computed tomography (CT);
    b. Selected patients should have CT sinuses with contrast, high-resolution CT chest, magnetic resonance imaging of orbit/brain with contrast and magnetic resonance imaging of spine with contrast;
    c. Selected patients for organ-specific ultrasound.
4. Laboratory evaluation
    a. Complete blood cell count, complete metabolic panel, erythrocyte sedimentation rate;
    b. Serum immunoglobulins;
    c. Coagulation studies, C-reactive protein, uric acid, and lactate dehydrogenase (LDH);
    d. Hemolysis panel (Coombs, haptoglobin, reticulocytes, and blood smear);
    e. Panel for autoimmune diseases (ALPS panel, antinuclear antibody, rheumatoid factor, HLA B27);
    f. NGS targeted gene mutations in RAF-RAS-MEK-ERK pathway;
    g. If familial form is suspected, then NGS test for *SLC29A3* (germline mutations);
    h. Bone-marrow biopsy (if cytopenia or abnormal peripheral blood smear are present);
    i. Lumbar puncture for CNS involvement.
5. Subspecialty consultation as needed
    a. Dermatology and ophthalmology evaluation before initiating MEK-inhibitor therapy.

6. RDD with Concurrent Disorders

Besides aforementioned lymphomas, MDS or rare solid tumors, it is not uncommon to accompany RDD with other histiocytic neoplasms and benign lymphoproliferative disorders. Herein, we only focus on the LCH, ECD, and IgG4 disorders that we will discuss here.

Diagnosis of IgG4 disease is based on recent consensus scoring made by the American College of Rheumatology and the European League Against Rheumatism [24]. Histologically IgG-4 related disease shows increased IgG4 plasma cells with a ratio of at least 0.4 IgG4: IgG plasma cells or more than 100 positive IgG4 plasma cells in a high-power field. There are five different morphologic variants (Multicentric Castleman disease–like, follicular hyperplasia, interfollicular expansion, progressive transformation of germinal centers, and inflammatory pseudotumor–like). A sixth variant has been suggested by Chen et al., yet it might be considered as an advanced case of interfollicular expansion type. Many studies have shown an increased number of IgG4 plasma cells and associated fibrosis in RDD; however, according to the criteria of the American College of Rheumatology and the European League Against Rheumatism, only from 10% to 30% of RDD concurrent IgG4-related disease [25–28]. Of note, nodal RDD tends to be slightly more affected than extranodal RDD by IgG4-related disease.

RDD can occasionally occur in patients with LCH [29,30]. There are mostly in case reports, with no case series being reported to the best of our knowledge. Immunohistochemical stains would be helpful to identify the two entities. Molecularly, LCH would often have *BRAF* V600E mutations, while RDD rarely has this kind of mutation. *MAP2K1* mutation is present in 1/3 of cases of RDD but uncommonly seen with LCH. *MAP2K1* and *BRAF* mutations in LCH are mutually exclusive.

ECD has been reported to be often associated with LCH with coincidence rate of 15% [31] and also occur with RDD, though less frequently. A multicenter study from Pitié-Salpêtrière Hospital, Memorial Sloan Kettering Cancer Center, and the Mayo Clinic referral centers showed that 11/353 (3.1%) had overlapping RDD with ECD, which is slightly more common than other histiocytic neoplasms overlapping with RDD. None of those cases had *BRAF V600E*; however, mutations were found in *MAP2K1* [32].

7. Histopathology and Immunochemistry

Histologic examination shows enlarged, matted, grossly involved lymph nodes and capsular fibrosis. In lymph nodes with subtotal involvement, dilation of sinuses causes severe architectural alterations. Sinuses are obstructed by a mixed population of cells, including histiocytes, lymphocytes, plasma cells, and histiocytes. The most distinctive cells are the histiocytes; hence, the name RDD histiocytes was coined. RDD histiocytes are usually large with round-to-oval nuclei, dispersed chromatin, prominent nucleoli, and abundant clear-to-foamy or vacuolated cytoplasm. The most unique feature of these histiocytes is emperipolesis (a Greek word meaning wandering in and around). During the process of emperipolesis, the histiocytes engulf intact cells and sometimes nuclear debris and lipids. The engulfed cells remain viable and can exit histiocytes in contrast to the process of phagocytosis (Figure 1). These findings are observed in both nodal and extranodal sites; however, there is a greater degree of fibrosis and RDD histiocytes with less frequent or absent emperipolesis on extranodal sites. Extranodal RDD also appears more frequently to be fibrosis and less frequently to be histiocytosis. RDD is often associated with abundant plasma cells in the medullary cords and around the venules [8].

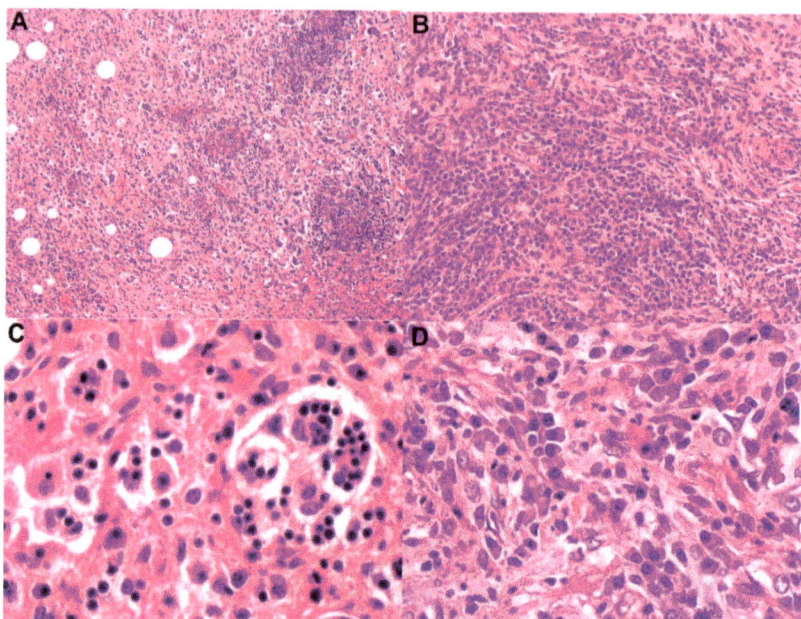

Figure 1. The selected images show a case of nodal Rosai–Dorfman disease with concurrent IgG4-related disease. (**A**) Low-power magnification shows effacement of normal lymph-node architecture by histiocytes (H & E, magnification 40×). (**B**) Higher-power magnification demonstrates increased plasma cells arranged in nests and singly associated with background fibrosis and histiocytes (immunoperoxidase, magnification 200×). (**C**) Loaded histiocytes with emperipolesis and (**D**) an increased number of plasma cells (immunoperoxidase, magnification 600× and 600×, respectively).

Fine-needle aspiration–smears and touch imprints are typically highly cellular with many histiocytes and engulfed lymphocytes (emperipolesis) against a background of mixed inflammatory cells, including plasma cells and lymphocytes. Histiocytes tend to be large with abundant cytoplasm and a round, vesicular nucleus with a small central nucleolus. In smear and imprint preparations, there tends to be a diagnostic dilemma; overlapping lymphocytes can be mistaken for emperipolesis as engulfed lymphocytes do not appear surrounded by a halo, as seen in tissue sections. In later stages of RDD, there tends to be increased plasma cells and cytoplasmic immunoglobulin inclusion (Russell bodies).

Studies have shown that RDD histiocytes express CD4, CD11c, CD14, CD68 (KP-1), and CD163 [33–35]. Uniquely, in RDD, the histiocytes express S100, which is a useful feature for visualizing the emperipolesis, as first described in a single case by Aoyama et al. [36] and confirmed in a larger series by Miettinen et al. [37] (see Figure 2). RDD is usually negative for pan B- or T-cell antigens, markers for Langerhans cells (CD1a and langerin/CD207), and follicular dendritic cell markers (CD21, CD23, CD35, and clusterin). RDD histiocytes are also reactive to α1-antichymotrypsin and α1-antitrypsin, which might suggest lysosomal activity.

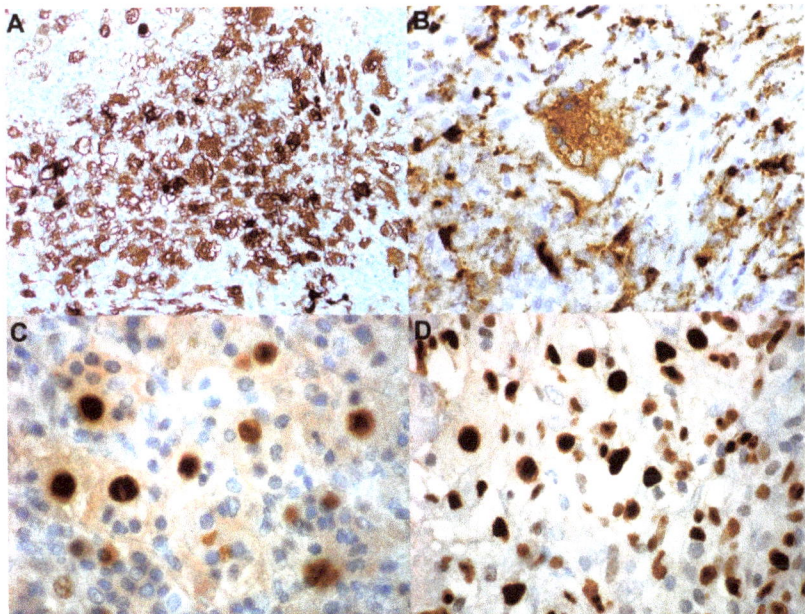

Figure 2. Routine immunohistochemical stains for Rosai–Dorfman disease. (**A**) S-100 immunohistochemical stain highlighting the histiocytes, which also demonstrates emperipolesis (immunoperoxidase, magnification 600×). (**B**) CD68 immunohistochemical stain highlighting the histiocytes (immunoperoxidase, magnification 600×). (**C,D**) BCL-1 and Oct2 immunohistochemical stains are positive for histiocytes of Rosai–Dorfman disease (immunoperoxidase, magnification 600×).

Recent studies have shown that 1/3 of RDD cases harboring mutations in the MAPK/ERK pathway that were found to be gain-of-function mutations leading to the upregulation of p-ERK and cyclin D1/BCL-1 in the histiocytes [38–40]. Cyclin D1/BCL-1, a key cell-cycle regulator, represents a major downstream target of the MAPK/ERK pathway. Expression that is positive for Cyclin D1/BCL-1 can be associated with phosphorylated -ERK (p-ERK), reflecting the constitutive activation of MAPK pathway [39]. However, some cases show cyclin D1 upregulation and absence of p-ERK expression; hence, cyclin D1 might be regulated by other oncogenic mechanisms bypassing the ERK pathway [40]. Positive cyclin D1/BCL-1 staining in RDD is not associated with an underlying translocation of the *CCND1* gene. Be cautious: some reactive histiocytes also express cyclin D1/BCL-1; however, this is usually dimly expressed. The marker becomes less specific for RDD if it is weakly expressed on histiocytes [41,42]. Besides cyclin D1/bcl-1, the Mayo group study showed a subset of RDD cases also expressed p16 (64%), Factor XIIIa (30%) and phosphorylated extracellular signal-related kinase (45%) [43]. The latter two parameters appeared to be associated with multifocality of RDD [43]. As Factor XIIIa is also seen with ECD, this should be interpreted with caution.

Another marker that was frequently expressed in many RDD cases is BCL-2. Since RDD cases usually have low Ki-67 proliferation index, the expression of BCL-2 might be caused by the activation of the anti-apoptotic process [40,43]. OCT2, a unique monocyte-macrophage marker, has also been found to be expressed in most cases of RDD, in contrast to other histiocytic disorders, such as LCH and ECD [43] (Figure 2). Plasma cell markers (IgG, IgG4, kappa and lambda) are used to identify concurrent IgG4 disease (Figure 3).

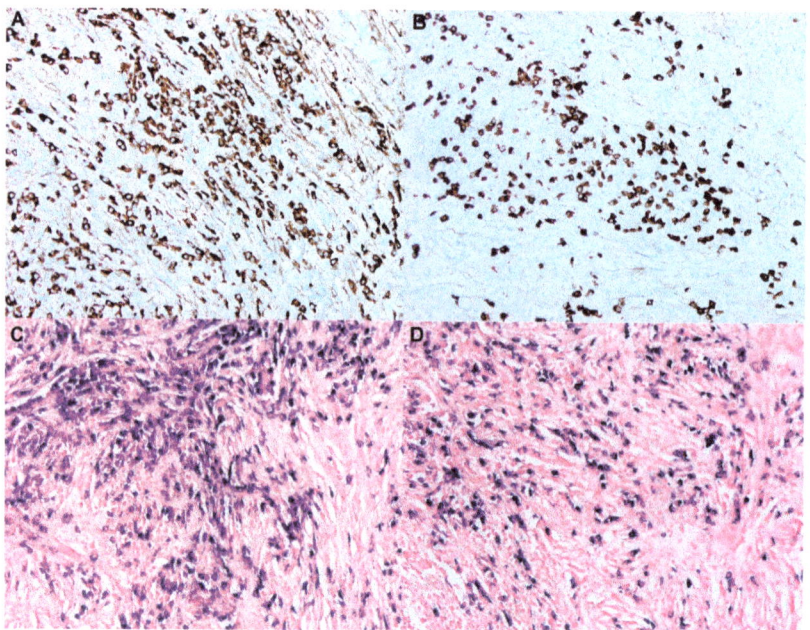

Figure 3. Representative images of IgG4 disease in a patient with Rosai–Dorfman disease (refer to Figure 1): increased plasma cells in a background of fibrosis. (**A**,**B**) Immunohistochemical stains demonstrate plasma cells positive for IgG and proportionally positive for IgG4 (**A**,**B**). immunoperoxidase 100×, respectively). (**C**,**D**) In situ hybridization using kappa and lambda light chain probes reveal the plasma cells to be polyclonal (in situ hybridization 100×, respectively).

Although RDD has many prominent features, which can help to distinguish this entity from other histiocytic disorders, certain features are nonspecific, e.g., emperipolesis can be identified in ECD, juvenile xanogranuloma, and malignant histiocytosis [6]. In addition to S100, histiocytic markers (Fascin, CD68, CD163, CD4, CD14) positive for RDD can be seen with numerous histiocytic disorders, especially when RDD concurs with other histiocytic lesions. Differentiation between RDD and other histiocytic disorders is sometimes challenging. For nodal RDD, differential diagnoses mainly include LCH-, ECD-, and ALK1-positive histiocytosis and infection or other malignancies associated with reactive histiocytosis.

7.1. Benign Disorders

1. Sinus histiocytosis, which is a benign nonspecific reaction in a reactive lymph node with increased histiocytes. This entity does not show emperipolesis, and few histiocytes stain for S100.
2. Toxoplasma lymphadenitis usually present with the diagnostic histologic triad of
   a. Sinusoidal expansion by monocytoid B cells;
   b. Follicular hyperplasia;
   c. Epithelioid histiocytes encroaching on reactive germinal centers differ from RDD, since these histiocytes usually occur in small groups with baby granulomatous changes;

   Serology test and special stains would be helpful for diagnosis.
3. Hemophagocytic lymphohistiocytosis (HLH): The patients with HLH present with hemophophagocytosis that cytologically could mimic emperipolesis.

   However, clinically the patients with HLH are critically ill, with disseminated disease, often life threatening, and associated with severe pancytopenia, hepatosplenomegaly, high levels of ferritin, triglycine, and soluble IL25, distinguishing it from RDD. S100 stain on phagocytic histiocytes is negative.

7.2. Neoplastic Disorders

1. LCH can be easily differentiated from RDD. Unlike RDD, Langerhans cells in LCH usually show nuclear groves and thin nuclear membranes and are often associated with abundant eosinophils and necrosis. Langerhans cells are positive for CD1a and langerin (CD207), which are negative in RDD, yet both RDD and LCH are positive for S100 [44,45]. An electron microscope shows a specific feature in cytoplasm of the LCH cells, called Birkbeck granules. *BRAF* V600E is more frequently mutated in LCH than in RDD. Another immunohistochemical stain that can be used to detect underlying *BRAF* V600E is the BRAF VE1 clone [46]. PD-L1 is more commonly positive in LCH than RDD [46].
2. Diagnosing ECD requires a comprehensive study, including clinicopathologic, radiologic, and molecular assessment. Pathognomonic, radiologic features for diagnosis include symmetrical long-bone osteosclerotic lesion of lower limbs and sheathing of the aorta (coating of the aorta by fibrosis). Histologically, it presents with histiocytes with xanthogranulomatous changes and fibrosis against the background of inflammatory cells and Touton giant cells. Similar to RDD, the histiocytes in ECD are also positive for CD63 and CD168, a small subset positive for S-100 that could mimic RDD. However, unlike RDD, the histiocytes in ECD do not show emperiolopoiesis, and are positive for XIIIa and *BRAF* mutations (>50% of cases) [47];
3. Classic Hodgkin lymphoma can rarely be localized in lymph-node sinuses, which can create a diagnostic dilemma in some cases; however, the presence of Reed–Sternberg cells and Hodgkin cells makes the distinction from RDD easier. Hodgkin cells and Reed–Sternberg cells are positive for CD30, CD15, dim PAX5, fascin, and MUM1, and the background histiocytes are positive for CD68 but not S100;
4. Anaplastic large-cell lymphoma can present with a sinusoidal pattern, but the hallmark cells with horseshoe nuclei are very distinctive and diffusely positive for CD30 by IHC stains (≥75% of neoplastic cells). For the ALK-positive variant, it harbors *ALK* translocations and is positive for ALK immunostaining.
5. ALK-positive histiocytosis is first described in 3 infants [48]. This entity is divided into three groups: Group 1A (infants with hematopoietic and liver involvement); group 1B (multisystemic diseases); and group 2 (patients with single-organ involvement [49]. Similar to RDD, ALK-positive histiocytosis shows emperipolesis and stains for histiocytic markers (CD168, CD63, CD4, CD14). Many cases also express OCT2 (61%), pERK (46%) and cyclin-D1 (49%). However, this entity harbors many ALK

translocations, most commonly *KIF5B-ALK*, and stains positive for ALK1. S100 is variably expressed, unlike RDD, which is uniformly expressed [49];
6. Histiocytic sarcoma shows histiocytic proliferation and usually has marked cytologic atypia, brisk mitotic activity, and is negative for S100. Though emperipolesis could be occasionally identified, unlike RDD, it also has an aggressive clinical course;
7. Juvenile xanthogranuloma, most commonly present in children, with a predilection for the head-and-neck region. It is often cutaneous; however, rarely, it can be subcutaneous or intramuscular. Usually, it resolves spontaneously. Histologically, proliferation of numerous mononuclear and multinucleated cells with Touton-like features on a background of inflammatory cells (lymphocytes and eosinophils) are consistently present. There can be variable foamy histiocytes and lipids. Emperipolesis could be seen. Both diseases are positive for CD68 and CD4. However, unlike RDD, the histiocytes are negative for S100 and more frequently positive for Factor XIIIa [50];
8. Follicular dendritic cell sarcoma may involve lymph nodes or extranodal sites. Oval- to- spindle cells with eosinophilic cytoplasm forming syncytial sheets. Tumor cells are admixed with small lymphocytes and positive for CD21, CD23, CD35, and clusterin, distinguishing it from RDD. Some cases may express S100 focally.

8. Genetic and Mutational Profile

Approximately 50% of cases of RDD do not have a known distinct mutational profile. From 30% to 50% of patients with RDD-harboring somatic mutations are frequently involved in *ARAF, NRAS, KRAS, MAP2K1, CSF1,* and *CBL* genes, of which *MA2P2K1* and *KRAS* were the most frequent, making up 14% and 12.5% of all RDD, respectively (see Table 2) [51–55] (Table 2) Garces et al. showed mutually excluded *KRAS* and *MAP21* gene mutations in RDD, together making up 33% of cases [38]. *NRAS* mutation was detected in numerous cases of purely cutaneous RDD. A study of Wu et al. showed *NRAS* (A146T) mutation was the most common among point mutants, followed by *NRAS* G13S, suggesting that the mutations may play a role in pathogenesis of cutaneous RDD [56]. *PTPN11, NF1* mutations have also occasionally been reported [39]. *BRAF* mutations can occasionally occur in RDD, and not just V600E mutations; other mutations were reported (*BRAF* Y472C and *BRAF* R188G, deletion in exon 12 of *BRAF*) [57–59]. *BRAF* (V600E) is more common in RDD overlapped with LCH or ECD diseases [60]. Given the low frequency of *BRAF* mutations in cases of RDD, one should pay an attention to RDD-overlapping diseases.

Table 2. Certain gene mutations identified in RDD [6,38,55].

Gene	Molecular Alteration	References
ARAF	N217K	[51]
MAP2K1	F53V, L115V, P124R, G128D, V50M, D65M	[38,51,52]
KRAS	A146T, A146V, K117N, G12D, G12R, G13S, Q22K,	[38,51,53,55,56,61]
NRAS	G13D	[51]
CBL	C384Y, GNAQ Q209H	[55]
KDM5A	amplification	[55]
FBXW7	E113D	[55]
BRAF	V600E, deletion (p. 486–491), Y472C and R188G	[57–59]
SMAD4	T521I (variant of unknown significance, 1 case)	[62]

There are many other genes that are mutated in RDD, including *SNX24*, and are involved in intracellular trafficking. *INTS2, CIC, SFR1, BRD4,* and *PHOX2B* genes play roles in the transcriptional regulation as well as cell-cycle regulation genes (*PDS5A, MUC4*); ubiquitin-proteasome pathway (*USP35*); and DNA-mismatch repair genes (*BRCA1, LATS2, ATM*) [54,63].

Some gene mutations frequently identified in myeloid or lymphoid neoplasms have also been observed in RDD, e.g., *ASXL1, TET2,* and *DNMT3A* [39]. A large cohort of

28 patients reported many mutations, which are implicated in other myeloid malignancies, e.g., *TET2*, *MLL4*, *NF1*, *ALK*, and *ASXL1*; many of these genes are driver mutations in different myeloid and lymphoid neoplasms [59]. Whether they might play a role in the pathogenesis of RDD or if they might cause transformation or transdifferentiation to these neoplasms has yet to be determined. Many other mutations have been reported: *SEC62*, *FCGBP*, *PIK3R2*, *PIK3CA*, *VCL*, *EGFR*, *ERBB2* and *TLR8* (minimum variable allele frequency in these mutations is 2%) [59]. The exact roles of these genes are of further exploration.

Cytogenetic testing usually does not have a role in RDD; however, testing can be conducted to rule out a neoplastic process. One case was reported to have a normal karyotype with a minor clone lacking chromosome 20 [64].

Familial RDD has been reported in patients with germline mutations of *SLC29A3* [65]. Two mutations have been reported to date: p.G427S and p.G437R. The spectrum of diseases associated with a mutation in the *SLC29A3* gene mainly include the following three diseases:

1. Familial or Faisalabad histiocytosis: Children present with sensorineural deafness and joint contractures. It is autosomal recessive disorder [65,66]. Histologically, it resembles RDD; therefore, obtaining a clinical history along with a genetic consultation is an important step;
2. H syndrome: Children present with hypogonadism, indurated, hyperpigmented, hypertrichotic skin plaques, hepatomegaly, cardiac abnormalities, and hearing loss [67,68]. Skin lesions share histologic features with RDD;
3. Pigmented hypertrichotic dermatosis with insulin-dependent diabetes syndrome: Children present with insulin-dependent diabetes mellitus and pigmented hypertrichosis [67].

All these diseases are described as histiocytosis-lymphadenopathy plus syndrome. A recent study confirmed that, despite sharing a missense mutation c.1088 G > A [p.Arg363Gln] of the SLC29A3 gene, the clinical phenotype of the intrafamilial SLC29A3 disorders could be heterogeneous [69].

Another cause of familial RDD is heterozygous germline mutations in the FAS and TNFRSF genes, which also cause ALPS. Patients with ALPS tend to have a male predominance, more aggressive disease behavior, and an earlier age of disease onset [70].

9. Prognosis

Nodal RDD has a good prognosis, which correlates with the number of nodal groups; however, this is according to an article published in 1990 [5]. To date, there has not been a large case series monitoring the prognosis of RDD patients. In extranodal RDD forms, prognosis also correlated with the number of organ systems that were involved. Prognosis is usually favorable for cutaneous, nodal, and bone RDD; however, CNS involvement with RDD has variable outcomes [13,16,71]. In most cases, it has a good prognosis; however, some patients have a progressive and fatal course. Regarding gastrointestinal involvement by RDD, a case series reported approximately 20% mortality. GU-system involvement has a worse prognosis of approximately 40% mortality in RDD involving the kidney. The largest series of RDD was reported by Foucar et al. in 1990 [5]; it showed that 17 (7%) of 238 patients died because of direct complications of their disease, infections, or amyloidosis.

10. Treatment

1. No standard therapy has been established for patients with RDD based on results of prospective clinical studies due to the rarity of this disorder. Treatment algorithms are based on retrospective case series, case reports, disease-registry analyses, and expert opinions. Most recently, the NCCN Clinical Practice Guidelines in Oncology, Histiocytic Neoplasms, Version 2.2021, proposed diagnostic and treatment algorithms for patients with RDD [23]. Observation, watch and wait, is considered for asymptomatic or mildly symptomatic patients as 40% of cases with nodal/cutaneous involvement will have spontaneous remission [72];

2. Complete surgical resection is used for patients with unifocal areas of involvement. Surgical therapy can also be useful for patients with spinal cord compression or upper-airway obstruction or with large lesions which might cause end-organ damage. Regarding cutaneous RDD, surgery has been found to be the most effective line of treatment for localized disease [73]. Endoscopic resection of sinonasal RDD can help with symptomatic relief [74];

3. External-beam radiation therapy can play a role in patients with localized unresectable symptomatic steroid-refractory masses, especially in extranodal locations. The most frequently administered doses ranged from 20 to 30 Gy with 2 Gy per fraction, but higher disease levels have also been reported. Overall response rate (ORR) was approximately 40% in patients treated with doses ranging from 30 to 49 Gy and 27% with doses <30 Gy;

4. Corticosteroids have been used in RDD as it was found that steroids decrease the nodal size and symptoms. The optimal dose and duration for this line treatment is ambiguous; however, prednisone (40–70 mg per day) demonstrated variable responses, ranging from failure–no response to complete response in cases with bone, orbit, CNS, and autoimmune-related RDD [75]. According to the consensus recommendations published in 2018, steroids alone do not lead to a stable response among patients with extranodal RDD. It has been found that patients with RDD require a higher dose of prednisone (>0.5 mg/kg per day). Similarly, dexamethasone is effective in RDD with nodal and intracranial lesions [76,77]. A case series of 57 patients reported by Mayo Clinic group showed that corticosteroid treatment was associated with 56% ORR in treatment-naïve patients. Relapses occurred in 53% of patients. When steroids were used as a second-line therapy, the ORR was 67% [15];

5. Sirolimus is frequently used for treating ALPS [78], which suggested a potential benefit for patients with RDD. This agent was effective in a case report of a child with resistant RDD and recurrent autoimmune cytopenias [79];

6. Chemotherapy and immunotherapy have been used to treat RDD with many different chemotherapeutic agents, leading to a mixed treatment responses and adverse events. Some agents were ineffective, such as anthracyclines and alkylating agents; however, vinca alkaloids have shown variable results. Many different regimens have been postulated to have good responses in RDD. A case series on 15 patients with massive lymphadenopathy was reported by the University of Pennsylvania group. The patients were treated with rituximab monotherapy, resulting in 64% progression-free survival at 24 months [80]. Other chemotherapy agents used in refractory RDD with promising activities were nucleoside analogs, such as cladribine (2.1–5 mg/m^2 per day for 5 days every 28 days for 6 months) and clofarabine (25 mg/m^2 per day for 5 days every 28 days for 6 months) [81–83];

7. Immunotherapy such as TNF-α inhibitors. thalidomide and lenalidomide were used due to the increased levels of TNF-α and interleukin-6 in patients with RDD. A case report of the patient treated with a low dose (50 mg/day) thalidomide with a dose escalation to 100 mg/day demonstrated promising results [84]. On the one hand, the results of thalidomide therapy have been mixed, and the side effects associated with administration of this agent are not negligible. Lenalidomide, on the other hand, has shown very good responses in patients with refractory nodal and bone RDD and overall better tolerance with fewer side effects, except myelosuppression compared to thalidomide [85]. Rituximab has also been used to treat autoimmune RDD; however, some cases show recurrence or become refractory [86–88];

8. Targeted therapy with imatinib has been used in a case report with refractory RDD. Imatinib could be an option for systemic involvement by non-LCH disorders [89]. Interestingly, the lesional histiocytes were positive for expression of PDGFRB and KIT/CD117 by immunohistochemical stain, but no underlying mutations in genes coding for these tyrosine kinases were identified. *BRAF* mutations have rarely been observed in RDD. BRAF inhibitor (dabrafenib) was reported to be used in a patient

with concurrent RDD and LCH with clinical and radiological response but increased *BRAF*-V600E post 13-month therapy; additional MEK inhibitor (trametinib) was added with limited follow-up time [60]. MEK inhibitor (cobimetinib) has shown good results in a patient with *KRAS* (p.G12R) mutated RDD [53]. Moyon et al. reported that two RDD patients received cobimetinib showed significant pulmonary response with regard to metabolism and tumor size [19].

11. Conclusions

In the past, RDD was thought to be a benign histiocytic proliferative disorder of unknown etiopathogenesis. Most recently, based on molecular and genetic data, a consensus has been reached defining RDD as a neoplastic myeloproliferative process with causative mutations in the MAPK pathway in a subset of cases. Additional IHC markers have been found to help refine the diagnosis of RDD, such as cyclin-D1 and OCT2. Even though standard therapy based on prospective clinical trials has not been well established to date, the discovery of novel driver mutations could be useful for the development of novel targeted therapy, resulting in better tolerance and outcomes.

Author Contributions: I.E.Y.: data collection, investigation, visualization, outlining, writing the original manuscript. L.S.: resources, data curation, Writing—Review and editing L.Z.: conceptualization, data collection, visualization, outlining, Writing—Review and editing. All authors have read and agreed to the published version of the manuscript.

Funding: This research received no external funding.

Institutional Review Board Statement: The study of histiocytosis and dendritic neoplasms has been approved by the Institutional Review Board (MCC 21376).

Informed Consent Statement: Not applicable.

Data Availability Statement: Not applicable.

Acknowledgments: Editorial assistance was provided by Daley Drucker and Gerard Hebert; no compensation was given beyond their regular salaries.

Conflicts of Interest: The authors declare no conflict of interest.

References

1. Destombes, P. Adenitis with lipid excess, in children or young adults, seen in the Antilles and in Mali. (4 cases). *Bull. Soc. Pathol. Exot. Fil.* **1965**, *58*, 1169–1175.
2. Azoury, F.J.; Reed, R.J. Histiocytosis. Report of an unusual case. *N. Engl. J. Med.* **1966**, *274*, 928–930. [CrossRef]
3. Rosai, J.; Dorfman, R.F. Sinus histiocytosis with massive lymphadenopathy. A newly recognized benign clinicopathological entity. *Arch. Pathol.* **1969**, *87*, 63–70. [PubMed]
4. Rosai, J.; Dorfman, R.F. Sinus histiocytosis with massive lymphadenopathy: A pseudolymphomatous benign disorder. Analysis of 34 cases. *Cancer* **1972**, *30*, 1174–1188. [CrossRef]
5. Foucar, E.; Rosai, J.; Dorfman, R. Sinus histiocytosis with massive lymphadenopathy (Rosai-Dorfman disease): Review of the entity. *Semin. Diagn. Pathol.* **1990**, *7*, 19–73. [PubMed]
6. Abla, O.; Jacobsen, E.; Picarsic, J.; Krenova, Z.; Jaffe, R.; Emile, J.F.; Durham, B.H.; Braier, J.; Charlotte, F.; Donadieu, J.; et al. Consensus recommendations for the diagnosis and clinical management of Rosai-Dorfman-Destombes disease. *Blood* **2018**, *131*, 2877–2890. [CrossRef]
7. Tsang, W.Y.; Yip, T.T.; Chan, J.K. The Rosai-Dorfman disease histiocytes are not infected by Epstein-Barr virus. *Histopathology* **1994**, *25*, 88–90. [CrossRef]
8. Kismet, E.; Koseoglu, V.; Atay, A.A.; Deveci, S.; Demirkaya, E.; Tuncer, K. Sinus histiocytosis with massive lymphadenopathy in three brothers. *Pediatr. Int.* **2005**, *47*, 473–476. [CrossRef]
9. Emile, J.F.; Abla, O.; Fraitag, S.; Horne, A.; Haroche, J.; Donadieu, J.; Requena-Caballero, L.; Jordan, M.B.; Abdel-Wahab, O.; Allen, C.E.; et al. Revised classification of histiocytoses and neoplasms of the macrophage-dendritic cell lineages. *Blood* **2016**, *127*, 2672–2681. [CrossRef]
10. Khoury, J.D.; Solary, E.; Abla, O.; Akkari, Y.; Alaggio, R.; Apperley, J.F.; Bejar, R.; Berti, E.; Busque, L.; Chan, J.K.C.; et al. The 5th edition of the World Health Organization Classification of Haematolymphoid Tumours: Myeloid and Histiocytic/Dendritic Neoplasms. *Leukemia* **2022**, *36*, 1703–1719. [CrossRef]

11. Frater, J.L.; Maddox, J.S.; Obadiah, J.M.; Hurley, M.Y. Cutaneous Rosai-Dorfman disease: Comprehensive review of cases reported in the medical literature since 1990 and presentation of an illustrative case. *J. Cutan. Med. Surg.* **2006**, *10*, 281–290. [CrossRef]
12. Ragotte, R.J.; Dhanrajani, A.; Pleydell-Pearce, J.; Del Bel, K.L.; Tarailo-Graovac, M.; van Karnebeek, C.; Terry, J.; Senger, C.; McKinnon, M.L.; Seear, M.; et al. The importance of considering monogenic causes of autoimmunity: A somatic mutation in KRAS causing pediatric Rosai-Dorfman syndrome and systemic lupus erythematosus. *Clin. Immunol.* **2017**, *175*, 143–146. [CrossRef] [PubMed]
13. Vaiselbuh, S.R.; Bryceson, Y.T.; Allen, C.E.; Whitlock, J.A.; Abla, O. Updates on histiocytic disorders. *Pediatr. Blood Cancer* **2014**, *61*, 1329–1335. [CrossRef] [PubMed]
14. Campo, E.; Jaffe, E.S.; Cook, J.R.; Quintanilla-Martinez, L.; Swerdlow, S.H.; Anderson, K.C.; Brousset, P.; Cerroni, L.; de Leval, L.; Dirnhofer, S.; et al. The International Consensus Classification of Mature Lymphoid Neoplasms: A Report from the Clinical Advisory Committee. *Blood* **2022**, *140*, 1229–125310. [CrossRef] [PubMed]
15. Goyal, G.; Ravindran, A.; Young, J.R.; Shah, M.V.; Bennani, N.N.; Patnaik, M.M.; Nowakowski, G.S.; Thanarajasingam, G.; Habermann, T.M.; Vassallo, R.; et al. Clinicopathological features, treatment approaches, and outcomes in Rosai-Dorfman disease. *Haematologica* **2020**, *105*, 348–357. [CrossRef]
16. Papo, M.; Cohen-Aubart, F.; Trefond, L.; Bauvois, A.; Amoura, Z.; Emile, J.F.; Haroche, J. Systemic Histiocytosis (Langerhans Cell Histiocytosis, Erdheim-Chester Disease, Destombes-Rosai-Dorfman Disease): From Oncogenic Mutations to Inflammatory Disorders. *Curr. Oncol. Rep.* **2019**, *21*, 62. [CrossRef]
17. Demicco, E.G.; Rosenberg, A.E.; Bjornsson, J.; Rybak, L.D.; Unni, K.K.; Nielsen, G.P. Primary Rosai-Dorfman disease of bone: A clinicopathologic study of 15 cases. *Am. J. Surg. Pathol.* **2010**, *34*, 1324–1333. [CrossRef]
18. Sandoval-Sus, J.D.; Sandoval-Leon, A.C.; Chapman, J.R.; Velazquez-Vega, J.; Borja, M.J.; Rosenberg, S.; Lossos, A.; Lossos, I.S. Rosai-Dorfman disease of the central nervous system: Report of 6 cases and review of the literature. *Medicine* **2014**, *93*, 165–175. [CrossRef]
19. Moyon, Q.; Boussouar, S.; Maksud, P.; Emile, J.F.; Charlotte, F.; Aladjidi, N.; Prevot, G.; Donadieu, J.; Amoura, Z.; Grenier, P.; et al. Lung Involvement in Destombes-Rosai-Dorfman Disease: Clinical and Radiological Features and Response to the MEK Inhibitor Cobimetinib. *Chest* **2020**, *157*, 323–333. [CrossRef]
20. Baker, J.C.; Kyriakos, M.; McDonald, D.J.; Rubin, D.A. Primary Rosai-Dorfman disease of the femur. *Skeletal. Radiol.* **2017**, *46*, 129–135. [CrossRef]
21. Taufiq, M.; Khair, A.; Begum, F.; Akhter, S.; Shamim Farooq, M.; Kamal, M. Isolated Intracranial Rosai-Dorfman Disease. *Case Rep. Neurol. Med.* **2016**, *2016*, 1972594. [CrossRef]
22. Cohen Aubart, F.; Idbaih, A.; Emile, J.F.; Amoura, Z.; Abdel-Wahab, O.; Durham, B.H.; Haroche, J.; Diamond, E.L. Histiocytosis and the nervous system: From diagnosis to targeted therapies. *Neuro-Oncology* **2021**, *23*, 1433–1446. [CrossRef] [PubMed]
23. Go, R.S.; Jacobsen, E.; Baiocchi, R.; Buhtoiarov, I.; Butler, E.B.; Campbell, P.K.; Coulter, D.W.; Diamond, E.; Flagg, A.; Goodman, A.M.; et al. Histiocytic Neoplasms, Version 2.2021, NCCN Clinical Practice Guidelines in Oncology. *J. Natl. Compr. Cancer Netw.* **2021**, *19*, 1277–1303. [CrossRef] [PubMed]
24. Wallace, Z.S.; Naden, R.P.; Chari, S.; Choi, H.K.; Della-Torre, E.; Dicaire, J.F.; Hart, P.A.; Inoue, D.; Kawano, M.; Khosroshahi, A.; et al. The 2019 American College of Rheumatology/European League Against Rheumatism classification criteria for IgG4-related disease. *Ann. Rheum. Dis.* **2020**, *79*, 77–87. [CrossRef] [PubMed]
25. Kuo, T.T.; Chen, T.C.; Lee, L.Y.; Lu, P.H. IgG4-positive plasma cells in cutaneous Rosai-Dorfman disease: An additional immunohistochemical feature and possible relationship to IgG4-related sclerosing disease. *J. Cutan. Pathol.* **2009**, *36*, 1069–1073. [CrossRef]
26. Menon, M.P.; Evbuomwan, M.O.; Rosai, J.; Jaffe, E.S.; Pittaluga, S. A subset of Rosai-Dorfman disease cases show increased IgG4-positive plasma cells: Another red herring or a true association with IgG4-related disease? *Histopathology* **2014**, *64*, 455–459. [CrossRef]
27. Zhang, X.; Hyjek, E.; Vardiman, J. A subset of Rosai-Dorfman disease exhibits features of IgG4-related disease. *Am. J. Clin. Pathol.* **2013**, *139*, 622–632. [CrossRef] [PubMed]
28. Liu, L.; Perry, A.M.; Cao, W.; Smith, L.M.; Hsi, E.D.; Liu, X.; Mo, J.Q.; Dotlic, S.; Mosunjac, M.; Talmon, G.; et al. Relationship between Rosai-Dorfman disease and IgG4-related disease: Study of 32 cases. *Am. J. Clin. Pathol.* **2013**, *140*, 395–402. [CrossRef]
29. O'Malley, D.P.; Duong, A.; Barry, T.S.; Chen, S.; Hibbard, M.K.; Ferry, J.A.; Hasserjian, R.P.; Thompson, M.A.; Richardson, M.S.; Jaffe, R.; et al. Co-occurrence of Langerhans cell histiocytosis and Rosai-Dorfman disease: Possible relationship of two histiocytic disorders in rare cases. *Mod. Pathol.* **2010**, *23*, 1616–1623. [CrossRef]
30. Cohen-Barak, E.; Rozenman, D.; Schafer, J.; Krausz, J.; Dodiuk-Gad, R.; Gabriel, H.; Shani-Adir, A. An unusual co-occurrence of Langerhans cell histiocytosis and Rosai-Dorfman disease: Report of a case and review of the literature. *Int. J. Dermatol.* **2014**, *53*, 558–563. [CrossRef]
31. Hervier, B.; Haroche, J.; Arnaud, L.; Charlotte, F.; Donadieu, J.; Neel, A.; Lifermann, F.; Villabona, C.; Graffin, B.; Hermine, O.; et al. Association of both Langerhans cell histiocytosis and Erdheim-Chester disease linked to the BRAFV600E mutation. *Blood* **2014**, *124*, 1119–1126. [CrossRef] [PubMed]
32. Razanamahery, J.; Diamond, E.L.; Cohen-Aubart, F.; Plate, K.H.; Lourida, G.; Charlotte, F.; Helias-Rodzewicz, Z.; Goyal, G.; Go, R.S.; Dogan, A.; et al. Erdheim-Chester disease with concomitant Rosai-Dorfman like lesions: A distinct entity mainly driven by MAP2K1. *Haematologica* **2020**, *105*, e5–e8. [CrossRef] [PubMed]

33. Bonetti, F.; Chilosi, M.; Menestrina, F.; Scarpa, A.; Pelicci, P.G.; Amorosi, E.; Fiore-Donati, L.; Knowles, D.M., 2nd. Immunohistological analysis of Rosai-Dorfman histiocytosis. A disease of S-100 + CD1-histiocytes. *Virchows Arch. A* **1987**, *411*, 129–135. [CrossRef]
34. Eisen, R.N.; Buckley, P.J.; Rosai, J. Immunophenotypic characterization of sinus histiocytosis with massive lymphadenopathy (Rosai-Dorfman disease). *Semin. Diagn Pathol.* **1990**, *7*, 74–82.
35. Paulli, M.; Rosso, R.; Kindl, S.; Boveri, E.; Marocolo, D.; Chioda, C.; Agostini, C.; Magrini, U.; Facchetti, F. Immunophenotypic characterization of the cell infiltrate in five cases of sinus histiocytosis with massive lymphadenopathy (Rosai-Dorfman disease). *Hum. Pathol.* **1992**, *23*, 647–654. [CrossRef]
36. Aoyama, K.; Terashima, K.; Imai, Y.; Katsushima, N.; Okuyama, Y.; Niikawa, K.; Mukada, T.; Takahashi, K. Sinus histiocytosis with massive lymphadenopathy. A histogenic analysis of histiocytes found in the fourth Japanese case. *Acta Pathol. Jpn.* **1984**, *34*, 375–388. [CrossRef] [PubMed]
37. Miettinen, M.; Paljakka, P.; Haveri, P.; Saxen, E. Sinus histiocytosis with massive lymphadenopathy. A nodal and extranodal proliferation of S-100 protein positive histiocytes? *Am. J. Clin. Pathol.* **1987**, *88*, 270–277. [CrossRef]
38. Garces, S.; Medeiros, L.J.; Patel, K.P.; Li, S.; Pina-Oviedo, S.; Li, J.; Garces, J.C.; Khoury, J.D.; Yin, C.C. Mutually exclusive recurrent KRAS and MAP2K1 mutations in Rosai-Dorfman disease. *Mod. Pathol.* **2017**, *30*, 1367–1377. [CrossRef]
39. Baraban, E.; Sadigh, S.; Rosenbaum, J.; Van Arnam, J.; Bogusz, A.M.; Mehr, C.; Bagg, A. Cyclin D1 expression and novel mutational findings in Rosai-Dorfman disease. *Br. J. Haematol.* **2019**, *186*, 837–844. [CrossRef]
40. Garces, S.; Medeiros, L.J.; Marques-Piubelli, M.L.; Coelho Siqueira, S.A.; Miranda, R.N.; Cuglievan, B.; Sriganeshan, V.; Medina, A.M.; Garces, J.C.; Saluja, K.; et al. Cyclin D1 expression in Rosai-Dorfman disease: A near-constant finding that is not invariably associated with mitogen-activated protein kinase/extracellular signal-regulated kinase pathway activation. *Hum. Pathol.* **2022**, *121*, 36–45. [CrossRef]
41. Abdulla, Z.; Turley, H.; Gatter, K.; Pezzella, F. Immunohistological recognition of cyclin D1 expression by non-lymphoid cells among lymphoid neoplastic cells. *APMIS* **2014**, *122*, 183–191. [CrossRef] [PubMed]
42. Wu, J.; Zhang, Y.; Sun, L.; Zhai, Q. Cyclin D1 expression by histiocytes may mimic cyclin D1-positive proliferation centres of chronic lymphocytic leukaemia/small lymphocytic lymphoma. *Pathol.-Res. Pract.* **2018**, *214*, 72–75. [CrossRef]
43. Ravindran, A.; Goyal, G.; Go, R.S.; Rech, K.L.; Mayo Clinic Histiocytosis Working, G. Rosai-Dorfman Disease Displays a Unique Monocyte-Macrophage Phenotype Characterized by Expression of OCT2. *Am. J. Surg. Pathol.* **2021**, *45*, 35–44. [CrossRef] [PubMed]
44. Favara, B.E.; Feller, A.C.; Pauli, M.; Jaffe, E.S.; Weiss, L.M.; Arico, M.; Bucsky, P.; Egeler, R.M.; Elinder, G.; Gadner, H.; et al. Contemporary classification of histiocytic disorders. The WHO Committee On Histiocytic/Reticulum Cell Proliferations. Reclassification Working Group of the Histiocyte Society. *Med. Pediatr. Oncol.* **1997**, *29*, 157–166. [CrossRef]
45. Orkin, S.H.; Nathan, D.G.; Ginsburg, D.; Look, A.T.; Fisher, D.E.; Lux, S. Lymphohistiocytic disorders. In *Nathan and Oski's Hematology of Infancy and Childhood*; WB Saunders: Philadelphia, PA, USA, 2003.
46. Ballester, L.Y.; Cantu, M.D.; Lim, K.P.H.; Sarabia, S.F.; Ferguson, L.S.; Renee Webb, C.; Allen, C.E.; McClain, K.L.; Mohila, C.A.; Punia, J.N.; et al. The use of BRAF V600E mutation-specific immunohistochemistry in pediatric Langerhans cell histiocytosis. *Hematol. Oncol.* **2018**, *36*, 307–315. [CrossRef] [PubMed]
47. Diamond, E.L.; Dagna, L.; Hyman, D.M.; Cavalli, G.; Janku, F.; Estrada-Veras, J.; Ferrarini, M.; Abdel-Wahab, O.; Heaney, M.L.; Scheel, P.J.; et al. Consensus guidelines for the diagnosis and clinical management of Erdheim-Chester disease. *Blood* **2014**, *124*, 483–492. [CrossRef]
48. Chan, J.K.; Lamant, L.; Algar, E.; Delsol, G.; Tsang, W.Y.; Lee, K.C.; Tiedemann, K.; Chow, C.W. ALK+ histiocytosis: A novel type of systemic histiocytic proliferative disorder of early infancy. *Blood* **2008**, *112*, 2965–2968. [CrossRef]
49. Kemps, P.G.; Picarsic, J.; Durham, B.H.; Helias-Rodzewicz, Z.; Hiemcke-Jiwa, L.; van den Bos, C.; van de Wetering, M.D.; van Noesel, C.J.M.; van Laar, J.A.M.; Verdijk, R.M.; et al. ALK-positive histiocytosis: A new clinicopathologic spectrum highlighting neurologic involvement and responses to ALK inhibition. *Blood* **2022**, *139*, 256–280. [CrossRef]
50. McClain, K.L. Histiocytic Diseases of Neonates: Langerhans Cell Histiocytosis, Rosai-Dorfman Disease, and Juvenile Xanthogranuloma. *Clin. Perinatol.* **2021**, *48*, 167–179. [CrossRef]
51. Diamond, E.L.; Durham, B.H.; Haroche, J.; Yao, Z.; Ma, J.; Parikh, S.A.; Wang, Z.; Choi, J.; Kim, E.; Cohen-Aubart, F.; et al. Diverse and Targetable Kinase Alterations Drive Histiocytic Neoplasms. *Cancer Discov.* **2016**, *6*, 154–165. [CrossRef] [PubMed]
52. Matter, M.S.; Bihl, M.; Juskevicius, D.; Tzankov, A. Is Rosai-Dorfman disease a reactve process? Detection of a MAP2K1 L115V mutation in a case of Rosai-Dorfman disease. *Virchows Arch.* **2017**, *471*, 545–547. [CrossRef]
53. Jacobsen, E.; Shanmugam, V.; Jagannathan, J. Rosai-Dorfman Disease with Activating KRAS Mutation—Response to Cobimetinib. *N. Engl. J. Med.* **2017**, *377*, 2398–2399. [CrossRef]
54. Durham, B.H.; Lopez Rodrigo, E.; Picarsic, J.; Abramson, D.; Rotemberg, V.; De Munck, S.; Pannecoucke, E.; Lu, S.X.; Pastore, A.; Yoshimi, A.; et al. Activating mutations in CSF1R and additional receptor tyrosine kinases in histiocytic neoplasms. *Nat. Med.* **2019**, *25*, 1839–1842. [CrossRef] [PubMed]
55. Lee, L.H.; Gasilina, A.; Roychoudhury, J.; Clark, J.; McCormack, F.X.; Pressey, J.; Grimley, M.S.; Lorsbach, R.; Ali, S.; Bailey, M.; et al. Real-time genomic profiling of histiocytoses identifies early-kinase domain BRAF alterations while improving treatment outcomes. *JCI Insight* **2017**, *2*, e89473. [CrossRef]

56. Wu, K.J.; Li, S.H.; Liao, J.B.; Chiou, C.C.; Wu, C.S.; Chen, C.C. NRAS Mutations May Be Involved in the Pathogenesis of Cutaneous Rosai Dorfman Disease: A Pilot Study. *Biology* **2021**, *10*, 396. [CrossRef]
57. Fatobene, G.; Haroche, J.; Helias-Rodzwicz, Z.; Charlotte, F.; Taly, V.; Ferreira, A.M.; Abdo, A.N.R.; Rocha, V.; Emile, J.F. BRAF V600E mutation detected in a case of Rosai-Dorfman disease. *Haematologica* **2018**, *103*, e377–e379. [CrossRef] [PubMed]
58. Richardson, T.E.; Wachsmann, M.; Oliver, D.; Abedin, Z.; Ye, D.; Burns, D.K.; Raisanen, J.M.; Greenberg, B.M.; Hatanpaa, K.J. BRAF mutation leading to central nervous system rosai-dorfman disease. *Ann. Neurol.* **2018**, *84*, 147–152. [CrossRef]
59. Chen, J.; Zhao, A.L.; Duan, M.H.; Cai, H.; Gao, X.M.; Liu, T.; Sun, J.; Liang, Z.Y.; Zhou, D.B.; Cao, X.X.; et al. Diverse kinase alterations and myeloid-associated mutations in adult histiocytosis. *Leukemia* **2022**, *36*, 573–576. [CrossRef] [PubMed]
60. Mastropolo, R.; Close, A.; Allen, S.W.; McClain, K.L.; Maurer, S.; Picarsic, J. BRAF-V600E-mutated Rosai-Dorfman-Destombes disease and Langerhans cell histiocytosis with response to BRAF inhibitor. *Blood Adv.* **2019**, *3*, 1848–1853. [CrossRef] [PubMed]
61. Shanmugam, V.; Margolskee, E.; Kluk, M.; Giorgadze, T.; Orazi, A. Rosai-Dorfman Disease Harboring an Activating KRAS K117N Missense Mutation. *Head Neck Pathol.* **2016**, *10*, 394–399. [CrossRef]
62. Gatalica, Z.; Bilalovic, N.; Palazzo, J.P.; Bender, R.P.; Swensen, J.; Millis, S.Z.; Vranic, S.; Von Hoff, D.; Arceci, R.J. Disseminated histiocytoses biomarkers beyond BRAFV600E: Frequent expression of PD-L1. *Oncotarget* **2015**, *6*, 19819–19825. [CrossRef] [PubMed]
63. Bruce-Brand, C.; Schneider, J.W.; Schubert, P. Rosai-Dorfman disease: An overview. *J. Clin. Pathol.* **2020**, *73*, 697–705. [CrossRef] [PubMed]
64. Sacchi, S.; Artusi, T.; Selleri, L.; Temperani, P.; Zucchini, P.; Vecchi, A.; Emilia, G.; Torelli, U. Sinus histiocytosis with massive lymphadenopathy: Immunological, cytogenetic and molecular studies. *Blut* **1990**, *60*, 339–344. [CrossRef] [PubMed]
65. Morgan, N.V.; Morris, M.R.; Cangul, H.; Gleeson, D.; Straatman-Iwanowska, A.; Davies, N.; Keenan, S.; Pasha, S.; Rahman, F.; Gentle, D.; et al. Mutations in SLC29A3, encoding an equilibrative nucleoside transporter ENT3, cause a familial histiocytosis syndrome (Faisalabad histiocytosis) and familial Rosai-Dorfman disease. *PLoS Genet.* **2010**, *6*, e1000833. [CrossRef]
66. Moynihan, L.M.; Bundey, S.E.; Heath, D.; Jones, E.L.; McHale, D.P.; Mueller, R.F.; Markham, A.F.; Lench, N.J. Autozygosity mapping, to chromosome 11q25, of a rare autosomal recessive syndrome causing histiocytosis, joint contractures, and sensorineural deafness. *Am. J. Hum. Genet.* **1998**, *62*, 1123–1128. [CrossRef]
67. Cliffe, S.T.; Kramer, J.M.; Hussain, K.; Robben, J.H.; de Jong, E.K.; de Brouwer, A.P.; Nibbeling, E.; Kamsteeg, E.J.; Wong, M.; Prendiville, J.; et al. SLC29A3 gene is mutated in pigmented hypertrichosis with insulin-dependent diabetes mellitus syndrome and interacts with the insulin signaling pathway. *Hum. Mol. Genet.* **2009**, *18*, 2257–2265. [CrossRef]
68. Bolze, A.; Abhyankar, A.; Grant, A.V.; Patel, B.; Yadav, R.; Byun, M.; Caillez, D.; Emile, J.F.; Pastor-Anglada, M.; Abel, L.; et al. A mild form of SLC29A3 disorder: A frameshift deletion leads to the paradoxical translation of an otherwise noncoding mRNA splice variant. *PLoS ONE* **2012**, *7*, e29708. [CrossRef]
69. Chouk, H.; Ben Rejeb, M.; Boussofara, L.; Elmabrouk, H.; Ghariani, N.; Sriha, B.; Saad, A.; H'Mida, D.; Denguezli, M. Phenotypic intrafamilial variability including H syndrome and Rosai-Dorfman disease associated with the same c.1088G > A mutation in the SLC29A3 gene. *Hum. Genom.* **2021**, *15*, 63. [CrossRef]
70. Maric, I.; Pittaluga, S.; Dale, J.K.; Niemela, J.E.; Delsol, G.; Diment, J.; Rosai, J.; Raffeld, M.; Puck, J.M.; Straus, S.E.; et al. Histologic features of sinus histiocytosis with massive lymphadenopathy in patients with autoimmune lymphoproliferative syndrome. *Am. J. Surg. Pathol.* **2005**, *29*, 903–911. [CrossRef] [PubMed]
71. Paryani, N.N.; Daugherty, L.C.; O'Connor, M.I.; Jiang, L. Extranodal rosai-dorfman disease of the bone treated with surgery and radiotherapy. *Rare Tumors* **2014**, *6*, 5531. [CrossRef]
72. Pulsoni, A.; Anghel, G.; Falcucci, P.; Matera, R.; Pescarmona, E.; Ribersani, M.; Villiva, N.; Mandelli, F. Treatment of sinus histiocytosis with massive lymphadenopathy (Rosai-Dorfman disease): Report of a case and literature review. *Am. J. Hematol.* **2002**, *69*, 67–71. [CrossRef] [PubMed]
73. Al-Khateeb, T.H. Cutaneous Rosai-Dorfman Disease of the Face: A Comprehensive Literature Review and Case Report. *J. Oral Maxillofac. Surg.* **2016**, *74*, 528–540. [CrossRef] [PubMed]
74. Chen, H.H.; Zhou, S.H.; Wang, S.Q.; Teng, X.D.; Fan, J. Factors associated with recurrence and therapeutic strategies for sinonasal Rosai-Dorfman disease. *Head Neck* **2012**, *34*, 1504–1513. [CrossRef] [PubMed]
75. Shulman, S.; Katzenstein, H.; Abramowsky, C.; Broecker, J.; Wulkan, M.; Shehata, B. Unusual presentation of Rosai-Dorfman disease (RDD) in the bone in adolescents. *Fetal Pediatr. Pathol.* **2011**, *30*, 442–447. [CrossRef]
76. McPherson, C.M.; Brown, J.; Kim, A.W.; DeMonte, F. Regression of intracranial rosai-dorfman disease following corticosteroid therapy. Case report. *J. Neurosurg.* **2006**, *104*, 840–844. [CrossRef] [PubMed]
77. Adeleye, A.O.; Amir, G.; Fraifeld, S.; Shoshan, Y.; Umansky, F.; Spektor, S. Diagnosis and management of Rosai-Dorfman disease involving the central nervous system. *Neurol. Res.* **2010**, *32*, 572–578. [CrossRef]
78. Teachey, D.T.; Greiner, R.; Seif, A.; Attiyeh, E.; Bleesing, J.; Choi, J.; Manno, C.; Rappaport, E.; Schwabe, D.; Sheen, C.; et al. Treatment with sirolimus results in complete responses in patients with autoimmune lymphoproliferative syndrome. *Br. J. Haematol.* **2009**, *145*, 101–106. [CrossRef]
79. Cooper, S.L.; Arceci, R.J.; Gamper, C.J.; Teachey, D.T.; Schafer, E.S. Successful Treatment of Recurrent Autoimmune Cytopenias in the Context of Sinus Histiocytosis With Massive Lymphadenopathy Using Sirolimus. *Pediatr. Blood Cancer* **2016**, *63*, 358–360. [CrossRef]

80. Namoglu, E.C.; Hughes, M.E.; Plastaras, J.P.; Landsburg, D.J.; Maity, A.; Nasta, S.D. Management and outcomes of sinus histiocytosis with massive lymphadenopathy (Rosai Dorfman Disease). *Leuk. Lymphoma* **2020**, *61*, 905–911. [CrossRef]
81. Simko, S.J.; Tran, H.D.; Jones, J.; Bilgi, M.; Beaupin, L.K.; Coulter, D.; Garrington, T.; McCavit, T.L.; Moore, C.; Rivera-Ortegon, F.; et al. Clofarabine salvage therapy in refractory multifocal histiocytic disorders, including Langerhans cell histiocytosis, juvenile xanthogranuloma and Rosai-Dorfman disease. *Pediatr. Blood Cancer* **2014**, *61*, 479–487. [CrossRef]
82. Aouba, A.; Terrier, B.; Vasiliu, V.; Candon, S.; Brousse, N.; Varet, B.; Hermine, O. Dramatic clinical efficacy of cladribine in Rosai-Dorfman disease and evolution of the cytokine profile: Towards a new therapeutic approach. *Haematologica* **2006**, *91*, ECR52. [PubMed]
83. Sasaki, K.; Pemmaraju, N.; Westin, J.R.; Wang, W.L.; Khoury, J.D.; Podoloff, D.A.; Moon, B.; Daver, N.; Borthakur, G. A single case of rosai-dorfman disease marked by pathologic fractures, kidney failure, and liver cirrhosis treated with single-agent cladribine. *Front. Oncol.* **2014**, *4*, 297. [CrossRef] [PubMed]
84. Chen, E.; Pavlidakey, P.; Sami, N. Rosai-Dorfman disease successfully treated with thalidomide. *JAAD Case Rep.* **2016**, *2*, 369–372. [CrossRef] [PubMed]
85. Rubinstein, M.; Assal, A.; Scherba, M.; Elman, J.; White, R.; Verma, A.; Strakhan, M.; Mohammadi, F.; Janakiram, M. Lenalidomide in the treatment of Rosai Dorfman disease–a first in use report. *Am. J. Hematol.* **2016**, *91*, E1. [CrossRef] [PubMed]
86. Petschner, F.; Walker, U.A.; Schmitt-Graff, A.; Uhl, M.; Peter, H.H. ["Catastrophic systemic lupus erythematosus" with Rosai-Dorfman sinus histiocytosis. Successful treatment with anti-CD20/rutuximab]. *Dtsch. Med. Wochenschr.* **2001**, *126*, 998–1001. [CrossRef] [PubMed]
87. Maklad, A.M.; Bayoumi, Y.; Tunio, M.; Alshakweer, W.; Dahar, M.A.; Akbar, S.A. Steroid-resistant extranodal rosai-dorfman disease of cheek mass and ptosis treated with radiation therapy. *Case Rep. Hematol.* **2013**, *2013*, 428297. [CrossRef]
88. Nadal, M.; Kervarrec, T.; Machet, M.C.; Petrella, T.; Machet, L. Cutaneous Rosai-Dorfman Disease Located on the Breast: Rapid Effectiveness of Methotrexate After Failure of Topical Corticosteroids, Acitretin and Thalidomide. *Acta Derm. Venereol.* **2015**, *95*, 758–759. [CrossRef]
89. Utikal, J.; Ugurel, S.; Kurzen, H.; Erben, P.; Reiter, A.; Hochhaus, A.; Nebe, T.; Hildenbrand, R.; Haberkorn, U.; Goerdt, S.; et al. Imatinib as a treatment option for systemic non-Langerhans cell histiocytoses. *Arch. Dermatol.* **2007**, *143*, 736–740. [CrossRef]

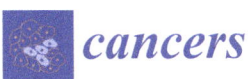

Review

Genetics Abnormalities with Clinical Impact in Primary Cutaneous Lymphomas

Fernando Gallardo [1,2,*] and Ramon M. Pujol [1,3]

[1] Department of Dermatology, Hospital del Mar, Parc de Salut Mar, Passeig Maritim 25-29, 08003 Barcelona, Spain
[2] Department of Medicine and Life Sciences, Universitat Pompeu Fabra, 08003 Barcelona, Spain
[3] Department of Medicine, Universitat Autònoma de Barcelona, 08003 Barcelona, Spain
* Correspondence: fgallardo@psmar.cat; Tel.: +34-932483380

Simple Summary: The genetic landscape of cutaneous T-cell lymphomas analyzed by sequencing high throughput techniques shows a heterogeneous somatic mutational profile and genomic copy number variations in the TCR signaling effectors, the NF-κB elements, DNA damage/repair elements, JAK/STAT pathway elements and epigenetic modifiers. A mutational and genomic stratification of these patients provides new opportunities for the development or repurposing of (personalized) therapeutic strategies. The genetic heterogeneity in cutaneous B-cell lymphoma parallels with the specific subtype. Damaging mutations in primary cutaneous diffuse large B-cell lymphoma of the leg type, involving MYD88 gene, or BCL6 and MYC translocations or CDKN2A deletions are useful for diagnostic purposes. The more indolent forms, as the primary cutaneous lymphoma of follicle center cell (somatic mutations in TNFRSF14 and 1p36 deletions) and the cutaneous lymphoproliferative disorder of the marginal zone cells (FAS gene), present with a more restricted pattern of genetic alterations.

Abstract: Primary cutaneous lymphomas comprise a heterogeneous group of extranodal non-Hodgkin lymphomas (NHL) that arise from skin resident lymphoid cells and are manifested by specific lymphomatous cutaneous lesions with no evidence of extracutaneous disease at the time of diagnosis. They may originate from mature T-lymphocytes (70% of all cases), mature B-lymphocytes (25–30%) or, rarely, NK cells. Cutaneous T-cell lymphomas (CTCL) comprise a heterogeneous group of T-cell malignancies including Mycosis Fungoides (MF) the most frequent subtype, accounting for approximately half of CTCL, and Sézary syndrome (SS), which is an erythrodermic and leukemic subtype characterized by significant blood involvement. The mutational landscape of MF and SS by NGS include recurrent genomic alterations in the TCR signaling effectors (i.e., PLCG1), the NF-κB elements (i.e., CARD11), DNA damage/repair elements (TP53 or ATM), JAK/STAT pathway elements or epigenetic modifiers (DNMT3). Genomic copy number variations appeared to be more prevalent than somatic mutations. Other CTCL subtypes such as primary cutaneous anaplastic large cell lymphoma also harbor genetic alterations of the JAK/STAT pathway in up to 50% of cases. Recently, primary cutaneous aggressive epidermotropic T-cell lymphoma, a rare fatal subtype, was found to contain a specific profile of JAK2 rearrangements. Other aggressive cytotoxic CTCL (primary cutaneous γδ T-cell lymphomas) also show genetic alterations in the JAK/STAT pathway in a large proportion of patients. Thus, CTCL patients have a heterogeneous genetic/transcriptional and epigenetic background, and there is no uniform treatment for these patients. In this scenario, a pathway-based personalized management is required. Cutaneous B-cell lymphoma (CBCL) subtypes present a variable genetic profile. The genetic heterogeneity parallels the multiple types of specialized B-cells and their specific tissue distribution. Particularly, many recurrent hotspot and damaging mutations in primary cutaneous diffuse large B-cell lymphoma of the leg type, involving MYD88 gene, or BCL6 and MYC translocations and BLIMP1 or CDKN2A deletions are useful for diagnostic and prognostic purposes for this aggressive subtype from other indolent CBCL forms.

Citation: Gallardo, F.; Pujol, R.M. Genetics Abnormalities with Clinical Impact in Primary Cutaneous Lymphomas. *Cancers* **2022**, *14*, 4972. https://doi.org/10.3390/cancers14204972

Academic Editor: Francesc Solé

Received: 2 September 2022
Accepted: 4 October 2022
Published: 11 October 2022

Publisher's Note: MDPI stays neutral with regard to jurisdictional claims in published maps and institutional affiliations.

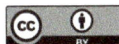

Copyright: © 2022 by the authors. Licensee MDPI, Basel, Switzerland. This article is an open access article distributed under the terms and conditions of the Creative Commons Attribution (CC BY) license (https://creativecommons.org/licenses/by/4.0/).

Keywords: cutaneous lymphoma; genetics

1. Introduction

Primary cutaneous lymphomas (CL) comprise a heterogeneous group of T and B-cell non-Hodgkin lymphomas (NHL) that arise from skin resident lymphoid cells and may extend to the lymph nodes, peripheral blood, and eventually extranodal sites [1]. The different clinical variants of CL have been recognized in the recent WHO classification of hematopoietic and lymphoid tissue neoplasms [1,2]

Primary cutaneous T-cell lymphomas (CTCL) are the most important group, accounting for 70% of CL, and have an estimated incidence of up to 10 new cases per million people per year [1,3]. Mycosis Fungoides (MF) and Sézary syndrome (SS) are the most representative entities and show a heterogeneous mutational landscape that comprises elements of the TCR signaling, NF-κB and the DNA damage/repair pathways, being copy number variations (CNV) more common than somatic mutations in the JAK/STAT pathway. Primary cutaneous anaplastic large cell lymphomas (pcALCL) have rearrangements at the IRF4/DUSP22 locus and common genetic alterations of the JAK/STAT pathway. Recently, recurrent JAK2 rearrangements have been reported in primary cutaneous CD8+ aggressive epidermotropic cytotoxic T-cell lymphoma (pcAETCL), a rare lethal subtype of CTCL, and may represent a new targeted therapeutic approach. In addition, other aggressive cytotoxic CTCL (primary cutaneous γδ T-cell lymphoma [pcGDTL]) show mutations in the JAK/STAT pathways in a large proportion of patients [1,2,4].

There is no curative treatment for MF, SS and other CTCL, and there is an urgent need for new effective well-tolerated treatments with a safe profile and that maintain long-term activity. In recent years the knowledge of specific therapeutic targets has allowed for the design of immunotherapies (both cytotoxic and immunoregulatory) such as brentuximab, mogamulizumab, or check-point inhibitors (PD1/PDL1 inhibitors), which have modified the disease-free survival of these patients in the short term. Given the heterogeneity of these CTCL tumours, it is essential to obtain personalized therapies (precision medicine) adapted to the different mechanisms and subtypes of CTCL and the characteristics of each patient in particular. The identification of new associated biomarkers will be relevant for the stratification of patients and in defining which ones will benefit from onco-specific drugs or pathway inhibitors. It can also be useful to establish prognostic value markers that allow for the adapting of the therapeutic attitude [4].

Primary cutaneous B-cell lymphomas (CBCL) form a present a variable genetic profile according its specialized B-cells and their specific tissue distribution. Primary cutaneous lymphoma of the follicle center cells presents common somatic mutations in TNFRSF14 and CREBBP or associates 1p36 deletions, but at lower frequencies than in systemic follicular lymphomas. Genetic alterations in the FAS gene have been described in a high percentage of cases and, although other translocations specific to extranodal (non-cutaneous) marginal zone lymphomas of the MALT (mucosa-associated lymphoid tissue) type can be observed, such as t(1;14)(p22;q32), t(11;18)(q21;q21), or t(14;18)(q32;q21)-IgH/MALT, the number of cases is very limited and they are of little diagnostic value. Primary cutaneous diffuse large B-cell lymphoma of the leg type involves characteristic mutations in the MYD88 gene or CDKN2A deletions [1,2].

Many of these genomic alterations in CL, being present in other mature NHL, may represent opportunities for the development of monitoring and therapeutic strategies that are currently in use or under investigation in other hematological malignancies.

2. Primary Cutaneous T-Cell Lymphomas: Mycosis Fungoides and Sézary Syndrome

MF accounts for 50% of all CL and is clinically manifested by a slow progression of the disease over years or decades from cutaneous macules to infiltrated plaques, until patients develop skin tumors or lymph node involvement, which significantly worsens the prognosis. SS is an aggressive disease that almost exclusively affects adults or elderly patients (mainly males) and is classically manifested by pruritic erythroderma, generalized lymphadenopathy, and atypical circulating of large mononuclear cells with convoluted nuclei (Sézary cells). The overall survival of SS is similar to that of advanced-stage MF, approximately 30% at 5 years [5–7].

MF/SS are generally malignant neoplasms of CD4+ T cells that exhibit a T-helper memory phenotype (CD45RO). The clonal expansion of malignant T cells in advanced stages occurs together with a loss or restriction of the diversity of the repertoire of T cell receptors (TCR), an increased activity or regulatory function by the same malignant cells, and a decrease in the number of CD8+ T cells. Malignant SS T cells co-express circulating receptor molecules such as CCR7, CD62L, L-selectin, and the central memory T cell marker CD27. In contrast, MF cells present a skin-resident effector memory T cell phenotype lacking CCR7/L-selectin, CD103, or CD27. They express CCR4, CD69, and the cutaneous lymphocyte antigen (CLA). Whole exome sequencing (WES) studies suggest that malignant clonotypes in MF develop in T-cell progenitors prior to TCRβ or TCRα rearrangements [8–10].

2.1. Genetic and Epigenetics Abnormalitites in MF/SS

Next-generation sequencing (NGS) approaches have been successfully applied, looking at the MF/SS mutational landscape and have identified putative genomic alterations and driver mutations in genes involved in the development and progression of these diseases. A significant proportion of studies have been focused on SS since homogeneous sampling is easier to analyze under NGS platforms. MF and SS harbor complex and heterogeneous (non disease-specific) genetic and epigenetic alterations. Many of the identified driver genes are shared by both diseases, and it remains open to discussion whether they represent extremes of the same spectrum of diseases or are different disorders [11–25]. Broad similarities across disease stages have been observed, although more structural variants have been detected in leukemic disease, leading to highly recurrent deletions of putative tumor suppressors that are uncommon in early-stage skin-centered MF (i.e., TP53 gene). Fusion genes play an important role in tumor development because they might result in disruption of either tumor suppressor genes or the activation of proto-oncogenes [11,25–28]. C>T transitions represent the main mechanism of mutations and the possibility of a contribution of UV exposure to MF/SS has been discussed [13,14,26]. On the other hand, alkylating-related signatures seem to be restricted to early MFs, and age-related signatures are enriched, but not exclusively, in SS. Many driver mutations are present in both forms of the mutations but are more prevalent in late-MF and in SS compared with skin-limited CTCL [26,27]. Different alterations on T-cell activation and NF-κB signaling, apoptosis, chromatin remodeling, DNA damage response together with signaling pathways including JAK/Signal Transducer and Activator of Transcription (STAT) and cell-cycle checkpoints have been most commonly detected [26,28].

2.1.1. Spectrum of Somatic Point Mutations

Recurrent mutations in the DNA damage/repair elements TP53 (18%) and splice-site mutation affecting the FAT (FRAP, TRAPP) domain of ATM are commonly detected [19,26]. The TCR/NF-κB signaling effectors carrying somatic mutations include PLCG1 (9–21%), TNFRSF1B or CARD11 (5–7%) and GLI3, which may interact with BCL10, a positive regulator of cell apoptosis and NF-κB activation [11,13,16,17,26]. Interesting hotspot point mutations in other oncogenes from this pathway such as NFKB1 (p.H67Y), KLF2 (p.H346Q/N/Y), and JUNB (p.A282V) and damaging mutations in the tumor suppressor genes FUBP1 and ANO6 have been newly identified in a large number of samples from diverse MF/SS stages [26,29]. Other interesting recurrent genes affected by somatic point mutations (but with a low prevalence of less than 5%) include stop-gain mutations in ITPR1/2 (a functional partner of the anti-apoptotic BCL2 gene), DSC1 and PKHD1L1 (cellular immunity) genes [11]. Singleton somatic mutations in RIPK2 and IL6 (CD4+ cells activation, TCRα/β differentiation), missense mutation in the (recombination activity) RAG2 gene and mutations in STAT5B gene have been reported in CTCL [12,13]. Interestingly, the status of PD1 mutations vs deletions seems to predict the patient survival in CTCL. Neoplastic T-cells in SS frequently express PD-1, and although gene mutations in CTCL commonly promote TCR-dependent proliferation, most CTCL cases show the "T-cell exhaustion" phenotype (PD1, TGT1 and CXCL13-positive) and could not proliferate after TCR stimulation. However, cases showing loss of PD-1 (deletion) may reverse this phenotype, increasing cell proliferation and prompting a worse clinical course [13,16,26]. Table 1 summarizes many of these genetic abnormalities reported in MF/SS.

Table 1. Summary of genetic abnormalities reported in MF/SS [11–28].

Signaling	Mutations	CNVs (Deletions/Gains)	Druggable Pathway
Cell cycle	TP53 (19%), FAS (6%), RHOA (3%)	TP53 (83%), CDKN2A (40%), RB1 (39%), ATM (30%), CDKN1A (11%) MYC (35%)	Cell cycle regulators BET-inhibitors
JAK/STAT	STAT5B (4%), JAK3 (3%) JAK1 (1%), STAT3 (1%)	STAT3 (60%), STAT5B (60%), JAK2 (13%)	JAK/STAT inhibitors
MAPK	KRAS, NRAS, BRAF, MAP2K1, MAPK1 (<1–2%)	BRAF (18%)	MAPK inhibitors Tirosin-Kinase inhibitors
TCR/NF-κB	PLCγ1 (10%), CARD11 (5%), CCR4 (5%) CD28 (4%), PRKCQ (<1%), TNFRSF1B (2%)	TNFAIP3 (25%), NF-κB2 (25%) PRKCQ (30%), CARD11 (23%), TNFRSF1B (15%), PLCγ1 (5%)	Check-point inhibitors Calcineurine inhibitors NF-κB inhibitors PI3K inhibitors IKK inhibitors
Chromatin	POT1 (6%), DNMT3A (4%), TET2 (4%), KMT2C/KMT2D (3%), CREBBP (3%), NCOR1 (3%), BCOR (3%), TRRAP (5%), KDM6A (1%)	NCOR1 (80%), ARID1A (58%), DNMT3A (38%), ARID5B (29%), SETDB2 (28%), SMARCC1 (21%) TRRAP (10%)	HDAC inhibitors

As many of these genetic abnormalities are shared by other different hematological neoplasms, they may represent clear candidates for genetic screening panel designs of T-cell NHL to improve diagnosis or monitoring (Table 2) [30].

Table 2. Proposal for an ampliseq panel of genes for mature T-cell malignant neoplasms [30].

Mature T-Cell Malignat Lymphoid Neoplasms: Candidate Genes for Amplification				
TP53	FAS	MAP3K5	PLCG1	STAT5A
DNM3TA	GLI3	MAPK14	PTEN	NFATC2
BCOR	IDH2	NLRP2	RASA1	TET2
CARD11	IL6ST	NRAS	RB1	TNFRSF1B
CCR4	ARID1A	STAT3	PDCD1	JAK3
TRRAP	JAK1	RHOA	RELB	TRAF3
CD79A	CREBBP	KRAS	NFκB1/2	TRAF6
SOCS1	JUNB	PIK3C2B	NF1	POT1
CTCF	NCOR1	KDM6A	SMARCB1	ZEB1

2.1.2. Genomic Copy Number Variants

Former approaches using comparative genomic hybridization array techniques detected recurrent large genomic and chromosome imbalances in tumor stage MF and SS that have now been confirmed by NGS. CNV particularly involve the 17p, 9p21 and 10q deletions and 17q amplification [31,32].

The landscape of somatic duplications in CTCL includes large chromosome bands in 8p23.3–q24.3 and 17p11.2–q23.2, 10p15.3–p12.2, and several focal somatic duplications that may encompass genes that play a role in tumorigenesis (ANKRD26, BCL7C, CRIP3, RAMP3 or TRBG4) [11–14,16,18,19,26].

On the other hand, somatic deletions at 10p11.1–q26.3, 11q23.3–q25, 19p13.2–p13.3, or 17p12–p13.3 encompass several interesting genes, such as loss of the tumor suppressor TP53 or DAD1 (pro-apoptosis). Genomic gains of RASA2, a mitogenic-activated protein kinase (MAPK) signaling pathway proto-oncogene or CBLB (proto-oncogene that activates T cells by inhibiting PLCG1) are very interesting candidates for further studies [11,19].

In addition, genetic CNV gains in DNMT3A, ARID1A, CTCF, NCOR1, KDM6A, SMARCB1, ZEB1, PRKCB, PTPRN2, and RLTPR are more frequent than somatic mutations, and occur in TNFAIP3, CSNK1A1 [12,13,18,24,25], and in various elements of the JAK/STAT pathway (STAT5B, STAT3) [11–14,22,24,26]. Deletions in GRAP (TCR signaling), AGAP6, ZBTB7A, and SBNO2 (cytokine signaling) also point to possible candidate genes in the pathogenesis of MF/SS [26,27]. The most prevalent and relevant CNVs are represented in Table 1.

2.1.3. Complex Chromosomal Rearrangements

Complex chromosomal rearrangements or fusion events are rare and also highly heterogeneous (TYK2-UPF1, COL25A1-NFKB2, FASN-SGMS1, SGMS1-ZEB1, SPATA21-RASA2, PITRM1-HK1, or BCR-NDUFAF6, among others) but they represent interesting candidates as potential biomarkers or therapeutic targets in CTCL. FASN (fatty acid protein synthase) together with SGMS1 (sphingomyelin synthase 1) are involved in several types of cancer and are regulated by the ABL proto-oncogene. ZEB1 encodes a zinc finger transcription factor and acts as a transcriptional repressor of IL2 (T-cell differentiation) [12–14,17]. TYK2 is essential for the differentiation and function of different immune cells. NFKB1, KLF2 or NFKB2 as well as other translocations that affect genes of the T cell differentiation pathway (TCR/NF-κB) have been repeatedly implicated in CTCL pathogenesis [11,13,16]. The elevated level of hexokinase 1 (PITRM1-HK1 fusion event) causes tumor cells to avoid apoptosis; the fusion of BCR-NDUFAF6 (ABL) is amenable to targeting in patients with SS as well as that of CTLA4 and CD28 fusion [16,33].

2.1.4. Epigenetics in CTCL

Some mutated genes in CTCL are epigenetic modifiers. The methylation of cytosine residues to 5-methocytosine is mediated by DNA methyltransferases (DNMTs), so gain-of-function mutations and CNVs of DNMT3A represent an interesting mechanism of genomic/epigenomic cooperation that can explain many changes in functions of many genes in CTCL. Furthermore, they have been identified with a high frequency in MF/SS, as occurs in many other hematological malignancies, which increases their relevance. Other alterations in epigenetic regulatory genes are the loss of DNA (hydroxy-) methylation mediated by the family of translocations ten-eleven (TET), mutations in isocitrate dehydrogenases, which inhibit TET proteins, and ARID1A/B (which form part of the chromatin patterning complexes) and the MLL genes, which mediate histone methyltransferases [12,26].

Epigenetic abnormalities complement the genomic landscape of MF/SS. Whole genome DNA methylation status has been scarcely deciphered in SS studies. Methylation status of CMTM2, C2orf40, G0S2, HSPB6, PROM1, o PAM genes have been identified as potential diagnostic epigenetic markers to differentiate SS from inflammatory erythrodermas [34].

The tumor suppressor genes CDKN2A and CDKN2B, which encode the cell cycle proteins p16, p14ARF and p15, are located in the 9p21.3 region, and are frequently lost in MF in tumor stages or in transformation, and are associated with a poor prognosis [35,36]. The genetic loss in this locus can be homozygous but often is associated with promoter hypermethylation of the other allele [37].

Differentially expressed microRNAs have been identified between inflammatory processes and/or normal skin and in MF in early stages. Thus, it has been observed that the microRNAs, miR-155, miR-146a, 146b-5p, miR-342-3p and let-7i were overexpressed, and the microRNAs, miR-203 and miR-205 decreased in MF. The group of microRNAs, miR-NAs 26a, miR-222, miR-181a and miR-146a, likewise, are differentially expressed between tumor and inflammatory cases. Table 3 brings together the main microRNAs differentially expressed in the different forms of CTCL [38,39].

Table 3. Differentially expressed microRNAs in CTCL.

miRNA profile in CTCL Cases	Upregulated miRNAs	Downregulated miRNAs
CTCL global expression pattern	miR-155, miR-326, miR-663b, miR-711, miR-130b, miR-142-3p, miR-93-5p, miR-181a, miR-34a, miR-106b-5p, miR-148a-3p, miR-338-3p	miR-200b, and miR-203
Advanced MF	miR-155, miR-146a, miR-146b-5p, miR-342-3p, let-7i, miR-17~92 cluster, miR-106b~25, miR-106a~363 clusters, miR-181a/b, miR-21, miR-142-3p/5p	miR-200ab/429 cluster, miR-10b, miR-193b, miR-23b/27b, miR-203, miR-205, miR-141/200c
Sézary syndrome	miR-21, miR-214, miR-486	miR-23b, miR-31, miR-132
pcALCL	miR-155, miR-27b, miR-30c and miR-29b, miR-21, miR-142-3p/5p	miR-141/200c

2.1.5. Current and Potential Therapeutic Implications: Towards a Personalized Medicine in CTCL

CTCL are malignant neoplasms that are genetically heterogeneous even within each clinical subtype, so a single therapy may not be suitable for all patients. Determining the specific profile of the specific mutations of each patient or subtype of CTCL is clearly a challenge with direct implications in the diagnosis, monitoring and design of (personalized) therapies. With knowledge of the (heterogeneous) genetics of CTCL and the stratification of patients by altered signaling pathways, different targeted therapeutic approaches can be proposed and are illustrated in Table 4. Therapies targeting the PI3K pathway (duvelisib), NF-κB inhibitors (bortezomib), alisertib (oral Aurora A kinase inhibitor), or JAK/STAT inhibitors, widely used in inflammatory conditions or hematologic malignancies, may show promise in CTCL and are awaiting efficacy and tolerance results from clinical trials. The presence of gene alterations related to immune evasion that lead to abnormal expression of PD1, PD-L1 and PD-L2 and co-stimulatory elements, such as CD28-ICOS, have prompted research on the use of anti-PD1/PD-L1 antibodies [22]. Finally, unraveling the epigenetics in CTCL may also have therapeutic implications. Thus, histone deacetylase (HDAC) inhibitors, such as vorinostat or romidepsin, are already approved in the US for use in CTCL, and resminostat is in clinical trials in Europe. In addition, cobomarsen, an oligonucleotide inhibitor of miR-155, is currently being investigated for use in CTCL [40].

Table 4. Selective/Personalized targeted approaches in MF/SS.

Signaling	Gene/Function	Targeted Therapy
TCR	PLCG1(+)	Calcineurine-inhibitors
	PTEN(−)	PI3K- inhibitors (duvelisib, idelalisib), mTOR- inhibitors
	RhoA(−)	Lenalidomide
	PRKG1(−)	MAPK- inhibitors
	PRKCQ(+)	MAPK-inh.
	CARD11(+)	Proteasome- inhibitors (bortezomib)
	TNFAIP3(−)	Proteasome- inhibitors
	NFKB2(+)	Proteasome- inhibitors
Membrane receptors/ Cytotoxicity or co-stimulation	CD30, CCR4, CD52, CD158	Brentuximab, Mogamulizumab, Alemtuzumab
	CD28(+) FusionCD28-CTLA4, CD28-ICOS(+)	Anti-CD80/CD86 Ipilimumab
	PD1/PDL1 (PDCD1(+/−))	PD1/PDL1 checkpoint- inhibitors

Table 4. Cont.

Signaling		Gene/Function	TargetedTherapy
Cytokines regulation, metabolism, transcription, cell differentiation		TNFRSF1B(TNFR2)(+) TNFRSF6(−) JAK1(+) JAK3(+) STAT3(+) STAT5B(+) RFC-1, PARP Notch(+)	Protesome- inhibitors Lenalidomide JAK- inhibitors (ruxolitinib) PARP- inhibitors γ-secretase- inhibitors
Chromatin remodeling		ARID1A(−), ARID5B(−), SMARCC1(−), ARID1B, ARID4A, ARID2, ARID3A, SMARCA4, HD3(−)	HDAC- inhibitors
Transcription signaling		ZEB1(−) IRF4(+) MYC(+)	MDM2- inhibitors Lenalidomide BET- inhibitors
Histones methylation	Histones methyltranspherases	MLL2(+), MLL3(+), MLL4(+), SETD1A(−), SETD1B(−), SETDB2(−), SETD6(−), EZH2	ZH2- inhibitors (Tazemetostat)
	Histones demethylases	KDM6B(−)	HDAC- inhibitors
Histones acethylation	Histones acetiltranspherases	CREBBP(−)	HDAC- inhibitors
	Histones deacethylases	HDAC6(+)	HDAC- inhibitors (Vorinostat, romidepsine, resminostat, panobinostat, belinostat)
DNA methylation	DNA methyltranspherases	DNMT3A, DNMT3B	Hypomethylants (5-azacitidine, decitabine)
	DNA demethylation	TET1(−), TET2(−)	Protesome- inhibitors
Cell cycle		CDKN1B(−), CDKN2A(−) RB1(−), RPS6KA1(−), ATR(−) TP53(−)	CDK- inhibitors Aurora kinase A- inhibitors MDM2- inhibitors
miRNA (Oligonucleotide antagonist)		miR155(+)	Cobomarsen
Apoptosis (BH3 mimetic antagonist)		BCL2(+)	Venetoclax

3. Other Cutaneous T-Cell Lymphomas Distinct from Mycosis Fungoides and Sézary Syndrome

Other clinical variants of CTCL have been recognized in the WHO classification that include the indolent primary cutaneous CD30(+) lymphoproliferative disorders, extranodal natural killer T-cell lymphoma (ENKTCL), pcGDTL, pcAETCL, subcutaneous panniculitis-like T-cell lymphoma (SPTCL), and primary cutaneous T-cell lymphoma, not otherwise specified (pcPTCL-NOS) [1,2].

3.1. Cutaneous CD30(+) Lymphoproliferative Disorders

The group of CD30(+) cutaneous lymphoproliferative disorders represents a spectrum of processes ranging from lymphomatoid papulosis (LyP), characterized by the presence of spontaneously regressing papules, to pcALCL, presenting as single or multiple cutaneous tumors with a low propensity to spread. Cases of pcALCL lack the common genetic alterations found in systemic CD30(+) ALCL, but up to 20% of pcALCL have rearrangements at the IRF4/DUSP22 locus. NGS technology detected mutations that affect the IL6-JAK1-STAT3 pathway in approximately 15–30% of cases, which places JAK/STAT as a candidate target for new personalized treatments in this CTCL subtype. Other genetic alterations include mutations in DNMT3A and TP53, and the PI3K or MAPK pathways. Other recurrent events affecting cancer-associated genes include the deletion of PRDM1 or TNFRSF14, the gain of EZH2 and TNFRSF8, mutations in LRP1B, PDPK1, and PIK3R1, and rearrangements of GPS2, LINC-PINT, or TNK1 [41–45]. Additionally, for pcALCL, array-CGH analyses have revealed chromosomal imbalances in CTSB (8p22), RAF1 (3p25), REL (2p12) and JUNB (19p13.2) and allelic deletion at 9p21–22, causing inactivation of CDKN2A tumor suppressor gene [46].Therefore, inhibition of these proliferation-promoting pathways should also be explored as potential alternative therapies.

Clinical behavior, phenotypical and genetic profile allow differentiation of pcALCL from systemic CD30(+) ALCL. Systemic CD30+/ALK+ ALCL has ALK gene rearrangements, and the combined nuclear and cytoplasmic expression of ALK protein strongly suggests an underlying t(2;5) translocation of ALK with nucleophosmin. The cytoplasmic expression of the ALK protein is associated with other fusion partners of the ALK gene such as TRAF1, ATIC or TPM3. Systemic CD30+/ALK− ALCL lack an ALK gene rearrangement and subsequently any ALK expression, but has other alterations, such as 6p25 rearrangements involving the IRF4/DUSP22 locus (the same as pcALCL which are negative for ALK expression, as well). Cases with IRF4/DUSP22 rearrangement have a more favorable clinical course than those systemic CD30+/ALK− ALCL which do not carry the IRF4/DUSP22 rearrangement, and similar to CD30+/ALK+ ALCL or pcALCL. On the other hand, patients with systemic CD30+/ALK− ALCL with TP63 rearrangements have a poor prognosis, while the absence of ALK, DUSP22, and TP63 rearrangements (triple negative) results in an intermediate prognosis. Finally, ALCL associated with breast implants is a rare subset of CD30+ALK− ALCL with an overall favorable prognosis. Deletions on chromosome 20q13.13 have been identified in two-thirds of cases of this latter subtype of ALCL [47]. The molecular alteration at the IRF4/DUSP22 locus is less frequent in LyP than in pcALCL and accounts for fewer than 5% of cases [48]. LyP may be associated withother T-cell lymphomas, particularly MF and pcALCL, being clonally related, which suggests that a non-random genetic event initiates the disease [49]. The management of LyP is that of an indolent CL, based on its excellent prognosis; however, this good prognosis is altered if LyP is associated with other lymphomas (up to 40% of cases in some series) [50,51]. The main genetic alterations reported in cutaneous and systemic ALCL are represented in Table 5.

Table 5. Summary of genetic abnormalities reported in cutaneous lymphomas other than MF/SS [41–47].

Other Cutaneous T-Cell Lymphomas	Gene/Translocation Target
Anaplastic Large cell lymphoma	t(2;5)(p23;q35)—ALK/NPM (ALK+ systemic) 6p25.3 — DUSP22/IRF4 3q28—TP63 NPM1-TYK2—JAK/STAT IL6-JAK-STAT mutation DNMT3A, TP53 mutation
Breast Implant-Associated Anaplastic Large cell lymphoma	20q13.13 loss
Primary cutaneous γ/δ T-cell lymphoma	STAT5B mutation—JAK/STAT SETD2 mutation
Subcutaneous Panniculitis-like T-cell lymphoma	HAVCR2 mutation—TIM-3
Primary cutaneous aggressive epidermotropic CD8(+) T-cell lymphoma	CAPRIN1-JAK2—JAK/STAT SELENOI-ABL1

3.2. Subcutaneous Panniculitis-like T-Cell Lymphoma

SPTCL is a rare primary cutaneous lymphoma composed of αβ CD8 cytotoxic T cells with a much less aggressive course than pcGDTL, although 15–20% of cases can develop hemophagocytic syndrome (HPS) and a fatal course. In approximately 20% of cases, the concomitant association or an overlapping presentation with lupus panniculitis has been described. Loss-of-function mutations in the HAVCR2 gene (encoding T-cell immunoglobulin mucin 3 [TIM-3]) have been described in up to 60–80% of cases, either as somatic or germline mutations, as a factor that predisposes to SPTCL development. Mutations in HAVCR2 alter highly conserved residues of TIM-3, an immune response modulator and, consequently, giving rise to an uncontrolled activation of the immune system. In patients of East Asian and Polynesian background, the pathogenic variant c.245A>G (HAVCR2Y82C) is usually detected, whereas for patients of European background, the c.291A>G (HAVCR2T101I) variant is usually demonstrated. Patients with mutated HAVCR2 (HAVCR2Y82C) seemed to be associated with younger age, the development of HPS or hemophagocytic lymphohistiocytosis-like systemic illness, and short relapse-free survival. Mutations in UNC13D, PIAS3, and KMT2D, and the upregulation of CCR4 were more frequent in non-mutated HAVCR2 SPTCL, and enrichment in genes involving IL6-JAK-STAT3 signaling and TNF-α signaling via NF-κB have also been reported [52,53].

3.3. Primary Cutaneous γδ T-Cell Lymphoma

The pcGDTL is a poor prognosis neoplasm with a 5-year overall survival of 10% which often shows systemic symptoms with features of HPS. NGS and TCR sequencing indicated that the cells-of-origin of pcGDTL are Vδ1 cells predominant in the epidermimotropic and dermal variants and Vδ2 cells in the panniculitic counterpart. Vδ1 and Vδ2 lymphomas show similar targetable mutations more commonly affecting the JAK/STAT, MAPK, MYC, and chromatin editing pathways [54].

3.4. Primary Cutaneous CD8(+) Aggressive Epidermotropic Cytotoxic T-Cell Lymphoma

Primary cutaneous CD8(+) aggressive epidermotropic lymphoma pcAETCL is a rare fatal subtype of T-cell NHL presenting complex karyotype and clonal evolution that reflects genomic instability. Gains of 7q, 8q24.3, 17q and losses of 9p21.3 (CDKN2A-CDKN2B) and 17p including the TP53 gene have been reported;however, very recently, the pcAETCL carries JAK2 gene fusions that may render them especially susceptible to JAK inhibitors [55–58].

3.5. Extranodal NK/T-Cells Lymphoma, Nasal Type

ENKTCL is an aggressive lymphoma associated with Epstein-Barr virus (EBV) infection that typically but not exclusively presents in the nasal and paranasal areas. It develops in adult patients from Caribbean or East Asian countries. The genetic profile of ENKTCL is characterized by mutations in JAK/STAT components, tumor suppressor genes (TP53 or MGA), epigenetic modifiers (KMT2D, ARID1A), and BCOR corepressor loss-of-function mutations. Gains in 8q24 [MYC], 2q gain and losses on chromosomes 6q16–q27, 6q21, or 11q22–q23 have also been described in ENKTCL [59]. Hydroa vacciniforme lymphoproliferative disease, formerly referred to as hydroa vacciniforme-like, encompasses a EBV-associated process that may harbor driver mutations in STAT3 and KMT2D among others genes, similar to ENKTCL, and may also represent future targets for therapy, as well [60].

3.6. Primary Cutaneous T-Cell Lymphoma, Not Otherwise Specified

The pcPTCL-NOS are a heterogeneous group of CTCL showing variable clinical (often aggressive) and immunohistochemical features giving rise to some difficulties with regard to classification among the CTCL variants, and may even exhibit T-cell helper follicular (THF) markers such as PD-1, CD10, CXCL13, BCL6, and ICOS and share pathologic characteristics with angioimmunoblastic T-cell and THF lymphomas [61]. Similarly to other non-cutaneous recurrent mutations that have been described in cases of PTCL-NOS affecting epigenetic regulators (KMT2C and ARID1A) and in TCR signaling molecules (PLCG1 and CD28). Mutations of TET2, RHOA (which induces THF lineage specification and promotes T-cell lymphomas in cooperation with loss of TET2), DNMT3A, and IDH2 are also detected. Non-THF, PTCL-NOS subtypes carry mutations and deletions of TP53 and/or CDKN2A. The identification of some cases with mTOR mutations raises the benefit of targeted therapy [62,63].

4. Primary Cutaneous B-Cell Lymphomas

Primary cutaneous B-cell lymphomas (CBCL) represent approximately 30% of the primary cutaneous lymphomas. They include a heterogeneous group of entities with different clinicopathological and evolutionary characteristics. They usually present as papules, nodules or tumors, solitary or multiple, occasionally appearing grouped or as multifocal generalized lesions. Three well-defined groups can be distinguished: primary cutaneous lymphoma of follicle center cells (pcBCLf), primary cutaneous lymphoma of marginal zone cells (pcBCLm), now proposed under the terminology of cutaneous lymphoproliferative disorder of the marginal zone cells, and primary cutaneous diffuse large B-cell lymphoma of the leg type (pcDLBCL). Intravascular large B-cell lymphoma (IVLBCL) and several provisional entities are also included in the WHO/EORTC classification [1,2].

pcBCLm and pcBCLf are lymphoproliferative processes with indolent clinical behavior and are usually manifested as non-ulcerated stable plaques or nodules while pcDLBCL of the leg type is more frequent in older individuals, appearing as fast-growing plaques or nodules with a tendency to ulceration, and represents a process of aggressive evolution. The therapeutic approach of pcDLBCL is similar to that of a systemic DLBCL [64].

CBCL are characterized histopathologically by nodular (pcBCLm and pcBCLf) or diffuse dermal infiltrates (pcDLBCL), occasionally extending into subcutaneous tissue without epidermal involvement and sparing a superficial band of the papillary dermis. Occasionally, expanded large lymphoid follicles (in pcBCLf) or residual follicles colonized by the underlying lymphoid proliferation (in pcBCLm) can be observed. The morphological characteristics of the infiltrating cells are variable depending on the CBCL subtype, either small or medium sized cells (in pcBCLm and pcBCLf) or large cells and immunoblasts (in pcDLBCL, leg type). Neoplastic cells usually express mature B-cell antigens and the diagnostic procedure includes the demonstration of a monoclonal rearrangement of the immunoglobulin heavy or light chain genes or the restriction of immunoglobulin light chain expression by immunohistochemical or in situ hybridization techniques [1,2,64].

4.1. Primary Cutaneous Follicular B-Cell Lymphoma

Neoplastic cells in pcBCLf correspond to mature B lymphocytes (CD19+, CD20+, CD79a+, PAX-5+), which express markers of germinal center cells (BCL-6, CD10) and, in contrast to nodal centrofollicular lymphomas, are usually BCL2-. Neoplastic cells do not express activated B cell markers (MUM1 or FOXP1), which makes it possible to differentiate them from pcDLCBL of the leg type [1,2].

A monoclonal B cell proliferation is detected in the majority of cases. Unfortunately, no specific genetic alterations have been identified. Translocation (14;18)(q32; q21) involving IgH/BCL2 genes, characteristic of systemic follicular lymphomas, is usually not detected. In rare instances, pcBCLf cases expressing BCL2 as a consequence of BCL2 gene breaks or 1p36 deletion have been reported. Occasionally, translocations between IgH and BCL6 genes, amplifications in 2p16.31-REL or deletions of 14q32.32 have also been described (see Table 6) [65]. Somatic mutations detected in pcBCLf were TNFRSF14 (40%, plus 10% with 1p36 deletions), followed by CREBBP, TNFAIP3 or KMT2D (20%). KMT2D, CREBBP, and BCL2 were significantly less commonly mutated in PCFCL than in systemic follicular lymphomas [66]. Recently, BCL2 rearrangement, chromatin-modifying gene mutations (CREBBP, KMT2D, EZH2, EP300) and the proliferation index have been proposed to classify pcBCLf specimens based on the likelihood of concurrent or future systemic spread. Since imaging may miss low-burden internal disease in some cases of systemic follicular lymphomas with cutaneous spread, many of these cases may represent systemic lymphomas misclassified as pcBCLf [67].

Table 6. Summary of genetic abnormalities reported in primary cutaneous B-cell lymphomas.

Cutaneous B-Cell Lymphoma Subtype	Gene/Trasnslocation	Target/Gene
Marginal zone lymphoma (ccutaneous counterpart)	t(14;18)(q32;q21)	IgH/MALT
	t(3;14)(p14.1;q32)	FOXP1/IGH
	18q trisomy	FAS muations
Follicular lymphoma	t(14;18)(q32;q21)	IgH/BCL2 (rare in cutaneous counterpart)
	2p16.31 (amp REL)	
	14q32.32 del	
	1p36 del	TNFRS14 mutations
DLBCL, leg type	9p21	CDKN2A (or hypermethytation)
	3p.14.1	FOXP1
	6q del	BIMP1
	8q24	MYC
	3q27.3, 14q32	BCL6, IgH
		MYD88-mut, CD79B, CARD11,TNFAIP3/A20 (NF-κB)
	PDL1/PDL2-transl.	
	18q21.31–q21 ampl.	BCL2

4.2. Primary Cutaneous Lymphoma of Marginal Zone Cells (Cutaneous Lymphoproliferative Disorder of the Marginal Zone Cells)

Primary cutaneous marginal zone cell lymphoma (pcBCLm) is included in the group of MALT-type lymphomas. MALT lymphomas are indolent neoplasms that develop in extranodal or mucosal locations such as the stomach, salivary glands, orbit, thyroid, breast, or lung. The pcBCLm could be considered the cutaneous variant of MALT-type extranodal lymphoma [1,2,68,69]. The term "cutaneous lymphoproliferative disorder of the marginal zone cells" has been proposed in the latest WHO classification.

These cells seem to develop in tissues where there is persistent lymphoid activation as a result of chronic antigenic stimulation (*Borrelia burgdorferi* infection, vaccines, tattoos). When the marginal zone lymphoid infiltrate becomes genetically unstable, that is, it acquires genetic alterations such as trisomy 3, trisomy 18, t(1;14)(p22;q32), t(11;18)(q21;q21), t(14;18)(q32;q21)-IgH/MALT, t(3;14)(q27;q32), t(3;14)(p14.1;q32) or FAS mutations, the lymphomatous transformation occurs. Such cytogenetic alterations observed in all MALT lymphomas are detected in a limited number of pBCLm cases (see Table 6) [70,71].

Neoplastic cells are small to medium-sized lymphocytes with a monocytoid-like appearance and a variable number of lymphocytes with plasmacytic morphology and plasma cells that are often observed in the periphery of lymphoid aggregates. Neoplastic cells show an immunophenotypic profile of mature B lymphocytes (CD20+, CD22+, CD70a+), are BCL2+ and negative for CD10 and BCL6 (follicular center cell antigens). Class-switched immunoglobulin expression IgG+/CXCR3- (expressing also IgG4) appears to be more common that non-class switch IgM+/CXCR3+ expression similar to other MALT-type lymphomas. Monotypic expression of immunoglobulin light chains can be demonstrated in a majority of cases [68].

4.3. Diffuse Large B-Cell Lymphoma of the Leg Type

Diffuse large B-cell lymphoma of the leg type (pcDLBCL) is a lymphoproliferative process composed of large lymphoid cells (centroblasts, immunoblasts) lacking germinal center formationand presentingan activated B cell phenotype, with the expression of BCL2, MUM1, and FOXP1 antigens. Neoplastic lymphoid cells generally do not express CD10, are occasionally BCL6+, and usually express MYC, IgM, and p63 [1,2,72].

NGS approaches have identified an original mutational landscape of pcDLBCL with a very restricted set of highly recurrent (up to 60–75%) mutations, CNV or neutral loss of heterozygosity, particularly involving MYD88 (p.L265P variant), CARD11, PIM1, and CD79B. Other genes involved in B-cell signaling, NFκB activation or DNA remodeling have also been found to be altered, notably TBL1XR1 (33%), MYC (26%), CREBBP (26%), IRF4

(21%) or HIST1H1E (41%). Amplifications or translocations in IgH, BCL6 or FOXP1 genes, genetic losses and hotspot mutations involving genes of the same pathway as well such as CDKN2A/2B, TNFAIP3/A20, PRDM1, TCF3, and CIITA provide a rationale for using selective inhibitors of the B-cell receptor to treat pcDLBCL of the leg type. The main genetic features in pcDLBCL are illustrated in Table 6. MYC and BCL2 are commonly expressed in cDLBCL of the leg type but double hits involving the MYC gene are rare and the prognostic value of MYC rearrangements seems debatable. However, mutations involving the BCR pathway (see above) may contribute to the resistance to first-line Rituximab-CHOP and deletions or hypermethylation of the p16 promoter appear to be associated with a poor prognosis as well [72–74].

Other Disorders Classified as Cutaneous Diffuse Large B-Cell Lymphomas

Intravascular large B-cell lymphoma (IVLBCL) is a rare subtype of DLBCL which often presents with characteristic cutaneous livedoid lesions andcentral nervous system involvement. Large atypical lymphoid cells are characteristically observed within the vascular lumens and corresponded to mature B lymphocytes (CD20+, CD79+) with an activated ABC phenotype MUM-1+/BCL2+/CD5+/PDL1+ and that are negative for CD10, with a high prevalence of MYD88 and CD79B mutations [75].

Several entities classified as diffuse large B-cell lymphoproliferative disorders with cutaneous presentation may represent a diagnostic challenge to differentiate from pcDLBCL. Here, the genetic/molecular profile described above takes on paramount importance in reaching the diagnosis. Among these clinical situations can be included some EBV-driven conditions that present primarily in the skin, or involving other extranodal sites such as EBV-positive mucocutaneous ulcer, lymphomatoid granulomatosis or plasmablastic lymphoma. Finally, some cases that do not fit any of the aforementioned well-characterized disorders can be considered as DLBCL not otherwise specified.

5. Concluding Remarks

CTCL carry a complex genomic landscape with several somatic point mutations, CNVs, and fusion events that could contribute to the pathogenesis of the disease. This genetic heterogeneity parallels the different subtypes of specialized T-cells. However, some recurrent hotspots and damaging mutations as well as CNV are shared by the different CTCL subtypes. Pathways that are repeatedly altered include the JAK/STAT, cell cycle/PI3K, TCR activation or NF-κB signaling.

Based on the evidence from different studies, it is likely that different genes such as PLCG1, CARD11, STAT5B, STAT3, FASN, NFKB1 or ZEB1, among many others, could be detected in a variable proportion of patients. Overlapping genomic features are present in multiple non-cutaneous T-cell neoplasms, also including genetic alterations in chromatin regulators such as TET, IDH or DNMT3.

The identification of recurrent alterations in CTCL will allow the design of genetic screening panels improving the diagnosis and better monitoring of the patients. In addition, a number of somatic deletions and duplications identified suggest that chromosomal instability is a feature of CTCL and should be further explored with additional genomic technology. Finally, a mutational and genomic (CNVs and fusion genes) stratification of CTCL patients provides new opportunities for the development or repurposing of therapeutic strategies to face the different entities included with the group of CTCL.

In the case of CBCL, genetic profiling has made possible the improvement in the diagnosis of aggressive forms. However, there are still scenarios that pose diagnostic difficulties. Genetic diagnosis will help to distinguish between primary and secondary cutaneous presentation, as well as between some pcBCLf and pcDLBCL forms.

Author Contributions: Conceptualization, F.G. and R.M.P.; methodology, F.G. and R.M.P.; software, F.G. and R.M.P.; validation, F.G. and R.M.P.; formal analysis, F.G. and R.M.P.; investigation, F.G. and R.M.P.; resources, F.G. and R.M.P.; data curation, F.G. and R.M.P.; writing—original draft preparation, F.G. and R.M.P.; writing—review and editing, F.G. and R.M.P.; visualization, F.G. and R.M.P.; supervision, F.G. and R.M.P.; project administration, F.G. and R.M.P.; funding acquisition, F.G. and R.M.P. All authors have read and agreed to the published version of the manuscript.

Funding: This research was funded by Instituto de Salud Carlos III (ISCIII). Project FI21/00390.

Conflicts of Interest: The authors declare that they have no conflict of interest.

References

1. Willemze, R.; Cerroni, L.; Kempf, W.; Berti, E.; Facchetti, F.; Swerdlow, S.H.; Jaffe, E.S. The 2018 update of the WHO-EORTC classifi-cation for primary cutaneous lymphomas. *Blood* **2019**, *133*, 1703–1714. [CrossRef] [PubMed]
2. Campo, E.; Jaffe, E.S.; Cook, J.R.; Quintanilla-Martinez, L.; Swerdlow, S.H.; Anderson, K.C.; Brousset, P.; Cerroni, L.; de Leval, L.; Dirnhofer, S.; et al. The International Consensus Classification of Mature Lymphoid Neoplasms: A Report from the Clinical Advisory Committee. *Blood* **2022**, *140*, 1229–1253. [CrossRef] [PubMed]
3. Dobos, G.; Pohrt, A.; Ram-Wolff, C.; Lebbé, C.; Bouaziz, J.-D.; Battistella, M.; Bagot, M.; De Masson, A. Epidemiology of Cutaneous T-Cell Lymphomas: A Systematic Review and Meta-Analysis of 16,953 Patients. *Cancers* **2020**, *12*, 2921. [CrossRef] [PubMed]
4. Quaglino, P.; Fava, P.; Pileri, A.; Grandi, V.; Sanlorenzo, M.; Panasiti, V.; Guglielmo, A.; Alberti-Violetti, S.; Novelli, M.; Astrua, C.; et al. Phenotypical Markers, Molecular Mutations, and Immune Microenvironment as Targets for New Treatments in Patients with Mycosis Fungoides and/or Sézary Syndrome. *J. Investig. Dermatol.* **2021**, *141*, 484–495. [CrossRef]
5. Scarisbrick, J.J. The PROCLIPI international registry, an important tool to evaluate the prognosis of cutaneous T cell lympho-mas. *Presse Med.* **2022**, *51*, 104123. [CrossRef]
6. Scarisbrick, J.J.; Prince, H.M.; Vermeer, M.; Quaglino, P.; Horwitz, S.; Porcu, P.; Stadler, R.; Wood, G.S.; Beylot-Barry, M.; Pham-Ledard, A.; et al. Cutaneous Lymphoma International Consortium Study of Outcome in Advanced Stages of Mycosis Fungoides and Sézary Syndrome: Effect of Specific Prognostic Markers on Survival and Development of a Prognostic Model. *J. Clin. Oncol.* **2015**, *33*, 3766–3773. [CrossRef]
7. Agar, N.S.; Wedgeworth, E.; Crichton, S.; Mitchell, T.J.; Cox, M.; Ferreira, S.; Robson, A.; Calonje, E.; Stefanato, C.M.; Wain, E.M.; et al. Sur-vival outcomes and prognostic factors in mycosis fungoides/Sézary syndrome: Validation of the revised International Society for Cutaneous Lymphomas/European Organisation for Research and Treatment of Cancer staging proposal. *J. Clin. Oncol.* **2010**, *28*, 4730–4739. [CrossRef]
8. Iyer, A.; Hennessey, D.; O'Keefe, S.; Patterson, J.; Wang, W.; Wong, G.K.-S.; Gniadecki, R. Branched evolution and genomic intratumor heterogeneity in the pathogenesis of cutaneous T-cell lymphoma. *Blood Adv.* **2020**, *4*, 2489–2500. [CrossRef]
9. Rassek, K.; Iżykowska, K. Single-Cell Heterogeneity of Cutaneous T-Cell Lymphomas Revealed Using RNA-Seq Technologies. *Cancers* **2020**, *12*, 2129. [CrossRef]
10. Herrera, A.; Cheng, A.; Mimitou, E.P.; Seffens, A.; George, D.; Bar-Natan, M.; Heguy, A.; Ruggles, K.V.; Scher, J.U.; Hymes, K.; et al. Mul-timodal single-cell analysis of cutaneous T-cell lymphoma reveals distinct subclonal tissue-dependent signatures. *Blood* **2021**, *138*, 1456–1464. [CrossRef]
11. Prasad, A.; Rabionet, R.; Espinet, B.; Zapata, L.; Puiggros, A.; Melero, C.; Puig, A.; Sarria-Trujillo, Y.; Ossowski, S.; Garcia-Muret, M.P.; et al. Identification of Gene Mutations and Fusion Genes in Patients with Sézary Syndrome. *J. Investig. Dermatol.* **2016**, *136*, 1490–1499. [CrossRef] [PubMed]
12. Kiel, M.J.; Sahasrabuddhe, A.A.; Rolland, D.C.M.; Velusamy, T.; Chung, F.; Schaller, M.; Bailey, N.G.; Betz, B.L.; Miranda, R.N.; Porcu, P.; et al. Genomic analyses reveal recurrent mutations in epigenetic modifiers and the JAK–STAT pathway in Sézary syndrome. *Nat. Commun.* **2015**, *6*, 8370. [CrossRef] [PubMed]
13. Choi, J.; Goh, G.; Walradt, T.; Hong, B.S.; Bunick, C.G.; Chen, K.; Bjornson, R.D.; Maman, Y.; Wang, T.; Tordoff, J.; et al. Genomic landscape of cutaneous T cell lymphoma. *Nat. Genet.* **2015**, *47*, 1011–1019. [CrossRef] [PubMed]
14. McGirt, L.Y.; Jia, P.; Baerenwald, D.A.; Duszynski, R.J.; Dahlman, K.B.; Zic, J.A.; Zwerner, J.P.; Hucks, D.; Dave, U.; Zhao, Z.; et al. Whole-genome sequencing reveals oncogenic mutations in mycosis fungoides. *Blood* **2015**, *126*, 508–519. [CrossRef] [PubMed]
15. Pérez, C.; González-Rincón, J.; Onaindia, A.; Almaráz, C.; García-Díaz, N.; Pisonero, H.; Curiel-Olmo, S.; Gómez, S.; Cereceda, L.; Madureira, R.; et al. Mutated JAK kinases and deregulated STAT activity are potential therapeutic targets in cutaneous T-cell lymphoma. *Haematologica* **2015**, *100*, e450–e453. [CrossRef] [PubMed]
16. Ungewickell, A.; Bhaduri, A.; Rios, E.J.; A Reuter, J.; Lee, C.S.; Mah, A.; Zehnder, A.M.; Ohgami, R.S.; Kulkarni, S.; Armstrong, R.; et al. Genomic analysis of mycosis fungoides and Sézary syndrome identifies recurrent alterations in TNFR2. *Nat. Genet.* **2015**, *47*, 1056–1060. [CrossRef] [PubMed]
17. Vaqué, J.P.; López, G.G.; Monsálvez, V.; Varela, I.; Martinez, N.; Pérez, C.; Domínguez, O.; Graña, O.; Rodriguez-Peralto, J.L.; Rodríguez-Pinilla, S.M.; et al. PLCG1 mutations in cutaneous T-cell lymphomas. *Blood* **2014**, *123*, 2034–2043. [CrossRef]
18. Wang, L.; Ni, X.; Covington, K.R.; Yang, B.Y.; Shiu, J.; Zhang, X.; Xi, L.; Meng, Q.; Langridge, T.; Drummond, J.; et al. Genomic profiling of Sézary syndrome identifies alterations of key T cell signaling and differentiation genes. *Nat. Genet.* **2015**, *47*, 1426–1434. [CrossRef]

19. da Silva Almeida, A.C.; Abate, F.; Khiabanian, H.; Martinez-Escala, E.; Guitart, J.; Tensen, C.P.; Vermeer, M.H.; Rabadan, R.; Ferrando, A.; Palomero, T. The mutational landscape of cutaneous T cell lymphoma and Sezary syndrome. *Nat. Genet.* **2015**, *47*, 1465–1470. [CrossRef]
20. Woollard, W.J.; Pullabhatla, V.; Lorenc, A.; Patel, V.M.; Butler, R.M.; Bayega, A.; Begum, N.; Bakr, F.; Dedhia, K.; Fisher, J.; et al. Candidate driver genes involved in genome maintenance and DNA repair in Sézary syndrome. *Blood* **2016**, *127*, 3387–3397. [CrossRef]
21. Garaicoa, F.H.; Roisman, A.; Arias, M.; Trila, C.; Fridmanis, M.; Abeldaño, A.; Vanzulli, S.; Narbaitz, M.; Slavutsky, I. Genomic imbalances and microRNA transcriptional profiles in patients with mycosis fungoides. *Tumor Biol.* **2016**, *37*, 13637–13647. [CrossRef] [PubMed]
22. Torres, A.N.B.; Cats, D.; Mei, H.; Szuhai, K.; Willemze, R.; Vermeer, M.H.; Tensen, C.P. Genomic analysis reveals recurrent dele-tion of JAK-STAT signaling in- hibitors HNRNPK and SOCS1 in mycosis fungoides. *Genes Chromosom. Cancer* **2018**, *57*, 653–664. [CrossRef] [PubMed]
23. Boonk, S.E.; Zoutman, W.H.; Marie-Cardine, A.; van der Fits, L.; Out-Luiting, J.J.; Mitchell, T.; Tosi, I.; Morris, S.L.; Moriarty, B.; Booken, N.; et al. Evaluation of Immunophenotypic and Molecular Biomarkers for Sézary Syndrome Using Standard Operating Procedures: A Multicenter Study of 59 Patients. *J. Investig. Dermatol.* **2016**, *136*, 1364–1372. [CrossRef] [PubMed]
24. Perez, C.; Mondejar, R.; Garcia-Diaz, N.; Cereceda, L.; Leon, A.; Montes, S.; Durán Vian, C.; Pérez Paredes, M.G.; González-Morán, A.; Alegre de Miguel, V.; et al. Advanced-stage mycosis fungoides: Role of the signal transducer and activator of transcription 3, nuclear factor-kB and nuclear factor of activated T cells pathways. *Br. J. Dermatol.* **2020**, *182*, 147–155. [CrossRef]
25. Caprini, E.; Bresin, A.; Cristofoletti, C.; Citterich, M.H.; Tocco, V.; Scala, E.; Monopoli, A.; Benucci, R.; Narducci, M.G.; Russo, G. Loss of the candidate tumor suppressor ZEB1 (TCF8, ZFHX1A) in Sézary syndrome. *Cell Death Dis.* **2018**, *9*, 1178. [CrossRef]
26. Park, J.; Yang, J.; Wenzel, A.T.; Ramachandran, A.; Lee, W.J.; Daniels, J.C.; Kim, J.; Martinez-Escala, E.; Amankulor, N.; Pro, B.; et al. Genomic analysis of 220 CTCLs identifies a novel recurrent gain-of-function alteration in RLTPR (p.Q575E). *Blood* **2017**, *130*, 1430–1440. [CrossRef]
27. Park, J.; Daniels, J.; Wartewig, T.; Ringbloom, K.G.; Martinez-Escala, M.E.; Choi, S.; Thomas, J.J.; Doukas, P.G.; Yang, J.; Snowden, C.; et al. Integrated genomic analyses of cutaneous T-cell lymphomas reveal the molecular bases for disease heterogeneity. *Blood* **2021**, *138*, 1225–1236. [CrossRef]
28. Chang, L.-W.; Patrone, C.C.; Yang, W.; Rabionet, R.; Gallardo, F.; Espinet, B.; Sharma, M.K.; Girardi, M.; Tensen, C.P.; Vermeer, M.; et al. An Integrated Data Resource for Genomic Analysis of Cutaneous T-Cell Lymphoma. *J. Investig. Dermatol.* **2018**, *138*, 2681–2683. [CrossRef]
29. Sánchez-Beato, M. PD-1 loss and T-cell exhaustion in CTCL tumoral T cells. *Blood* **2021**, *138*, 1201–1203. [CrossRef]
30. Bigas, A.; Rodriguez-Sevilla, J.J.; Espinosa, L.; Gallardo, F. Recent advances in T-cell lymphoid neoplasms. *Exp. Hematol.* **2021**, *106*, 3–18. [CrossRef]
31. van Doorn, R.; van Kester, M.S.; Dijkman, R.; Vermeer, M.H.; Mulder, A.A.; Szuhai, K.; Knijnenburg, J.; Boer, J.M.; Willemze, R.; Tensen, C.P. Oncogenomic analysis of mycosis fungoides reveals major differences with Sezary syndrome. *Blood* **2009**, *113*, 127–136. [CrossRef] [PubMed]
32. Salgado, R.; Servitje, O.; Gallardo, F.; Vermeer, M.H.; Ortiz-Romero, P.L.; Karpova, M.B.; Zipser, M.C.; Muniesa, C.; García-Muret, M.P.; Estrach, T.; et al. Oligonucleotide Array-CGH Identifies Genomic Subgroups and Prognostic Markers for Tumor Stage Mycosis Fungoides. *J. Investig. Dermatol.* **2010**, *130*, 1126–1135. [CrossRef] [PubMed]
33. Sekulic, A.; Liang, W.S.; Tembe, W.; Izatt, T.; Kruglyak, S.; Kiefer, J.A.; Cuyugan, L.; Zismann, V.; Legendre, C.; Pittelkow, M.R.; et al. Personalized treatment of Sézary syndrome by targeting a novel CTLA4:CD28 fusion. *Mol. Genet. Genomic Med.* **2015**, *3*, 130–136. [CrossRef]
34. van Doorn, R.; Slieker, R.C.; Boonk, S.E.; Zoutman, W.H.; Goeman, J.J.; Bagot, M.; Michel, L.; Tensen, C.P.; Willemze, R.; Heijmans, B.T.; et al. Epigenomic Analysis of Sézary Syndrome Defines Patterns of Aberrant DNA Methylation and Identifies Diagnostic Markers. *J. Investig. Dermatol.* **2016**, *136*, 1876–1884. [CrossRef]
35. Gallardo, F.; Esteller, M.; Pujol, R.M.; Costa, C.; Estrach, T.; Servitje, O. Methylation status of the p15, p16 and MGMT promoter genes in primary cutaneous T-cell lymphomas. *Haematologica* **2004**, *89*, 1401–1403.
36. van Doorn, R. Mycosis fungoides: Promoter hypermethylation predicts disease progression. *Br. J. Dermatol.* **2004**, *170*, 1216. [CrossRef] [PubMed]
37. Sandoval, J.; Díaz-Lagares, A.; Salgado, R.; Servitje, O.; Climent, F.; Ortiz-Romero, P.L.; Pérez-Ferriols, A.; Garcia-Muret, M.P.; Estrach, T.; Garcia, M.; et al. MicroRNA Expression Profiling and DNA Methylation Signature for Deregulated MicroRNA in Cutaneous T-Cell Lymphoma. *J. Investig. Dermatol.* **2015**, *135*, 1128–1137. [CrossRef] [PubMed]
38. Ralfkiaer, U.; Lindahl, L.M.; Lindal, L.; Litman, T.; Gjerdrum, L.M.R.; Ahler, C.B.; Gniadecki, R.; Marstrand, T.; Fredholm, S.; Iversen, L.; et al. MicroRNA expression in early mycosis fungoides is distinctly different from atopic dermatitis and advanced cutaneous T-cell lymphoma. *Anticancer Res.* **2014**, *34*, 7207–7217.
39. Manso, R.; Martínez-Magunacelaya, N.; Eraña-Tomás, I.; Monsálvez, V.; Rodríguez-Peralto, J.L.; Ortiz-Romero, P.-L.; Santonja, C.; Cristóbal, I.; A Piris, M.; Rodriguez-Pinilla, S.M. Mycosis fungoides progression could be regulated by microRNAs. *PLoS ONE* **2018**, *13*, e0198477. [CrossRef]
40. Zinzani, P.L.; Bonthapally, V.; Huebner, D.; Lutes, R.; Chi, A.; Pileri, S. Panoptic clinical review of the current and future treatment of relapsed/refractory T-cell lymphomas: Cutaneous T-cell lymphomas. *Crit. Rev. Oncol.* **2016**, *99*, 228–240. [CrossRef]

41. Prieto-Torres, L.; Rodriguez-Pinilla, S.M.; Onaindia, A.; Ara, M.; Requena, L.; Piris, M.Á. CD30-positive primary cutaneous lym-phoproliferative disorders: Molecular alterations and targeted therapies. *Haematologica* **2019**, *104*, 226–235. [CrossRef] [PubMed]
42. Torres, A.N.B.; Melchers, R.C.; Van Grieken, L.; Out-Luiting, J.J.; Mei, H.; Agaser, C.; Kuipers, T.B.; Quint, K.D.; Willemze, R.; Vermeer, M.H.; et al. Whole-genome profiling of primary cutaneous anaplastic large cell lymphoma. *Haematologica* **2021**, *107*, 1619–1632. [CrossRef]
43. Melchers, R.C.; Willemze, R.; van de Loo, M.; van Doorn, R.; Jansen, P.M.; Cleven, A.H.G.; Solleveld, N.; Bekkenk, M.W.; van Kester, M.S.; Diercks, G.F.H.; et al. Clinical, Histologic, and Molecular Characteristics of Anaplastic Lymphoma Kinase-positive Primary Cu-taneous Anaplastic Large Cell Lymphoma. *Am. J. Surg. Pathol.* **2020**, *44*, 776–781. [CrossRef]
44. Maurus, K.; Appenzeller, S.; Roth, S.; Brändlein, S.; Kneitz, H.; Goebeler, M.; Rosenwald, A.; Geissinger, E.; Wobser, M. Recurrent On-cogenic JAK and STAT Alterations in Cutaneous CD30-Positive Lymphoproliferative Disorders. *Journal Invest Dermatol.* **2020**, *140*, 2023–2031. [CrossRef] [PubMed]
45. Velusamy, T.; Kiel, M.J.; Sahasrabuddhe, A.A.; Rolland, D.; Dixon, C.A.; Bailey, N.G.; Betz, B.L.; Brown, N.A.; Hristov, A.C.; Wilcox, R.A.; et al. A novel recurrent NPM1-TYK2 gene fusion in cutaneous CD30-positive lymphoproliferative disorders. *Blood* **2014**, *124*, 3768–3771. [CrossRef]
46. Mao, X.; Orchard, G.; Lillington, D.M.; Russell-Jones, R.; Young, B.D.; Whittaker, S. Genetic alterations in primary cutaneous CD30+ anaplastic large cell lymphoma. *Genes Chromosom. Cancer* **2003**, *37*, 176–185. [CrossRef]
47. Pina-Oviedo, S.; Ortiz-Hidalgo, C.; Carballo-Zarate, A.A.; Zarate-Osorno, A. ALK-Negative Anaplastic Large Cell Lymphoma: Current Concepts and Molecular Pathogenesis of a Heterogeneous Group of Large T-Cell Lymphomas. *Cancers* **2021**, *13*, 4667. [CrossRef]
48. Karai, L.J.; Kadin, M.E.; Hsi, E.D.; Sluzevich, J.C.; Ketterling, R.P.; Knudson, R.A.; Feldman, A.L. Chromosomal Rearrangements of 6p25.3 Define a New Subtype of Lymphomatoid Papulosis. *Am. J. Surg. Pathol.* **2013**, *37*, 1173–1181. [CrossRef]
49. Chott, A.; Vonderheid, E.C.; Olbricht, S.; Miao, N.-N.; Balk, S.P.; Kadin, M.E. The Same Dominant T Cell Clone Is Present in Multiple Regressing Skin Lesions and Associated T Cell Lymphomas of Patients with Lymphomatoid Papulosis. *J. Investig. Dermatol.* **1996**, *106*, 696–700. [CrossRef]
50. Cordel, N.; Tressières, B.; D'Incan, M.; Machet, L.; Grange, F.; Estève, É.; Dalac, S.; Ingen-Housz-Oro, S.; Bagot, M.; Beylot-Barry, M.; et al. Frequency and Risk Factors for Associated Lymphomas in Patients with Lymphomatoid Papulosis. *Oncologist* **2015**, *21*, 76–83. [CrossRef]
51. de Souza, A.; el-Azhary, R.; Camilleri, M.F.; Wada, D.A.; Appert, D.L.; Gibson, L.E. In search of prognostic indicators for lymphomatoid papulosis: A retrospective study of 123 patients. *J. Am. Acad. Dermatol.* **2012**, *66*, 928–937. [CrossRef] [PubMed]
52. Gayden, T.; Sepulveda, F.E.; Khuong-Quang, D.-A.; Pratt, J.; Valera, E.T.; Garrigue, A.; Kelso, S.; Sicheri, F.; Mikael, L.G.; Hamel, N.; et al. Germline HAVCR2 mutations altering TIM-3 characterize subcutaneous panniculitis-like T cell lymphomas with hemopha-gocytic lymphohistiocytic syndrome. *Nat. Gen.* **2018**, *50*, 1650–1657. [CrossRef] [PubMed]
53. Koh, J.; Jang, I.; Mun, S.; Lee, C.; Cha, H.J.; Oh, Y.H.; Kim, J.M.; Han, J.H.; Paik, J.H.; Cho, J.; et al. Genetic profiles of subcutaneous pannicu-litis-like T-cell lymphoma and clinicopathological impact of HAVCR2 mutations. *Blood Adv.* **2021**, *5*, 3919–3930. [CrossRef]
54. Daniels, J.; Doukas, P.G.; Escala, M.E.M.; Ringbloom, K.G.; Shih, D.J.H.; Yang, J.; Tegtmeyer, K.; Park, J.; Thomas, J.J.; Selli, M.E.; et al. Cellular origins and genetic landscape of cutaneous gamma delta T cell lymphomas. *Nat. Commun.* **2020**, *11*, 1806. [CrossRef]
55. Berti, E.; Tomasini, D.; Vermeer, M.H.; Meijer, C.J.; Alessi, E.; Willemze, R. Primary Cutaneous CD8-Positive Epidermotropic Cytotoxic T Cell Lymphomas: A Distinct Clinicopathological Entity with an Aggressive Clinical Behavior. *Am. J. Pathol.* **1999**, *155*, 483–492. [CrossRef]
56. Fanoni, D.; Corti, L.; Alberti-Violetti, S.; Tensen, C.P.; Venegoni, L.; Vermeer, M.; Willemze, R.; Berti, E. Array-based CGH of primary cutaneous CD8+ aggressive EPIDERMO-tropic cytotoxic T-cell lymphoma. *Genes Chromosom. Cancer* **2018**, *57*, 622–629. [CrossRef] [PubMed]
57. Lee, K.; Evans, M.G.; Yang, L.; Ng, S.; Snowden, C.; Khodadoust, M.S.; A Brown, R.; Trum, N.A.; Querfeld, C.; Doan, L.T.; et al. Primary Cytotoxic T Cell Lymphomas Harbor Recurrent Targetable Alterations in the JAK-STAT Pathway. *Blood* **2021**, *138*, 2435–2440. [CrossRef]
58. Bastidas-Torres, A.N.; Cats, D.; Out-Luiting, J.J.; Fanoni, D.; Mei, H.; Venegoni, L.; Willemze, R.; Vermeer, M.H.; Berti, E.; Tensen, C.P. De-regulation of JAK2 signaling underlies primary cutaneous CD8+ aggressive epidermotropic cytotoxic T-cell lymphoma. *Haematologica* **2022**, *107*, 702–714.
59. Lee, S.; Park, H.Y.; Kang, S.Y.; Kim, S.J.; Hwang, J.; Lee, S.; Kwak, S.H.; Park, K.S.; Yoo, H.Y.; Kim, W.S.; et al. Genetic alterations of JAK/STAT cascade and histone modification in extranodal NK/T-cell lymphoma nasal type. *Oncotarget* **2015**, *6*, 17764–17776. [CrossRef]
60. Xie, Y.; Wang, T.; Wang, L. Hydroa vacciniforme-like lymphoproliferative disorder: A study of clinicopathology and whole-exome sequencing in Chinese patients. *J. Dermatol. Sci.* **2020**, *99*, 128–134. [CrossRef]
61. Kempf, W.; Mitteldorf, C.; Battistella, M.; Willemze, R.; Cerroni, L.; Santucci, M.; Geissinger, E.; Jansen, P.; Vermeer, M.H.; Marschalko, M.; et al. Primary cutaneous peripheral T-cell lymphoma, not otherwise specified: Results of a multicentre European

Organization for Research and Treatment of Cancer (EORTC) cutaneous lymphoma taskforce study on the clinico-pathological and prog-nostic features. *J. Eur. Acad. Dermatol. Venereol.* **2021**, *35*, 658–668. [CrossRef] [PubMed]
62. Palomero, T.; Couronné, L.; Khiabanian, H.; Kim, M.Y.; Ambesi-Impiombato, A.; Perez-Garcia, A.; Carpenter, Z.; Abate, F.; Allegretta, M.; Haydu, J.E.; et al. Recurrent mutations in epigenetic regulators, RHOA and FYN kinase in peripheral T cell lymphomas. *Nat. Genet.* **2014**, *46*, 166–170. [CrossRef] [PubMed]
63. Watatani, Y.; Sato, Y.; Miyoshi, H.; Sakamoto, K.; Nishida, K.; Gion, Y.; Nagata, Y.; Shiraishi, Y.; Chiba, K.; Tanaka, H.; et al. Molecular heterogeneity in peripheral T-cell lymphoma, not otherwise specified revealed by comprehensive genetic profiling. *Leukemia* **2019**, *33*, 2867–2883. [CrossRef] [PubMed]
64. Senff, N.J.; Noordijk, E.M.; Kim, Y.H.; Bagot, M.; Berti, E.; Cerroni, L.; Dummer, R.; Duvic, M.; Hoppe, R.T.; Pimpinelli, N.; et al. European Organization for Research and Treatment of Cancer and International Society for Cutaneous Lymphoma consensus recom-mendations for the management of cutaneous B-cell lymphomas. *Blood* **2008**, *112*, 1600–1609. [CrossRef]
65. Szablewski, V.; Ingen-Housz-Oro, S.; Baia, M.; Delfau-Larue, M.H.; Copie-Bergman, C.; Ortonne, N. Primary Cutaneous Follicle Center Lymphomas Expressing BCL2 Protein Frequently Harbor BCL2 Gene Break and May Present 1p36 Deletion: A Study of 20 Cases. *Am. J. Surg. Pathol.* **2016**, *40*, 127–136. [CrossRef]
66. Barasch, N.J.; Liu, Y.-C.; Ho, J.; Bailey, N.; Aggarwal, N.; Cook, J.R.; Swerdlow, S.H. The molecular landscape and other distinctive features of primary cutaneous follicle center lymphoma. *Hum. Pathol.* **2020**, *106*, 93–105. [CrossRef]
67. Zhou, X.A.; Yang, J.; Ringbloom, K.G.; Martinez-Escala, M.E.; Stevenson, K.E.; Wenzel, A.T.; Fantini, D.; Martin, H.K.; Moy, A.P.; Morgan, E.A.; et al. Genomic landscape of cutaneous follicular lymphomas reveals 2 subgroups with clinically predictive molecular features. *Blood Adv.* **2021**, *5*, 649–661. [CrossRef]
68. Edinger, J.T.; Kant, J.A.; Swerdlow, S.H. Cutaneous Marginal Zone Lymphomas Have Distinctive Features and Include 2 Subsets. *Am. J. Surg. Pathol.* **2010**, *34*, 1830–1841. [CrossRef]
69. Servitje, O.; Muniesa, C.; Benavente, Y.; Monsálvez, V.; Garcia-Muret, M.P.; Gallardo, F.; Domingo-Domenech, E.; Lucas, A.; Climent, F.; Rodriguez-Peralto, J.L.; et al. Primary cutaneous marginal zone B-cell lymphoma: Response to treatment and disease-free sur-vival in a series of 137 patients. *J. Am. Acad. Dermatol.* **2013**, *69*, 357–365. [CrossRef]
70. Rodríguez-Sevilla, J.J.; Salar, A. Recent Advances in the Genetic of MALT Lymphomas. *Cancers* **2021**, *14*, 176. [CrossRef]
71. Vela, V.; Juskevicius, D.; Dirnhofer, S.; Menter, T.; Tzankov, A. Mutational landscape of marginal zone B-cell lymphomas of various origin: Organotypic alterations and diagnostic potential for assignment of organ origin. *Virchows Arch.* **2021**, *480*, 403–413. [CrossRef] [PubMed]
72. Gros, A.; Menguy, S.; Bobée, V.; Ducharme, O.; Cassaigne, I.C.; Vergier, B.; Parrens, M.; Beylot-Barry, M.; Pham-Ledard, A.; Ruminy, P.; et al. Integrative diagnosis of primary cutaneous large B-cell lymphomas supports the relevance of cell of origin profiling. *PLoS ONE* **2022**, *17*, e0266978. [CrossRef] [PubMed]
73. Menguy, S.; Gros, A.; Pham-Ledard, A.; Battistella, M.; Ortonne, N.; Comoz, F.; Balme, B.; Szablewski, V.; Lamant, L.; Carlotti, A.; et al. MYD88 Somatic Mutation Is a Diagnostic Criterion in Primary Cutaneous Large B-Cell Lymphoma. *J. Investig. Dermatol.* **2016**, *136*, 1741–1744. [CrossRef]
74. Mareschal, S.; Pham-Ledard, A.; Viailly, P.J.; Dubois, S.; Bertrand, P.; Maingonnat, C.; Fontanilles, M.; Bohers, E.; Ruminy, P.; Tournier, I.; et al. Identification of Somatic Mutations in Primary Cutaneous Diffuse Large B-Cell Lymphoma, Leg Type by Massive Parallel Sequencing. *J. Investig. Dermatol.* **2017**, *137*, 1984–1994. [CrossRef] [PubMed]
75. Schrader, A.M.R.; Jansen, P.M.; Willemze, R.; Vermeer, M.; Cleton-Jansen, A.-M.; Somers, S.F.; Veelken, H.; van Eijk, R.; Kraan, W.; Kersten, M.J.; et al. High prevalence of MYD88 and CD79B mutations in intravascular large B-cell lymphoma. *Blood* **2018**, *131*, 2086–2089. [CrossRef]

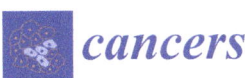

Review

Beyond Pathogenic *RUNX1* Germline Variants: The Spectrum of Somatic Alterations in RUNX1-Familial Platelet Disorder with Predisposition to Hematologic Malignancies

Alisa Förster [†], Melanie Decker [†], Brigitte Schlegelberger and Tim Ripperger *

Department of Human Genetics, Hannover Medical School, Carl-Neuberg-Str. 1, 30625 Hannover, Germany; foerster.alisa@mh-hannover.de (A.F.); decker.melanie@mh-hannover.de (M.D.); schlegelberger.brigitte@mh-hannover.de (B.S.)
* Correspondence: ripperger.tim@mh-hannover.de
† These authors contributed equally to this work.

Simple Summary: Pathogenic germline variants affecting *RUNX1* are associated with qualitative and/or quantitative platelet defects, and predispose to hematologic malignancies. The latter manifests in approximately 44% of carriers and can occur from early childhood to late adulthood. In addition to the predisposing *RUNX1* germline variant, the acquisition of somatic genetic alterations is presumed to drive leukemic transformation in an inflammatory bone marrow niche. The spectrum of somatic mutations occurs heterogeneously between individuals, even within families, and there is no clear genotype–phenotype correlation. In this review, we summarize previously published patients harboring (likely) pathogenic *RUNX1* germline alterations in whom somatic alterations were additionally analyzed. We provide an overview of their phenotypes and the most frequent somatic genetic alterations.

Abstract: Pathogenic loss-of-function *RUNX1* germline variants cause autosomal dominantly-inherited familial platelet disorder with predisposition to hematologic malignancies (RUNX1-FPD). RUNX1-FPD is characterized by incomplete penetrance and a broad spectrum of clinical phenotypes, even within affected families. Heterozygous *RUNX1* germline variants set the basis for leukemogenesis, but, on their own, they are not transformation-sufficient. Somatically acquired secondary events targeting *RUNX1* and/or other hematologic malignancy-associated genes finally lead to MDS, AML, and rarely other hematologic malignancies including lymphoid diseases. The acquisition of different somatic variants is a possible explanation for the variable penetrance and clinical heterogeneity seen in RUNX1-FPD. However, individual effects of secondary variants are not yet fully understood. Here, we review 91 cases of RUNX1-FPD patients who predominantly harbor somatic variants in genes such as *RUNX1*, *TET2*, *ASXL1*, *BCOR*, *PHF6*, *SRSF2*, *NRAS*, and *DNMT3A*. These cases illustrate the importance of secondary events in the development and progression of RUNX1-FPD-associated hematologic malignancies. The leukemia-driving interplay of predisposing germline variants and acquired variants remain to be elucidated to better understand clonal evolution and malignant transformation and finally allow risk-adapted surveillance and targeted therapeutic measures to prevent leukemia.

Keywords: *RUNX1* germline variants; RUNX1-FPD; leukemia predisposition; hematologic malignancies; somatic mutations

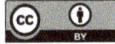

1. Introduction

Over the past decades, it has become evident that the RUNX family transcription factor 1 (RUNX1) is a key player in embryogenesis and hematopoiesis [1]. RUNX1 is encoded by on the long arm of chromosome 21 (i.e., 21q22.12). It was previously also known as acute myeloid leukemia 1 (*AML1*), core-binding factor A2 (*CBFA2*), and Runt-related transcription factor 1. Three major protein isoforms of RUNX1 are known (i.e., RUNX1a, RUNX1b, and RUNX1c). Their expression is regulated by two different promoters [2,3]. The distal P1 promotor initiates the generation of transcription variant 1, which is translated to isoform RUNX1c [3]. The proximal P2 promotor and an alternative splicing mechanism drive the expression of transcription variant 2 and 3, encoding for isoform RUNX1b and RUNX1a, respectively [2]. All RUNX1 isoforms can form heterodimers with core-binding factor beta (CBFB). As a core-binding factor complex, they function as transcriptional regulators [4]. Binding to CBFB significantly enhances the DNA-binding ability of RUNX1 [5,6] and protects RUNX1 from ubiquitin-mediated proteasomal degradation [7]. The best-studied function of RUNX1 is the activation of transcription of its target genes [5,8]. Through its interplay with many cofactors and interaction partners, RUNX1 can also lead to the repression of transcription [9,10]. The essential role of RUNX1 in stem cell differentiation, especially in hematopoiesis, is highlighted by the absence of definitive hematopoietic stem cells in homozygous *Runx1* knock-out mice and their hemorrhagic death at day E.12.5 of development [11–14]. RUNX1 is involved in the differentiation of lymphoid and myeloid lineage cells, especially in the megakaryocytic lineage. Moreover, RUNX1 promotes gene expression for megakaryocyte development, while genes important for erythropoiesis are suppressed [11,15].

Somatic *RUNX1* aberrations are recurrently detected in various myeloid malignancies, such as myelodysplastic syndrome (MDS), acute myeloid leukemia (AML) [16], and myeloproliferative neoplasms. Characteristic *RUNX1* translocations (i.e., t(12;21), t(8;21), and t(3;21)), are considered as common events in hematologic malignancies (HM) [17]. To date, about 70 chromosomal translocations encompassing *RUNX1* have been reported in patients with HM [18,19]. Noteworthy, acquired mono- or biallelic somatic *RUNX1* variants, including deletions, missense, splice site, frameshift, and nonsense variants, correlate with worse prognosis in sporadic AML, MDS, and T-cell acute lymphoblastic leukemia (T-ALL) [20–23]. Therefore, AML with somatic *RUNX1* variants is considered a biologically distinct AML subtype associated with poor outcomes in the 2016 revision of the World Health Organization (WHO) classification of myeloid neoplasms and acute leukemia [24].

Regarding germline mutations, *RUNX1* was first associated with leukemia predisposition in 1999 [25]. Nowadays, pathogenic germline loss-of-function *RUNX1* variants are known to be causative of autosomal dominantly inherited familial platelet disorder with a predisposition to hematologic malignancies (RUNX1-FPD, FPDMM, FPD/AML, ORPHA: 71290, MIM: 601399), also recognized in the 2016 WHO classification of myeloid neoplasms and acute leukemia [24]. Patients with RUNX1-FPD often suffer from mild to moderate thrombocytopenia and/or platelet aggregation defects [25–27]. Remarkably, about 44% of individuals will develop HM, usually MDS or AML [28]. The age of onset of HM ranges from 6 to 76 years with an average age at diagnosis of 33 years [29,30]. Notably, several groups identified (likely) pathogenic germline *RUNX1* variants in up to 3% of AML patients [31–33]. Others reported about 8% of germline *RUNX1*-mutated cases in their AML study cohorts, although they were not solely (likely) pathogenic [34]. Future investigations based on proper germline material and variant classification are required to elucidate the impact of (likely) pathogenic *RUNX1* variants on sporadically appearing HM. In general, the incidence of (likely) pathogenic germline *RUNX1* variants might be underestimated due to no or mild non-malignant symptoms and/or late disease onset. Additionally, *RUNX1* copy number alterations (CNAs) are not always properly investigated in routine diagnostics and some next-generation sequencing (NGS) approaches are hampered by insufficient coverage of *RUNX1*. To date, more than 200 families with RUNX1-FPD have been reported [35]. However, the penetrance is incomplete and the expressivity is variable as the spectrum of clinical phenotypes, even within families, is broad [36,37]. *RUNX1* germline variants are classified as either (likely) benign, variant of uncertain significance (VUS), or (likely) pathogenic based on specific guidelines proposed by the ClinGen Myeloid Malignancy Variant Curation Expert Panel (MM-VCEP) [38], which was recently updated (https://www.clinicalgenome.org/affiliation/50034/, accessed on 7 June 2022).

Yet, regarding these guidelines, many *RUNX1* variants are classified as VUS hence their probable pathogenicity needs further evaluation for classification such as functional assays, including DNA binding, hetero-dimerization with CBFB and transactivation, as performed by Decker and colleagues [39,40].

As genetic analyses have evolved from single-gene testing to NGS, different HM-associated and candidate genes can be simultaneously investigated. These advantages have not only led to the application of NGS in the identification of germline predispositions but, moreover, its implementation in analyzing the somatic mutation profile of blood and bone marrow. Somatically acquired mutations reported in HM-patients with germline *RUNX1* variants are suspected to be the cause of clonal transformation [15,41,42]. For example, Gaidzik et al. reported germline and somatic *RUNX1* variants predominantly co-occurring with a complex pattern of somatic gene mutations frequently involving mutations in epigenetic modifiers (e.g., *ASXL1*, *IDH2*, *KMT2A*, and *EZH2*), components of the spliceosome complex (e.g., *SRSF2* and *SF3B1*) and, moreover, *STAG2*, *PHF6*, and *BCOR* [43]. Additionally, acquired variants in the RAS-pathway genes (e.g., *HRAS*, *KRAS*, and *NRAS*) and other genes such as *CBL*, *CDC25C*, *FLT3*, *NFE2*, and *WT1* were described [36,44]. Loss of *RUNX1* heterozygosity and trisomy 21 with duplication of the mutant allele are also common secondary events [45]. Recently, evidence arose that the inflammatory milieu may promote progression to HM in individuals with germline susceptibility [46]. This supports the notion that germline *RUNX1* mutations are not solely sufficient to develop neoplasia, but favor the acquisition of additional somatic mutations in an inflammatory environment required for the development of overt leukemia [15]. Apart from this, the acquisition of different somatic variants may explain the variable penetrance and clinical heterogeneity seen in RUNX1-FPD. Nevertheless, understanding the clonal evolution of hematopoietic cells in germline *RUNX1*-mutated patients leading to HM remains to be elucidated [36,47].

2. Methods

To better define the spectrum of acquired variants in individuals with (likely) pathogenic *RUNX1* germline variants, we performed an extended systematic literature search in the PubMed database using the terms "RUNX1 germline", "RUNX1 predisposition", and "familial leukemia". In this review, we initially included only patients with *RUNX1* germline variants in which somatic variants were investigated irrespective of variant findings. However, we excluded two cases in total, as these samples were not comparable to the other reviewed cases: one was described as a therapy-related AML that developed after T-ALL in a patient with the RUNX1 alteration p.(Gln335Argfs*259) [45,48] whereas the other individual harboring the *RUNX1* variant c.611G>A p.(Arg204Gln) was diagnosed with T-ALL, MDS, and secondary AML at age 22, 23, and 24, respectively [36].

If necessary, nomenclature of *RUNX1* variants was adapted to transcript variant 1 (NM_001754.4) encoding for isoform RUNX1c. All reported *RUNX1* germline variants were (re)classified using current recommendations according to the second version of the ClinGen MM-VCEP specifications of the ACMG/AMP variant interpretation guidelines [38] (https://www.clinicalgenome.org/affiliation/50034/, accessed on 7 June 2022). For further evaluation, we selected only patients with (likely) pathogenic *RUNX1* germline variants based on the current guidelines as only these were considered as confirmed RUNX1-FPD cases in the present study. Following this approach, we retrospectively enrolled 91 individuals out of 60 families reported in the original publications listed in Appendix A. To gain insights into the molecular mechanisms leading to malignant transformation and disease heterogeneity in RUNX1-FPD, we compared and evaluated the potential interplay of germline *RUNX1* variants, acquired somatic alterations and reported clinical phenotypes.

3. Disease-Causing *RUNX1* Germline Variants and Associated Phenotypes in RUNX1-FPD

The integrated results of 91 included patients are given in Table 1 summarizing their clinical and genetic features. The cohort of enrolled patients mirrored the known broad phenotypic heterogeneity of patients with RUNX1-FPD. Of 91 individuals, 30 (33%) cases had no signs of HM (Figure 1). Out of these, the majority of individuals (i.e., 28, 93%) were reported with cytopenia. Two individuals (6%) had no FPD-related symptoms. This is in line with previous findings reporting thrombocytopenia as the most common phenotypic feature seen in individuals with (likely) pathogenic germline *RUNX1* variant and no HM [38]. In contrast to the previously reported HM risk of 44% [28], 61 out of the 91 enrolled patients (67%) were reported with HM. However, this high percentage is biased by our inclusion criteria focusing on patients with reported screenings for somatic alterations being a general standard in HM diagnostics but yet not in individuals with a genetic predisposition to HM. Regarding the type of malignant neoplasms, 37 individuals were diagnosed with AML (61%), nine with MDS (15%), seven with MDS/AML (11%), four with lymphoblastic HM (i.e., B- and T-ALL, 7%), and four with other myeloid malignancies (i.e., myeloproliferative neoplasm, chronic myelomonocytic leukemia, juvenile myelomonocytic leukemia, 7%) (Figure 1), which resembles the distribution of malignancy types in the RUNX1 database (RUNX1db) [35]. Recently, evidence emerged that besides T-ALL also lymphoid malignancies of B-cell origin are part of the phenotypic spectrum, even though *RUNX1* germline variants are primarily associated with myeloid malignancies [47,49]. Yet, larger cohorts are needed to evaluate this assumption.

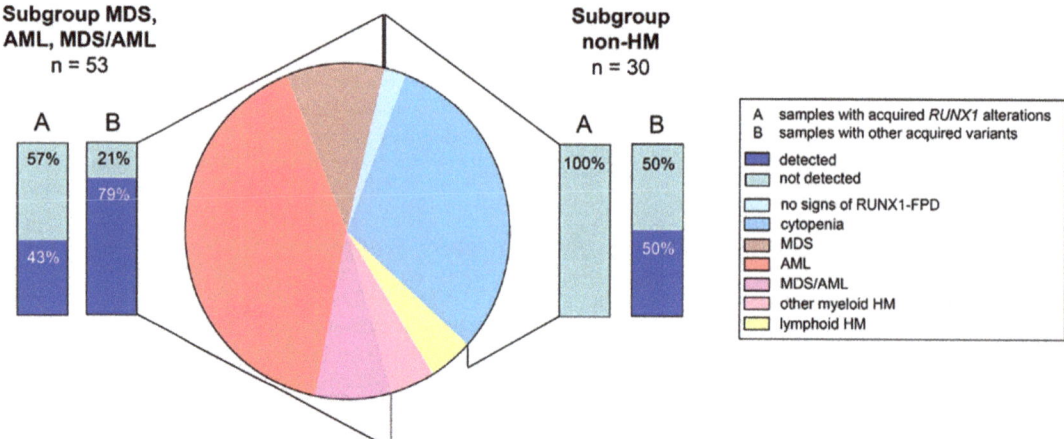

Figure 1. Phenotype and somatic variant status of our retrospective RUNX1-FPD cohort. Distribution of phenotypic subgroups within the retrospective RUNX1-FPD cohort including ratios of cases with somatic RUNX1 variants and ratios of other acquired variants. AML—acute myeloid leukemia, HM—hematologic malignancies, MDS—myelodysplastic syndrome, MDS/AML—patients who developed myelodysplastic syndrome and subsequently acute myeloid leukemia, non-HM—cases without reported hematologic malignancies, RUNX1-FPD—familial platelet disorder with predisposition to hematologic malignancies.

Among the herein analyzed 60 families, 17 (28%) carried frameshift variants, 15 (25%) nonsense variants, and 14 (23%) whole gene or exonic deletions. Therefore, frameshift variants, nonsense variants and deletions were found to be the most common variant types among all (likely) pathogenic germline *RUNX1* alterations. Further germline variant types comprise 13 (17%) missense variants and one (3%) splice site variant (Table 1, Figure 2). The most common disease-causing variant type in the RUNX1db are missense variants and deletions, followed by *RUNX1* frameshift and nonsense variants [35]. Noteworthy, Homan et al. reported (likely) pathogenic splice site variants in 11% of RUNX1-FPD families, whereas only one splice site variant could be included in the present study. This difference in the occurrence of *RUNX1* germline splice site variants indicates that the analyzed cohort underlies a certain bias. All 27 germline *RUNX1* missense variants are located within the Runt homology domain (RHD, amino acid 77-204), whereas nonsense and frameshift variants are evenly distributed over the gene (Figure 2), which is in line with published studies investigating type and location of germline and somatic *RUNX1* variants [36,50,51]. Additionally, all identified (likely) pathogenic germline *RUNX1* frameshift variants are unique to the affected families in the RUNX1db [35] and in the herein analyzed cohort. Other germline variant types occur in more than one individual and/or family. Arg166, Arg201 and Arg204 are the most frequently mutated RUNX1 amino acid (aa) positions in RUNX1-FPD in the RUNX1db [35] as well as in the present cohort (Figure 2). Among 30 individuals without HM, germline *RUNX1* missense and nonsense variants were reported in 37% and 10% of cases, respectively. In contrast, patients with MDS, AML or MDS/AML had missense and nonsense variants in 23% and 38% of cases, respectively. These findings may suggest that nonsense rather than missense germline *RUNX1* variants might promote progression to MDS and/or AML in the analyzed cohort. However, Brown and colleagues did not find a significant correlation between the type of variant and the risk of HM by analyzing 82 *RUNX1* germline variants [36]. Previous studies suggested that germline *RUNX1* variants causing dominant-negative effects rather than variants leading to haploinsufficiency might more potently drive the malignant transformation towards HM [27,52,53]. This hypothesis could not be supported by the analyzed RUNX1-FPD patients herein. *RUNX1* haploinsufficiency variants due to nonsense and frameshift mutations predicted to undergo nonsense-mediated decay (i.e., affecting positions before codon 304 of RUNX1c, [38]), as well as whole gene deletions, are not predominantly found in the pre-HM group of our analyses. Of note, information (i.e., functional data) on *RUNX1* missense variants regarding their dominant-negative effect is not given for most alterations. In summary, larger and unbiased cohorts are necessary to specify possible genotype-phenotype correlations in RUNX1-FPD. Available data does not justify variant type-specific risk stratifications regarding HM. The ongoing NIH Natural History Study of Hematologic and Premalignant Conditions Associated with RUNX1 Mutation will provide further insights into the natural cause of the disease and may show correlations between variant type and HM risk, as *RUNX1* germline carriers are intensively monitored over time independent of their clinical phenotype (study number 19-HG-0059, https://www.genome.gov/Current-NHGRI-Clinical-Studies/hematologic-and-premalignant-conditions-associated-with-RUNX1-mutation, accessed on 7 June 2022).

The median age of RUNX1-FPD diagnosis was highly variable ($n = 63$, median 42 years, range 0.08–74). Relevant information was not given for 28 patients (Table 1). The median age at diagnosis was lower for patients with MDS (median 33 years, range 7–58) compared to patients diagnosed with AML (median 43 years, range 0.08–74). This might illustrate the notion that in some patients, MDS might transform into AML later on. Previously, the median age at diagnosis of HM was reported as 29–35 years among *RUNX1* germline carriers [37,54]. In the RUNX1db, the median age at diagnosis is 43 (range 3–69) and for pre-leukemic patients 34 (range 1–76) [35]. In 20% of RUNX1-FPD patients, a childhood-onset malignancy was observed [37]. In line with this, our retrospective cohort encompasses 15% of cases of minors including six AML, two MDS, one B-ALL, one chronic myelomonocytic leukemia, and one juvenile myelomonocytic leukemia. Conclusively, the age of onset in our retrospective cohort and the ratio of childhood-onset cases are comparable to other RUNX1-FPD cohorts. However, it should be noted that the definition of "age at diagnosis" may vary from study to study, as some authors used this term at the time of first reported symptoms and others at the time of genetic diagnosis. Additionally, caution should be taken when comparing simplex RUNX1-FPD patients and individuals from RUNX1-FPD families, since healthy family members of index patients diagnosed by predictive testing might get earlier investigations regarding their symptoms and the presence of clonal hematopoiesis than diseased individuals without any family history of HM diagnosed due to their own phenotype.

A further limitation of the retrospective analyses in the present study was the different approaches in the included publications in order to determine the germline origin of a detected *RUNX1* variant. Authors considered variants to be of germline origin via segregation analysis, analysis of DNA derived from buccal swabs, fibroblasts, or remission material as well as approaches comparing tumor and normal tissues. When molecular profiling reveals a pathogenic variant in hematologic tissues with a variant allele fraction of at least 30% in a gene known to confer inherited cancer risk, a germline origin should be suspected and subsequently verified [55]. This and germline testing, in general, can be carried out by analysis of DNA extracted from cultured fibroblasts [56] or by segregation analyses. For the latter, however, the germline origin of the respective variant cannot be excluded if the variant is not detected in family members. Notably, genetic testing must also include analysis of copy number changes by NGS or array-CGH in order to pinpoint *RUNX1* CNAs. Taken together, we want to point out that the method (i.e., Sanger sequencing or NGS), as well as tissue (i.e., bone marrow, buccal swabs, peripheral blood, fibroblasts, fingernails), is important in terms of detection of a potential germline variant.

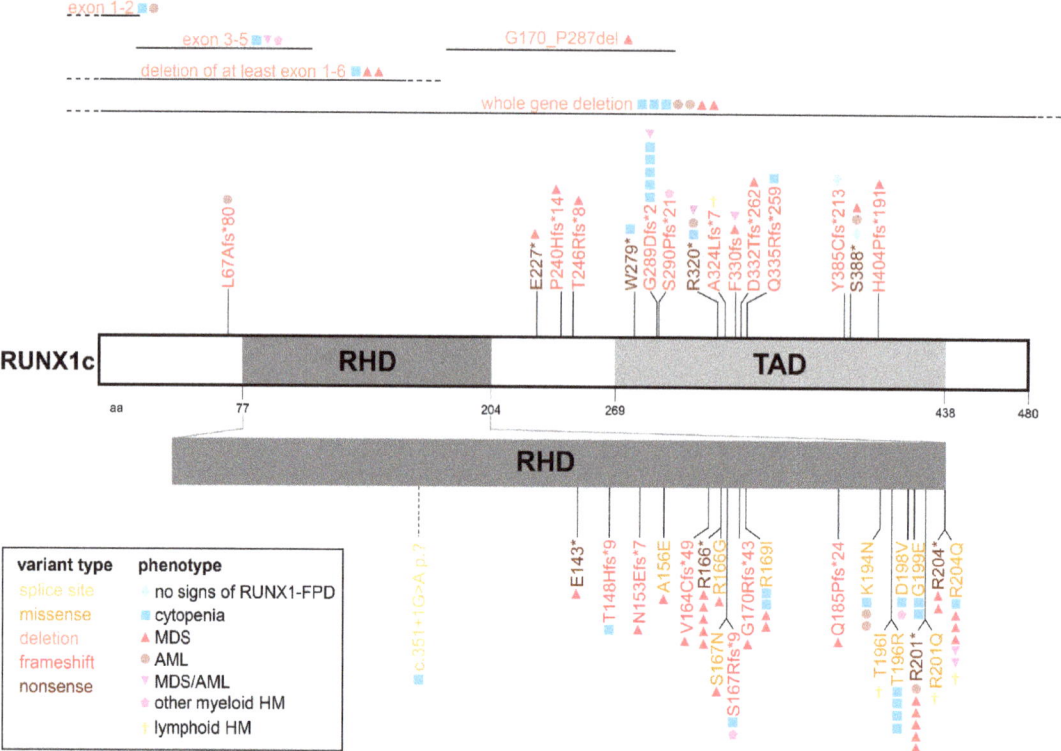

Figure 2. *RUNX1* germline variants in the retrospective RUNX1-FPD cohort. Schematic visualization of germline *RUNX1* variants included in the retrospective RUNX1-FPD cohort including variant type and patients' phenotype. Nomenclature refers to transcript variant 1 (NM_001754.4) encoding for isoform RUNX1c. AML—acute myeloid leukemia, HM—hematologic malignancies, MDS—myelodysplastic syndrome, MDS/AML—patients who developed MDS and subsequently AML, RHD—runt-homology domain, RUNX1-FPD—familial platelet disorder with predisposition to hematologic malignancies, TAD—transactivation domain.

Table 1. Comparison of clinical and genetic characteristics of the retrospectively reviewed cohort of 91 patients with RUNX1-FPD.

	All Cases (n = 91): Number (Range or %)	No Signs of RUNX1-FPD (n = 2): Number (Range or %)	Cytopenia (n = 28): Number (Range or %)	MDS (n = 9): Number (Range or %)	AML (n = 37): Number (Range or %)	MDS/AML (n = 7): Number (Range or %)	Other Myeloid HM [a] (n = 4): Number (Range or %)	Lymphoid HM [b] (n = 4): Number (Range or %)
Characteristics								
median age at diagnosis (years) [c]	42 (0.08–74)	35.5 (18–53)	52.5 (3–71)	29 (7–58)	42 (0.08–74)	55 (37–65)	37.5 (10–63)	29 (16–42)
age at diagnosis, NA	28 (31%)	0 (0%)	18 (64%)	2 (22%)	7 (19%)	1 (14%)	0 (0%)	0 (0%)
Germline RUNX1 variant type								
missense	27 (30%)	0 (0%)	11 (39%)	2 (22%)	8 (22%)	2 (29%)	1 (25%)	3 (75%)
nonsense	23 (25%)	1 (50%)	2 (7%)	3 (33%)	15 (41%)	2 (29%)	0 (0%)	0 (0%)
frameshift	24 (26%)	1 (50%)	8 (29%)	1 (11%)	9 (24%)	2 (29%)	2 (50%)	1 (25%)
deletion [d]	16 (18%)	0 (0%)	6 (21%)	3 (33%)	5 (14%)	1 (14%)	1 (25%)	0 (0%)
splice site	1 (1%)	0 (0%)	1 (4%)	0 (0%)	0 (0%)	0 (0%)	0 (0%)	0 (0%)
Karyotype								
normal	25 (27%)	0 (0%)	9 (32%)	2 (22%)	9 (24%)	2 (29%)	1 (25%)	1 (25%)
abnormal	31 (34%)	0 (0%)	0 (0%)	6 (67%)	19 (51%)	2 (25%)	1 (25%)	3 (75%)
NA	35 (38%)	2 (100%)	19 (68%)	1 (11%)	9 (24%)	3 (43%)	2 (50%)	0 (0%)
Somatic RUNX1 alteration								
detected	23 (25%)	0 (0%)	0 (0%)	2 (22%)	20 (54%)	1 (14%)	0 (0%)	0 (0%)
not detected	66 (73%)	2 (100%)	28 (100%)	7 (78%)	17 (46%)	6 (86%)	4 (100%)	4 (100%)
NA	2 (2%)	0 (0%)	0 (0%)	0 (0%)	0 (0%)	0 (0%)	0 (0%)	0 (0%)
Additional somatic variants								
median number of analyzed genes	28 (1–51)	27 (21–33)	33 (1–43)	23 (2–38)	27 (1–51)	38 (17–48)	16.5 (3–33)	35 (1–43)
median number of somatic variants	2 (0–32)	3 (0–6)	0.5 (0–6)	2 (0–20)	2 (0–12)	2 (0–10)	2.5 (1–3)	2 (1–32)
no variants detected	25 (27%)	1 (50%)	14 (50%)	3 (33%)	6 (16%)	1 (29%)	0 (0%)	0 (0%)

Abbreviations: AML—acute myeloid leukemia; HM—hematologic malignancies; MDS—myelodysplastic syndrome; NA—not available; RUNX1-FPD—familial platelet disorder with predisposition to hematologic malignancies. [a] including two chronic myelomonocytic leukemia, one juvenile myelomonocytic leukemia, and one myeloproliferative neoplasm not further specified. [b] including one B-cell acute lymphoblastic leukemia, one T-cell acute lymphoblastic leukemia, one T-cell non-Hodgkin lymphoma, and one acute lymphoblastic leukemia not further specified. [c] some authors refer to the time of first reported symptoms and others at the time of genetic diagnosis. [d] includes whole gene deletions as well as exonic deletions (for details please refer to Figure 2).

4. Spectrum of Somatic Variants and Affected Genes in RUNX1-FPD

Our retrospective analyses included 91 previously published individuals carrying (likely) pathogenic *RUNX1* germline variants, who were analyzed for additional somatic gene variants regardless of whether a somatic variant was identified or not. Somatic alterations were investigated by karyotyping, array-CGH, and/or DNA sequencing (i.e., mainly NGS panels). Overall, 31 of 56 (55%) cases with given karyotype information showed a somatically abnormal karyotype, all of which were associated with HM. Interestingly, of 19 patients with acquired somatic *RUNX1* mutations, 15 had an abnormal karyotype (79%). In four of these cases chromosome 21 was affected, leading to duplication of the mutated *RUNX1* allele, detected via karyotyping and variant allele fraction of the *RUNX1* germline variant. In contrast, only 14 (41%) cases were reported with an abnormal karyotype in 34 cases without somatic *RUNX1* alterations and available karyotype information. Noteworthy, *RUNX1* somatic status was not analyzed in two cases with abnormal karyotype. A summary of frequently investigated and mutated genes is given in Figures 3 and 4. Additional detailed information on all detected somatic variants and analyzed genes can be found in Supplementary Table S1. Collectively, a median of 28 (range 1–51) genes was analyzed per sample (n = 91). Overall, *RUNX1* represents the most frequently analyzed gene (i.e., investigated in 89 of 91 cases, 98%). Other commonly analyzed genes were *GATA2, PTPN11, CEBPA, JAK2, IDH1, IDH2, KIT, KRAS, NRAS, NPM1, ASXL1, CBL,* and *MPL*. On a median, two (range 0–32) somatic variants were detected per sample. Among all 91 reported cases, the most common somatically altered genes were *RUNX1, TET2, ASXL1, BCOR, PHF6,* and *SRSF2*, while variants in other genes were uniquely reported in specific malignancies. Remarkably, no additional acquired variants were detected in 21 (23%) of 91 samples. These cases were primarily associated with a pre-leukemic phenotype corroborating the notion that acquisition of somatic alterations is correlated with disease progression, particularly malignant transformation. The mutational signature of the four enrolled lymphoblastic HMs differed from myeloid samples as somatic variants were recurrently found in *NOTCH1, PHF6,* and *TET2*. Somatic *RUNX1* alterations were found in 23 of all cases (25%) and in 23 of 53 patients (43%) with reported MDS, AML, or MDS/AML. None of the 30 non-HM patients had a secondary somatically acquired *RUNX1* variant. *RUNX1* being the most frequently investigated gene was also the most frequently mutated gene. This high frequency was significantly higher than in patients with assumed sporadic AML and is in line with data from previous reports, as somatic alterations of *RUNX1* were reported as the most common somatic mutation in patients with RUNX1-FPD (i.e., 36%) [36]. Noteworthy, the authors of studies included in our retrospective analysis did not investigate if *RUNX1* germline and somatic variants appear in *cis* or *trans*. All 23 carriers of an additional *RUNX1* somatic variant were diagnosed with MDS and/or AML. In these patients, the median number of additionally acquired variants was two variants per sample (range 0–10) with only four cases without any additionally acquired variant besides *RUNX1*. Additional alterations were frequently found in *FLT3, IDH1, SRSF2, WT1,* and *BCOR*. On the contrary, a median of one variant per sample (range 0–20) (e.g., in *TET2, ASXL1, SRSF2, PDS5B,* and *NUP214*) was detected among 66 individuals who harbored no somatic *RUNX1* variant and included 36 with and 30 without a reported HM. Of note, no somatic *RUNX1* variants were reported in subgroups with lymphoid or other myeloid HM. In summary, the most frequently mutated genes differ from those that were frequently analyzed, except for *RUNX1*. Thus, future sequencing panels need adaptation to include, at least, the most common somatically altered genes in RUNX1-FPD to improve monitoring of clonal hematopoiesis and malignant transformation in these patients. All RUNX1-FPD patients harboring somatic *RUNX1* variants were diagnosed with MDS, MDS/AML, or AML, the majority of them had clonal cytogenetic alterations and carried additional somatic alterations in genes despite *RUNX1*. This indicates that in RUNX1-FPD, somatic acquisition of additional *RUNX1* variants was only present in HM but not in premalignant stages. Thus, somatic *RUNX1* alterations may serve as a genetic indicator of malignant transformation.

Our retrospective analyses included 91 previously published individuals carrying (likely) pathogenic *RUNX1* germline variants, who were analyzed for additional somatic gene variants regardless of whether a somatic variant was identified or not. Somatic alterations were investigated by karyotyping, array-CGH, and/or DNA sequencing (i.e., mainly NGS panels). Overall, 31 of 56 (55%) cases with given karyotype information showed a somatically abnormal karyotype, all of which were associated with HM. Interestingly, of 19 patients with acquired somatic *RUNX1* mutations, 15 had an abnormal karyotype (79%). In four of these cases chromosome 21 was affected, leading to duplication of the mutated *RUNX1* allele, detected via karyotyping and variant allele fraction of the *RUNX1* germline variant. In contrast, only 14 (41%) cases were reported with an abnormal karyotype in 34 cases without somatic *RUNX1* alterations and available karyotype information. Noteworthy, *RUNX1* somatic status was not analyzed in two cases with abnormal karyotype.

A summary of frequently investigated and mutated genes is given in Figures 3 and 4. Additional detailed information on all detected somatic variants and analyzed genes can be found in Supplementary Table S1. Collectively, a median of 28 (range 1–51) genes was analyzed per sample (n = 91). Overall, *RUNX1* represents the most frequently analyzed gene (i.e., investigated in 89 of 91 cases, 98%). Other commonly analyzed genes were *GATA2*, *PTPN11*, *CEBPA*, *JAK2*, *IDH1*, *IDH2*, *KIT*, *KRAS*, *NRAS*, *NPM1*, *ASXL1*, *CBL*, and *MPL*. On a median, two (range 0–32) somatic variants were detected per sample. Among all 91 reported cases, the most common somatically altered genes were *RUNX1*, *TET2*, *ASXL1*, *BCOR*, *PHF6*, and *SRSF2*, while variants in other genes were uniquely reported in specific malignancies. Remarkably, no additional acquired variants were detected in 21 (23%) of 91 samples. These cases were primarily associated with a pre-leukemic phenotype corroborating the notion that acquisition of somatic alterations is correlated with disease progression, particularly malignant transformation. The mutational signature of the four enrolled lymphoblastic HMs differed from myeloid samples as somatic variants were recurrently found in *NOTCH1*, *PHF6*, and *TET2*. Somatic *RUNX1* alterations were found in 23 of all cases (25%) and in 23 of 53 patients (43%) with reported MDS, AML, or MDS/AML. None of the 30 non-HM patients had a secondary somatically acquired *RUNX1* variant. *RUNX1* being the most frequently investigated gene was also the most frequently mutated gene. This high frequency was significantly higher than in patients with assumed sporadic AML and is in line with data from previous reports, as somatic alterations of *RUNX1* were reported as the most common somatic mutation in patients with RUNX1-FPD (i.e., 36%) [36]. Noteworthy, the authors of studies included in our retrospective analysis did not investigate if *RUNX1* germline and somatic variants appear in *cis* or *trans*. All 23 carriers of an additional *RUNX1* somatic variant were diagnosed with MDS and/or AML. In these patients, the median number of additionally acquired variants was two variants per sample (range 0–10) with only four cases without any additionally acquired variant besides *RUNX1*. Additional alterations were frequently found in *FLT3*, *IDH1*, *SRSF2*, *WT1*, and *BCOR*. On the contrary, a median of one variant per sample (range 0–20) (e.g., in *TET2*, *ASXL1*, *SRSF2*, *PDS5B*, and *NUP214*) was detected among 66 individuals who harbored no somatic *RUNX1* variant and included 36 with and 30 without a reported HM. Of note, no somatic *RUNX1* variants were reported in subgroups with lymphoid or other myeloid HM. In summary, the most frequently mutated genes differ from those that were frequently analyzed, except for *RUNX1*. Thus, future sequencing panels need adaptation to include, at least, the most common somatically altered genes in RUNX1-FPD to improve monitoring of clonal hematopoiesis and malignant transformation in these patients. All RUNX1-FPD patients harboring somatic *RUNX1* variants were diagnosed with MDS, MDS/AML, or AML, the majority of them had clonal cytogenetic alterations and carried additional somatic alterations in genes despite *RUNX1*. This indicates that in RUNX1-FPD, somatic acquisition of additional *RUNX1* variants was only present in HM but not in premalignant stages. Thus, somatic *RUNX1* alterations may serve as a genetic indicator of malignant transformation.

We compared the groups of MDS, AML, and MDS/AML (n = 53) with the non-HM group (n = 30) in our retrospective analyses (Figures 3 and 4). With a median of 27 (range 1–51) and 33 (range 1–43), the number of analyzed genes per sample was comparable in MDS and/or AML and non-HM samples, respectively. In MDS, AML, and MDS/AML patients the median number of detected somatic variants was two (range 0–20) whereas in non-HM patients a median number of 0.5 (range 0–6) variants was detected per sample. Conclusively, MDS and/or AML cases had a maximum number of 20 somatic variants per sample, whereas the maximum number of somatic variants in non-HM cases was six. One or no somatic variant was identified in 67% of non-HM cases, whereas 60% of the MDS, AML, MDS/AML subgroup carried two or more acquired variants. This highlights the association between the number of acquired variants and disease progression. In MDS, AML, MDS/AML, 27 (51%) of cases presented with an abnormal karyotype particularly encompassing the *RUNX1* locus, 23 (43%) showed a somatic *RUNX1* alteration, and 42 (79%) had additionally acquired variants (Figure 1). On the contrary, across all non-HM samples, only one of 10 investigated karyotypes (10%) was abnormal, none of 30 cases had acquired a *RUNX1* alteration, and only 15 (50%) harbored any acquired variants besides *RUNX1* (Figure 1). High-throughput sequencing studies have shown that approximately 78–89% of sporadic MDS patients exhibit at least one pathogenic variant in a variety of genes [57,58]. The occurrence and number of pathogenic variants are further associated with disease severity, which is also seen in our comparison between non-HM and MDS, AML, MDS/AML in RUNX1-FPD cases. Interestingly, in MDS and/or AML, *RUNX1*, *BCOR*, *TET2*, *SRSF2*, and *NRAS* were frequently mutated genes. In the non-malignant samples, *TET2*, *ASXL1*, *PDS5B*, *NUP214*, and *SMC1A* were recurrently mutated underlining that some variants may occur as early events (e.g., *TET2*) providing growth advantage possibly leading to overt leukemia [15]. Next, we subdivided 53 MDS, AML, MDS/AML patients into subgroups (i) with acquired *RUNX1* alterations and, (ii) without acquired *RUNX1* alterations. Thereby, we identified that in the group with acquired *RUNX1* alterations, especially *FLT3*, *BCOR*, *SRSF2*, *IDH1*, and *WT1* variants were frequently detected whereas recurrent variants in the group without acquired *RUNX1* alteration were found in *BCOR*, *NRAS*, *TET2*, *PHF6*, and *CDC25C*. Previously, Brown et al. observed somatic variants affecting *NRAS*, *SRSF2*, *DNMT3A* and other genes associated with epigenetic regulation in RUNX1-FPD patients with AML [36]. Here, we observed somatic *DNMT3A* variants in four (11%) out of 37 RUNX1-FPD AMLs, one RUNX1-FPD myeloproliferative neoplasm, and one RUNX1-FPD thrombocytopenia patient. However, *DNMT3A* was not analyzed in seven of 37 RUNX1-FPD AML cases. Moreover, Brown et al. observed that somatic *RUNX1* and somatic *DNMT3A* variants do not co-occur in RUNX1-FPD patients [36]. However, our retrospective analyses identified one RUNX1-FPD patient who developed AML and carried acquired variants in *RUNX1* and *DNMT3A*.

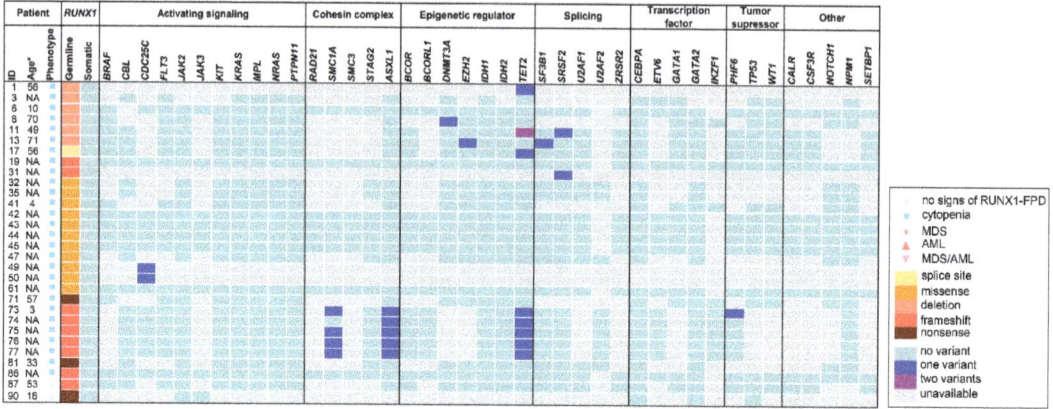

Figure 3. Frequently investigated and affected genes within the subgroup non-hematologic malignancy. Illustration of age, phenotype, type of *RUNX1* germline variant and analyzed somatic variants for 30 non-HM cases. For references to the individual patients please refer to the supplementary data. AML—acute myeloid leukemia, HM—hematologic malignancies, MDS—myelodysplastic syndrome, MDS/AML—patients who developed MDS and subsequently AML, NA—not available, RUNX1-FPD—familial platelet disorder with predisposition to hematologic malignancies * some authors refer to the age of first reported symptoms and others to the age of genetic diagnosis.

Somatic variants in *CDC25C* and *GATA2* were reported to be altered in RUNX1-FPD patients. Somatic variants in the *CDC25C* gene were recurrently mutated in 13 individuals from seven Japanese RUNX1-FPD families [44]. However, we found that *CDC25C* was investigated in 34 cases and only found variants in Japanese patients by Yoshimi and colleagues. Since US and European studies have not confirmed this data [48,59,60], an ethnicity effect on the acquisition of somatic variants is assumed [61]. A previously published comparison of the somatic mutational signatures between the familial and sporadic *RUNX1*-mutated AML patients showed enrichment for somatic mutations affecting the second *RUNX1* allele and *GATA2* [36]. In our retrospective cohort, we identified *GATA2* variants only in two samples (i.e., one MDS/AML, and one AML), although *GATA2* gene was investigated in 76% of all 91 samples. In conclusion, our retrospective analyses do not support the hypotheses, that *CDC25C* and *GATA2* are among the most frequently somatically affected genes in RUNX1-FPD.

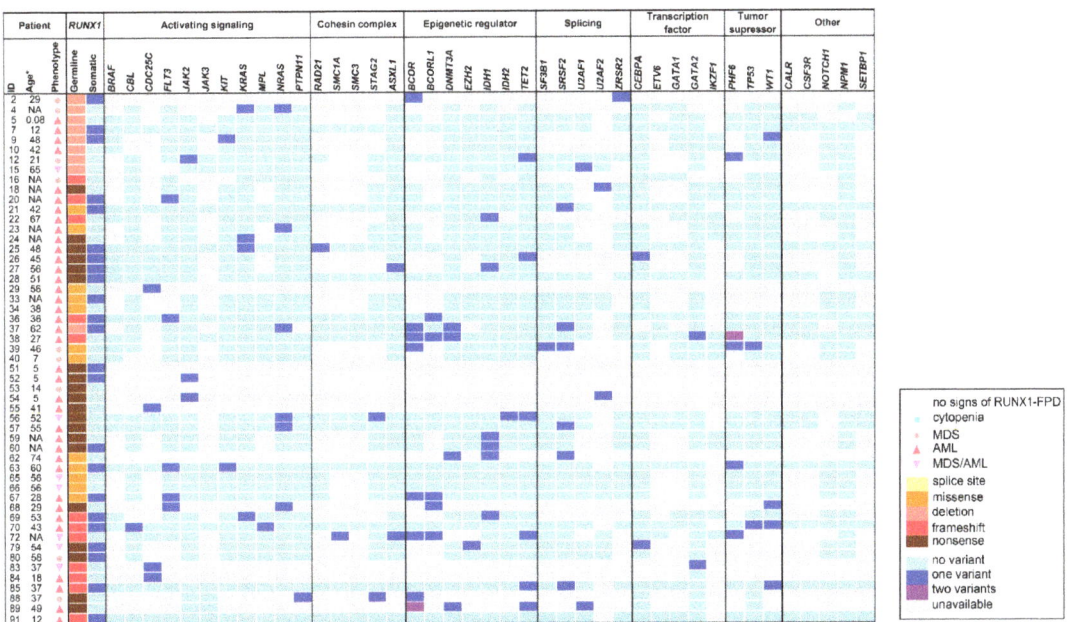

Figure 4. Frequently investigated and affected genes within the subgroups MDS, AML, and MDS/AML. Illustration of age, phenotype, type of *RUNX1* germline variant and analyzed somatic variants for 53 HM cases with MDS and/or AML. For references to the individual patients please refer to the supplementary data. AML—acute myeloid leukemia, HM—hematologic malignancies, MDS—myelodysplastic syndrome, MDS/AML—patients who developed MDS and subsequently AML, NA—not available, RUNX1-FPD—familial platelet disorder with predisposition to hematologic malignancies. * some authors refer to the age of first reported symptoms and others to the age of genetic diagnosis.

Next, we compared the identified somatic variants in RUNX1-FPD to those found in a patient with sporadic HM. Somatic mutations in *TET2* occur in about 15–30% of patients with various sporadic myeloid malignancies [16,62,63]. Moreover, alterations of the *TET2* gene commonly occur biallelic in the context of sporadic hematologic neoplasms. Interestingly, we observed *TET2* alterations in 15 out of 91 patients (16%). In one of the patients with cytopenia, two *TET2* variants were identified. However, information was not given on whether these variants occurred in *cis* or in *trans*. *TET2* variants were found in six MDS, AML and MDS/AML RUNX1-FPD cases (n = 53, 11%). Therefore, *TET2* variants in the analyzed RUNX1-FPD cohort appear to be less frequent than in sporadic leukemia. Since *TET2* variants were concomitantly observed with variants in *NPM1*, *FLT3*, *JAK2*, *RUNX1*, *CEBPA*, *CBL*, and *KRAS* in sporadic AML patients [64], we evaluated these genes in *TET2*-mutated AML samples. Thereby, we only found two acquired *RUNX1* alterations and one *CEBPA* variant co-occurring in patients with *TET2* variants. In sporadic HM,

DNMT3A variants occur in about 20% of AML [65], 8% of MDS [66], and 17% of T-ALL patients [67]. Variants in TET2, JAK2, and SRSF2 occur in 10–60% of patients with sporadic chronic myelomonocytic leukemia [68]. Here, a JAK2, an SRSF2, and an ASXL1 variant were detected in a patient with chronic myelomonocytic leukemia [50]. Pathogenic variants in one of the three core genes (i.e., CALR, MPL, and JAK2) are characteristic in the context of sporadic myeloproliferative neoplasms [69–71]. The only myeloproliferative neoplasm included in this review presented with a JAK2 and a DNMT3A variant. Additionally, IDH1, FLT3, NPM1, and RASopathy-associated genes including NRAS, KRAS, and PTPN11 are frequently altered in sporadic HM [72,73]. Despite IDH1, FLT3 was the most frequently altered gene in the RUNX1-FPD AML subgroup ($n = 37$). However, no acquired variant was found in NPM1 [63]. Mutational analyses of the PTPN11 gene in 70 out of 91 samples (77%) revealed only one sample carrying a variant in this gene. Taken together, several frequently affected genes in sporadic HM are also affected by alterations in the analyzed retrospective RUNX1-FPD cohort. Besides different frequencies of additionally occurring genetic variants and the predominance of somatic RUNX1 variants, there are no characteristic differences between somatic variants detected in sporadic HM and RUNX1-FPD-associated HM.

Our retrospective analyses of somatic variants including 91 RUNX1-FPD cases had several limitations regarding sequencing panels, type and choice of samples, and differences in the provided information. Most of the literature focused on single genes or gene panels consisting of candidate genes already associated with HM leading to a data bias. Thus, it should be acknowledged that such approaches might overlook somatic variants in other genes not yet associated with HM. Noteworthy, variants with low variant allele fractions might also be sequencing artifacts. Moreover, it should be kept in mind that different tissues (e.g., peripheral blood, bone marrow) investigated at different time points (e.g., pre-symptomatic, during cytopenia, during HM, after chemotherapy, at relapse) might lead to divergent somatic signatures.

5. Prospective Surveillance Strategies for RUNX1-FPD Patients

The diagnosis of RUNX1-FPD is of clinical interest for future management of the index patient and relatives at risk. It is currently not possible to predict an individual RUNX1-FPD patient's risk of developing HM or the time of malignant transformation [74], because there are no genotype–phenotype correlations in RUNX1-FPD [36]. Specific somatic signatures identified in RUNX1-FPD patients may indicate progression to HM, but the impact of individual variants or specific combinations of them are not yet well understood. Early clonal evolution with the development of pre-leukemic and subsequent leukemic clones is common in patients with germline RUNX1 mutations [75]. Mutations in hematopoietic stem cells that initiate sporadic leukemia generally occur in genes encoding epigenetic regulatory proteins such as DNMT3A, ASXL1, IDH2, and TET2 whereas secondary, driver mutations involve genes encoding several functional categories of proteins including transcription factors (e.g., CEBPA, RUNX1, GATA2, and ETV6), signaling molecules (e.g., FLT3, NRAS, PTPN11, KRAS, KIT, CBL, and NF1), splicing factors (e.g., SRSF2, SF3B1, and U2AF1), and proteins with other functions (e.g., NPM1, SMC1A) [15,76]. In sporadic AML, somatic mutations in RUNX1 are usually secondary events, whereas, in FPD/AML, RUNX1 germline mutations are initiating or predisposing events [15]. Of note, variants in the TET2, DNMT3A, and ASLX1 genes are also frequently detected in hematopoietic stem cells from non-diseased elderly individuals and are associated with age-related clonal hematopoiesis of indeterminate potential (CHIP) linked with an increased risk of HM and cardiovascular disease [77,78]. Interestingly, Brown et al. observed a decreased number of somatic mutations in genes associated with CHIP among familial compared to sporadic cases with RUNX1-mutated AML [36]. Moreover, they found mutations in known-CHIP-associated genes, including DNMT3A and TET2, in 22% of preleukemic RUNX1-FPD patients and 40% of patients with myeloid malignancy [36], which is more frequently than within the general population [79].

Monitoring RUNX1-FPD patients by sequencing panels to detect clonal hematopoiesis and/or alterations by variant allele fractions of already known variants may offer the opportunity to intervene at the pre-leukemic stage, prior to the appearance of overt MDS or frank leukemia. Previous data highlight the promise of surveillance and future potential for early intervention prior to the development of an overt HM in the at-risk population [75]. However, this requires the knowledge of which acquired variants are associated with malignant transformation [15]. So far, likely due to the rarity of RUNX1-FPD, only a few studies and cases were reported yielding ambiguous results. Improved knowledge of the genetic landscape and its non-HM-associated variability as well as its malignant transformation-associated alterations may translate into improved diagnostics and risk stratification in the future. The goal is to monitor RUNX1-FPD patients allowing early detection of disease progression to MDS or AML that would allow timely clinical intervention. RUNX1-FPD patients with progressive cytopenia, immunophenotypic abnormalities by flow cytometry, karyotypic abnormalities, and/or abnormal bone marrow features may have a higher risk of progression and need closer follow-up including complete blood count every six months and/or NGS-based mutational analysis of relevant gene panels [74]. Kanagal-Shamanna and colleagues recommend an initial bone marrow examination in all individuals with *RUNX1* germline variant in order to assess baseline changes and exclude occult malignancy [74]. Following initial bone marrow examination, patients must be closely monitored for progression to HM by regular bone marrow examination if complete blood count or NGS studies show abnormalities [74]. However, the process of disease progression in HM is complex and the spectrum of implicated genes and pathways is vast. Furthermore, therapeutic approaches that directly target genetic alterations and subsequently aberrant signaling pathways might be of interest. So far, only some recurrent driver mutations in AML including *FLT3*, *NPM1*, *DNMT3A*, *IDH1/2*, and *TET2*, can be therapeutically targeted [80]. Presently, we lack information about somatic variants that drive progression to overt leukemia that, moreover, predict malignancy risk for individual RUNX1-FPD patients. In the future, knowledge about somatic mutation patterns may precisely predict the disease progression of RUNX1-FPD. Further studies are needed to better define the mutation signature in the preleukemic and leukemic clones, as well as their dynamics over time, to finally determine the prognostic value of such investigations. The ongoing NIH Natural History Study of Hematologic and Premalignant Conditions Associated with RUNX1 Mutation will provide further insights into the potential correlations between the spectrum of acquired variants and disease progression (study number 19-HG-0059, https://www.genome.gov/Current-NHGRI-Clinical-Studies/hematologic-and-premalignant-conditions-associated-with-RUNX1-mutation, accessed on 7 June 2022).

6. Conclusions

Retrospective analysis supports the theory of stepwise malignant transformation in RUNX1-FPD. A correlation between the number of acquired variants and disease progression was identified. Moreover, somatic *RUNX1* variants were clearly associated with MDS and/or AML in RUNX1-FPD patients and may serve as a genetic indicator of malignant transformation. The acquisition of different somatic variants may explain the clinical heterogeneity seen in RUNX1-FPD, even within affected families. However, the process of disease progression in RUNX1-FPD is complex since the pathogenesis cannot be explained merely by a single acquired variant. The spectrum of somatic variants and genes implicated in the progression is vast. It highlights the importance of somatic mutations in the development of frank leukemia. Recent advantages in NGS technologies reveal the entire picture of genetic alterations involved in tumorigenesis piece by piece. Applied panels should be adapted to cover all relevant genes. In addition, it is worth considering that not all acquired variants are necessarily attributed to disease progression and we need to distinguish between driver and passenger variants. Prospectively, synergistic effects of *RUNX1* germline variants together with acquired variants should be evaluated with functional assays. Additionally, sharing identified germline and somatic variants with phenotypic information in appropriate databases in a standardized way, e.g., within the RUNX1db [35] or the database of the natural history study, will lead to a growing body of knowledge being the prerequisite for evidence-based care in the future. Taken together, upcoming detailed and unbiased analyses can provide insights into the synergistic effects of germline and somatic variants including their prognostic value. This is key to enabe better risk stratification during surveillance and, in the future, may allow tailored chemoprevention studies to avoid malignant transformation in RUNX1-FPD.

Supplementary Materials: The following supporting information can be downloaded at: https://www.mdpi.com/article/10.3390/cancers14143431/s1, Table S1: Detailed information of all retrospectively enrolled 91 individuals out of 60 families reported in the original publications listed in Appendix A.

Author Contributions: Conceptualization, T.R.; data acquisition, writing original draft, figure design: A.F., M.D. and T.R.; supervision: T.R. and B.S. All authors have read and agreed to the published version of the manuscript.

Funding: This research was funded by the BMBF grant *MyPred Network for young individuals with syndromes predisposing to myeloid malignancies* (01GM1911B).

Conflicts of Interest: The authors declare no conflict of interest.

Appendix A

In this review, we retrospectively enrolled 91 individuals out of 60 families reported in the following publications: [31,36,44,45,48–50,54,59–61,73–75,81–90]. Additional detailed information on all patients including original patient IDs and their genetic information can be found in Supplementary Table S1.

References

1. Sood, R.; Kamikubo, Y.; Liu, P. Role of RUNX1 in hematological malignancies. *Blood* **2017**, *129*, 2070–2082. [CrossRef]
2. Miyoshi, H.; Ohira, M.; Shimizu, K.; Mitani, K.; Hirai, T.; Imai, T.; Yokoyama, K.; Soeda, E.; Ohki, M. Alternative splicing and genomic structure of the AML1 gene involved in acute myeloid leukemia. *Nucleic Acids Res.* **1995**, *23*, 2762–2769. [CrossRef]
3. Kagoshima, H.; Shigesada, K.; Satake, M.; Ito, Y.; Miyoshi, H.; Ohki, M.; Pepling, M.; Gergen, P. The Runt domain identifies a new family of heteromeric transcriptional regulators. *Trends Genet.* **1993**, *9*, 338–341. [CrossRef]
4. Wang, S.; Wang, Q.; Crute, B.E.; Melnikova, I.N.; Keller, S.R.; Speck, N.A. Cloning and characterization of subunits of the T-cell receptor and murine leukemia virus enhancer core-binding factor. *Mol. Cell Biol.* **1993**, *13*, 3324–3339. [CrossRef]
5. Ogawa, E.; Inuzuka, M.; Maruyama, M.; Satake, M.; Naito-Fujimoto, M.; Ito, Y.; Shigesada, K. Molecular cloning and characterization of PEBP2 beta, the heterodimeric partner of a novel Drosophila runt-related DNA binding protein PEBP2 alpha. *Virology* **1993**, *194*, 314–331. [CrossRef]
6. Bravo, J.; Li, Z.; Speck, N.A.; Warren, A.J. The leukemia-associated AML1 (Runx1)—CBF beta complex functions as a DNA-induced molecular clamp. *Nat. Struct. Biol.* **2001**, *8*, 371–378. [CrossRef]
7. Huang, G.; Shigesada, K.; Ito, K.; Wee, H.J.; Yokomizo, T.; Ito, Y. Dimerization with PEBP2beta protects RUNX1/AML1 from ubiquitin-proteasome-mediated degradation. *Embo J.* **2001**, *20*, 723–733. [CrossRef]
8. Kanno, T.; Kanno, Y.; Chen, L.F.; Ogawa, E.; Kim, W.Y.; Ito, Y. Intrinsic transcriptional activation-inhibition domains of the polyomavirus enhancer binding protein 2/core binding factor alpha subunit revealed in the presence of the beta subunit. *Mol. Cell Biol.* **1998**, *18*, 2444–2454. [CrossRef]
9. Lutterbach, B.; Westendorf, J.J.; Linggi, B.; Isaac, S.; Seto, E.; Hiebert, S.W. A mechanism of repression by acute myeloid leukemia-1, the target of multiple chromosomal translocations in acute leukemia. *J. Biol. Chem.* **2000**, *275*, 651–656. [CrossRef]
10. Durst, K.L.; Hiebert, S.W. Role of RUNX family members in transcriptional repression and gene silencing. *Oncogene* **2004**, *23*, 4220–4224. [CrossRef]
11. Hong, D.; Fritz, A.J.; Gordon, J.A.; Tye, C.E.; Boyd, J.R.; Tracy, K.M.; Frietze, S.E.; Carr, F.E.; Nickerson, J.A.; Van Wijnen, A.J.; et al. RUNX1-dependent mechanisms in biological control and dysregulation in cancer. *J. Cell Physiol.* **2019**, *234*, 8597–8609. [CrossRef]
12. Okuda, T.; van Deursen, J.; Hiebert, S.W.; Grosveld, G.; Downing, J.R. AML1, the target of multiple chromosomal translocations in human leukemia, is essential for normal fetal liver hematopoiesis. *Cell* **1996**, *84*, 321–330. [CrossRef]
13. Yzaguirre, A.D.; de Bruijn, M.F.; Speck, N.A. The Role of Runx1 in Embryonic Blood Cell Formation. *Adv. Exp. Med. Biol.* **2017**, *962*, 47–64. [CrossRef]
14. Wang, Q.; Stacy, T.; Binder, M.; Marin-Padilla, M.; Sharpe, A.H.; Speck, N.A. Disruption of the Cbfa2 gene causes necrosis and hemorrhaging in the central nervous system and blocks definitive hematopoiesis. *Proc. Natl. Acad. Sci. USA* **1996**, *93*, 3444–3449. [CrossRef]

15. Bellissimo, D.C.; Speck, N.A. RUNX1 Mutations in Inherited and Sporadic Leukemia. *Front. Cell Dev. Biol.* **2017**, *5*, 111. [CrossRef]
16. Metzeler, K.H.; Herold, T.; Rothenberg-Thurley, M.; Amler, S.; Sauerland, M.C.; Görlich, D.; Schneider, S.; Konstandin, N.P.; Dufour, A.; Bräundl, K.; et al. Spectrum and prognostic relevance of driver gene mutations in acute myeloid leukemia. *Blood* **2016**, *128*, 686–698. [CrossRef]
17. Hayashi, Y.; Harada, Y.; Huang, G.; Harada, H. Myeloid neoplasms with germ line RUNX1 mutation. *Int. J. Hematol.* **2017**, *106*, 183–188. [CrossRef]
18. Hayashi, Y.; Harada, Y.; Harada, H. Myeloid neoplasms and clonal hematopoiesis from the RUNX1 perspective. *Leukemia* **2022**, *36*, 1203–1214. [CrossRef]
19. Huret, J.L.; Ahmad, M.; Arsaban, M.; Bernheim, A.; Cigna, J.; Desangles, F.; Guignard, J.C.; Jacquemot-Perbal, M.C.; Labarussias, M.; Leberre, V.; et al. Atlas of genetics and cytogenetics in oncology and haematology in 2013. *Nucleic Acids Res.* **2013**, *41*, D920–D924. [CrossRef]
20. Stengel, A.; Kern, W.; Meggendorfer, M.; Nadarajah, N.; Perglerovà, K.; Haferlach, T.; Haferlach, C. Number of RUNX1 mutations, wild-type allele loss and additional mutations impact on prognosis in adult RUNX1-mutated AML. *Leukemia* **2018**, *32*, 295–302. [CrossRef]
21. Yamato, G.; Shiba, N.; Yoshida, K.; Hara, Y.; Shiraishi, Y.; Ohki, K.; Okubo, J.; Park, M.J.; Sotomatsu, M.; Arakawa, H.; et al. RUNX1 mutations in pediatric acute myeloid leukemia are associated with distinct genetic features and an inferior prognosis. *Blood* **2018**, *131*, 2266–2270. [CrossRef]
22. Mendler, J.H.; Maharry, K.; Radmacher, M.D.; Mrózek, K.; Becker, H.; Metzeler, K.H.; Schwind, S.; Whitman, S.P.; Khalife, J.; Kohlschmidt, J.; et al. RUNX1 mutations are associated with poor outcome in younger and older patients with cytogenetically normal acute myeloid leukemia and with distinct gene and MicroRNA expression signatures. *J. Clin. Oncol.* **2012**, *30*, 3109–3118. [CrossRef]
23. Grossmann, V.; Kern, W.; Harbich, S.; Alpermann, T.; Jeromin, S.; Schnittger, S.; Haferlach, C.; Haferlach, T.; Kohlmann, A. Prognostic relevance of RUNX1 mutations in T-cell acute lymphoblastic leukemia. *Haematologica* **2011**, *96*, 1874–1877. [CrossRef]
24. Arber, D.A.; Orazi, A.; Hasserjian, R.; Thiele, J.; Borowitz, M.J.; Le Beau, M.M.; Bloomfield, C.D.; Cazzola, M.; Vardiman, J.W. The 2016 revision to the World Health Organization classification of myeloid neoplasms and acute leukemia. *Blood* **2016**, *127*, 2391–2405. [CrossRef]
25. Song, W.J.; Sullivan, M.G.; Legare, R.D.; Hutchings, S.; Tan, X.; Kufrin, D.; Ratajczak, J.; Resende, I.C.; Haworth, C.; Hock, R.; et al. Haploinsufficiency of CBFA2 causes familial thrombocytopenia with propensity to develop acute myelogenous leukaemia. *Nat. Genet.* **1999**, *23*, 166–175. [CrossRef]
26. Deuitch, N.; Broadbridge, E.; Cunningham, L.; Liu, P. RUNX1 Familial Platelet Disorder with Associated Myeloid Malignancies. In *GeneReviews*®; Adam, M.P., Ardinger, H.H., Pagon, R.A., Wallace, S.E., Bean, L.J.H., Gripp, K.W., Mirzaa, G.M., Amemiya, A., Eds.; University of Washington: Seattle, WA, USA, 1993.
27. Latger-Cannard, V.; Philippe, C.; Bouquet, A.; Baccini, V.; Alessi, M.C.; Ankri, A.; Bauters, A.; Bayart, S.; Cornillet-Lefebvre, P.; Daliphard, S.; et al. Haematological spectrum and genotype-phenotype correlations in nine unrelated families with RUNX1 mutations from the French network on inherited platelet disorders. *Orphanet J. Rare Dis.* **2016**, *11*, 49. [CrossRef]
28. Godley, L.A. Inherited predisposition to acute myeloid leukemia. *Semin. Hematol.* **2014**, *51*, 306–321. [CrossRef]
29. Churpek, J.E.; Lorenz, R.; Nedumgottil, S.; Onel, K.; Olopade, O.I.; Sorrell, A.; Owen, C.J.; Bertuch, A.A.; Godley, L.A. Proposal for the clinical detection and management of patients and their family members with familial myelodysplastic syndrome/acute leukemia predisposition syndromes. *Leuk. Lymphoma* **2013**, *54*, 28–35. [CrossRef]
30. West, A.H.; Godley, L.A.; Churpek, J.E. Familial myelodysplastic syndrome/acute leukemia syndromes: A review and utility for translational investigations. *Ann. N. Y. Acad. Sci.* **2014**, *1310*, 111–118. [CrossRef]
31. Simon, L.; Spinella, J.F.; Yao, C.Y.; Lavallée, V.P.; Boivin, I.; Boucher, G.; Audemard, E.; Bordeleau, M.E.; Lemieux, S.; Hébert, J.; et al. High frequency of germline RUNX1 mutations in patients with RUNX1-mutated AML. *Blood* **2020**, *135*, 1882–1886. [CrossRef]
32. Feurstein, S.; Zhang, L.; DiNardo, C.D. Accurate germline RUNX1 variant interpretation and its clinical significance. *Blood Adv.* **2020**, *4*, 6199–6203. [CrossRef]
33. Bąk, A.; Skonieczka, K.; Jaśkowiec, A.; Junkiert-Czarnecka, A.; Heise, M.; Pilarska-Deltow, M.; Potoczek, S.; Czyżewska, M.; Haus, O. Searching for germline mutations in the RUNX1 gene among Polish patients with acute myeloid leukemia. *Leuk. Lymphoma* **2021**, *62*, 1749–1755. [CrossRef]
34. Ernst, M.P.T.; Kavelaars, F.G.; Löwenberg, B.; Valk, P.J.M.; Raaijmakers, M. RUNX1 germline variants in RUNX1-mutant AML: How frequent? *Blood* **2021**, *137*, 1428–1431. [CrossRef]
35. Homan, C.C.; King-Smith, S.L.; Lawrence, D.M.; Arts, P.; Feng, J.; Andrews, J.; Armstrong, M.; Ha, T.; Dobbins, J.; Drazer, M.W.; et al. The RUNX1 database (RUNX1db): Establishment of an expert curated RUNX1 registry and genomics database as a public resource for familial platelet disorder with myeloid malignancy. *Haematologica* **2021**, *106*, 3004–3007. [CrossRef]
36. Brown, A.L.; Arts, P.; Carmichael, C.L.; Babic, M.; Dobbins, J.; Chong, C.E.; Schreiber, A.W.; Feng, J.; Phillips, K.; Wang, P.P.S.; et al. RUNX1-mutated families show phenotype heterogeneity and a somatic mutation profile unique to germline predisposed AML. *Blood Adv.* **2020**, *4*, 1131–1144. [CrossRef]
37. Brown, A.L.; Hahn, C.N.; Scott, H.S. Secondary leukemia in patients with germline transcription factor mutations (RUNX1, GATA2, CEBPA). *Blood* **2020**, *136*, 24–35. [CrossRef]

38. Luo, X.; Feurstein, S.; Mohan, S.; Porter, C.C.; Jackson, S.A.; Keel, S.; Chicka, M.; Brown, A.L.; Kesserwan, C.; Agarwal, A.; et al. ClinGen Myeloid Malignancy Variant Curation Expert Panel recommendations for germline RUNX1 variants. *Blood Adv.* **2019**, *3*, 2962–2979. [CrossRef]
39. Decker, M.; Lammens, T.; Ferster, A.; Erlacher, M.; Yoshimi, A.; Niemeyer, C.M.; Ernst, M.P.T.; Raaijmakers, M.; Duployez, N.; Flaum, A.; et al. Functional classification of RUNX1 variants in familial platelet disorder with associated myeloid malignancies. *Leukemia* **2021**, *35*, 3304–3308. [CrossRef]
40. Decker, M.; Agarwal, A.; Benneche, A.; Churpek, J.E.; Duployez, N.; DuVall, A.; Ernst, M.P.T.; Förster, A.; Høberg Vetti, H.; Nash, M.; et al. Validation and clinical application of transactivation assays for RUNX1 variant classification. *Blood Adv.* **2022**, *6*, 3195–3200. [CrossRef]
41. Ripperger, T.; Steinemann, D.; Göhring, G.; Finke, J.; Niemeyer, C.M.; Strahm, B.; Schlegelberger, B. A novel pedigree with heterozygous germline RUNX1 mutation causing familial MDS-related AML: Can these families serve as a multistep model for leukemic transformation? *Leukemia* **2009**, *23*, 1364–1366. [CrossRef]
42. Osato, M.; Yanagida, M.; Shigesada, K.; Ito, Y. Point mutations of the RUNx1/AML1 gene in sporadic and familial myeloid leukemias. *Int. J. Hematol.* **2001**, *74*, 245–251. [CrossRef] [PubMed]
43. Gaidzik, V.I.; Teleanu, V.; Papaemmanuil, E.; Weber, D.; Paschka, P.; Hahn, J.; Wallrabenstein, T.; Kolbinger, B.; Köhne, C.H.; Horst, H.A.; et al. RUNX1 mutations in acute myeloid leukemia are associated with distinct clinico-pathologic and genetic features. *Leukemia* **2016**, *30*, 2160–2168. [CrossRef] [PubMed]
44. Yoshimi, A.; Toya, T.; Kawazu, M.; Ueno, T.; Tsukamoto, A.; Iizuka, H.; Nakagawa, M.; Nannya, Y.; Arai, S.; Harada, H.; et al. Recurrent CDC25C mutations drive malignant transformation in FPD/AML. *Nat. Commun.* **2014**, *5*, 4770. [CrossRef] [PubMed]
45. Preudhomme, C.; Renneville, A.; Bourdon, V.; Philippe, N.; Roche-Lestienne, C.; Boissel, N.; Dhedin, N.; André, J.M.; Cornillet-Lefebvre, P.; Baruchel, A.; et al. High frequency of RUNX1 biallelic alteration in acute myeloid leukemia secondary to familial platelet disorder. *Blood* **2009**, *113*, 5583–5587. [CrossRef]
46. Meisel, M.; Hinterleitner, R.; Pacis, A.; Chen, L.; Earley, Z.M.; Mayassi, T.; Pierre, J.F.; Ernest, J.D.; Galipeau, H.J.; Thuille, N.; et al. Microbial signals drive pre-leukaemic myeloproliferation in a Tet2-deficient host. *Nature* **2018**, *557*, 580–584. [CrossRef]
47. Avagyan, S.; Brown, A.L. To T or not to B: Germline RUNX1 mutation preferences in pediatric ALL predisposition. *J. Clin. Invest.* **2021**, *131*. [CrossRef]
48. Antony-Debré, I.; Duployez, N.; Bucci, M.; Geffroy, S.; Micol, J.B.; Renneville, A.; Boissel, N.; Dhédin, N.; Réa, D.; Nelken, B.; et al. Somatic mutations associated with leukemic progression of familial platelet disorder with predisposition to acute myeloid leukemia. *Leukemia* **2016**, *30*, 999–1002. [CrossRef]
49. Six, K.A.; Gerdemann, U.; Brown, A.L.; Place, A.E.; Cantor, A.B.; Kutny, M.A.; Avagyan, S. B-cell acute lymphoblastic leukemia in patients with germline RUNX1 mutations. *Blood Adv.* **2021**, *5*, 3199–3202. [CrossRef]
50. DiFilippo, E.C.; Coltro, G.; Carr, R.M.; Mangaonkar, A.A.; Binder, M.; Khan, S.P.; Rodriguez, V.; Gangat, N.; Wolanskyj, A.; Pruthi, R.K.; et al. Spectrum of abnormalities and clonal transformation in germline RUNX1 familial platelet disorder and a genomic comparative analysis with somatic RUNX1 mutations in MDS/MPN overlap neoplasms. *Leukemia* **2020**, *34*, 2519–2524. [CrossRef]
51. Harada, H.; Harada, Y.; Niimi, H.; Kyo, T.; Kimura, A.; Inaba, T. High incidence of somatic mutations in the AML1/RUNX1 gene in myelodysplastic syndrome and low blast percentage myeloid leukemia with myelodysplasia. *Blood* **2004**, *103*, 2316–2324. [CrossRef]
52. Michaud, J.; Wu, F.; Osato, M.; Cottles, G.M.; Yanagida, M.; Asou, N.; Shigesada, K.; Ito, Y.; Benson, K.F.; Raskind, W.H.; et al. In vitro analyses of known and novel RUNX1/AML1 mutations in dominant familial platelet disorder with predisposition to acute myelogenous leukemia: Implications for mechanisms of pathogenesis. *Blood* **2002**, *99*, 1364–1372. [CrossRef] [PubMed]
53. Matheny, C.J.; Speck, M.E.; Cushing, P.R.; Zhou, Y.; Corpora, T.; Regan, M.; Newman, M.; Roudaia, L.; Speck, C.L.; Gu, T.L.; et al. Disease mutations in RUNX1 and RUNX2 create nonfunctional, dominant-negative, or hypomorphic alleles. *Embo J.* **2007**, *26*, 1163–1175. [CrossRef] [PubMed]
54. Fenwarth, L.; Caulier, A.; Lachaier, E.; Goursaud, L.; Marceau-Renaut, A.; Fournier, E.; Lebon, D.; Boyer, T.; Berthon, C.; Marolleau, J.P.; et al. Hereditary Predisposition to Acute Myeloid Leukemia in Older Adults. *Hemasphere* **2021**, *5*, e552. [CrossRef] [PubMed]
55. Feurstein, S.; Drazer, M.; Godley, L.A. Germline predisposition to hematopoietic malignancies. *Hum. Mol. Genet.* **2021**, *30*, R225–R235. [CrossRef]
56. DeRoin, L.; Cavalcante de Andrade Silva, M.; Petras, K.; Arndt, K.; Phillips, N.; Wanjari, P.; Subramanian, H.P.; Montes, D.; McElherne, J.; Theissen, M.; et al. Feasibility and limitations of cultured skin fibroblasts for germline genetic testing in hematologic disorders. *Hum. Mutat.* **2022**, *43*, 950–962. [CrossRef]
57. Papaemmanuil, E.; Gerstung, M.; Malcovati, L.; Tauro, S.; Gundem, G.; Van Loo, P.; Yoon, C.J.; Ellis, P.; Wedge, D.C.; Pellagatti, A.; et al. Clinical and biological implications of driver mutations in myelodysplastic syndromes. *Blood* **2013**, *122*, 3616–3627; quiz 3699. [CrossRef]
58. Haferlach, T.; Nagata, Y.; Grossmann, V.; Okuno, Y.; Bacher, U.; Nagae, G.; Schnittger, S.; Sanada, M.; Kon, A.; Alpermann, T.; et al. Landscape of genetic lesions in 944 patients with myelodysplastic syndromes. *Leukemia* **2014**, *28*, 241–247. [CrossRef]
59. Churpek, J.E.; Pyrtel, K.; Kanchi, K.L.; Shao, J.; Koboldt, D.; Miller, C.A.; Shen, D.; Fulton, R.; O'Laughlin, M.; Fronick, C.; et al. Genomic analysis of germ line and somatic variants in familial myelodysplasia/acute myeloid leukemia. *Blood* **2015**, *126*, 2484–2490. [CrossRef]

60. Haslam, K.; Langabeer, S.E.; Hayat, A.; Conneally, E.; Vandenberghe, E. Targeted next-generation sequencing of familial platelet disorder with predisposition to acute myeloid leukaemia. *Br. J. Haematol.* **2016**, *175*, 161–163. [CrossRef]
61. Tawana, K.; Wang, J.; Király, P.A.; Kállay, K.; Benyó, G.; Zombori, M.; Csomor, J.; Al Seraihi, A.; Rio-Machin, A.; Matolcsy, A.; et al. Recurrent somatic JAK-STAT pathway variants within a RUNX1-mutated pedigree. *Eur. J. Hum. Genet.* **2017**, *25*, 1020–1024. [CrossRef]
62. Delhommeau, F.; Dupont, S.; Della Valle, V.; James, C.; Trannoy, S.; Massé, A.; Kosmider, O.; Le Couedic, J.P.; Robert, F.; Alberdi, A.; et al. Mutation in TET2 in myeloid cancers. *N. Engl. J. Med.* **2009**, *360*, 2289–2301. [CrossRef] [PubMed]
63. Döhner, H.; Estey, E.; Grimwade, D.; Amadori, S.; Appelbaum, F.R.; Büchner, T.; Dombret, H.; Ebert, B.L.; Fenaux, P.; Larson, R.A.; et al. Diagnosis and management of AML in adults: 2017 ELN recommendations from an international expert panel. *Blood* **2017**, *129*, 424–447. [CrossRef] [PubMed]
64. Weissmann, S.; Alpermann, T.; Grossmann, V.; Kowarsch, A.; Nadarajah, N.; Eder, C.; Dicker, F.; Fasan, A.; Haferlach, C.; Haferlach, T.; et al. Landscape of TET2 mutations in acute myeloid leukemia. *Leukemia* **2012**, *26*, 934–942. [CrossRef] [PubMed]
65. Ley, T.J.; Ding, L.; Walter, M.J.; McLellan, M.D.; Lamprecht, T.; Larson, D.E.; Kandoth, C.; Payton, J.E.; Baty, J.; Welch, J.; et al. DNMT3A mutations in acute myeloid leukemia. *N. Engl. J. Med.* **2010**, *363*, 2424–2433. [CrossRef] [PubMed]
66. Walter, M.J.; Ding, L.; Shen, D.; Shao, J.; Grillot, M.; McLellan, M.; Fulton, R.; Schmidt, H.; Kalicki-Veizer, J.; O'Laughlin, M.; et al. Recurrent DNMT3A mutations in patients with myelodysplastic syndromes. *Leukemia* **2011**, *25*, 1153–1158. [CrossRef] [PubMed]
67. Grossmann, V.; Haferlach, C.; Weissmann, S.; Roller, A.; Schindela, S.; Poetzinger, F.; Stadler, K.; Bellos, F.; Kern, W.; Haferlach, T.; et al. The molecular profile of adult T-cell acute lymphoblastic leukemia: Mutations in RUNX1 and DNMT3A are associated with poor prognosis in T-ALL. *Genes Chromosomes Cancer* **2013**, *52*, 410–422. [CrossRef] [PubMed]
68. Itzykson, R.; Fenaux, P.; Bowen, D.; Cross, N.C.P.; Cortes, J.; De Witte, T.; Germing, U.; Onida, F.; Padron, E.; Platzbecker, U.; et al. Diagnosis and Treatment of Chronic Myelomonocytic Leukemias in Adults: Recommendations From the European Hematology Association and the European LeukemiaNet. *Hemasphere* **2018**, *2*, e150. [CrossRef]
69. Tefferi, A. Primary myelofibrosis: 2017 update on diagnosis, risk-stratification, and management. *Am. J. Hematol.* **2016**, *91*, 1262–1271. [CrossRef]
70. Vannucchi, A.M.; Lasho, T.L.; Guglielmelli, P.; Biamonte, F.; Pardanani, A.; Pereira, A.; Finke, C.; Score, J.; Gangat, N.; Mannarelli, C.; et al. Mutations and prognosis in primary myelofibrosis. *Leukemia* **2013**, *27*, 1861–1869. [CrossRef]
71. Tefferi, A.; Vannucchi, A.M. Genetic Risk Assessment in Myeloproliferative Neoplasms. *Mayo Clin. Proc.* **2017**, *92*, 1283–1290. [CrossRef]
72. Bolouri, H.; Farrar, J.E.; Triche, T., Jr.; Ries, R.E.; Lim, E.L.; Alonzo, T.A.; Ma, Y.; Moore, R.; Mungall, A.J.; Marra, M.A.; et al. The molecular landscape of pediatric acute myeloid leukemia reveals recurrent structural alterations and age-specific mutational interactions. *Nat. Med.* **2018**, *24*, 103–112. [CrossRef] [PubMed]
73. Pastor, V.; Hirabayashi, S.; Karow, A.; Wehrle, J.; Kozyra, E.J.; Nienhold, R.; Ruzaike, G.; Lebrecht, D.; Yoshimi, A.; Niewisch, M.; et al. Mutational landscape in children with myelodysplastic syndromes is distinct from adults: Specific somatic drivers and novel germline variants. *Leukemia* **2017**, *31*, 759–762. [CrossRef] [PubMed]
74. Kanagal-Shamanna, R.; Loghavi, S.; DiNardo, C.D.; Medeiros, L.J.; Garcia-Manero, G.; Jabbour, E.; Routbort, M.J.; Luthra, R.; Bueso-Ramos, C.E.; Khoury, J.D. Bone marrow pathologic abnormalities in familial platelet disorder with propensity for myeloid malignancy and germline RUNX1 mutation. *Haematologica* **2017**, *102*, 1661–1670. [CrossRef] [PubMed]
75. Lachowiez, C.; Bannon, S.; Loghavi, S.; Wang, F.; Kanagal-Shamanna, R.; Mehta, R.; Daver, N.; Borthakur, G.; Pemmaraju, N.; Ravandi, F.; et al. Clonal evolution and treatment outcomes in hematopoietic neoplasms arising in patients with germline RUNX1 mutations. *Am. J. Hematol.* **2020**, *95*, E313–E315. [CrossRef]
76. Papaemmanuil, E.; Gerstung, M.; Bullinger, L.; Gaidzik, V.I.; Paschka, P.; Roberts, N.D.; Potter, N.E.; Heuser, M.; Thol, F.; Bolli, N.; et al. Genomic Classification and Prognosis in Acute Myeloid Leukemia. *N. Engl. J. Med.* **2016**, *374*, 2209–2221. [CrossRef]
77. Jaiswal, S.; Fontanillas, P.; Flannick, J.; Manning, A.; Grauman, P.V.; Mar, B.G.; Lindsley, R.C.; Mermel, C.H.; Burtt, N.; Chavez, A.; et al. Age-related clonal hematopoiesis associated with adverse outcomes. *N. Engl. J. Med.* **2014**, *371*, 2488–2498. [CrossRef]
78. Marnell, C.S.; Bick, A.; Natarajan, P. Clonal hematopoiesis of indeterminate potential (CHIP): Linking somatic mutations, hematopoiesis, chronic inflammation and cardiovascular disease. *J. Mol. Cell Cardiol.* **2021**, *161*, 98–105. [CrossRef]
79. Cook, E.K.; Luo, M.; Rauh, M.J. Clonal hematopoiesis and inflammation: Partners in leukemogenesis and comorbidity. *Exp. Hematol.* **2020**, *83*, 85–94. [CrossRef]
80. Falini, B.; Sportoletti, P.; Brunetti, L.; Martelli, M.P. Perspectives for therapeutic targeting of gene mutations in acute myeloid leukaemia with normal cytogenetics. *Br. J. Haematol.* **2015**, *170*, 305–322. [CrossRef]
81. Sakurai, M.; Kasahara, H.; Yoshida, K.; Yoshimi, A.; Kunimoto, H.; Watanabe, N.; Shiraishi, Y.; Chiba, K.; Tanaka, H.; Harada, Y.; et al. Genetic basis of myeloid transformation in familial platelet disorder/acute myeloid leukemia patients with haploinsufficient RUNX1 allele. *Blood Cancer J.* **2016**, *6*, e392. [CrossRef]
82. Béri-Dexheimer, M.; Latger-Cannard, V.; Philippe, C.; Bonnet, C.; Chambon, P.; Roth, V.; Grégoire, M.J.; Bordigoni, P.; Lecompte, T.; Leheup, B.; et al. Clinical phenotype of germline RUNX1 haploinsufficiency: From point mutations to large genomic deletions. *Eur. J. Hum. Genet.* **2008**, *16*, 1014–1018. [CrossRef] [PubMed]

83. Bluteau, D.; Gilles, L.; Hilpert, M.; Antony-Debré, I.; James, C.; Debili, N.; Camara-Clayette, V.; Wagner-Ballon, O.; Cordette-Lagarde, V.; Robert, T.; et al. Down-regulation of the RUNX1-target gene NR4A3 contributes to hematopoiesis deregulation in familial platelet disorder/acute myelogenous leukemia. *Blood* **2011**, *118*, 6310–6320. [CrossRef] [PubMed]
84. Duarte, B.K.L.; Yamaguti-Hayakawa, G.G.; Medina, S.S.; Siqueira, L.H.; Snetsinger, B.; Costa, F.F.; Rauh, M.J.; Ozelo, M.C. Longitudinal sequencing of RUNX1 familial platelet disorder: New insights into genetic mechanisms of transformation to myeloid malignancies. *Br. J. Haematol.* **2019**, *186*, 724–734. [CrossRef]
85. Bagla, S.; Regling, K.A.; Wakeling, E.N.; Gadgeel, M.; Buck, S.; Zaidi, A.U.; Flore, L.A.; Chicka, M.; Schiffer, C.A.; Chitlur, M.B.; et al. Distinctive phenotypes in two children with novel germline RUNX1 mutations-one with myeloid malignancy and increased fetal hemoglobin. *Pediatr. Hematol. Oncol.* **2021**, *38*, 65–79. [CrossRef] [PubMed]
86. Ng, I.K.; Lee, J.; Ng, C.; Kosmo, B.; Chiu, L.; Seah, E.; Mok, M.M.H.; Tan, K.; Osato, M.; Chng, W.J.; et al. Preleukemic and second-hit mutational events in an acute myeloid leukemia patient with a novel germline RUNX1 mutation. *Biomark. Res.* **2018**, *6*, 16. [CrossRef]
87. Manchev, V.T.; Bouzid, H.; Antony-Debré, I.; Leite, B.; Meurice, G.; Droin, N.; Prebet, T.; Costello, R.T.; Vainchenker, W.; Plo, I.; et al. Acquired TET2 mutation in one patient with familial platelet disorder with predisposition to AML led to the development of pre-leukaemic clone resulting in T2-ALL and AML-M0. *J. Cell Mol. Med.* **2017**, *21*, 1237–1242. [CrossRef] [PubMed]
88. Rajpal, S.; Jain, A.; Jamwal, M.; Jain, N.; Sachdeva, M.U.S.; Malhotra, P.; Varma, N.; Das, R. A novel germline RUNX1 mutation with co-occurrence of somatic alterations in a case of myeloid neoplasm with familial thrombocytopenia: First report from India. *Leuk. Lymphoma* **2019**, *60*, 2568–2571. [CrossRef] [PubMed]
89. Staňo Kozubík, K.; Radová, L.; Pešová, M.; Réblová, K.; Trizuljak, J.; Plevová, K.; Fiamoli, V.; Gumulec, J.; Urbánková, H.; Szotkowski, T.; et al. C-terminal RUNX1 mutation in familial platelet disorder with predisposition to myeloid malignancies. *Int. J. Hematol.* **2018**, *108*, 652–657. [CrossRef]
90. Shiba, N.; Hasegawa, D.; Park, M.J.; Murata, C.; Sato-Otsubo, A.; Ogawa, C.; Manabe, A.; Arakawa, H.; Ogawa, S.; Hayashi, Y. CBL mutation in chronic myelomonocytic leukemia secondary to familial platelet disorder with propensity to develop acute myeloid leukemia (FPD/AML). *Blood* **2012**, *119*, 2612–2614. [CrossRef]

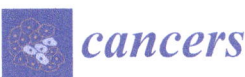

Review

Comprehensive Analysis of Acquired Genetic Variants and Their Prognostic Impact in Systemic Mastocytosis

Oscar González-López [1,2], Javier I. Muñoz-González [1,2], Alberto Orfao [1,2], Iván Álvarez-Twose [2,3] and Andrés C. García-Montero [1,2,*]

[1] Cancer Research Center (IBMCC, USAL/CSIC), Department of Medicine, Universidad de Salamanca, Biomedical Research Institute of Salamanca and Spanish Network on Mastocytosis (REMA), 37007 Salamanca, Spain; oscar_villa_93@usal.es (O.G.-L.); jmunogon@usal.es (J.I.M.-G.); orfao@usal.es (A.O.)

[2] Centro de Investigación Biomédica en Red Cáncer (CIBERONC), 28029 Madrid, Spain; ivana@sescam.jccm.es

[3] Instituto de Estudios de Mastocitosis de Castilla La Mancha (CLMast, Virgen del Valle Hospital) and REMA, 45071 Toledo, Spain

* Correspondence: angarmon@usal.es

Simple Summary: Systemic mastocytosis (SM) is a clonal haematopoietic stem cell disease typically characterized by the expansion and accumulation of neoplastic mast cells carrying the activating *KIT* D816V as a driver mutation. Multilineage involvement of haematopoiesis by this *KIT* mutation, particularly in a multi-mutated context, also involving other genes (e.g., *SRSF2*, *ASXL1*, *DNMT3A*, *RUNX1*, *EZH2*, *CBL* and *NRAS*) found to be frequently mutated in other myeloid neoplasms, have recently emerged as a genetic background associated with malignant transformation of SM. Therefore, assessment of multilineage involvement of haematopoiesis by *KIT* D816V and additional mutations in genes known to be associated with the prognosis of SM have become of great help to identify good vs. poor-prognosis SM patients who could benefit from a closer follow-up and, eventually, also early cytoreductive treatment.

Abstract: Systemic mastocytosis (SM) is a rare clonal haematopoietic stem cell disease in which activating *KIT* mutations (most commonly *KIT* D816V) are present in virtually every (>90%) adult patient at similar frequencies among non-advanced and advanced forms of SM. The *KIT* D816V mutation is considered the most common pathogenic driver of SM. Acquisition of this mutation early during haematopoiesis may cause multilineage involvement of haematopoiesis by *KIT* D816V, which has been associated with higher tumour burden and additional mutations in other genes, leading to an increased rate of transformation to advanced SM. Thus, among other mutations, alterations in around 30 genes that are also frequently mutated in other myeloid neoplasms have been reported in SM cases. From these genes, 12 (i.e., *ASXL1*, *CBL*, *DNMT3A*, *EZH2*, *JAK2*, *KRAS*, *NRAS*, *SF3B1*, *RUNX1*, *SF3B1*, *SRSF2*, *TET2*) have been recurrently reported to be mutated in SM. Because of all the above, assessment of multilineage involvement of haematopoiesis by the *KIT* D816V mutation, in the setting of multi-mutated haematopoiesis as revealed by a limited panel of genes (i.e., *ASXL1*, *CBL*, *DNMT3A*, *EZH2*, *NRAS*, *RUNX1* and *SRSF2*) and associated with a poorer patient outcome, has become of great help to identify SM patients at higher risk of disease progression and/or poor survival who could benefit from closer follow-up and eventually also early cytoreductive treatment.

Keywords: systemic mastocytosis; prognostic; mutations; *KIT*; D816V; *ASXL1*; *DNMT3A*; *EZH2*; *RUNX1*; *SRSF2*

Citation: González-López, O.; Muñoz-González, J.I.; Orfao, A.; Álvarez-Twose, I.; García-Montero, A.C. Comprehensive Analysis of Acquired Genetic Variants and Their Prognostic Impact in Systemic Mastocytosis. *Cancers* **2022**, *14*, 2487. https://doi.org/10.3390/cancers14102487

Academic Editor: Steven Knapper

Received: 4 April 2022
Accepted: 15 May 2022
Published: 18 May 2022

Publisher's Note: MDPI stays neutral with regard to jurisdictional claims in published maps and institutional affiliations.

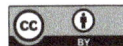

Copyright: © 2022 by the authors. Licensee MDPI, Basel, Switzerland. This article is an open access article distributed under the terms and conditions of the Creative Commons Attribution (CC BY) license (https://creativecommons.org/licenses/by/4.0/).

1. Introduction

Systemic mastocytosis (SM) is a rare hematologic disease characterized by an abnormal expansion and accumulation of pathological mast cells (MCs) in skin and/or other several extracutaneous tissues such as bone marrow (BM) and the gastro-intestinal tract. Currently,

SM is divided into five different diagnostic subtypes according to the World Health Organization (WHO) 2016 classification [1]. These include indolent SM (ISM), smouldering SM (SSM), aggressive SM (ASM), SM with associated haematological neoplasms (SM-AHN) and MC leukaemia (MCL). Additionally, the inclusion of two new subtypes of SM into the classification of the disease is currently under consideration: a variant of ISM known as BM mastocytosis (BMM) [2,3], which is characterized by a low BM MC burden in the absence of skin lesions, and a very rare (<5%) variant of mastocytosis, which shows tumour mast cells (MCs) with a well-differentiated morphology together with a CD25$^-$ CD2$^-$ immunophenotype and unique clinical, biological and molecular features, termed well-differentiated SM (WDSM) [4]. From a prognostic point of view, all these diagnostic subtypes of SM can be grouped into (i) non-advanced forms of SM (Non-AdvSM), which include BMM, ISM and SSM, typically characterized by a more stable and indolent course of the disease and a life expectancy similar or close to that of a sex- and age-matched population; and (ii) advanced SM (AdvSM) including ASM, SM-AHN and MCL, which typically display an adverse prognosis associated with a significantly shortened life expectancy requiring cytoreductive therapy [1]. Despite this, some ISM patients (<5%) can eventually evolve to SSM and AdvSM [5]. Conversely, a small proportion of AdvSM patients may also show a relatively stable disease course over years or even decades [6,7].

Currently, the aetiopathogenic mechanisms involved in malignant transformation of SM remain largely unknown. However, from an ontogenetic point of view, it is known that pathological MCs from the vast majority of patients (>90%) carries the D816V mutation in the *KIT* protooncogene [8,9] regardless of the diagnostic subtype of SM and its clinical course (e.g., Non-AdvSM or AdvSM). Despite this, multilineage involvement of hematopoietic cells other than MCs by *KIT* D816V, together with the existence of additional mutations in genes other than *KIT* (e.g., *SRSF2*, *ASXL1*, *RUNX1*, *EZH2*) have been demonstrated in recent years to mostly affect (but not only) AdvSM patients [10–12]. It is noteworthy that most of the latter mutations involve genes that are also recurrently mutated in other (myeloid) haematological malignancies [10,11,13], suggesting a tendency for their acquisition in haematopoietic cells that have an appropriate altered genetic background (i.e., *KIT* D816V-positive cells) that could favour malignant transformation and a more aggressive disease behaviour.

2. *KIT* Mutations in Systemic Mastocytosis

The *KIT* gene is a proto-oncogene encoding for a trans-membrane receptor (mast/stem cell growth factor receptor (KIT)) with tyrosine kinase (TK) activity located on the long arm of human chromosome 4 [14]. When the KIT ligand—stem cell growth factor (SCF)—binds to KIT, conformational changes occur that lead to dimerization of the receptor and its activation by autophosphorylation [15]. Of note, intracellular signalling triggered upon activation of the KIT receptor is key to the normal development of haematopoiesis and the survival of haematopoietic stem cells (HSC) [16]. Except for MCs and some natural killer (NK) cells, *KIT* is no longer expressed by other mature myeloid and lymphoid haematopoietic cells [17]. In MCs, *KIT* expression remains at high levels throughout maturation [18,19], playing a critical role in MC proliferation, differentiation and survival [15,20]. Therefore, the acquisition of mutations that could impair the normal function of KIT (e.g., activating *KIT* mutations) has pro-oncogenic effects associated with inhibition of apoptosis and increased MC proliferation and survival [21,22].

2.1. KIT D816V Mutation

The D816V mutation of *KIT* is located at exon 17 within the tyrosine kinase (TK) 2 domain of the *KIT* gene. This mutation causes constitutive activation of the KIT receptor in the absence of SCF binding and represents the most frequent genetic alteration in SM (>90% of adult SM patients) [9,15]. In fact, constitutive activation of KIT causes preferential differentiation of HSC toward cell lines regulated by *KIT* expression and signalling (mainly MCs and to a large extent also other myeloid lineages). The fact that MCs are the only haematopoietic cells that express *KIT* throughout their maturation [18,19] would explain why this *KIT*-activating mutation induces the expansion and accumulation of pathological MCs in different organs and tissues, as typically observed in SM and other *KIT*-mutated MC diseases [23]. Of note, the prevalence of the *KIT* D816V mutation is very similar among adult patients diagnosed with Non-AdvSM and AdvSM [9]. Therefore, the *KIT* D816V mutation is considered as a (specific) diagnostic marker of SM, regardless of the subtype of the disease, its presence being one of the four minor criteria required by WHO for the diagnosis of SM [1,24,25]. However, the presence of this mutation cannot explain by itself the wide spectrum of disease behaviour observed among SM patients, ranging from stable and even pauci-symptomatic to progressive and even highly-aggressive disease [5].

2.2. Other KIT Mutations

Overall, *KIT* mutations other than *KIT* D816V can be found in up to 4–5% adults and one third of children with mastocytosis [9]. In adults, these mutations are mostly located at codons 814–822 within exon 17 [9,26–31], including several mutant variants at codon 816 [9,32–46] (Table 1). *KIT* mutations located outside exon 17 include rare mutations that mostly affect exons 2 [29], 5 [40], 7–11 [29,32,40,46–58], 13 [29,59] and 18 [29]. Of note, most mutations other than *KIT* D816V correspond to isolated cases of SM-AHN, MCL or WDSM (Table 1). Interestingly, MCL patients with *KIT* mutations other than D816V often lack additional somatic high-risk mutations [46]. Although the vast majority of *KIT* mutations defined above are acquired (somatic) genetic variants, a few mutations typically located in exons 8 to 10 of *KIT* (e.g., delD419 [60], S451C [61], K509C [62,63] or F522C [54]) correspond to germinal mutations that frequently show a familial aggregation pattern.

From a clinical point of view, the exact location of the mutations in the *KIT* gene is of great relevance, since those mutations that occur within the transmembrane or juxtamembrane domains of the *KIT* gene (exons 9–11) induce spontaneous receptor dimerization, making pathological MCs sensitive to conventional TK inhibitor therapies (e.g., imatinib) [52–55,62,64], while *KIT* mutations involving the catalytic domain (exons 13–18) cause a conformational change of the protein, which confers intrinsic resistance to imatinib and other TK inhibitors commonly used to treat other human tumours [65,66].

Table 1. *KIT* mutations other than D816V described in adult patients with systemic mastocytosis (SM).

Domain	Exon	Mutation	Subtype SM
Extracellular: Ligand (SCF) binding domain	2	R49C	SM-u [29]
	5	Y269C	SM-AHN [40]
Extracellular: Dimerization domain	7	V399I	SM-u [29]
	8	D419del	ISM [47]
	9	S451C S476I S501_A502dup A502_Y503dup Y503_F504InsAY F504_N505delIns5 K509R K509I	SM-u [61] MCL [48] ASM [50] MCL [49] SM-u [29] MCL [51,52] ASM [40] SM-AHN [51] SM-u [29] ISM [62] ASM [53] MCL [62] WDSM [63]
Transmembrane domain	10	F522C	WDSM [32,54,55] MCL [46]
Juxta-membrane domain	11	V559I V560G	ASM [56] SM-u [40] ISM [57] MCL [58]
TK1 domain	13	K642E V654A	ASM [29,40] MCL [59]

Table 1. Cont.

Domain	Exon	Mutation	Subtype SM
TK2 domain	17	A814S	SM-AHN [26]
		A814T	SM-AHN [27]
		I815-V816Ins	ISM [9]
		D816H	AdvSM [32,33] SM-AHN [26,34–36] MCL [46,67,68]
		D816Y	ISM [37] AdvSM [32,33] SM-AHN [26,27,36,38,39] MCL [9,46]
		D816I	SM-AHN [40]
		D816A	SM-AHN [41,45] ASM [42]
		D816G	MCL [43]
		D816T	SM-u [44]
		I817V	WDSM [9]
		D820G	ASM [28]
		N822K	SM-u [30] SM-AHN [31]
	18	V852G	SM-u [29]

Abbreviations: AdvSM: advanced systemic mastocytosis (SM); ASM: aggressive SM; ISM: indolent SM; MCL: mast cell leukaemia; SM-AHN: SM with an associated haematological neoplasm; SM-u: SM unclassified; WDSM: well-differentiated SM.

3. Clonal Haematopoiesis in Systemic Mastocytosis

SM is considered a clonal HSC disease characterized by the expansion and accumulation of neoplastic MCs [69–71]. As a neoplasm involving the HSC compartment, the *KIT* D816V (and other *KIT*) mutations can be found in both neoplastic MCs and CD34$^+$ BM HSC, as well as in other myeloids (e.g., neutrophils [9,72–74], monocytes [9,70,72–74], basophils [70,72,74] and/or eosinophils [9,74]) and/or lymphoid (e.g., T and B lymphocytes [9,70,73,74]) cells. In such cases presenting multilineage involvement of haematopoiesis, clonal myeloid (MM) or myeloid plus lymphoid (MML) cells are found, which derive from the expansion and differentiation of D816V-mutated HSCs to different myeloid and/or lymphoid cell lineages [5,75]. Moreover, *KIT* D816V-mutated BM mesenchymal stem cells (MSCs) are also frequently detected in MML-mutated cases [36,76,77]. Overall, multilineage involvement of haematopoiesis by the *KIT* D816V mutation is found in virtually all ASM and SSM patients, in around one third of ISM cases and in a small proportion ($\leq$10%) of BMM patients [9,78]. In SM-AHN, the frequency of patients that show a multilineage *KIT* D816V mutation may vary significantly [36] depending on the specific subtypes of SM and AHN [9]. Thus, *KIT* D816V-mutated AHN cells have been found in 89% of SM associated with chronic myelomonocytic leukaemia (SM-CMML), while this would only occur in 20% of SM associated with myeloproliferative neoplasms (MPN) and 30% of SM associated with acute myeloblastic leukaemia (AML); in turn, the *KIT* mutation is almost systematically restricted to the MC compartment in patients with SM associated with lymphoid neoplasms [36].

4. Mutations in Genes Other Than *KIT*

Emergence of the *KIT* D816V mutation in an HSC during the development of haematopoietic cells would potentially lead to multilineage involvement of haematopoiesis [77]. This would favour the expansion of neoplastic MCs and an increasing tumour burden; in addition, it might also lead to an increased genomic instability that may facilitate acquisition and accumulation of additional genetic alterations (Table 2 and Table S1) in the *KIT*-mutated or unmutated HSC and contribute to the malignant transformation of the disease via distinct molecular mechanisms, e.g., activation/repression of anti-/pro-apoptotic mechanisms [79].

Table 2. Mutations in genes other than *KIT* reported in systemic mastocytosis.

Gene	Exon	Gene Mutations				
ASXL1	6	S135C [12]				
	8	G219V [12]				
	12	Y591* [80]	I641fs [13]	P698Afs* [32]	I919Yfs* [29]	H1008Tfs* [29]
		E602* [29]	G642fs [12]	R786Efs* [29]	P920Tfs* [80]	G1026Dfs* [29]
		A611T [29]	G643Wfs* [13]	D820Mfs* [29]	R965_G966del [12]	I1220F [80]
		I617Pfs* [32]	G646Wfs* [29,81]	T844fs [12]	Y974* [32]	G1397S [29]
		H630fs [12]/Gfs* [29]	G646Afs* [29]	S846Vfs* [81]	I980Kfs* [32]	A1521S [12]
		E635Rfs* [13,29,32]	R693* [13]	P849Lfs* [29]	E997* [29]	*1542fs [13]
CBL	8	Q367dup [80]	Y371C [29]/H [29]/S [29]		M374K [29]	L380P [10,29,82]
		C384R [12]/Y [29]	M400K [10,32]	C404Y [10,29]	W408C [10,32]	
	9	G413D [29]	R420Q [10,29]	I423N [29]		
	11	R550W [12]				
DNMT3A	3	E30A [80]				
	4	N90S [12]				
	8	R320* [12,29]				
	10	A380V [12]	K420* [12]			
	15	W581C [12]	L594Cfs* [29]	R598* [29]	D600Afs* [29]	
	16	S638C [12]				
	17	S663L [12]				
	18	S714F [12]	R720L [12]			
	19	E733G [29]	F755S [12]	R771G [29]/Q [80]		
	23	N879D [13]	R882C [12,13]/H [12,13,80]			
EZH2	3	L50Wfs* [13]				
	5	I146T [13]				
	7	S220F [32]				
	8	R288* [32]				
	14	Q545* [13]				
	15	R583Q [13]	N608K [13]			
	17	F672L [29]				
	18	R690C [29]	H694R [40]			
JAK2	14	V617F [12,29,32]	S605Y [12]			
KRAS	2	V14I [83]				
	3	Q70H [12]				
	5	I187N [12]				
NRAS	2	G12S [29]	G12D [29,84]	G13D [84]		
	3	Q61L [29]				
RUNX1	4	L56S [29]	P86fs [13]		E88Rfs* [13]	S94I [29]
		D96Gfs [85]	R107C [13]		N109T [13]/del [29]	F116L [12]
	5	S141L [29]	A142T [13]		N146K [12,13]	R162K [13,29]
	7	V238Gfs* [13]				
SF3B1	5	Y141C [12]				
	14	R625C [29]	W658C [29]	T663I [29]	K666N [29]/T [13,32]	
	15	K700E [13,29,83]	A711D [86]			
SRSF2	1	V18L [10]	P95 A [13]/H [10,32,85]/L [10]/R [12,13]/T [87]			

Table 2. Cont.

Gene	Exon	Gene Mutations				
TET2	3	L34F [29] H192Y [13] V218Wfs* [32] Y234* [51] R248Q [29] S254Rfs* [51] E259Gfs* [29] N275Ifs* [12,13] Q278* [29] T279fs [12] N281* [29] R282G [29]	Q321* [83] E368* [13] Q373Rfs* [51] P409Lfs* [80] G429R [29] L431* [51] E452Rfs* [29,88] D527Gfs* [29] Q530* [29] E537Sfs* [29] R550* [29] H558Lfs* [51]	P562Tfs* [29] N595Ifs* [51] P612fs [12] L615Sfs* [29] Y620fs [12] Y634* [29] Q652* [29] Q652Sfs* [80] Q659Rfs* [29] Q684Nfs* [29] Q705Sfs* [29] A727S [12]	Q729* [32] Q731* [51] Q734* [51] Q752_fs* [29] L757Tfs* [29] L806Rfs* [29] Q810* [29,88] N837Yfs* [32] L840* [51] T849Hfs* [89] Y867H [29] V872Cfs* [29]	Q933* [51] Q939* [29] K948Nfs* [83] W954* [29] Q958Tfs* [29] Q963* [29] S972Ffs* [29] C1016Wfs* [29,88] Q1020* [80] I1024Qfs* [51] P1061Qfs* [51] Q1084P [29]
	4	D1143Mfs* [32,51]				
	5	Q1170* [88]				
	6	H1219D [32]	Y1245Lfs [85]	S1246* [51]	Y1255fs [12]	
	8	Y1337* [80]	A1341E [85]			
	9	Y1351* [51] Q1389* [51]	R1359 C [88]/H [29] T1393I [29]	S1369L [29]	H1380Y [29]	D1384V [29]
	10	R1465* [29]	R1467G_fs* [29]	K1493fs [12]		
	11	L1515Ffs* [51] L1531A_fs* [29,88] K1533* [29] E1555R_fs* [29] Y1598Sfs* [29] S1611Y [12]	M1615* [89] Q1652Hfs* [29] Y1679L_fs* [29] Q1680* [29] S1688_fs* [29,51,88] M1701I [29]	V1718L [29] P1723S [29] D1750Efs* [51] N1765* [29] M1800Dfs* [51] H1817Pfs* [29]	L1819* [29] I1873T [80] E1879* [29] H1881L [29]/R [29,51,88] T1884A [29] L1886S [29]	N1890S [12] R1891G [29] F1901Lfs* [51] Y1902C [29] H1904R [80] H1912Y [13]

*: Stop codon resulting in an incomplete protein.

In line with this hypothesis, mutations in genes which are also frequently mutated in other myeloid malignancies are also present at relatively high frequencies in AdvSM patients [10,11,13,90–92] (Figure 1). In this regard, it has been recently described that certain DNA methylation patterns may be relevant in the pathogenesis of systemic diseases associated with MC activation [93]. Moreover, a significant number of somatic mutations has been identified in a broad number of genes involved in epigenetic regulatory mechanisms, which have been associated, at least in part, with the pathogenesis, clinical behaviour and evolution of different myeloid neoplasms, including SM [94,95]. Thus, around 30–40% of AdvSM present with an associated myeloid haematological neoplasm already at diagnosis [69], suggesting a close relationship between both malignancies. In line with this, next generation sequencing (NGS) studies have confirmed the presence of recurrent mutations in genes involved in post-transcriptional mRNA processing, epigenetic modification of DNA and transcription and signal transduction factors, in both SM and other myeloid neoplasms [10,11,51,81,87]. Among others, mutations have been recurrently reported in AdvSM in the *ASXL1*, *CBL*, *DNMT3A*, *NRAS*, *RUNX1*, *SRSF2* and *TET2* genes in AdvSM [10,12,13,29,32,46,50,51,68,80,81,87,96,97]. In contrast, the presence of these additional mutations is a relatively infrequent finding in BMM and ISM patients [10,29,51,80,87].

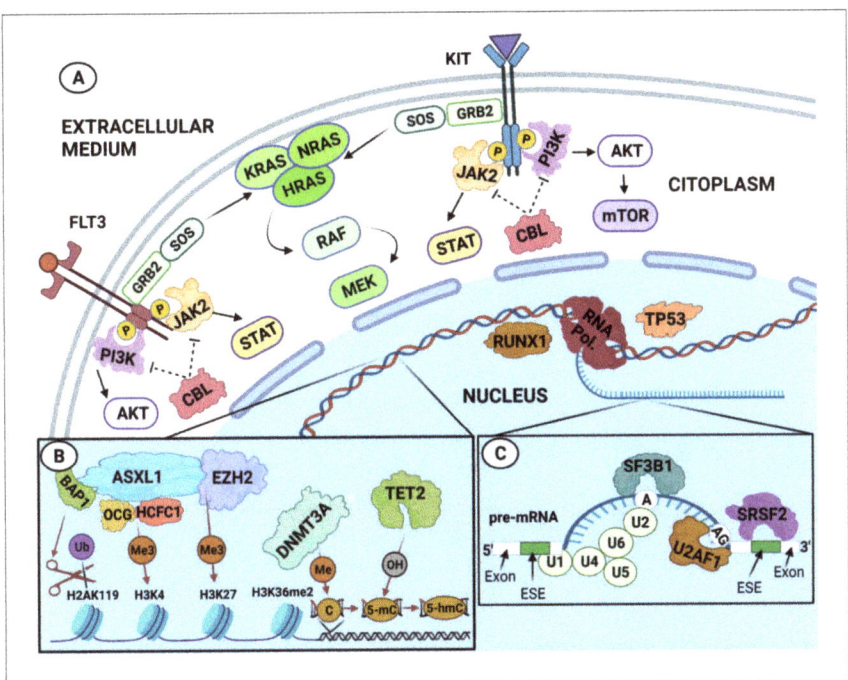

Figure 1. Genes recurrently mutated in systemic mastocytosis categorized by cellular functions. (**A**) Signal transduction and transcription regulation. Extracellular signals are received and transmitted effectively into the cell by activation of cell-surface receptors such as tyrosine kinase receptors TKR (e.g., FLT3 or KIT), resulting in the activation of intracellular signalling cascades, including the MAPK (i.e., RAS), STATs (i.e., JAK2) and PI3K pathways, which promote cell proliferation, survival and apoptosis by inducing gene transcription and/or DNA epigenetic modifications [98]. Activation/repression of these pathways require appropriate regulation of the activity and/or quantity of specific proteins. As an example, CBL proteins negatively regulate TKR (e.g., FLT3, KIT) and non-TKR (e.g., PI3K, JAK2) proteins through their ubiquitination and proteasomal degradation [99]. (**B**) Epigenetic regulation. ASXL1 and *EZH2* are members of the Polycomb group (PcG) of proteins, which are considered necessary to disrupt chromatin compaction in localized areas by activating/repressing specific histone markers. *EZH2* is involved in transferring methyl groups to histone H3 lysine 27 (H3K27), whereas ASXL1, associated with BAP1, is involved in de-ubiquitinating mono-ubiquitinated histone H2AK119 and, when associated with the OGT/HCFC1 complex, in the methylation (Me3) of H3K4 [100]. The DNMT3A protein is recruited by the histone mark H3K36me2 [101] to be involved in the methylation of cytosines (5mC), whereas the TET protein family is involved in active demethylation through oxidation of 5mC to 5hmC [102]. Overall, this mechanism results in enhancing transcription of certain genes while repressing the transcription of other genes. (**C**) RNA splicing. At the pre-mRNA level, the SF3B1, SRSF2 and U2AF1 proteins cooperate with U1–U6 small nuclear ribonucleoproteins (sn-RNPs), forming the U2-dependent splicing complex that brings the two intronic ends together by attaching the two exons and removing the intron [103]. This process transforms the pre-mRNA into mRNA, which can be transduced into a protein by ribosomes. Abbreviations: A, branch site; AG, splice receptor site; BAP1, BRCA-1-associated protein 1; ESE, exonic splicing enhancer; 5mC, 5 methyl cytosine; H, histone; HCFC1, host cell factor C1; Me, methylation; OH, hydroxylation; OGT, O-linked *N*-acetylglucosamine (GlcNAc) transferase; pre-mRNA, precursor messenger RNA; PcG, polycomb group; RTKs, receptor tyrosine kinases; Ub, ubiquitin; U1-U6, small nuclear ribonucleoproteins (snRNPs). Created using BioRender.

4.1. Mutations Affecting Transcription Factors and Signalling Pathways

The correct function and development of the human organism strongly relies on the precise regulation and appropriate production of specific sets of proteins. Gene expression is largely regulated by transcription factors and the activation of processes involved in various intracellular signalling pathways. In this regard, alterations in genes involved in these processes, such as the *CBL*, *JAK2*, *K/NRAS* and/or *RUNX1* genes [104], have been associated with several haematological malignancies. To date, mutations in a total of 11 genes related to transcription factors and signalling pathways have been described in patients with different subtypes of SM; of note, while some of these genes have been sporadically reported to be mutated in SM (*EPHA7* [12,13], *FLT3* [29], *IKZF1* [13], *PIK3CD* [12,13], *ROS1* [12,13] and *TP53* [29]) (Tables S1 and S2), others (e.g., *CBL*, *JAK2*, *K/NRAS* and *RUNX1*) are recurrently found to be altered in SM, particularly among SM-AHN patients (Table 3).

Table 3. Frequency of mutations in genes affecting transcription factors and signalling pathways found to be recurrently altered in systemic mastocytosis.

Gene	SM Diagnostic Subgroup	Mutated Cases/Total Cases (%)	Overall Frequency	WHO Subtype	Mutated Cases/ Total Cases (%)		Overall Frequency
CBL	Non-AdvSM	1/12 (0) [10] 1/216 (0.5) [12] 0/6 (0) [13] 0/44 (0) [29] 0/1 (0) [50] 1/29 (3.4) [51] 0/26 (0) [68] 0/15 (0) [80] 0/6 (0) [85]	1%	BMM	0/65 (0) [12]		0%
				ISM	1/10 (10) [10] 0/3 (0) [13] 0/1 (0) [50] 0/26 (0) [68] 0/4 (0) [85]	1/144 (1) [12] 0/44 (0) [29] 1/28 (4) [51] 0/15 (0) [80]	1%
				SSM	0/2 (0) [10] 0/3 (0) [13] 0/2 (0) [85]	0/7 (0) [12] 0/1 (0) [51]	0%
	AdvSM	7/27 (26) [10] 1/13 (8) [12] 0/14 (0) [13] 16/106 (15) [29] 25/272 (9) [32] 1/25 (4) [50] 0/35 (0) [51] 10/83 (12) [68] 1/10 (10) [80] 3/26 (12) [81] 2/13 (15) [85] 4/19 (21) [90]	11%	ASM	0/1 (0) [10] 0/9 (0) [13] 0/2 (0) [50] 0/3 (0) [68] 0/1 (0) [85]	0/9 (0) [12] 1/25 (4) [29] 0/9 (0) [51] 0/2 (0) [80] 0/6 (0) [90]	2%
				SM-AHN	6/23 (26) [10] 0/5 (0) [13] 1/21 (5) [50] 10/72 (14) [68] 2/12 (17) [85]	1/4 (25) [12] 15/80 (19) [29] 0/23 (0) [51] 3/26 (12) [81] 4/13 (31) [90]	15%
				MCL	2/7 (29) [10] 0/2 (0) [50] 0/8 (0) [68]	0/1 (0) [29] 0/3 (0) [51]	10%
JAK2	Non-AdvSM	0/12 (0) [10] 2/97 (2) [12] 0/6 (0) [13] 0/44 (0) [29] 0/1 (0) [50] 0/29 (0) [51] 2/26 (8) [68] 0/6 (0) [85] 0/13 (0) [88]	2%	BMM	1/23 (4) [12]		4%
				ISM	0/10 (0) [10] 0/3 (0) [13] 0/1 (0) [50] 2/26 (8) [68] 0/13 (0) [88]	1/70 (1) [12] 0/44 (0) [29] 0/28 (0) [51] 0/4 (0) [85]	2%
				SSM	0/2 (0) [10] 0/3 (0) [13] 0/2 (0) [85]	0/4 (0) [12] 0/1 (0) [51]	0%
	AdvSM	2/27 (7) [10] 0/14 (0) [13] 9/106 (9) [29] 25/213 (12) [32] 3/25 (12) [50] 3/35 (9) [51] 12/83 (15) [68] 3/47 (6) [81] 1/13 (8) [85] 2/29 (7) [88]	10%	ASM	0/1 (0) [10] 0/9 (0) [13] 0/2 (0) [50] 0/3 (0) [68] 0/5 (0) [88]	0/7 (0) [12] 0/25 (0) [29] 0/9 (0) [51] 0/1 (0) [85]	0%
				SM-AHN	2/23 (9) [10] 0/5 (0) [13] 3/21 (14) [50] 12/72 (17) [68] 1/12 (8) [85]	0/3 (0) [12] 9/80 (11) [29] 3/23 (13) [51] 3/47 (6) [81] 2/23 (9) [88]	11%
				MCL	0/3 (0) [10] 0/1 (0) [50] 0/8 (0) [68]	0/1 (0) [29] 0/3 (0) [51] 0/1 (0) [88]	0%

Table 3. Cont.

Gene	SM Diagnostic Subgroup	Mutated Cases/Total Cases (%)	Overall Frequency	WHO Subtype	Mutated Cases/Total Cases (%)		Overall Frequency
KRAS	Non-AdvSM	0/12 (0) [10] 2/97 (2) [12] 0/6 (0) [13] 0/29 (0) [51] 0/36 (0) [84]	1%	BMM	0/23 (0) [12]		0%
				ISM	0/10 (0) [10] 0/3 (0) [13] 0/27 (0) [84]	2/70 (3) [12] 0/28 (0) [51]	1%
				SSM	0/2 (0) [10] 0/3 (0) [13] 0/9 (0) [84]	0/4 (0) [12] 0/1 (0) [51]	0%
	AdvSM	4/27 (15) [10] 0/10 (0) [12] 0/14 (0) [13] 0/35 (0) [51] 2/16 (13) [68]	6%	ASM	0/1 (0) [10] 0/9 (0) [13]	0/7 (0) [12] 0/9 (0) [51]	0%
				SM-AHN	4/23 (17) [10] 0/5 (0) [13] 2/16 (13) [68]	0/3 (0) [12] 0/23 (0) [51]	9%
				MCL	0/3 (0) [10]	0/2 (0) [51]	0%
NRAS	Non-AdvSM	0/12 (0) [10] 0/6 (0) [13] 0/44 (0) [29] 0/1 (0) [50] 0/23 (0) [51] 0/36 (0) [84] 1/298 (0.3) [97]	0.2%	BMM			
				ISM	0/10 (0) [10] 0/44 (0) [29] 0/22 (0) [51]	0/3 (0) [13] 0/1 (0) [50] 0/27 (0) [84]	0%
				SSM	0/2 (0) [10] 0/1 (0) [51]	0/3 (0) [13] 0/9 (0) [84]	0%
	AdvSM	2/27 (7) [10] 0/14 (0) [13] 3/105 (3) [29] 1/25 (4) [50] 1/25 (4) [51] 2/16 (13) [68] 3/173 (2) [97]	3%	ASM	0/1 (0) [10] 0/25 (0) [29] 0/7 (0) [51]	0/9 (0) [13] 0/2 (0) [50]	0%
				SM-AHN	2/23 (9) [10] 3/80 (4) [29] 1/16 (6) [51]	0/5 (0) [13] 1/21 (5) [50] 2/16 (13) [68]	6%
				MCL	0/3 (0) [10] 0/2 (0) [50]	1/1 (100) [29] 0/2 (0) [51]	13%
RUNX1	Non-AdvSM	0/12 (0) [10] 1/309 (0.3) [12] 2/10 (20) [13] 0/44 (0) [29] 0/26 (0) [68] 0/6 (0) [85] 1/530 (0.2) [97]	0.4%	BMM	1/90 (1) [12]		1%
				ISM	0/10 (0) [10] 0/3 (0) [13] 0/26 (0) [68]	0/211 (0) [12] 0/44 (0) [29] 0/4 (0) [85]	0%
				SSM	0/2 (0) [10] 2/7 (29) [13]	0/8 (0) [12] 0/2 (0) [85]	11%
	AdvSM	9/27 (33) [10] 0/13 (0) [12] 7/24 (29) [13] 5/106 (5) [29] 66/329 (20) [32] 15/83 (18) [68] 1/13 (8) [85] 38/210 (18) [97]	18%	ASM	1/1 (100) [10] 2/11 (18) [13] 1/3 (33) [68]	0/9 (0) [12] 0/25 (0) [29] 0/1 (0) [85]	8%
				SM-AHN	8/23 (35) [10] 5/13 (39) [13] 14/72 (19) [68]	0/4 (0) [12] 5/80 (6) [29] 1/12 (8) [85]	16%
				MCL	0/3 (0) [10] 0/8 (0) [68]	0/1 (0) [29]	0%

Overall frequencies represent the weighted average of the percentage of patients with at least one mutation in that gene. out of the total number of patients studied within the different cohorts, for each SM subgroup. Abbreviations: AdvSM: advanced systemic mastocytosis (SM); ASM: aggressive SM; BMM: bone marrow mastocytosis; ISM: indolent SM; MCL: mast cell leukaemia; Non-AdvSM: non-advanced SM; SM-AHN: SM with an associated haematological neoplasm; SSM: smouldering SM.

The *CBL* (Casitas B-lineage lymphoma proto-oncogene) gene is located on chromosome 11 and encodes for a protein involved in the functional regulation (via competitive blockade) of tyrosine kinase (TK) receptors; in addition, the CBL product also acts in ubiquitination-mediated protein degradation in the proteasome [105,106]. Overall, mutations affecting the *CBL* gene in myeloid malignancies show a predominance of deletions involving the exon 8 of this gene [107] at frequencies that vary from 15% of patients diagnosed with juvenile myelomonocytic leukaemia, to 13% of CMML (mostly the *CBL* Y371 mutation) [108,109], 10% of AML and 8% of atypical chronic myeloid leukaemia cases [109–111]. Similarly, *CBL* mutations are found in a variable percentage of SM patients [10,11,29,46,68,80,81], where they are predominantly located at exon 8 (frequently also at codon Y371) (Table 2), their frequency ranging from <1% in Non-AdvSM patients to >10% of AdvSM cases [10,29,80,81,90], including >25% of SM-AHN patients in some cohorts [10,90] (average of 15%) (Table 3).

In contrast to other myeloid neoplasms in which the impact of *CBL* mutations remains unclear [106,109,110,112], their presence in SM has been associated with poorer outcomes [90].

The *JAK2* (Janus Kinase 2) gene is located on human chromosome 9 and encodes a protein that acts as an intracellular (non-receptor) TK that is associated with various cell surface receptors for transducing activating signals through relevant pathways such as the mitogen-activated protein kinase (MAPK) and signal transducer and activator of transcription (STATs) pathways [98,113,114]. The most common *JAK2* activating mutation, the *JAK2* V617F mutation, has been reported in several diagnostic subtypes of MPN [115], which can explain its high incidence (about 11%) in SM-AHN patients [29,50,51,81,88] as compared to other diagnostic subtypes of SM [10,12,29,51,88] (Table 3 and Table S3). A recent study in SM-AHN patients showed that *KIT* D816V and *JAK2* V617F mutations probably arise in two independent clones in most patients, in which the presence of *JAK2* mutations appears to have a low prognostic impact [116].

The *KRAS* (Kirsten Rat Sarcoma Viral Oncogene Homolog) and *NRAS* (Neuroblastoma RAS Viral Oncogene Homolog) genes are both located on chromosome 12, and they encode proteins involved in signalling pathways associated with growth factor membrane receptors through their interaction with membrane GTPases. A large number of somatic mutations involving the *KRAS*/*NRAS* genes have been identified, mostly associated with solid tumours such as lung cancer, pancreatic cancer and colorectal cancer, among other prevalent tumours [117,118]; in some of these tumours such as metastatic colorectal cancer, *KRAS* and *NRAS* mutations have also been associated with a poorer prognosis [119]. In myeloid neoplasms, *NRAS* mutations have been associated with the development of AML (7–13%) secondary to different subtypes of MPN; however, it remains unclear whether these mutations directly promote progression to leukaemia [111]. With regards to SM, *KRAS* and/or *NRAS* mutations have been sporadically reported in ISM [12,97] and MCL cases [10,29], while they are more frequently found among SM-AHN patients, particularly in cases associated with poor-prognosis myeloid neoplasms (i.e., AML) [10,29,46,50,51,68,84] (Table 3 and Table S3); in this setting, some authors have suggested that these mutations might have an adverse prognostic impact [120].

RUNX1 (Runt-Related Transcription Factor 1) is a gene located on human chromosome 21 that encodes a functional protein that acts as a transcription factor involved in the development of HSC [121]. The most frequent *RUNX1* mutations have been associated with progression from MPN to AML [122], which could explain the high frequency of these mutations (up to 37%) among patients with secondary AML [105,111]. In line with these findings, the presence of *RUNX1* mutations in patients with MDS is associated with resistance to specific chemotherapeutic drugs and shortened survival [123,124]. In SM, *RUNX1* mutations are preferentially located at exons 4 and 5 of the gene [10–13,29,32,68,97,125] (Table 2), with a frequency that ranges from <1% of Non-AdvSM patients to up to 18% of AdvSM cases, the highest frequency being detected in SM-AHN patients [10,13] (Table 3). From a prognostic point of view, *RUNX1*-mutated cases have been associated with an adverse outcome, both among Non-AdvSM and AdvSM patients [11–13,97,126].

4.2. Mutations in Genes Involved in Epigenetic Regulatory Mechanisms

Although the specific role of each individual epigenetic alteration detected in SM remains unknown [127–130], recurrent mutations in genes involved in epigenetic modifications of DNA (i.e., *ASXL1*, *CILK1*, *DNMT3A*, *EZH2*, *IDH1*, *IDH2*, *KAT6B*, *NPM1*, *SETBP1* and *TET2* genes) have been recurrently identified (Table 2, Tables S1 and S2); among these, mutations involving the *ASXL1*, *DNMT3A*, *EZH2* and *TET2* genes are the most commonly reported ones (Table 4).

Table 4. Frequency of mutations in genes involved in epigenetic regulatory mechanisms found to be recurrently altered in systemic mastocytosis.

Gene	SM Diagnostic Subgroup	Mutated Cases/Total Cases (%)	Overall Frequency	WHO Subtype	Mutated Cases/Total Cases (%)		Overall Frequency
ASXL1	Non-AdvSM	0/12 (0) [10] 6/309 (2) [12] 0/10 (0) [13] 0/44 (0) [29] 0/1 (0) [50] 0/26 (0) [68] 1/15 (7) [80] 0/6 (0) [85] 6/530 (1) [97]	1%	BMM	1/90 (1) [12]		1%
				ISM	0/10 (0) [10] 0/3 (0) [13] 0/1 (0) [50] 1/15 (7) [80] 6/530 (1) [97]	4/211 (2) [12] 0/44 (0) [29] 0/26 (0) [68] 0/4 (0) [85]	1%
				SSM	0/2 (0) [10] 0/7 (0) [13]	1/8 (13) [12] 0/2 (0) [85]	5%
	AdvSM	8/27 (30) [10] 2/13 (15) [12] 2/24 (8) [13] 25/106 (24) [29] 66/229 (29) [32] 12/25 (48) [50] 21/83 (25) [68] 2/10 (20) [80] 6/43 (14) [81] 5/13 (39) [85] 5/19 (26) [90] 35/210 (17) [97]	24%	ASM	0/1 (0) [10] 1/11 (9) [13] 0/2 (0) [50] 0/2 (0) [80] 1/6 (17) [90]	1/9 (11) [12] 4/25 (16) [29] 0/3 (0) [68] 0/1 (0) [85]	9%
				SM-AHN	8/23 (35) [10] 1/13 (8) [13] 4/21 (19) [50] 6/43 (14) [81] 4/13 (31) [90]	1/4 (25) [12] 21/80 (26) [29] 21/72 (29) [68] 5/12 (42) [85]	25%
				MCL	0/3 (0) [10] 0/2 (0) [50]	0/1 (0) [29] 0/8 (0) [68]	0%
DNMT3A	Non-AdvSM	14/309 (5) [12] 0/10 (0) [13] 2/44 (5) [29] 0/26 (0) [68] 2/15 (13) [80] 20/530 (4) [97]	4%	BMM	2/90 (2) [12]		2%
				ISM	10/211 (0.5) [12] 2/44 (5) [29] 2/15 (13) [80]	0/3 (0) [13] 0/26 (0) [68]	5%
				SSM	2/8 (25) [12]	0/7 (0) [13]	13%
	AdvSM	4/13 (31) [12] 3/24 (13) [13] 7/106 (7) [29] 1/83 (1) [68] 1/10 (10) [80] 2/19 (11) [90] 9/210 (4) [97]	6%	ASM	3/9 (33) [12] 0/25 (0) [29] 0/2 (0) [80]	3/11 (27) [13] 0/3 (0) [68] 0/6 (0) [90]	11%
				SM-AHN	1/4 (25) [12] 7/80 (9) [29] 1/8 (13) [80]	0/13 (0) [13] 1/72 (1) [68] 2/13 (15) [90]	6%
				MCL	0/1 (0) [29]	0/8 (0) [68]	0%
EZH2	Non-AdvSM	0/12 (0) [10] 0/309 (0) [12] 1/10 (10) [13] 0/44 (0) [29] 0/26 (0) [68] 0/15 (0) [80] 0/6 (0) [85]	0.2%	BMM	0/90 (0) [12]		0%
				ISM	0/10 (0) [10] 0/3 (0) [13] 0/26 (0) [68] 0/4 (0) [85]	0/211 (0) [12] 0/44 (0) [29] 0/15 (0) [80]	0%
				SSM	0/2 (0) [10] 1/7 (14) [13]	0/8 (0) [12] 0/2 (0) [85]	5%
	AdvSM	2/27 (7) [10] 0/13 (0) [12] 4/24 (17) [13] 3/106 (3) [29] 17/305 (6) [32] 2/83 (2) [68] 0/10 (0) [80] 2/13 (15) [85]	5%	ASM	0/1 (0) [10] 2/11 (18) [13] 0/3 (0) [68] 0/1 (0) [85]	0/9 (0) [12] 1/25 (4) [29] 0/2 (0) [80]	6%
				SM-AHN	2/23 (9) [10] 2/13 (15) [13] 2/72 (3) [68] 2/12 (17) [85]	0/4 (0) [12] 2/80 (3) [29] 0/8 (0) [80]	5%
				MCL	0/3 (0) [10] 0/8 (0) [68]	0/1 (0) [29]	0%

Table 4. Cont.

Gene	SM Diagnostic Subgroup	Mutated Cases/Total Cases (%)	Overall Frequency	WHO Subtype	Mutated Cases/ Total Cases (%)		Overall Frequency
TET2	Non-AdvSM	0/12 (0) [10] 7/309 (2) [12] 0/10 (0) [13] 0/1 (0) [50] 2/29 (7) [51] 1/26 (4) [68] 1/15 (7) [80] 0/6 (0) [85] 2/13 (15) [88]	3%	BMM	2/90 (2) [12]		2%
				ISM	0/10 (0) [10] 0/3 (0) [13] 1/28 (4) [51] 1/15 (7) [80] 2/13 (15) [88]	5/211 (2) [12] 0/1 (0) [50] 1/26 (4) [68] 0/4 (0) [85]	3%
				SSM	0/2 (0) [10] 0/7 (0) [13] 0/2 (0) [85]	0/8 (0) [12] 1/1 (100) [51]	5%
	AdvSM	15/27 (56) [10] 2/13 (15) [12] 3/24 (13) [13] 137/329 (42) [32] 12/25 (48) [50] 12/35 (34) [51] 33/83 (40) [68] 5/10 (50) [80] 12/32 (38) [81] 6/13 (46) [85] 10/29 (35) [88] 5/19 (26) [90]	39%	ASM	0/1 (0) [10] 0/11 (0) [13] 3/9 (33) [51] 0/2 (0) [80] 2/5 (40) [88]	1/9 (11) [12] 2/2 (100) [50] 0/3 (0) [68] 0/1 (0) [85] 1/6 (17) [90]	21%
				SM-AHN	15/23 (65) [10] 3/13 (23) [13] 9/23 (39) [51] 5/8 (63) [80] 6/12 (50) [85] 4/13 (31) [90]	1/4 (25) [12] 9/21 (43) [50] 33/72 (46) [68] 12/32 (38) [81] 8/23 (35) [88]	43%
				MCL	0/3 (0) [10] 0/3 (0) [51] 0/1 (0) [88]	1/2 (50) [50] 0/8 (0) [68]	6%

Overall frequencies represent the weighted average of the percentage of patients with at least one mutation in that gene out of the total number of patients studied in the different cohorts for each SM subgroup. Abbreviations: AdvSM: advanced systemic mastocytosis (SM); ASM: aggressive SM; BMM: bone marrow mastocytosis; ISM: indolent SM; MCL: mast cell leukaemia; Non-AdvSM: non-advanced SM; SM-AHN: SM with an associated haematological neoplasm; SSM: smouldering SM.

The *ASXL1* (ASXL transcriptional regulator 1) gene encodes for a protein that interacts with the retinoic acid receptor involved in chromatin remodelling, although its precise function remains largely unknown [131]. The most frequent *ASXL1* mutations found in myeloid neoplasms are located at exon 12 [132], with an overall incidence that ranges from <7% of patients with essential thrombocytopenia (ET) or polycythaemia vera (PV), to almost 40% of primary myelofibrosis cases [133]. *ASXL1* is also the second most frequently mutated gene in MDS and CMML, and it is altered in up to 30% of AML patients [132,134]. Most reported *ASXL1* mutations in SM are also located at exon 12 [12,13,29,32,80,81] (Table 2) with a highly variable frequency that ranges from 1% of BMM cases to >20% of AdvSM patients, particularly of SM-AHN cases (Table 4). Similarly to other myeloid neoplasms [124,133,135], *ASXL1* mutations have been also (recurrently) associated with a worse prognosis in SM [11,29,68,80,81,85].

The *DNMT3A* (DNA Methyltransferase 3 Alpha) gene located on chromosome 2, encodes for an enzyme responsible for the methylation of CpG islands, which is critical in various physiological processes during embryogenesis and/or in the inactivation of the X chromosome [136]. The most frequently described mutation in the *DNMT3A* gene occurs at codon R882 [137], being present in 8–13% of MDS, 26% of AML secondary to MDS and 2% of CMML patients [137,138]. In general, the presence of *DNMT3A* mutations in patients with myeloid malignancies has been associated with a higher number of blasts in BM and greater leukocyte counts in blood [124,134] in the absence of a clear prognostic impact [134,137–139]. Although *DNMT3A* mutations have been described at relatively similarly low frequencies in Non-AdvSM and AdvSM (4% vs. 6%, respectively) (Table 4), their presence has been associated with a significantly poorer prognosis in some patient cohorts [12,80].

The *EZH2* (Enhancer of Zeste 2 polycomb repressive complex 2 subunit) gene encodes a protein of the PRC2 complex involved in proliferation, differentiation, ageing and maintenance of the chromatin structure through methylation, acting as both a tumour suppressor gene and an oncogene [105]. The *EZH2* gene is coded in chromosome 7, and its mutations have been described in both myeloid and lymphoid malignancies, as well as in solid tumours, where they have been recurrently associated with more advanced tumour stages and metastatic disease [140]. In myeloid neoplasms, *EZH2* mutations have been described in patients with PV (3%), myelofibrosis (13%), CMML (6%), AML (6%) and MDS (10%) [105,134,139,141,142]; in MDS they have been associated with a worse prognosis [124,142]. In SM, *EZH2* mutations have been reported almost exclusively within AdvSM patients [10,13,29,32,85], particularly among ASM and SM-AHN cases (Table 4).

The *TET2* (Ten–eleven translocation methylcytosine dioxygenase 2) gene is located on chromosome 4 and encodes for a protein that catalyses the conversion of 5-methylcytosine (5-mc) to 5-hydroxymethylcytosine (5-hmc) in the DNA [143]. It is believed that 5-hmc may initiate DNA demethylation by preventing binding to the CpG islands of DNA methyltransferases characteristic of these sequences [144]. To date, *TET2* mutations have been described in every exon of the gene, and sometimes mutations involving both alleles coexist in the same cell [13,145]. *TET2* mutations are considered to be early events in the development of haematological malignancies such as MPN, MDS, CMML and different subtypes of leukaemia and lymphoma, as well as in SM [145]. Overall, *TET2* mutations have been described in about 14% of MPN, 23% of MDS (in which they usually occur together with mutations in *SF3B1*, *U2AF1*, *ASXL1*, *SRSF2* and/or *DNMT3A* and also a normal karyotype [124]) and 30% of CMML patients (often associated with mutations in the *SRSF2* and *U2AF1* genes) [10,91,124,134,146]. In SM, *TET2* is the most frequently mutated gene other than *KIT*. In these later patients, *TET2* mutations have been reported along the entire gene sequence but more frequently at exons 3, 9 and 11 (Table 2). As found also in MDS, the coexistence of *TET2* and *SRSF2* gene mutations has also been reported in SM [10,85]. Of note, in vitro studies suggest that in a significant proportion of patients with SM-AHN, *TET2* mutations may precede the *KIT* D816V mutation [85], similarly to what would also occur with *ASXL1* and *SRSF2* mutations. However, despite *TET2* mutations being significantly more frequently detected in AdvSM vs. Non-AdvSM patients (39% vs. 3% of the cases, respectively) [10,12,13,32,50,51,68,80,81,85,88,90] (Table 4), and their being associated with the presence of C-findings [51], they do not seem to have any prognostic impact in SM [10–13,29,68,80,81,97,139].

4.3. Mutations in Genes Involved in Alternative mRNA Splicing

The presence of mutations in genes associated with the spliceosome, responsible for alternative RNA processing, has been linked to different diagnostic subtypes of haematopoietic malignancies (e.g., MDS) and some solid tumours (e.g., ocular uveal melanoma or pulmonary fibrosis) [86,147]. These include mutations in the *SF3B1*, *SRSF2* and *U2AF1* genes, from which mutations in the former two genes have been described in SM at relatively high frequencies in SM (Table 5) and/or (i.e., *SRSF2*) in association with poorer outcomes [11,96].

Table 5. Frequency of mutations in genes involved in alternative mRNA splicing recurrently found in systemic mastocytosis.

Gene	SM Prognostic Subgroup	Mutated Cases/ Total Cases (%)	Overall Frequency	WHO Subtype	Mutated Cases/ Total Cases (%)		Overall Frequency
SF3B1	Non-AdvSM	2/309 (0.6) [12] 0/10 (0) [13] 0/44 (0) [29] 0/26 (0) [68] 0/6 (0) [85]	0.5%	BMM	1/90 (1) [12]		1%
				ISM	1/211 (0.5) [12] 0/44 (0) [29] 10/4 (0) [85]	0/3 (0) [13] 0/26 (0) [68]	0.3%
				SSM	0/8 (0) [12] 0/2 (0) [85]	0/7 (0) [13]	0%
	AdvSM	0/13 (0) [12] 3/24 (13) [13] 9/106 (9) [29] 18/305 (6) [32] 2/83 (2) [68] 1/13 (8) [85]	7%	ASM	0/9 (0) [12] 1/25 (4) [29] 0/1 (0) [85]	2/11 (18) [13] 0/3 (0) [68]	6%
				SM-AHN	0/4 (0) [12] 7/80 (9) [29] 1/12 (8) [85]	1/13 (8) [13] 2/72 (3) [68]	6%
				MCL	1/1 (100) [29]	0/8 (0) [68]	13%
SRSF2	Non-AdvSM	0/12 (0) [10] 0/309 (0) [12] 0/10 (0) [13] 0/44 (0) [29] 0/1 (0) [50] 0/26 (0) [68] 0/6 (0) [85] 7/530 (1) [97]	0.7%	BMM	0/90 (0) [12]		0%
				ISM	0/10 (0) [10] 0/3 (0) [13] 0/1 (0) [50] 0/4 (0) [85]	0/211 (0) [12] 0/44 (0) [29] 0/26 (0) [68]	0%
				SSM	0/2 (0) [10] 0/7 (0) [13]	0/8 (0) [12] 0/2 (0) [85]	0%
	AdvSM	14/27 (52) [10] 2/13 (15) [12] 3/24 (13) [13] 1/106 (1) [29] 120/329 (37) [32] 8/25 (32) [50] 31/83 (37) [68] 4/13 (31) [85] 79/210 (38) [97]	32%	ASM	0/1 (0) [10] 0/11 (0) [13] 1/2 (50) [50] 0/1 (0) [85]	1/9 (11) [12] 0/25 (0) [29] 0/3 (0) [68]	4%
				SM-AHN	13/23 (57) [10] 3/13 (23) [13] 7/21 (33) [50] 4/12 (33) [85]	1/4 (25) [12] 1/80 (1) [29] 31/72 (43) [68]	27%
				MCL	1/3 (33) [10] 0/2 (0) [50]	0/1 (0) [29] 0/8 (0) [68]	7%

Overall frequencies represent the weighted average of the percentage of patients with at least one mutation in that gene out of the total number of patients studied within the different cohorts for each subgroup of SM. Abbreviations: AdvSM: advanced systemic mastocytosis (SM); ASM: aggressive SM; BMM: bone marrow mastocytosis; ISM: indolent SM; MCL: mast cell leukaemia; Non-AdvSM: non-advanced SM; SM-AHN: SM with an associated haematological neoplasm; SSM: smouldering SM.

The *SRSF2* (serine and arginine rich splicing factor 2) gene encodes for a protein that is critical for alternative mRNA processing at the post-transcriptional level [148], which also acts as an important regulator of DNA stability, being a key player in the DNA acetylation/phosphorylation network [149]. The most frequent somatic mutations of *SRSF2* found in SM patients are located at codon P95 [10,12,13,32,87] (Table 2). Among patients with other myeloid haematological neoplasms, *SRSF2* mutations are particularly frequent (28–30%) among CMML cases [150] and, to a less extent, MDS (11%) and AML (6%) patients [124,134,150]. Recent studies in SM patients show the presence of *SRSF2* mutations in a variable percentage of cases ranging from <1% of Non-AdvSM cases to around one third of AdvSM patients (Table 5), being one of the most frequently mutated genes in SM, particularly in SM-AHN cases [10–13,29,32,46,50,68,80,87,97]. In contrast to other haematological neoplasms [134,151–153], the presence of *SRSF2* mutations has been consistently associated with an adverse prognosis in patients with SM [13,97], particularly among AdvSM cases [11,46,68].

The *SF3B1* (splicing factor 3b subunit 1) gene is located in chromosome 2, and it encodes for the largest subunit of the SF3B complex, a core component of the U2 small nuclear ribonucleoprotein of the U2-dependent spliceosome [154]. *SF3B1* is the most commonly mutated splicing factor gene in MDS patients [155], in whom it is associated with a more favourable outcome [156]. In contrast to *SRSF2*, *SF3B1* mutations have been less frequently described in SM [12,13,29,32,83,86], with only the K666 codon found to be mutated in more than two patient series. Actually, *SF3B1* mutations are detected in <7% of AdvSM patients (most frequently in SM-MDS cases [13,68,85]) (Table S3), while they are rarely found in Non-AdvSM patients [10,12,29,68] (Table 5). Likewise, *U2AF1* mutations are also relatively rare in SM, with a higher incidence in AdvSM [10,29,50] vs. Non-AdvSM cases (6% vs. 1%, respectively) (Table S2); these mutations are mostly located at codons S34 [29,157,158] and Q157 [29] of the *U2AF1* gene (Table S1).

5. Prognostic Impact of Acquired Gene Mutations in Systemic Mastocytosis

Acquisition of the *KIT* D816V mutation in HSC during haematopoiesis leads to multi-lineage involvement by the *KIT* mutation [77], which is associated with a poor prognosis of Non-AdvSM cases due to an increased risk of progression to AdvSM [5,77]. Despite the relatively early onset of the *KIT* D816V mutation throughout life, in at least a fraction of (i.e., multilineal) SM patients [159], the most common clinical manifestations of the disease (e.g., urticaria pigmentosa and/or anaphylaxis) usually emerge at the third or fourth decades of life in the majority of SM cases [9,159,160]. Thus, from the constitutive activation of KIT in HSC until the development of an advanced form of SM, progressive expansion and accumulation of mutated cells is required to occur, probably in association with the acquisition of secondary genetic lesions, an increased capacity to maintain them (e.g., activation/repression of anti-/pro-apoptotic mechanisms) [79] and/or the cooperation with a specific genetic background [161]. Studies performed in murine models and in patients with SM have shown that the coexistence of the *KIT* D816V mutation and mutation(s) in genes other than *KIT* are probably necessary for the progression and transformation from pauci-symptomatic Non-AdvSM to advanced forms of the disease [10,51,159,162]. However, neither a specific mutation (or mutation profile) nor a specific genetic background shared by all AdvSM patients have been identified so far [10,11,13,51,80,81,85,87,88,137]. Instead, the number of mutated genes (other than *KIT*) significantly increases from ISM to ASM [13,46] and other subtypes of AdvSM [10,29,163]. Of note, the acquisition of these additional (somatic) mutations in ISM patients who present with the multilineage *KIT* D816V mutation is usually associated with progression of the disease to, e.g., SSM and/or ASM [12,32]. In fact, demonstration of multilineage involvement of haematopoiesis by the *KIT* D816V mutation has been shown to be an independent prognostic factor for predicting progression of ISM [5]. In line with these findings, most AdvSM cases carry the multilineage *KIT* D816V mutation associated with involvement of CD34$^+$ HSC, except for a minor fraction of SM-AHN patients that have the *KIT* D816V mutation restricted to the MC compartment in BM. Interestingly, in these latter cases, the SM and AHN components of the disease appear to derive from independent clones that coexist in the same individual [36]. Despite the prognostic relevance of the multilineage *KIT* mutation, access to BM cell purification techniques required to investigate the presence of the *KIT* mutation in different myeloid and lymphoid compartments of BM cells is still restricted to a limited number of diagnostic laboratories, which has hampered the use of the multilineage *KIT* mutation as a predictor for the progression of ISM to SSM and AdvSM in routine diagnostics [7,32,120]. In line with this, the use of high sensitivity (quantitative) methods for the identification of the *KIT* D816V mutation [164–166] has proven in recent years to be of great utility to identify ISM patients that present the multilineage *KIT* as those that display a high *KIT* D816V variant allele frequency (VAF) in unfractionated BM (i.e., VAF $\geq$ 1–2%) [12,167] and/or blood (VAF $\geq$ 6%). [78] In fact, these later ISM cases also carry a significantly higher probability of undergoing disease progression associated with a significantly shortened life expectancy [167]. These findings support the use of a high *KIT* D816V VAF (as assessed by allele-specific qPCR) as a surrogate marker of multilineage involvement of haematopoiesis by the *KIT* D816V mutation [168].

In parallel, several studies on the general adult population have shown that the presence of mutations in genes that are considered to be initiators (or "drivers") of clonal expansions of HSC [169,170], while exceptional among individuals <40 years of age [170], progressively increases from the fifth decade of life onwards [171,172], being recognized as age-related clonal haematopoiesis (ARCH). Of note, ARCH is characterized by the presence of somatic mutations in genes that are also frequently mutated in SM (e.g., *ASXL1*, *DNMT3A*, *EZH2*, *RUNX1*, *SF3B1*, *SRSF2* and *TET2*) and other myeloid neoplasms [92,173,174]. Some of these ARCH-related genetic mutations that are frequently reported in AdvSM cases have been confirmed to be directly associated with the development of haematopoietic neoplasms and are considered clonal haematopoiesis of oncogenic potential (CHOP) mutations [175] (e.g., *SRSF2* [11], *ASXL1* [11], *DNMT3A* [80], *RUNX1* [11], *EZH2* [13], *CBL* [90]). These findings may contribute to explain the higher prevalence of myeloid neoplasms among older individuals and would be in agreement with the observation that age ≥60 years at diagnosis of SM predicts an increased risk of (primary and secondary) AdvSM [7,32,120]. Therefore, acquisition of ARCH-related gene mutations is currently considered to be closely associated with (a higher risk for) more advanced forms of SM. Among AdvSM patients, mutations in most of these genes (e.g., *ASXL1*, *CBL*, *JAK2*, *KRAS*, *NRAS*, *RUNX1*, *SRSF2* and *TET2*) have been reported to be more frequently associated with SM-AHN than ASM, with only a few exceptions that involve genes that show similarly mutated frequencies in both subtypes of SM (i.e., *DNMT3A*, *EZH2* and *SF3B1*) (Tables 4 and 5). Moreover, for most of these mutated genes (e.g., *ASLXL1*, *DNMT3A*, *EZH2*, *IKZF1*, *RUNX1*, *SF3B1*, *SRSF2* and *TET2*) [12], a high VAF is usually detected in the BM of AdvSM patients, which might also reflect the presence of multilineage involvement of haematopoiesis by these mutations, similarly to what has been described above for *KIT* D816V [9,13,74]. In these multi-mutated SM patients, the exact sequence of acquisition of genetic mutations remains unclear; thus, in some patients, the *KIT* D816V appears to be the first acquired mutation [13], while another subgroup of SM cases carries the *KIT* D816V mutation and mutations in genes other than *KIT* in different cell clones [13,36,85], and in a third subgroup of SM patients, the *KIT* mutation appears to be a secondary event. Of note, the two later subgroups of patients are usually diagnosed with SM associated with another myeloid neoplasm (i.e., SM-AHN) [13,36,85].

Altogether, these observations suggest that in patients with Non-AdvSM, the disease is mostly driven by the *KIT* D816V mutation, while the occurrence of additional mutations in other genes would be required (prior to or after the *KIT* mutation) for the development of AdvSM. In order to elucidate whether any of these mutated genes confers an adverse prognosis, multiple studies have been conducted in SM [11–13,29,32,68,80,90,120,160,176], from which a few include medium to large patient cohorts ($n \geq 100$) [12,29,32,68,97]. Of note, the number of genes screened in these studies is highly variable, ranging from 9 genes [80] to 410 genes [13], with a few patients being investigated by whole-genome [13] or whole-exome [42,177–179] sequencing. Overall, these studies found a total of 30 different genes to be mutated in SM (Table 2 and Table S1), from which 11 (i.e., *ASXL1*, *CBL*, *DNMT3A*, *EZH2*, *JAK2*, *KRAS*, *NRAS*, *RUNX1*, *SF3B1*, *SRSF2*, *TET2*) are recurrently mutated genes in several SM cohorts (Tables 3–5). From these later 11 mutated genes, a few have (independent) prognostic implications as regards disease progression and/or overall patient survival (i.e., *SRSF2* [11,32], *ASXL1* [11,32], *DNMT3A* [12], *RUNX1* [11,32], *EZH2* [13], *CBL* [90] and *NRAS* [120]), particularly when mutation/s are present at high VAF [12]. Because of this, the presence of mutations in limited sets of genes has been included in several recently proposed risk stratification models for both AdvSM (i.e., *SRSF2/ASXL1/RUNX1* [11], *SRSF2/ASXL1/RUNX1/EZH2* [13], *ASXL1/RUNX1/NRAS* [120]) and Non-AdvSM (e.g., *ASXL1/RUNX1/DNMT3A* [12]). The recent development of SM-induced pluripotent stem cells (iPSCs) positive for *KIT* D816V and other concurrent mutations [180], which accurately reflect the genetic background of SM patients' multi-mutated pathological cells, may become a powerful tool to dissect the impact of these mutations on the aetiopathogenic mechanisms involved in disease progression [181]. Therefore, molecular characterization of the genetic background of AdvSM patients, including NGS as described above, VAF assessment of somatic mutations [125,182] and drug screening in patient-derived iPSCs [180,183], may lead to improved molecularly targeted treatment options in a context of personalized precision medicine.

6. Conclusions

At present it is well-established that SM is a clonal HSC disease characterized by the expansion and accumulation of neoplastic MCs, where the presence of activating *KIT* mutations (most commonly *KIT* D816V) is a hallmark of the disease, being present in most (>90%) adult patients, at similar frequencies in Non-AdvSM and AdvSM. Despite the *KIT* D816V mutation being currently considered the pathogenic driver of SM, it cannot explain by itself the heterogeneous clinical behaviour of this disease. In this regard, the presence of multilineage involvement of haematopoiesis by the *KIT* D816V mutation, particularly in the context of a multi-mutated disease in which additional myeloid-neoplasm-associated genes other than *KIT* are also mutated, emerges as the altered genetic background that might contribute to explain malignant transformation of SM. Because of this, assessment of multilineage involvement of haematopoiesis by the *KIT* D816V mutation should be performed in newly diagnosed SM patients to identify those cases at high risk of progression to AdvSM. In addition, identification of other pathogenic mutations in genes with known prognostic impacts in SM (i.e., *SRSF2*, *ASXL1*, *DNMT3A*, *RUNX1*, *EZH2*, *CBL* and *NRAS*) should also be performed in SM patients with multilineage involvement of haematopoiesis by *KIT* D816V for further identification of patients at higher risk of death who may benefit from a closer follow-up and eventually, also, early cytoreductive treatment. Just as nowadays the measurement of allele burden of the *KIT* D816V mutation has become an important predictor of treatment response assessment [182] and survival [125], further analysis of the VAF for these later genes might provide a more reliable marker for assessing tumour burden as compared to other clinical and/or laboratory parameters, which can be also altered by medication or intercurrent processes (e.g., infectious and/or allergic diseases) [184–186]. Importantly, all above molecular markers should be used in combination with other disease features for accurate risk stratification of SM patients [12,32,97,120].

Supplementary Materials: The following supporting information can be downloaded at: https://www.mdpi.com/article/10.3390/cancers14102487/s1, Table S1: Sporadic gene mutations reported in systemic mastocytosis patients; Table S2: Frequency of mutations involving genes other than KIT found to be sporadically mutated in systemic mastocytosis patients; Table S3: Frequency of mutations involving genes other than KIT in patients with systemic mastocytosis associated to another haematological neoplasm.

Author Contributions: Conceptualization: A.C.G.-M.; data curation and construction of tables and figure: O.G.-L. and A.C.G.-M.; writing, editing and reviewing of the manuscript: O.G.-L., J.I.M.-G., A.O., I.Á.-T. and A.C.G.-M. All authors have read and agreed to the published version of the manuscript.

Funding: Our laboratory is supported by grants from the Instituto de Salud Carlos III (ISCIII) and co-founded by the European Union through the European Regional Development Fund (FEDER; grant number PI19/01166), as well as from the Centro de Investigación Biomédica en Red en Cáncer (CIBERONC) programme (grant number CB16/12/00400). O.G.-L. was supported by a grant from ISCIII-FEDER (grant number FI20/00116).

Institutional Review Board Statement: Not applicable.

Informed Consent Statement: Not applicable.

Acknowledgments: Figure 1 was created with BioRender.com software (BioRender, Toronto, Canada).

Conflicts of Interest: The authors declare no conflict of interest.

References

1. Valent, P.; Akin, C.; Metcalfe, D.D. Mastocytosis: 2016 updated WHO classification and novel emerging treatment concepts. *Blood* **2017**, *129*, 1420–1427. [CrossRef] [PubMed]
2. Zanotti, R.; Bonifacio, M.; Lucchini, G.; Sperr, W.R.; Scaffidi, L.; van Anrooij, B.; Oude Elberink, H.N.; Rossignol, J.; Hermine, O.; Gorska, A.; et al. Refined diagnostic criteria for bone marrow mastocytosis: A proposal of the European competence network on mastocytosis. *Leukemia* **2022**, *36*, 516–524. [CrossRef] [PubMed]

3. Escribano, L.; Alvarez-Twose, I.; Garcia-Montero, A.; Sanchez-Munoz, L.; Jara-Acevedo, M.; Orfao, A. Indolent systemic mastocytosis without skin involvement vs. isolated bone marrow mastocytosis. *Haematologica* **2011**, *96*, e26; author reply e28. [CrossRef] [PubMed]
4. Álvarez-Twose, I.; Jara-Acevedo, M.; Morgado, J.M.; García-Montero, A.; Sánchez-Muñoz, L.; Teodósio, C.; Matito, A.; Mayado, A.; Caldas, C.; Mollejo, M.; et al. Clinical, immunophenotypic, and molecular characteristics of well-differentiated systemic mastocytosis. *J. Allergy Clin. Immunol.* **2016**, *137*, 168–178.e161. [CrossRef]
5. Escribano, L.; Alvarez-Twose, I.; Sanchez-Munoz, L.; Garcia-Montero, A.; Nunez, R.; Almeida, J.; Jara-Acevedo, M.; Teodosio, C.; Garcia-Cosio, M.; Bellas, C.; et al. Prognosis in adult indolent systemic mastocytosis: A long-term study of the Spanish Network on Mastocytosis in a series of 145 patients. *J. Allergy Clin. Immunol.* **2009**, *124*, 514–521. [CrossRef]
6. Valent, P.; Akin, C.; Hartmann, K.; Nilsson, G.; Reiter, A.; Hermine, O.; Sotlar, K.; Sperr, W.R.; Escribano, L.; George, T.I.; et al. Advances in the Classification and Treatment of Mastocytosis: Current Status and Outlook toward the Future. *Cancer Res.* **2017**, *77*, 1261–1270. [CrossRef]
7. Sperr, W.R.; Kundi, M.; Alvarez-Twose, I.; van Anrooij, B.; Oude Elberink, J.N.G.; Gorska, A.; Niedoszytko, M.; Gleixner, K.V.; Hadzijusufovic, E.; Zanotti, R.; et al. International prognostic scoring system for mastocytosis (IPSM): A retrospective cohort study. *Lancet Haematol.* **2019**, *6*, e638–e649. [CrossRef]
8. Longley, B.J.; Tyrrell, L.; Lu, S.Z.; Ma, Y.S.; Langley, K.; Ding, T.G.; Duffy, T.; Jacobs, P.; Tang, L.H.; Modlin, I. Somatic c-KIT activating mutation in urticaria pigmentosa and aggressive mastocytosis: Establishment of clonality in a human mast cell neoplasm. *Nat. Genet.* **1996**, *12*, 312–314. [CrossRef]
9. Garcia-Montero, A.C.; Jara-Acevedo, M.; Teodosio, C.; Sanchez, M.L.; Nunez, R.; Prados, A.; Aldanondo, I.; Sanchez, L.; Dominguez, M.; Botana, L.M.; et al. KIT mutation in mast cells and other bone marrow hematopoietic cell lineages in systemic mast cell disorders: A prospective study of the Spanish Network on Mastocytosis (REMA) in a series of 113 patients. *Blood* **2006**, *108*, 2366–2372. [CrossRef]
10. Schwaab, J.; Schnittger, S.; Sotlar, K.; Walz, C.; Fabarius, A.; Pfirrmann, M.; Kohlmann, A.; Grossmann, V.; Meggendorfer, M.; Horny, H.P.; et al. Comprehensive mutational profiling in advanced systemic mastocytosis. *Blood* **2013**, *122*, 2460–2466. [CrossRef]
11. Jawhar, M.; Schwaab, J.; Schnittger, S.; Meggendorfer, M.; Pfirrmann, M.; Sotlar, K.; Horny, H.P.; Metzgeroth, G.; Kluger, S.; Naumann, N.; et al. Additional mutations in SRSF2, ASXL1 and/or RUNX1 identify a high-risk group of patients with KIT D816V(+) advanced systemic mastocytosis. *Leukemia* **2016**, *30*, 136–143. [CrossRef] [PubMed]
12. Munoz-Gonzalez, J.I.; Alvarez-Twose, I.; Jara-Acevedo, M.; Henriques, A.; Vinas, E.; Prieto, C.; Sanchez-Munoz, L.; Caldas, C.; Mayado, A.; Matito, A.; et al. Frequency and prognostic impact of KIT and other genetic variants in indolent systemic mastocytosis. *Blood* **2019**, *134*, 456–468. [CrossRef] [PubMed]
13. Munoz-Gonzalez, J.I.; Jara-Acevedo, M.; Alvarez-Twose, I.; Merker, J.D.; Teodosio, C.; Hou, Y.; Henriques, A.; Roskin, K.M.; Sanchez-Munoz, L.; Tsai, A.G.; et al. Impact of somatic and germline mutations on the outcome of systemic mastocytosis. *Blood Adv.* **2018**, *2*, 2814–2828. [CrossRef] [PubMed]
14. Yarden, Y.; Kuang, W.J.; Yang-Feng, T.; Coussens, L.; Munemitsu, S.; Dull, T.J.; Chen, E.; Schlessinger, J.; Francke, U.; Ullrich, A. Human proto-oncogene c-kit: A new cell surface receptor tyrosine kinase for an unidentified ligand. *EMBO J.* **1987**, *6*, 3341–3351. [CrossRef]
15. Orfao, A.; Garcia-Montero, A.C.; Sanchez, L.; Escribano, L. Recent advances in the understanding of mastocytosis: The role of KIT mutations. *Br. J. Haematol.* **2007**, *138*, 12–30. [CrossRef]
16. Li, C.L.; Johnson, G.R. Stem cell factor enhances the survival but not the self-renewal of murine hematopoietic long-term repopulating cells. *Blood* **1994**, *84*, 408–414. [CrossRef]
17. Majumder, S.; Brown, K.; Qiu, F.H.; Besmer, P. c-kit protein, a transmembrane kinase: Identification in tissues and characterization. *Mol. Cell. Biol.* **1988**, *8*, 4896–4903. [CrossRef]
18. Orfao, A.; Matarraz, S.; Perez-Andres, M.; Almeida, J.; Teodosio, C.; Berkowska, M.A.; van Dongen, J.J.M.; EuroFlow. Immunophenotypic dissection of normal hematopoiesis. *J. Immunol. Methods* **2019**, *475*, 112684. [CrossRef]
19. Teodosio, C.; Mayado, A.; Sanchez-Munoz, L.; Morgado, J.M.; Jara-Acevedo, M.; Alvarez-Twose, I.; Garcia-Montero, A.C.; Matito, A.; Caldas, C.; Escribano, L.; et al. The immunophenotype of mast cells and its utility in the diagnostic work-up of systemic mastocytosis. *J. Leukoc. Biol.* **2015**, *97*, 49–59. [CrossRef]
20. Okayama, Y.; Kawakami, T. Development, migration, and survival of mast cells. *Immunol. Res.* **2006**, *34*, 97–115. [CrossRef]
21. Kitamura, Y.; Hirotab, S. Kit as a human oncogenic tyrosine kinase. *Cell. Mol. Life Sci. CMLS* **2004**, *61*, 2924–2931. [CrossRef] [PubMed]
22. Kitayama, H.; Tsujimura, T.; Matsumura, I.; Oritani, K.; Ikeda, H.; Ishikawa, J.; Okabe, M.; Suzuki, M.; Yamamura, K.; Matsuzawa, Y.; et al. Neoplastic transformation of normal hematopoietic cells by constitutively activating mutations of c-kit receptor tyrosine kinase. *Blood* **1996**, *88*, 995–1004. [CrossRef] [PubMed]
23. Munoz-Gonzalez, J.I.; Garcia-Montero, A.C.; Orfao, A.; Alvarez-Twose, I. Pathogenic and diagnostic relevance of KIT in primary mast cell activation disorders. *Ann. Allergy Asthma Immunol.* **2021**, *127*, 427–434. [CrossRef] [PubMed]
24. Akin, C.; Metcalfe, D.D. Systemic Mastocytosis. *Annu. Rev. Med.* **2004**, *55*, 419–432. [CrossRef]
25. Jaiswal, S.; Fontanillas, P.; Flannick, J.; Manning, A.; Grauman, P.V.; Mar, B.G.; Lindsley, R.C.; Mermel, C.H.; Burtt, N.; Chavez, A.; et al. Age-related clonal hematopoiesis associated with adverse outcomes. *N. Engl. J. Med.* **2014**, *371*, 2488–2498. [CrossRef]

26. Pullarkat, S.T.; Pullarkat, V.; Kroft, S.H.; Wilson, C.S.; Ahsanuddin, A.N.; Mann, K.P.; Thein, M.; Grody, W.W.; Brynes, R.K. Systemic mastocytosis associated with t(8;21)(q22;q22) acute myeloid leukemia. *J. Hematop.* **2009**, *2*, 27–33. [CrossRef]
27. Sotlar, K.; Horny, H.P.; Simonitsch, I.; Krokowski, M.; Aichberger, K.J.; Mayerhofer, M.; Printz, D.; Fritsch, G.; Valent, P. CD25 indicates the neoplastic phenotype of mast cells: A novel immunohistochemical marker for the diagnosis of systemic mastocytosis (SM) in routinely processed bone marrow biopsy specimens. *Am. J. Surg. Pathol.* **2004**, *28*, 1319–1325. [CrossRef]
28. Pignon, J.M.; Giraudier, S.; Duquesnoy, P.; Jouault, H.; Imbert, M.; Vainchenker, W.; Vernant, J.P.; Tulliez, M. A new c-kit mutation in a case of aggressive mast cell disease. *Br. J. Haematol.* **1997**, *96*, 374–376. [CrossRef]
29. Pardanani, A.; Lasho, T.; Elala, Y.; Wassie, E.; Finke, C.; Reichard, K.K.; Chen, D.; Hanson, C.A.; Ketterling, R.P.; Tefferi, A. Next-generation sequencing in systemic mastocytosis: Derivation of a mutation-augmented clinical prognostic model for survival. *Am. J. Hematol.* **2016**, *91*, 888–893. [CrossRef]
30. Baek, J.O.; Kang, H.K.; Na, S.Y.; Lee, J.R.; Roh, J.Y.; Lee, J.H.; Kim, H.J.; Park, S. N822K c-kit mutation in CD30-positive cutaneous pleomorphic mastocytosis after germ cell tumour of the ovary. *Br. J. Dermatol.* **2012**, *166*, 1370–1373. [CrossRef]
31. Arredondo, A.R.; Gotlib, J.; Shier, L.; Medeiros, B.; Wong, K.; Cherry, A.; Corless, C.; Arber, D.A.; Valent, P.; George, T.I. Myelomastocytic leukemia versus mast cell leukemia versus systemic mastocytosis associated with acute myeloid leukemia: A diagnostic challenge. *Am. J. Hematol.* **2010**, *85*, 600–606. [CrossRef] [PubMed]
32. Jawhar, M.; Schwaab, J.; Alvarez-Twose, I.; Shoumariyeh, K.; Naumann, N.; Lubke, J.; Perkins, C.; Munoz-Gonzalez, J.I.; Meggendorfer, M.; Kennedy, V.; et al. MARS: Mutation-Adjusted Risk Score for Advanced Systemic Mastocytosis. *J. Clin. Oncol.* **2019**, *37*, 2846–2856. [CrossRef] [PubMed]
33. Schwaab, J.; Cabral do, O.H.N.; Naumann, N.; Jawhar, M.; Weiss, C.; Metzgeroth, G.; Schmid, A.; Lubke, J.; Reiter, L.; Fabarius, A.; et al. Importance of Adequate Diagnostic Workup for Correct Diagnosis of Advanced Systemic Mastocytosis. *J. Allergy Clin. Immunol. Pract.* **2020**, *8*, 3121–3127.e3121. [CrossRef] [PubMed]
34. Pullarkat, V.A.; Pullarkat, S.T.; Calverley, D.C.; Brynes, R.K. Mast cell disease associated with acute myeloid leukemia: Detection of a new c-kit mutation Asp816His. *Am. J. Hematol.* **2000**, *65*, 307–309. [CrossRef]
35. Pullarkat, V.A.; Bueso-Ramos, C.; Lai, R.; Kroft, S.; Wilson, C.S.; Pullarkat, S.T.; Bu, X.; Thein, M.; Lee, M.; Brynes, R.K. Systemic mastocytosis with associated clonal hematological non-mast-cell lineage disease: Analysis of clinicopathologic features and activating c-kit mutations. *Am. J. Hematol.* **2003**, *73*, 12–17. [CrossRef]
36. Sotlar, K.; Colak, S.; Bache, A.; Berezowska, S.; Krokowski, M.; Bultmann, B.; Valent, P.; Horny, H.P. Variable presence of KITD816V in clonal haematological non-mast cell lineage diseases associated with systemic mastocytosis (SM-AHNMD). *J. Pathol.* **2010**, *220*, 586–595. [CrossRef]
37. Longley, B.J., Jr.; Metcalfe, D.D.; Tharp, M.; Wang, X.; Tyrrell, L.; Lu, S.Z.; Heitjan, D.; Ma, Y. Activating and dominant inactivating c-KIT catalytic domain mutations in distinct clinical forms of human mastocytosis. *Proc. Natl. Acad. Sci. USA* **1999**, *96*, 1609–1614. [CrossRef]
38. Horny, H.P.; Sotlar, K.; Sperr, W.R.; Valent, P. Systemic mastocytosis with associated clonal haematological non-mast cell lineage diseases: A histopathological challenge. *J. Clin. Pathol.* **2004**, *57*, 604–608. [CrossRef]
39. Nagai, S.; Ichikawa, M.; Takahashi, T.; Sato, H.; Yokota, H.; Oshima, K.; Izutsu, K.; Hangaishi, A.; Kanda, Y.; Motokura, T.; et al. The origin of neoplastic mast cells in systemic mastocytosis with AML1/ETO-positive acute myeloid leukemia. *Exp. Hematol.* **2007**, *35*, 1747–1752. [CrossRef]
40. Lasho, T.; Finke, C.; Zblewski, D.; Hanson, C.A.; Ketterling, R.P.; Butterfield, J.H.; Tefferi, A.; Pardanani, A. Concurrent activating KIT mutations in systemic mastocytosis. *Br. J. Haematol.* **2016**, *173*, 153–156. [CrossRef]
41. Yabe, M.; Masukawa, A.; Kato, S.; Yabe, H.; Nakamura, N.; Matsushita, H. Systemic mastocytosis associated with t(8;21) acute myeloid leukemia in a child: Detection of the D816A mutation of KIT. *Pediatric Blood Cancer* **2012**, *59*, 1313–1316. [CrossRef] [PubMed]
42. Tsutsumi, M.; Miura, H.; Inagaki, H.; Shinkai, Y.; Kato, A.; Kato, T.; Hamada-Tsutsumi, S.; Tanaka, K.; Kudo, K.; Yoshikawa, T.; et al. An aggressive systemic mastocytosis preceded by ovarian dysgerminoma. *BMC Cancer* **2020**, *20*, 1162. [CrossRef] [PubMed]
43. Nakamura, R.; Chakrabarti, S.; Akin, C.; Robyn, J.; Bahceci, E.; Greene, A.; Childs, R.; Dunbar, C.E.; Metcalfe, D.D.; Barrett, A.J. A pilot study of nonmyeloablative allogeneic hematopoietic stem cell transplant for advanced systemic mastocytosis. *Bone Marrow Transpl.* **2006**, *37*, 353–358. [CrossRef] [PubMed]
44. Heinrich, M.C.; Joensuu, H.; Demetri, G.D.; Corless, C.L.; Apperley, J.; Fletcher, J.A.; Soulieres, D.; Dirnhofer, S.; Harlow, A.; Town, A.; et al. Phase II, open-label study evaluating the activity of imatinib in treating life-threatening malignancies known to be associated with imatinib-sensitive tyrosine kinases. *Clin. Cancer Res.* **2008**, *14*, 2717–2725. [CrossRef]
45. Frederiksen, J.K.; Shao, L.; Bixby, D.L.; Ross, C.W. Shared clonal cytogenetic abnormalities in aberrant mast cells and leukemic myeloid blasts detected by single nucleotide polymorphism microarray-based whole-genome scanning. *Genes Chromosomes Cancer* **2016**, *55*, 389–396. [CrossRef]
46. Jawhar, M.; Schwaab, J.; Meggendorfer, M.; Naumann, N.; Horny, H.P.; Sotlar, K.; Haferlach, T.; Schmitt, K.; Fabarius, A.; Valent, P.; et al. The clinical and molecular diversity of mast cell leukemia with or without associated hematologic neoplasm. *Haematologica* **2017**, *102*, 1035–1043. [CrossRef]
47. Lanternier, F.; Cohen-Akenine, A.; Palmerini, F.; Feger, F.; Yang, Y.; Zermati, Y.; Barète, S.; Sans, B.; Baude, C.; Ghez, D.; et al. Phenotypic and Genotypic Characteristics of Mastocytosis According to the Age of Onset. *PLoS ONE* **2008**, *3*, e1906. [CrossRef]

48. Valent, P.; Berger, J.; Cerny-Reiterer, S.; Peter, B.; Eisenwort, G.; Hoermann, G.; Mullauer, L.; Mannhalter, C.; Steurer, M.; Bettelheim, P.; et al. Chronic mast cell leukemia (MCL) with KIT S476I: A rare entity defined by leukemic expansion of mature mast cells and absence of organ damage. *Ann. Hematol.* **2015**, *94*, 223–231. [CrossRef]
49. Georgin-Lavialle, S.; Lhermitte, L.; Suarez, F.; Yang, Y.; Letard, S.; Hanssens, K.; Feger, F.; Renand, A.; Brouze, C.; Canioni, D.; et al. Mast cell leukemia: Identification of a new c-Kit mutation, dup(501-502), and response to masitinib, a c-Kit tyrosine kinase inhibitor. *Eur. J. Haematol.* **2012**, *89*, 47–52. [CrossRef]
50. Rouet, A.; Aouba, A.; Damaj, G.; Soucie, E.; Hanssens, K.; Chandesris, M.O.; Livideanu, C.B.; Dutertre, M.; Durieu, I.; Grandpeix-Guyodo, C.; et al. Mastocytosis among elderly patients: A multicenter retrospective French study on 53 patients. *Medicine* **2016**, *95*, e3901. [CrossRef]
51. Soucie, E.; Hanssens, K.; Mercher, T.; Georgin-Lavialle, S.; Damaj, G.; Livideanu, C.; Chandesris, M.O.; Acin, Y.; Létard, S.; de Sepulveda, P.; et al. In aggressive forms of mastocytosis, TET2 loss cooperates with c-KITD816V to transform mast cells. *Blood* **2012**, *120*, 4846–4849. [CrossRef] [PubMed]
52. Mital, A.; Piskorz, A.; Lewandowski, K.; Wasag, B.; Limon, J.; Hellmann, A. A case of mast cell leukaemia with exon 9 KIT mutation and good response to imatinib. *Eur. J. Haematol.* **2011**, *86*, 531–535. [CrossRef] [PubMed]
53. Zhang, L.Y.; Smith, M.L.; Schultheis, B.; Fitzgibbon, J.; Lister, T.A.; Melo, J.V.; Cross, N.C.; Cavenagh, J.D. A novel K509I mutation of KIT identified in familial mastocytosis-in vitro and in vivo responsiveness to imatinib therapy. *Leuk. Res.* **2006**, *30*, 373–378. [CrossRef] [PubMed]
54. Akin, C.; Fumo, G.; Yavuz, A.S.; Lipsky, P.E.; Neckers, L.; Metcalfe, D.D. A novel form of mastocytosis associated with a transmembrane c-kit mutation and response to imatinib. *Blood* **2004**, *103*, 3222–3225. [CrossRef] [PubMed]
55. Broderick, V.; Waghorn, K.; Langabeer, S.E.; Jeffers, M.; Cross, N.C.P.; Hayden, P.J. Molecular response to imatinib in KIT F522C-mutated systemic mastocytosis. *Leuk. Res.* **2019**, *77*, 28–29. [CrossRef]
56. Nakagomi, N.; Hirota, S. Juxtamembrane-type c-kit gene mutation found in aggressive systemic mastocytosis induces imatinib-resistant constitutive KIT activation. *Lab. Investig.* **2007**, *87*, 365–371. [CrossRef]
57. Büttner, C.; Henz, B.M.; Welker, P.; Sepp, N.T.; Grabbe, J. Identification of Activating c-kit Mutations in Adult-, but not in Childhood-Onset Indolent Mastocytosis: A Possible Explanation for Divergent Clinical Behavior. *J. Investig. Dermatol.* **1998**, *111*, 1227–1231. [CrossRef]
58. Furitsu, T.; Tsujimura, T.; Tono, T.; Ikeda, H.; Kitayama, H.; Koshimizu, U.; Sugahara, H.; Butterfield, J.H.; Ashman, L.K.; Kanayama, Y.; et al. Identification of mutations in the coding sequence of the proto-oncogene c-kit in a human mast cell leukemia cell line causing ligand-independent activation of c-kit product. *J. Clin. Investig.* **1993**, *92*, 1736–1744. [CrossRef]
59. Spector, M.S.; Iossifov, I.; Kritharis, A.; He, C.; Kolitz, J.E.; Lowe, S.W.; Allen, S.L. Mast-cell leukemia exome sequencing reveals a mutation in the IgE mast-cell receptor beta chain and KIT V654A. *Leukemia* **2012**, *26*, 1422–1425. [CrossRef]
60. Hartmann, K.; Wardelmann, E.; Ma, Y.; Merkelbach-Bruse, S.; Preussner, L.M.; Woolery, C.; Baldus, S.E.; Heinicke, T.; Thiele, J.; Buettner, R.; et al. Novel germline mutation of KIT associated with familial gastrointestinal stromal tumors and mastocytosis. *Gastroenterology* **2005**, *129*, 1042–1046. [CrossRef]
61. Wang, H.J.; Lin, Z.M.; Zhang, J.; Yin, J.H.; Yang, Y. A new germline mutation in KIT associated with diffuse cutaneous mastocytosis in a Chinese family. *Clin. Exp. Dermatol.* **2014**, *39*, 146–149. [CrossRef] [PubMed]
62. de Melo Campos, P.; Machado-Neto, J.A.; Scopim-Ribeiro, R.; Visconte, V.; Tabarroki, A.; Duarte, A.S.; Barra, F.F.; Vassalo, J.; Rogers, H.J.; Lorand-Metze, I.; et al. Familial systemic mastocytosis with germline KIT K509I mutation is sensitive to treatment with imatinib, dasatinib and PKC412. *Leuk. Res.* **2014**, *38*, 1245–1251. [CrossRef] [PubMed]
63. Alvarez-Twose, I.; Matito, A.; Morgado, J.M.; Sanchez-Munoz, L.; Jara-Acevedo, M.; Garcia-Montero, A.; Mayado, A.; Caldas, C.; Teodosio, C.; Munoz-Gonzalez, J.I.; et al. Imatinib in systemic mastocytosis: A phase IV clinical trial in patients lacking exon 17 KIT mutations and review of the literature. *Oncotarget* **2017**, *8*, 68950–68963. [CrossRef] [PubMed]
64. Frost, M.J.; Ferrao, P.T.; Hughes, T.P.; Ashman, L.K. Juxtamembrane mutant V560GKit is more sensitive to Imatinib (STI571) compared with wild-type c-kit whereas the kinase domain mutant D816VKit is resistant. *Mol. Cancer Ther.* **2002**, *1*, 1115–1124. [PubMed]
65. Akin, C.; Brockow, K.; D'Ambrosio, C.; Kirshenbaum, A.S.; Ma, Y.; Longley, B.J.; Metcalfe, D.D. Effects of tyrosine kinase inhibitor STI571 on human mast cells bearing wild-type or mutated c-kit. *Exp. Hematol.* **2003**, *31*, 686–692. [CrossRef]
66. Ma, Y.; Zeng, S.; Metcalfe, D.D.; Akin, C.; Dimitrijevic, S.; Butterfield, J.H.; McMahon, G.; Longley, B.J. The c-KIT mutation causing human mastocytosis is resistant to STI571 and other KIT kinase inhibitors; kinases with enzymatic site mutations show different inhibitor sensitivity profiles than wild-type kinases and those with regulatory-type mutations. *Blood* **2002**, *99*, 1741–1744. [CrossRef]
67. Valent, P.; Blatt, K.; Eisenwort, G.; Herrmann, H.; Cerny-Reiterer, S.; Thalhammer, R.; Müllauer, L.; Hoermann, G.; Sadovnik, I.; Schwarzinger, I.; et al. FLAG-induced remission in a patient with acute mast cell leukemia (MCL) exhibiting t(7;10)(q22;q26) and KIT D816H. *Leuk. Res. Rep.* **2014**, *3*, 8–13. [CrossRef]
68. Naumann, N.; Jawhar, M.; Schwaab, J.; Kluger, S.; Lubke, J.; Metzgeroth, G.; Popp, H.D.; Khaled, N.; Horny, H.P.; Sotlar, K.; et al. Incidence and prognostic impact of cytogenetic aberrations in patients with systemic mastocytosis. *Genes Chromosomes Cancer* **2018**, *57*, 252–259. [CrossRef]
69. Valent, P.; Horny, H.P.; Escribano, L.; Longley, B.J.; Li, C.Y.; Schwartz, L.B.; Marone, G.; Nunez, R.; Akin, C.; Sotlar, K.; et al. Diagnostic criteria and classification of mastocytosis: A consensus proposal. *Leuk. Res.* **2001**, *25*, 603–625. [CrossRef]

70. Yavuz, A.S.; Lipsky, P.E.; Yavuz, S.; Metcalfe, D.D.; Akin, C. Evidence for the involvement of a hematopoietic progenitor cell in systemic mastocytosis from single-cell analysis of mutations in the c-kit gene. *Blood* **2002**, *100*, 661–665. [CrossRef]
71. Akin, C. Clonality and molecular pathogenesis of mastocytosis. *Acta Haematol.* **2005**, *114*, 61–69. [CrossRef] [PubMed]
72. Kocabas, C.N.; Yavuz, A.S.; Lipsky, P.E.; Metcalfe, D.D.; Akin, C. Analysis of the lineage relationship between mast cells and basophils using the c-kit D816V mutation as a biologic signature. *J. Allergy Clin. Immunol.* **2005**, *115*, 1155–1161. [CrossRef] [PubMed]
73. Akin, C.; Kirshenbaum, A.S.; Semere, T.; Worobec, A.S.; Scott, L.M.; Metcalfe, D.D. Analysis of the surface expression of c-kit and occurrence of the c-kit Asp816Val activating mutation in T cells, B cells, and myelomonocytic cells in patients with mastocytosis. *Exp. Hematol.* **2000**, *28*, 140–147. [CrossRef]
74. Mayado, A.; Teodosio, C.; Dasilva-Freire, N.; Jara-Acevedo, M.; Garcia-Montero, A.C.; Alvarez-Twose, I.; Sanchez-Munoz, L.; Matito, A.; Caldas, C.; Munoz-Gonzalez, J.I.; et al. Characterization of CD34(+) hematopoietic cells in systemic mastocytosis: Potential role in disease dissemination. *Allergy* **2018**, *73*, 1294–1304. [CrossRef] [PubMed]
75. Valent, P.; Akin, C.; Arock, M.; Bock, C.; George, T.I.; Galli, S.J.; Gotlib, J.; Haferlach, T.; Hoermann, G.; Hermine, O.; et al. Proposed Terminology and Classification of Pre-Malignant Neoplastic Conditions: A Consensus Proposal. *EBioMedicine* **2017**, *26*, 17–24. [CrossRef]
76. Taylor, M.L.; Sehgal, D.; Raffeld, M.; Obiakor, H.; Akin, C.; Mage, R.G.; Metcalfe, D.D. Demonstration that mast cells, T cells, and B cells bearing the activating kit mutation D816V occur in clusters within the marrow of patients with mastocytosis. *J. Mol. Diagn. JMD* **2004**, *6*, 335–342. [CrossRef]
77. Garcia-Montero, A.C.; Jara-Acevedo, M.; Alvarez-Twose, I.; Teodosio, C.; Sanchez-Munoz, L.; Muniz, C.; Munoz-Gonzalez, J.I.; Mayado, A.; Matito, A.; Caldas, C.; et al. KIT D816V-mutated bone marrow mesenchymal stem cells in indolent systemic mastocytosis are associated with disease progression. *Blood* **2016**, *127*, 761–768. [CrossRef]
78. Jara-Acevedo, M.; Teodosio, C.; Sanchez-Munoz, L.; Alvarez-Twose, I.; Mayado, A.; Caldas, C.; Matito, A.; Morgado, J.M.; Munoz-Gonzalez, J.I.; Escribano, L.; et al. Detection of the KIT D816V mutation in peripheral blood of systemic mastocytosis: Diagnostic implications. *Mod. Pathol.* **2015**, *28*, 1138–1149. [CrossRef]
79. Teodosio, C.; Garcia-Montero, A.C.; Jara-Acevedo, M.; Sanchez-Munoz, L.; Pedreira, C.E.; Alvarez-Twose, I.; Matarraz, S.; Morgado, J.M.; Barcena, P.; Matito, A.; et al. Gene expression profile of highly purified bone marrow mast cells in systemic mastocytosis. *J. Allergy Clin. Immunol.* **2013**, *131*, 1213–1224. [CrossRef]
80. Traina, F.; Visconte, V.; Jankowska, A.M.; Makishima, H.; O'Keefe, C.L.; Elson, P.; Han, Y.; Hsieh, F.H.; Sekeres, M.A.; Mali, R.S.; et al. Single nucleotide polymorphism array lesions, TET2, DNMT3A, ASXL1 and CBL mutations are present in systemic mastocytosis. *PLoS ONE* **2012**, *7*, e43090. [CrossRef]
81. Damaj, G.; Joris, M.; Chandesris, O.; Hanssens, K.; Soucie, E.; Canioni, D.; Kolb, B.; Durieu, I.; Gyan, E.; Livideanu, C.; et al. ASXL1 but not TET2 mutations adversely impact overall survival of patients suffering systemic mastocytosis with associated clonal hematologic non-mast-cell diseases. *PLoS ONE* **2014**, *9*, 85362. [CrossRef] [PubMed]
82. Shen, W.; Szankasi, P.; Sederberg, M.; Schumacher, J.; Frizzell, K.A.; Gee, E.P.; Patel, J.L.; South, S.T.; Xu, X.; Kelley, T.W. Concurrent detection of targeted copy number variants and mutations using a myeloid malignancy next generation sequencing panel allows comprehensive genetic analysis using a single testing strategy. *Br. J. Haematol.* **2016**, *173*, 49–58. [CrossRef] [PubMed]
83. Cross, N.C.P.; Hoade, Y.; Tapper, W.J.; Carreno-Tarragona, G.; Fanelli, T.; Jawhar, M.; Naumann, N.; Pieniak, I.; Lubke, J.; Ali, S.; et al. Recurrent activating STAT5B N642H mutation in myeloid neoplasms with eosinophilia. *Leukemia* **2019**, *33*, 415–425. [CrossRef] [PubMed]
84. Wilson, T.M.; Maric, I.; Simakova, O.; Bai, Y.; Chan, E.C.; Olivares, N.; Carter, M.; Maric, D.; Robyn, J.; Metcalfe, D.D. Clonal analysis of NRAS activating mutations in KIT-D816V systemic mastocytosis. *Haematologica* **2011**, *96*, 459–463. [CrossRef]
85. Jawhar, M.; Schwaab, J.; Schnittger, S.; Sotlar, K.; Horny, H.P.; Metzgeroth, G.; Muller, N.; Schneider, S.; Naumann, N.; Walz, C.; et al. Molecular profiling of myeloid progenitor cells in multi-mutated advanced systemic mastocytosis identifies KIT D816V as a distinct and late event. *Leukemia* **2015**, *29*, 1115–1122. [CrossRef]
86. Visconte, V.; Makishima, H.; Maciejewski, J.P.; Tiu, R.V. Emerging roles of the spliceosomal machinery in myelodysplastic syndromes and other hematological disorders. *Leukemia* **2012**, *26*, 2447–2454. [CrossRef]
87. Hanssens, K.; Brenet, F.; Agopian, J.; Georgin-Lavialle, S.; Damaj, G.; Cabaret, L.; Chandesris, M.O.; de Sepulveda, P.; Hermine, O.; Dubreuil, P.; et al. SRSF2-p95 hotspot mutation is highly associated with advanced forms of mastocytosis and mutations in epigenetic regulator genes. *Haematologica* **2014**, *99*, 830–835. [CrossRef]
88. Tefferi, A.; Levine, R.L.; Lim, K.H.; Abdel-Wahab, O.; Lasho, T.L.; Patel, J.; Finke, C.M.; Mullally, A.; Li, C.Y.; Pardanani, A.; et al. Frequent TET2 mutations in systemic mastocytosis: Clinical, KITD816V and FIP1L1-PDGFRA correlates. *Leukemia* **2009**, *23*, 900–904. [CrossRef]
89. Grinfeld, J.; Nangalia, J.; Baxter, E.J.; Wedge, D.C.; Angelopoulos, N.; Cantrill, R.; Godfrey, A.L.; Papaemmanuil, E.; Gundem, G.; MacLean, C.; et al. Classification and Personalized Prognosis in Myeloproliferative Neoplasms. *N. Engl. J. Med.* **2018**, *379*, 1416–1430. [CrossRef]
90. Pardanani, A.D.; Lasho, T.L.; Finke, C.; Zblewski, D.L.; Abdelrahman, R.A.; Wassie, E.A.; Gangat, N.; Hanson, C.A.; Ketterling, R.P.; Tefferi, A. ASXL1 and CBL mutations are independently predictive of inferior survival in advanced systemic mastocytosis. *Br. J. Haematol.* **2016**, *175*, 534–536. [CrossRef]

91. Papaemmanuil, E.; Gerstung, M.; Malcovati, L.; Tauro, S.; Gundem, G.; Van Loo, P.; Yoon, C.J.; Ellis, P.; Wedge, D.C.; Pellagatti, A.; et al. Clinical and biological implications of driver mutations in myelodysplastic syndromes. *Blood* **2013**, *122*, 3616–3699. [CrossRef] [PubMed]
92. Bejar, R. CHIP, ICUS, CCUS and other four-letter words. *Leukemia* **2017**, *31*, 1869–1871. [CrossRef] [PubMed]
93. Haenisch, B.; Frohlich, H.; Herms, S.; Molderings, G.J. Evidence for contribution of epigenetic mechanisms in the pathogenesis of systemic mast cell activation disease. *Immunogenetics* **2014**, *66*, 287–297. [CrossRef] [PubMed]
94. Itzykson, R.; Fenaux, P. Epigenetics of myelodysplastic syndromes. *Leukemia* **2014**, *28*, 497–506. [CrossRef]
95. Shih, A.H.; Abdel-Wahab, O.; Patel, J.P.; Levine, R.L. The role of mutations in epigenetic regulators in myeloid malignancies. *Nature reviews. Cancer* **2012**, *12*, 599–612. [CrossRef]
96. Jawhar, M.; Schwaab, J.; Hausmann, D.; Clemens, J.; Naumann, N.; Henzler, T.; Horny, H.P.; Sotlar, K.; Schoenberg, S.O.; Cross, N.C.; et al. Splenomegaly, elevated alkaline phosphatase and mutations in the SRSF2/ASXL1/RUNX1 gene panel are strong adverse prognostic markers in patients with systemic mastocytosis. *Leukemia* **2016**, *30*, 2342–2350. [CrossRef]
97. Munoz-Gonzalez, J.I.; Alvarez-Twose, I.; Jara-Acevedo, M.; Zanotti, R.; Perkins, C.; Jawhar, M.; Sperr, W.R.; Shoumariyeh, K.; Schwaab, J.; Greiner, G.; et al. Proposed global prognostic score for systemic mastocytosis: A retrospective prognostic modelling study. *Lancet Haematol* **2021**, *8*, e194–e204. [CrossRef]
98. Villarino, A.V.; Kanno, Y.; O'Shea, J.J. Mechanisms and consequences of Jak-STAT signaling in the immune system. *Nat. Immunol.* **2017**, *18*, 374–384. [CrossRef]
99. Leardini, D.; Messelodi, D.; Muratore, E.; Baccelli, F.; Bertuccio, S.N.; Anselmi, L.; Pession, A.; Masetti, R. Role of CBL Mutations in Cancer and Non-Malignant Phenotype. *Cancers* **2022**, *14*, 839. [CrossRef]
100. Chung, Y.R.; Schatoff, E.; Abdel-Wahab, O. Epigenetic alterations in hematopoietic malignancies. *Int. J. Hematol.* **2012**, *96*, 413–427. [CrossRef]
101. Weinberg, D.N.; Papillon-Cavanagh, S.; Chen, H.; Yue, Y.; Chen, X.; Rajagopalan, K.N.; Horth, C.; McGuire, J.T.; Xu, X.; Nikbakht, H.; et al. The histone mark H3K36me2 recruits DNMT3A and shapes the intergenic DNA methylation landscape. *Nature* **2019**, *573*, 281–286. [CrossRef] [PubMed]
102. Vainchenker, W.; Kralovics, R. Genetic basis and molecular pathophysiology of classical myeloproliferative neoplasms. *Blood* **2017**, *129*, 667–679. [CrossRef] [PubMed]
103. Sperling, A.S.; Gibson, C.J.; Ebert, B.L. The genetics of myelodysplastic syndrome: From clonal haematopoiesis to secondary leukaemia. *Nature reviews. Cancer* **2017**, *17*, 5–19. [CrossRef] [PubMed]
104. Latchman, D.S. Transcription-Factor Mutations and Disease. *N. Engl. J. Med.* **1996**, *334*, 28–33. [CrossRef]
105. Vainchenker, W.; Delhommeau, F.; Constantinescu, S.N.; Bernard, O.A. New mutations and pathogenesis of myeloproliferative neoplasms. *Blood* **2011**, *118*, 1723–1735. [CrossRef]
106. Kales, S.C.; Ryan, P.E.; Nau, M.M.; Lipkowitz, S. Cbl and human myeloid neoplasms: The Cbl oncogene comes of age. *Cancer Res.* **2010**, *70*, 4789–4794. [CrossRef]
107. Sargin, B.; Choudhary, C.; Crosetto, N.; Schmidt, M.H.; Grundler, R.; Rensinghoff, M.; Thiessen, C.; Tickenbrock, L.; Schwable, J.; Brandts, C.; et al. Flt3-dependent transformation by inactivating c-Cbl mutations in AML. *Blood* **2007**, *110*, 1004–1012. [CrossRef]
108. Caligiuri, M.A.; Briesewitz, R.; Yu, J.; Wang, L.; Wei, M.; Arnoczky, K.J.; Marburger, T.B.; Wen, J.; Perrotti, D.; Bloomfield, C.D.; et al. Novel c-CBL and CBL-b ubiquitin ligase mutations in human acute myeloid leukemia. *Blood* **2007**, *110*, 1022–1024. [CrossRef]
109. Reindl, C.; Quentmeier, H.; Petropoulos, K.; Greif, P.A.; Benthaus, T.; Argiropoulos, B.; Mellert, G.; Vempati, S.; Duyster, J.; Buske, C.; et al. CBL exon 8/9 mutants activate the FLT3 pathway and cluster in core binding factor/11q deletion acute myeloid leukemia/myelodysplastic syndrome subtypes. *Clin. Cancer Res.* **2009**, *15*, 2238–2247. [CrossRef]
110. Grand, F.H.; Hidalgo-Curtis, C.E.; Ernst, T.; Zoi, K.; Zoi, C.; McGuire, C.; Kreil, S.; Jones, A.; Score, J.; Metzgeroth, G.; et al. Frequent CBL mutations associated with 11q acquired uniparental disomy in myeloproliferative neoplasms. *Blood* **2009**, *113*, 6182–6192. [CrossRef]
111. Beer, P.A.; Delhommeau, F.; LeCouedic, J.P.; Dawson, M.A.; Chen, E.; Bareford, D.; Kusec, R.; McMullin, M.F.; Harrison, C.N.; Vannucchi, A.M.; et al. Two routes to leukemic transformation after a JAK2 mutation-positive myeloproliferative neoplasm. *Blood* **2010**, *115*, 2891–2900. [CrossRef] [PubMed]
112. Makishima, H.; Cazzolli, H.; Szpurka, H.; Dunbar, A.; Tiu, R.; Huh, J.; Muramatsu, H.; O'Keefe, C.; Hsi, E.; Paquette, R.L.; et al. Mutations of e3 ubiquitin ligase cbl family members constitute a novel common pathogenic lesion in myeloid malignancies. *J. Clin. Oncol.* **2009**, *27*, 6109–6116. [CrossRef]
113. Bader, M.S.; Meyer, S.C. JAK2 in Myeloproliferative Neoplasms: Still a Protagonist. *Pharmaceuticals* **2022**, *15*, 160. [CrossRef] [PubMed]
114. Guo, Y.J.; Pan, W.W.; Liu, S.B.; Shen, Z.F.; Xu, Y.; Hu, L.L. ERK/MAPK signalling pathway and tumorigenesis. *Exp. Ther. Med.* **2020**, *19*, 1997–2007. [CrossRef] [PubMed]
115. Szybinski, J.; Meyer, S.C. Genetics of Myeloproliferative Neoplasms. *Hematol. Oncol. Clin. N Am.* **2021**, *35*, 217–236. [CrossRef]
116. Naumann, N.; Lubke, J.; Shomali, W.; Reiter, L.; Horny, H.P.; Jawhar, M.; Dangelo, V.; Fabarius, A.; Metzgeroth, G.; Kreil, S.; et al. Clinical and histopathological features of myeloid neoplasms with concurrent Janus kinase 2 (JAK2) V617F and KIT proto-oncogene, receptor tyrosine kinase (KIT) D816V mutations. *Br. J. Haematol.* **2021**, *194*, 344–354. [CrossRef]
117. Chiosea, S.I.; Sherer, C.K.; Jelic, T.; Dacic, S. KRAS mutant allele-specific imbalance in lung adenocarcinoma. *Mod. Pathol.* **2011**, *24*, 1571–1577. [CrossRef]

118. Krasinskas, A.M.; Moser, A.J.; Saka, B.; Adsay, N.V.; Chiosea, S.I. KRAS mutant allele-specific imbalance is associated with worse prognosis in pancreatic cancer and progression to undifferentiated carcinoma of the pancreas. *Mod. Pathol.* **2013**, *26*, 1346–1354. [CrossRef]
119. Chang, Y.Y.; Lin, J.K.; Lin, T.C.; Chen, W.S.; Jeng, K.J.; Yang, S.H.; Wang, H.S.; Lan, Y.T.; Lin, C.C.; Liang, W.Y.; et al. Impact of KRAS mutation on outcome of patients with metastatic colorectal cancer. *Hepato Gastroenterol.* **2014**, *61*, 1946–1953.
120. Pardanani, A.; Shah, S.; Mannelli, F.; Elala, Y.C.; Guglielmelli, P.; Lasho, T.L.; Patnaik, M.M.; Gangat, N.; Ketterling, R.P.; Reichard, K.K.; et al. Mayo alliance prognostic system for mastocytosis: Clinical and hybrid clinical-molecular models. *Blood Adv.* **2018**, *2*, 2964–2972. [CrossRef]
121. Ichikawa, M.; Goyama, S.; Asai, T.; Kawazu, M.; Nakagawa, M.; Takeshita, M.; Chiba, S.; Ogawa, S.; Kurokawa, M. AML1/Runx1 Negatively Regulates Quiescent Hematopoietic Stem Cells in Adult Hematopoiesis. *J. Immunol.* **2008**, *180*, 4402–4408. [CrossRef] [PubMed]
122. Ding, Y.; Harada, Y.; Imagawa, J.; Kimura, A.; Harada, H. AML1/RUNX1 point mutation possibly promotes leukemic transformation in myeloproliferative neoplasms. *Blood* **2009**, *114*, 5201–5205. [CrossRef] [PubMed]
123. Gaidzik, V.I.; Bullinger, L.; Schlenk, R.F.; Zimmermann, A.S.; Rock, J.; Paschka, P.; Corbacioglu, A.; Krauter, J.; Schlegelberger, B.; Ganser, A.; et al. RUNX1 mutations in acute myeloid leukemia: Results from a comprehensive genetic and clinical analysis from the AML study group. *J. Clin. Oncol.* **2011**, *29*, 1364–1372. [CrossRef] [PubMed]
124. Bejar, R.; Stevenson, K.E.; Caughey, B.A.; Abdel-Wahab, O.; Steensma, D.P.; Galili, N.; Raza, A.; Kantarjian, H.; Levine, R.L.; Neuberg, D.; et al. Validation of a prognostic model and the impact of mutations in patients with lower-risk myelodysplastic syndromes. *J. Clin. Oncol.* **2012**, *30*, 3376–3382. [CrossRef]
125. Jawhar, M.; Schwaab, J.; Naumann, N.; Horny, H.-P.; Sotlar, K.; Haferlach, T.; Metzgeroth, G.; Fabarius, A.; Valent, P.; Hofmann, W.-K.; et al. Response and progression on midostaurin in advanced systemic mastocytosis: KIT D816V and other molecular markers. *Blood* **2017**, *130*, 137–145. [CrossRef]
126. Pardanani, A.; Lasho, T.; Barraco, D.; Patnaik, M.; Elala, Y.; Tefferi, A. Next generation sequencing of myeloid neoplasms with eosinophilia harboring the FIP1L1-PDGFRA mutation. *Am. J. Hematol.* **2016**, *91*, 10–11. [CrossRef]
127. Sharma, S.; Kelly, T.K.; Jones, P.A. Epigenetics in cancer. *Carcinogenesis* **2010**, *31*, 27–36. [CrossRef]
128. Figueroa, M.E.; Lugthart, S.; Li, Y.; Erpelinck-Verschueren, C.; Deng, X.; Christos, P.J.; Schifano, E.; Booth, J.; van Putten, W.; Skrabanek, L.; et al. DNA methylation signatures identify biologically distinct subtypes in acute myeloid leukemia. *Cancer Cell* **2010**, *17*, 13–27. [CrossRef]
129. Reszka, E.; Jablonska, E.; Wieczorek, E.; Valent, P.; Arock, M.; Nilsson, G.; Nedoszytko, B.; Niedoszytko, M. Epigenetic Changes in Neoplastic Mast Cells and Potential Impact in Mastocytosis. *Int. J. Mol. Sci.* **2021**, *22*, 2964. [CrossRef]
130. Gorska, A.; Jablonska, E.; Reszka, E.; Niedoszytko, M.; Lange, M.; Gruchala-Niedoszytko, M.; Jarczak, J.; Strapagiel, D.; Gorska-Ponikowska, M.; Bastian, P.; et al. DNA methylation profile in patients with indolent systemic mastocytosis. *Clin. Transl. Allergy* **2021**, *11*, e12074. [CrossRef]
131. Katoh, M. Functional and cancer genomics of ASXL family members. *Br. J. Cancer* **2013**, *109*, 299–306. [CrossRef] [PubMed]
132. Gelsi-Boyer, V.; Trouplin, V.; Adelaide, J.; Bonansea, J.; Cervera, N.; Carbuccia, N.; Lagarde, A.; Prebet, T.; Nezri, M.; Sainty, D.; et al. Mutations of polycomb-associated gene ASXL1 in myelodysplastic syndromes and chronic myelomonocytic leukaemia. *Br. J. Haematol.* **2009**, *145*, 788–800. [CrossRef] [PubMed]
133. Carbuccia, N.; Murati, A.; Trouplin, V.; Brecqueville, M.; Adelaide, J.; Rey, J.; Vainchenker, W.; Bernard, O.A.; Chaffanet, M.; Vey, N.; et al. Mutations of ASXL1 gene in myeloproliferative neoplasms. *Leukemia* **2009**, *23*, 2183–2186. [CrossRef] [PubMed]
134. Kar, S.A.; Jankowska, A.; Makishima, H.; Visconte, V.; Jerez, A.; Sugimoto, Y.; Muramatsu, H.; Traina, F.; Afable, M.; Guinta, K.; et al. Spliceosomal gene mutations are frequent events in the diverse mutational spectrum of chronic myelomonocytic leukemia but largely absent in juvenile myelomonocytic leukemia. *Haematologica* **2013**, *98*, 107–113. [CrossRef] [PubMed]
135. Tefferi, A. Novel mutations and their functional and clinical relevance in myeloproliferative neoplasms: JAK2, MPL, TET2, ASXL1, CBL, IDH and IKZF1. *Leukemia* **2010**, *24*, 1128–1138. [CrossRef]
136. Jia, Y.; Li, P.; Fang, L.; Zhu, H.; Xu, L.; Cheng, H.; Zhang, J.; Li, F.; Feng, Y.; Li, Y.; et al. Negative regulation of DNMT3A de novo DNA methylation by frequently overexpressed UHRF family proteins as a mechanism for widespread DNA hypomethylation in cancer. *Cell Discov.* **2016**, *2*, 16007. [CrossRef]
137. Walter, M.J.; Ding, L.; Shen, D.; Shao, J.; Grillot, M.; McLellan, M.; Fulton, R.; Schmidt, H.; Kalicki-Veizer, J.; O'Laughlin, M.; et al. Recurrent DNMT3A mutations in patients with myelodysplastic syndromes. *Leukemia* **2011**, *25*, 1153–1158. [CrossRef]
138. Tie, R.; Zhang, T.; Fu, H.; Wang, L.; Wang, Y.; He, Y.; Wang, B.; Zhu, N.; Fu, S.; Lai, X.; et al. Association between DNMT3A mutations and prognosis of adults with de novo acute myeloid leukemia: A systematic review and meta-analysis. *PLoS ONE* **2014**, *9*, e93353. [CrossRef]
139. Jankowska, A.M.; Makishima, H.; Tiu, R.V.; Szpurka, H.; Huang, Y.; Traina, F.; Visconte, V.; Sugimoto, Y.; Prince, C.; O'Keefe, C.; et al. Mutational spectrum analysis of chronic myelomonocytic leukemia includes genes associated with epigenetic regulation: UTX, EZH2, and DNMT3A. *Blood* **2011**, *118*, 3932–3941. [CrossRef]
140. Chase, A.; Cross, N.C.P. Aberrations of *EZH2* in Cancer. *Clinical Cancer Res.* **2011**, *17*, 2613–2618. [CrossRef]
141. Ernst, T.; Chase, A.J.; Score, J.; Hidalgo-Curtis, C.E.; Bryant, C.; Jones, A.V.; Waghorn, K.; Zoi, K.; Ross, F.M.; Reiter, A.; et al. Inactivating mutations of the histone methyltransferase gene EZH2 in myeloid disorders. *Nat. Genet* **2010**, *42*, 722–726. [CrossRef] [PubMed]

142. Nikoloski, G.; Langemeijer, S.M.C.; Kuiper, R.P.; Knops, R.; Massop, M.; Tonnissen, E.R.L.T.M.; van der Heijden, A.; Scheele, T.N.; Vandenberghe, P.; de Witte, T.; et al. Somatic mutations of the histone methyltransferase gene EZH2 in myelodysplastic syndromes. *Nat. Genet* **2010**, *42*, 665–667. [CrossRef] [PubMed]
143. Ito, S.; D'Alessio, A.C.; Taranova, O.V.; Hong, K.; Sowers, L.C.; Zhang, Y. Role of Tet proteins in 5mC to 5hmC conversion, ES-cell self-renewal and inner cell mass specification. *Nature* **2010**, *466*, 1129–1133. [CrossRef] [PubMed]
144. Tan, L.; Shi, Y.G. Tet family proteins and 5-hydroxymethylcytosine in development and disease. *Development* **2012**, *139*, 1895–1902. [CrossRef]
145. Holmfeldt, L.; Mullighan, C.G. The role of TET2 in hematologic neoplasms. *Cancer Cell* **2011**, *20*, 1–2. [CrossRef]
146. Delhommeau, F.; Dupont, S.; Della Valle, V.; James, C.; Trannoy, S.; Masse, A.; Kosmider, O.; Le Couedic, J.P.; Robert, F.; Alberdi, A.; et al. Mutation in TET2 in myeloid cancers. *N. Engl. J. Med.* **2009**, *360*, 2289–2301. [CrossRef]
147. Bejar, R. Splicing Factor Mutations in Cancer. *Adv. Exp. Med. Biol.* **2016**, *907*, 215–228. [CrossRef]
148. Fu, X.D. Specific commitment of different pre-mRNAs to splicing by single SR proteins. *Nature* **1993**, *365*, 82–85. [CrossRef]
149. Edmond, V.; Moysan, E.; Khochbin, S.; Matthias, P.; Brambilla, C.; Brambilla, E.; Gazzeri, S.; Eymin, B. Acetylation and phosphorylation of SRSF2 control cell fate decision in response to cisplatin. *EMBO J.* **2011**, *30*, 510–523. [CrossRef]
150. Yoshida, K.; Sanada, M.; Shiraishi, Y.; Nowak, D.; Nagata, Y.; Yamamoto, R.; Sato, Y.; Sato-Otsubo, A.; Kon, A.; Nagasaki, M.; et al. Frequent pathway mutations of splicing machinery in myelodysplasia. *Nature* **2011**, *478*, 64–69. [CrossRef]
151. Meggendorfer, M.; Roller, A.; Haferlach, T.; Eder, C.; Dicker, F.; Grossmann, V.; Kohlmann, A.; Alpermann, T.; Yoshida, K.; Ogawa, S.; et al. SRSF2 mutations in 275 cases with chronic myelomonocytic leukemia (CMML). *Blood* **2012**, *120*, 3080–3088. [CrossRef] [PubMed]
152. Thol, F.; Kade, S.; Schlarmann, C.; Loffeld, P.; Morgan, M.; Krauter, J.; Wlodarski, M.W.; Kolking, B.; Wichmann, M.; Gorlich, K.; et al. Frequency and prognostic impact of mutations in SRSF2, U2AF1, and ZRSR2 in patients with myelodysplastic syndromes. *Blood* **2012**, *119*, 3578–3584. [CrossRef] [PubMed]
153. Mian, S.A.; Smith, A.E.; Kulasekararaj, A.G.; Kizilors, A.; Mohamedali, A.M.; Lea, N.C.; Mitsopoulos, K.; Ford, K.; Nasser, E.; Seidl, T.; et al. Spliceosome mutations exhibit specific associations with epigenetic modifiers and proto-oncogenes mutated in myelodysplastic syndrome. *Haematologica* **2013**, *98*, 1058–1066. [CrossRef] [PubMed]
154. Will, C.L.; Luhrmann, R. Spliceosome structure and function. *Cold Spring Harb. Perspect. Biol.* **2011**, *3*, a003707. [CrossRef]
155. Pellagatti, A.; Armstrong, R.N.; Steeples, V.; Sharma, E.; Repapi, E.; Singh, S.; Sanchi, A.; Radujkovic, A.; Horn, P.; Dolatshad, H.; et al. Impact of spliceosome mutations on RNA splicing in myelodysplasia: Dysregulated genes/pathways and clinical associations. *Blood* **2018**, *132*, 1225–1240. [CrossRef]
156. Malcovati, L.; Papaemmanuil, E.; Bowen, D.T.; Boultwood, J.; Della Porta, M.G.; Pascutto, C.; Travaglino, E.; Groves, M.J.; Godfrey, A.L.; Ambaglio, I.; et al. Clinical significance of SF3B1 mutations in myelodysplastic syndromes and myelodysplastic/myeloproliferative neoplasms. *Blood* **2011**, *118*, 6239–6246. [CrossRef]
157. Graubert, T.A.; Shen, D.; Ding, L.; Okeyo-Owuor, T.; Lunn, C.L.; Shao, J.; Krysiak, K.; Harris, C.C.; Koboldt, D.C.; Larson, D.E.; et al. Recurrent mutations in the U2AF1 splicing factor in myelodysplastic syndromes. *Nat. Genet* **2011**, *44*, 53–57. [CrossRef]
158. Hirabayashi, S.; Flotho, C.; Moetter, J.; Heuser, M.; Hasle, H.; Gruhn, B.; Klingebiel, T.; Thol, F.; Schlegelberger, B.; Baumann, I.; et al. Spliceosomal gene aberrations are rare, coexist with oncogenic mutations, and are unlikely to exert a driver effect in childhood MDS and JMML. *Blood* **2012**, *119*, e96–e99. [CrossRef]
159. Broesby-Olsen, S.; Kristensen, T.K.; Møller, M.B.; Bindslev-Jensen, C.; Vestergaard, H. Adult-onset systemic mastocytosis in monozygotic twins with KIT D816V and JAK2 V617F mutations. *J. Allergy Clin. Immunol.* **2012**, *130*, 806–808. [CrossRef]
160. Lim, K.H.; Tefferi, A.; Lasho, T.L.; Finke, C.; Patnaik, M.; Butterfield, J.H.; McClure, R.F.; Li, C.Y.; Pardanani, A. Systemic mastocytosis in 342 consecutive adults: Survival studies and prognostic factors. *Blood* **2009**, *113*, 5727–5736. [CrossRef]
161. Galata, G.; Garcia-Montero, A.C.; Kristensen, T.; Dawoud, A.A.Z.; Munoz-Gonzalez, J.I.; Meggendorfer, M.; Guglielmelli, P.; Hoade, Y.; Alvarez-Twose, I.; Gieger, C.; et al. Genome-wide association study identifies novel susceptibility loci for KIT D816V positive mastocytosis. *Am. J. Hum. Genet.* **2021**, *108*, 284–294. [CrossRef] [PubMed]
162. De Vita, S.; Schneider, R.K.; Garcia, M.; Wood, J.; Gavillet, M.; Ebert, B.L.; Gerbaulet, A.; Roers, A.; Levine, R.L.; Mullally, A.; et al. Loss of Function of TET2 Cooperates with Constitutively Active KIT in Murine and Human Models of Mastocytosis. *PLoS ONE* **2014**, *9*, 96209. [CrossRef] [PubMed]
163. Bejar, R.; Stevenson, K.; Abdel-Wahab, O.; Galili, N.; Nilsson, B.; Garcia-Manero, G.; Kantarjian, H.; Raza, A.; Levine, R.L.; Neuberg, D.; et al. Clinical Effect of Point Mutations in Myelodysplastic Syndromes. *N. Engl. J. Med.* **2011**, *364*, 2496–2506. [CrossRef] [PubMed]
164. Kristensen, T.; Vestergaard, H.; Moller, M.B. Improved detection of the KIT D816V mutation in patients with systemic mastocytosis using a quantitative and highly sensitive real-time qPCR assay. *J. Mol. Diagn. JMD* **2011**, *13*, 180–188. [CrossRef]
165. Kristensen, T.; Vestergaard, H.; Bindslev-Jensen, C.; Moller, M.B.; Broesby-Olsen, S. Sensitive KIT D816V mutation analysis of blood as a diagnostic test in mastocytosis. *Am. J. Hematol.* **2014**, *89*, 493–498. [CrossRef]
166. Erben, P.; Schwaab, J.; Metzgeroth, G.; Horny, H.P.; Jawhar, M.; Sotlar, K.; Fabarius, A.; Teichmann, M.; Schneider, S.; Ernst, T.; et al. The KIT D816V expressed allele burden for diagnosis and disease monitoring of systemic mastocytosis. *Ann. Hematol.* **2014**, *93*, 81–88. [CrossRef]

167. Hoermann, G.; Gleixner, K.V.; Dinu, G.E.; Kundi, M.; Greiner, G.; Wimazal, F.; Hadzijusufovic, E.; Mitterbauer, G.; Mannhalter, C.; Valent, P.; et al. The KIT D816V allele burden predicts survival in patients with mastocytosis and correlates with the WHO type of the disease. *Allergy* **2014**, *69*, 810–813. [CrossRef]
168. Hoermann, G.; Sotlar, K.; Jawhar, M.; Kristensen, T.; Bachelot, G.; Nedoszytko, B.; Carter, M.C.; Horny, H.P.; Bonadonna, P.; Sperr, W.R.; et al. Standards of Genetic Testing in the Diagnosis and Prognostication of Systemic Mastocytosis in 2022: Recommendations of the EU-US Cooperative Group. *J. Allergy Clin. Immunol. Pract.* **2022**. [CrossRef]
169. Steensma, D.P.; Bejar, R.; Jaiswal, S.; Lindsley, R.C.; Sekeres, M.A.; Hasserjian, R.P.; Ebert, B.L. Clonal hematopoiesis of indeterminate potential and its distinction from myelodysplastic syndromes. *Blood* **2015**, *126*, 9–16. [CrossRef]
170. Zink, F.; Stacey, S.N.; Norddahl, G.L.; Frigge, M.L.; Magnusson, O.T.; Jonsdottir, I.; Thorgeirsson, T.E.; Sigurdsson, A.; Gudjonsson, S.A.; Gudmundsson, J.; et al. Clonal hematopoiesis, with and without candidate driver mutations, is common in the elderly. *Blood* **2017**, *130*, 742–752. [CrossRef]
171. Jacobs, K.B.; Yeager, M.; Zhou, W.; Wacholder, S.; Wang, Z.; Rodriguez-Santiago, B.; Hutchinson, A.; Deng, X.; Liu, C.; Horner, M.J.; et al. Detectable clonal mosaicism and its relationship to aging and cancer. *Nat. Genet.* **2012**, *44*, 651–658. [CrossRef] [PubMed]
172. Laurie, C.C.; Laurie, C.A.; Rice, K.; Doheny, K.F.; Zelnick, L.R.; McHugh, C.P.; Ling, H.; Hetrick, K.N.; Pugh, E.W.; Amos, C.; et al. Detectable clonal mosaicism from birth to old age and its relationship to cancer. *Nat. Genet.* **2012**, *44*, 642–650. [CrossRef]
173. Hall, J.; Al Hafidh, J.; Balmert, E.; Dabbas, B.; Vaupel, C.; El Hader, C.; McGinniss, M.; Beruti, S.; Bejar, R. Somatic Mutations Indicative of Clonal Hematopoiesis Are Present in a Large Fraction of Cytopenic Patients Who Lack Diagnostic Evidence of MDS. *Blood* **2014**, *124*, 3272. [CrossRef]
174. Shlush, L.I. Age-related clonal hematopoiesis. *Blood* **2018**, *131*, 496–504. [CrossRef]
175. Valent, P.; Kern, W.; Hoermann, G.; Milosevic Feenstra, J.D.; Sotlar, K.; Pfeilstöcker, M.; Germing, U.; Sperr, W.R.; Reiter, A.; Wolf, D.; et al. Clonal Hematopoiesis with Oncogenic Potential (CHOP): Separation from CHIP and Roads to AML. *Int. J. Mol. Sci.* **2019**, *20*, 789. [CrossRef] [PubMed]
176. Shah, S.; Pardanani, A.; Elala, Y.C.; Lasho, T.L.; Patnaik, M.M.; Reichard, K.K.; Hanson, C.A.; Ketterling, R.P.; Tefferi, A. Cytogenetic abnormalities in systemic mastocytosis: WHO subcategory-specific incidence and prognostic impact among 348 informative cases. *Am. J. Hematol.* **2018**, *93*, 1461–1466. [CrossRef] [PubMed]
177. Youk, J.; Koh, Y.; Kim, J.W.; Kim, D.Y.; Park, H.; Jung, W.J.; Ahn, K.S.; Yun, H.; Park, I.; Sun, C.H.; et al. A scientific treatment approach for acute mast cell leukemia: Using a strategy based on next-generation sequencing data. *Blood Res.* **2016**, *51*, 17–22. [CrossRef]
178. Li, P.; Biancon, G.; Patel, T.; Pan, Z.; Kothari, S.; Halene, S.; Prebet, T.; Xu, M.L. Comprehensive Clinicopathologic and Molecular Analysis of Mast Cell Leukemia With Associated Hematologic Neoplasm: A Report and In-Depth Study of 5 Cases. *Front. Oncol.* **2021**, *11*, 730503. [CrossRef]
179. Lasho, T.L.; Finke, C.M.; Zblewski, D.; Patnaik, M.; Ketterling, R.P.; Chen, D.; Hanson, C.A.; Tefferi, A.; Pardanani, A. Novel recurrent mutations in ethanolamine kinase 1 (ETNK1) gene in systemic mastocytosis with eosinophilia and chronic myelomonocytic leukemia. *Blood Cancer J.* **2015**, *5*, e275. [CrossRef]
180. Toledo, M.A.S.; Gatz, M.; Sontag, S.; Gleixner, K.V.; Eisenwort, G.; Feldberg, K.; Hamouda, A.E.I.; Kluge, F.; Guareschi, R.; Rossetti, G.; et al. Nintedanib targets KIT D816V neoplastic cells derived from induced pluripotent stem cells of systemic mastocytosis. *Blood* **2021**, *137*, 2070–2084. [CrossRef]
181. Dorrance, A. "Mast"ering drug discovery with iPSCs. *Blood* **2021**, *137*, 1993–1994. [CrossRef]
182. Shomali, W.; Gotlib, J. Response Criteria in Advanced Systemic Mastocytosis: Evolution in the Era of KIT Inhibitors. *Int. J. Mol. Sci.* **2021**, *22*, 2983. [CrossRef] [PubMed]
183. Rowe, R.G.; Daley, G.Q. Induced pluripotent stem cells in disease modelling and drug discovery. *Nat. Rev. Genet.* **2019**, *20*, 377–388. [CrossRef] [PubMed]
184. Andersohn, F.; Konzen, C.; Garbe, E. Systematic review: Agranulocytosis induced by nonchemotherapy drugs. *Ann. Intern. Med.* **2007**, *146*, 657–665. [CrossRef] [PubMed]
185. Schwartz, L.B.; Metcalfe, D.D.; Miller, J.S.; Earl, H.; Sullivan, T. Tryptase levels as an indicator of mast-cell activation in systemic anaphylaxis and mastocytosis. *N. Engl. J. Med.* **1987**, *316*, 1622–1626. [CrossRef] [PubMed]
186. Schwartz, L.B. Diagnostic value of tryptase in anaphylaxis and mastocytosis. *Immunol. Allergy Clin. N. Am.* **2006**, *26*, 451–463. [CrossRef] [PubMed]

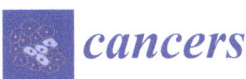

Review

Latest Contributions of Genomics to T-Cell Acute Lymphoblastic Leukemia (T-ALL)

Eulàlia Genescà * and Celia González-Gil

Institut d'Investigació Contra la Leucemia Josep Carreras (IJC), Campus ICO-Germans Trias i Pujol, Universitat Autònoma de Barcelona, 08916 Badalona, Spain; cgonzalez@carrerasresearch.org
* Correspondence: egenesca@carrerasresearch.org; Tel.: +34-935572800 (ext. 4150)

Simple Summary: Thanks to the use of high-resolution genetic techniques to detect cryptic aberrations present in T-ALL, we now have a clearer view of the genetic landscape that explains the particular oncogenetic processes taking place in each T-ALL. We also have begun to understand relapse-specific mechanisms. This review aims to summarize the latest advances in our knowledge of the genome in T-ALL and highlight the areas where the research on this ALL subtype is progressing, thereby identifying the key issues that need to be addressed in the medium-to-long term to move forward in the applicability of this knowledge into clinics.

Abstract: As for many neoplasms, initial genetic data about T-cell acute lymphoblastic leukemia (T-ALL) came from the application of cytogenetics. This information helped identify some recurrent chromosomal alterations in T-ALL at the time of diagnosis, although it was difficult to determine their prognostic impact because of their low incidence in the specific T-ALL cohort analyzed. Genetic knowledge accumulated rapidly following the application of genomic techniques, drawing attention to the importance of using high-resolution genetic techniques to detect cryptic aberrations present in T-ALL, which are not usually detected by cytogenetics. We now have a clearer appreciation of the genetic landscape of the different T-ALL subtypes at diagnosis, explaining the particular oncogenetic processes taking place in each T-ALL, and we have begun to understand relapse-specific mechanisms. This review aims to summarize the latest advances in our knowledge of the genome in T-ALL. We highlight areas where the research in this subtype of ALL is progressing with the aim of identifying key questions that need to be answered in the medium-long term if this knowledge is to be applied in clinics.

Keywords: T-cell acute lymphoblastic leukemia; genomics; non-coding; germline; aging; relapse

Citation: Genescà, E.; González-Gil, C. Latest Contributions of Genomics to T-Cell Acute Lymphoblastic Leukemia (T-ALL). *Cancers* **2022**, *14*, 2474. https://doi.org/10.3390/cancers14102474

Academic Editor: Ilaria Iacobucci

Received: 25 March 2022
Accepted: 12 May 2022
Published: 17 May 2022

Publisher's Note: MDPI stays neutral with regard to jurisdictional claims in published maps and institutional affiliations.

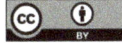

Copyright: © 2022 by the authors. Licensee MDPI, Basel, Switzerland. This article is an open access article distributed under the terms and conditions of the Creative Commons Attribution (CC BY) license (https://creativecommons.org/licenses/by/4.0/).

1. Introduction

Acute Lymphoblastic Leukemia (ALL) is an infrequent aggressive cancer with an age-standardized incidence of 0.68/100,000 individuals that is most common in children under 5 years of age [1]. ALL includes B- and T-cell lineage subtypes. While these diseases share many similarities, such as some general cancer genetic lesions in cell cycle regulators such as *CDKN2A/B* and *MYC* [2], their genetic background, origin, and outcome are distinct. The T-ALL subtype accounts for 10–15% of pediatric and 25% of adult ALL cases. It is more frequent in males than in females, and more often presents at younger ages, being considered an AYA (adolescent and young adult)-affecting disease [3]. Although intensive chemotherapy treatments have been crucial for increasing the survival rate of affected children up to 93% [4], globally, adult survival rates are still very poor, remaining below 50% [5]. The main cause of treatment failure and worse outcome is relapse [6,7]. In this scenario, T-ALL patients with primary-resistant or relapsed leukemia present a dismal prognosis, mainly due to the rapid progression of the recurrent course of the disease and the lack of effective therapeutic options [7,8].

Initial genetic studies based on the use of cytogenetics and FISH helped identify some recurrent chromosomal alterations in T-ALL at the time of diagnosis, but it proved difficult to determine their prognostic impact because of their low incidence in the specific T-ALL cohort analyzed. Genetic knowledge flourished with the application of genomic techniques, first with the analysis of gene expression profiles (GEPs), followed by the application of comparative genomic hybridization arrays (CGHas), and later, the next generation sequencing (NGS) technique. Consequently, we now have a clearer appreciation of the different T-ALL genetic subtypes at the time of diagnosis and are beginning to understand relapse-specific mechanisms.

The aim of this review is to summarize the latest scientific advances in our knowledge of the T-ALL genome. We will highlight the areas where the research on this ALL subtype is progressing, thereby identifying the key issues that need to be addressed in the medium-to-long term to move forward in the applicability of this knowledge into clinics.

2. T-ALL Classification by Differentiation Stage

The main contribution of genomic techniques in T-ALL has been to show that the blockade of the differentiation process that occurs in the lymphocyte is the consequence of specific genetic alterations occurring in pre-leukemic stages. From a historical perspective, the first studies to classify T-ALL aroused with the use of the gene expression array (GEa). This revealed that structural abnormalities, mainly rearrangements identified in T-ALL by karyotyping as a rare event [9–19], led to much overexpression of (1) basic helix-loop-helix (bHLH) transcription factor genes such as *TAL1*, *TAL2*, and *LYL1*; (2) LIM-only (*LMO*) domain genes such as *LMO1* and *LMO2*; and (3) homeobox genes such as *TLX1* (*HOX11*) and *TLX3* (*HOX11L2*). Supervised analysis of the expression data revealed a correlation between the expression of these transcription factors (TFs) and a lymphocyte-specific differentiation arrest time point. Three main groups (clusters) were obtained: (1) immature, (2) HOXA, and (3) TAL [20,21]. To describe this in more detail, HOXA samples cluster with the Pre-T1 (CD34 + CD1a+) and Pre-T2/Pre-T3 (CD4+, CD8αβ-, CD3- and TCR αβ-) sub-populations, together with the *TLX1*-expressing cases and some cases expressing *TLX3*. TAL samples cluster with subpopulations corresponding to thymocytes with a pre-TCR (Beta selection). Of note, samples from the immature group included some TLX3-expressing leukemic samples and clustered with the most immature early T-cell precursor and pro-T subpopulations [21]. Later on, the addition of copy number data, generated by CGHa, together with the use of NGS, yielded a clearer view of the genetic determinants that define these groups. Thus, according to the differentiation arrest time point of the blast cell we can differentiate the immature subtype, characterized by the absence of CD8 and CD1a immunomarkers, high levels of expression of *LYL1* [20] and *MEF2C* [22] TFs, and the absence of bi-allelic deletions in TCRγ [23]. Within the immature T-ALL leukemias, the early T-cell precursor ALL (ETP-ALL)—defined by the absence of CD1a and CD8 immunomarkers and the presence of stem cells or myeloid markers such as CD117, CD34, HLA-DR, CD13, CD33, CD11b, and CD65 [24], together with negative or dim CD5 expression, defined as expression in <75% of the blasts; rarely presents *CDKN2A/B* deletions and *NOTCH1/FBXW7* mutations [25–27]. In addition, mutations affecting epigenetic regulators and transcription factors governing hematopoietic and T-cell development are also frequently observed in this immature subtype [25,28–31]. We will discuss this subgroup in detail later. The cortical subtype is characterized by the expression of CD1a, and often both CD4 and CD8 immunomarkers are also found. At the genetic level, the group is characterized by aberrant expression of *TLX1*, *TLX3*, and *HOXA* genes (*HOXA5*, *HOXA9*, *HOXA10*) [20,21] and the overexpression of the *NKX2-1* rearranged gene [22]. Other specific alterations in this subset of T-ALL have been found in *PHF6*, *DNM2*, *BCL11B*, *CDKN1B*, and *RB1* [32]. The mature subtype is characterized by blasts expressing CD4 or CD8 and surface CD3 immunomarkers [20] and the presence of Tαβ cell-receptor rearrangements [21]. The genetic hallmark of the group is the activation of the

TAL oncogene [20], together with the presence of del(6)(q) [33] and mutations in *PIK3R* and *PTEN* [32]. Figure 1 summarizes these findings.

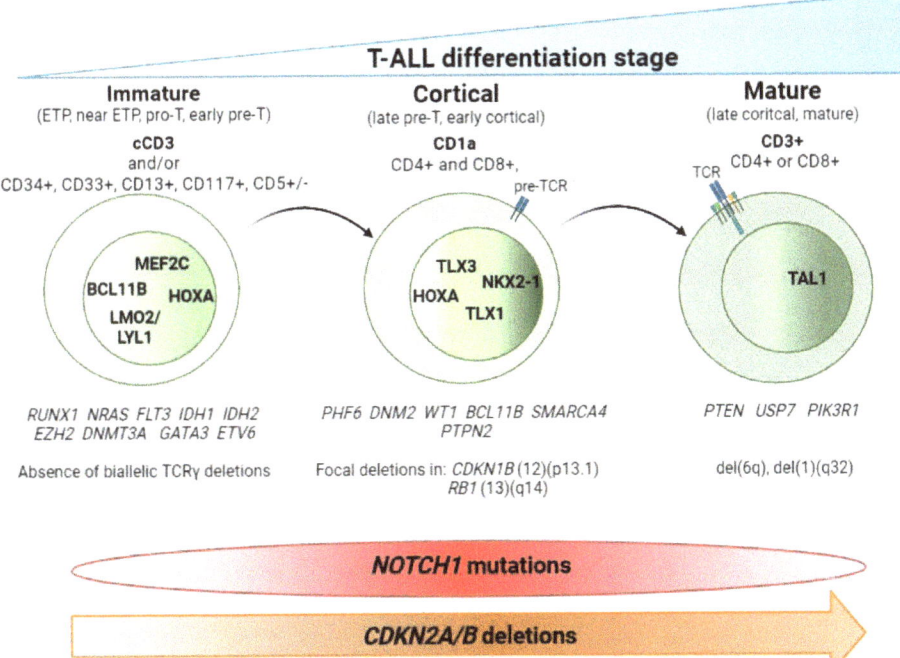

Figure 1. T-ALL classification by stage of differentiation arrest. Schematic representation of the three main T-ALL subtypes according to the blockade of the differentiation process. Hallmark immuno-markers of each subtype are highlighted in bold at the top. Other accompanying immunomarkers, for precise definition of the subtypes, are showed below. TCR maturation is represented in the blasts. Presence of TCR on the blast surface is also a hallmark in the mature subtype. Active transcription factors in each subtype of T-ALL are represented in the nucleus according to the maturation transition. The genes most frequently mutated in each subtype, followed by copy number alterations, are shown beneath. The distributions of *NOTCH1* mutations and *CDKN2A*/B deletions are indicated at the bottom.

Collectively, the data generated during twenty years of genomics research into T-ALL highlight the importance of using high-resolution genetic techniques. These not only make it possible to detect the cryptic aberrations present in T-ALL but also to define primary genetic events that determine the acquisition of the secondary genetic events necessary for transforming T-cell progenitors. This thereby explains the particular oncogenetic processes taking place in each T-ALL. We are moving towards an immuno-genetic T-ALL classification. One of the knowledge gaps here relates to T-ALL leukemias with unidentified primary events, although the driving TF is aberrantly expressed. In those cases, it is reasonable to argue that alterations in regulatory regions and/or in enhancers of the TF can alter its expression.

2.1. Non-Coding Mutations

Analysis of non-coding data generated by whole genome sequencing (WGS) or direct target sequencing is an emerging area of investigation, but recently published data have shown that small (or not) insertions and deletions generating novel regulatory sequences can explain the overexpression seen in TFs, such as *TAL1* and *LMO1*, that have no detectable primary rearrangements. Here we provide a summary of the non-coding alterations identified in *TAL1*, *LMO1/2*, and other important T-ALL oncogenes such as *MYC* and *PTEN*. Non-coding variants discovered in T-ALL are also summarized in Table 1.

Table 1. Non-coding mutations identified so far in T-ALL.

Gene	Affected Region	Variant	Alteration	Functional Impact	Frequency	Reference
MYC	1427 kb downstream of *MYC*	Focal duplications	Creation of binding site for NOTCH1	*MYC* expression	8/160 (5%) Adult and pediatric	[34]
TAL1	8 kb upstream of the transcription start site of *TAL1*	Heterozygous indel (2–18 bp)	Creation of binding motifs for the MYB TF	*TAL1* overexpression	8/146 (5.5%) pediatric	[35,36]
LMO1	4 kb upstream of the transcriptional start site of *LMO1*	SNV: C → T	Creation of binding motifs for the MYB TF	*LMO1* overexpression	4/187 (2.14%) pediatric	[36,37]
LMO2	Non-coding region of the exon 2 of *LMO2*	Heterozygous indel	Creation of binding motifs for the MYB TF	Activating *LMO2* function	6/160 (3.75%) pediatric 9/163 (5.52%) adult	[38]
PTEN	550 kb downstream of transcription start site of *PTEN*	Focal deletions	Deletion of *PTEN* enhancer region	Reduced levels of *PTEN*	5/398 (1.25%)	[39]

Abbreviations: *MYC*: MYC proto-oncogene, bHLH transcription factor; *TAL1*: T cell acute lymphocytic leukaemia 1; bp: base pair; *LMO1*: LIM domain only 1; SNV: single nucleotide variant; TF: transcription factor; *LMO2*: LIM domain only 1; *PTEN*: phosphatase and tensin homolog; PE: *PTEN* enhancer.

The first non-coding alterations found to affect T-ALL corresponded those affecting *MYC* TF activation by *NOTCH1* [34]. Recurrent focal duplications at chromosome 8q24 were identified in a CGH screening in 8/160 (5%) of the T-ALL cases analyzed. The amplification was located +1427 kb downstream of *MYC*. The alteration was named N-Me for NOTCH *MYC* enhancer. The region was shown to interact with the *MYC* proximal promoter and induced orientation-independent *MYC* expression in reporter assays. Analysis of N-Me knockout mice demonstrated a selective role of this regulatory element in the development T-ALL in a NOTCH1-induced T-ALL model [34].

Concomitant to this finding, a non-coding alteration located in a regulatory region of *TAL1* was also identified. A 12-bp indel that introduced two consecutive de novo binding motifs for the MYB TF, creating a super-enhancer, was identified using chromatin immunoprecipitation experiments and sequencing (CHIP-seq) in the Jurkat cell line [35]. The screening of 146 unselected pediatric primary T-ALL samples collected at diagnosis revealed that eight cases (5.5%) contained the 2–18-bp heterozygous indel, confirming the in vitro results. Sequencing DNA from remission bone marrow samples in two available cases showed wild-type sequences at this site, indicating that the mutations were somatically acquired in the blasts. The authors suggested that the initial mechanistic event in the aberrant super-enhancer formation was the recruitment of CBP by MYB, followed by abundant H3K27 acetylation, which facilitated the binding of a core complex composed of RUNX1, GATA-3, and *TAL1* itself [35]. These results were validated in a study that set out to identify non-coding mutations in 31 pediatric T-ALL cases from the available WGS data. Non-coding *TAL1* mutations were significantly associated with *TAL1* expression, implying a cis-regulating effect. Consistent with previous results, a similar, MYB binding-dependent *TAL1* promoter activation mechanism was described [36].

Subsequent studies used the same experimental procedure; (1) identification of a core sequence by CHIP-seq in T-ALL cell lines; (2) identification of epigenetic marks supporting transcriptional activity in the region and the transcriptional complex; and (3) validation of the alteration in a large cohort of pediatric T-ALL cases revealed a C-to-T single nucleotide transition occurring as a somatic mutation in the non-coding sequence

4 kb upstream of the transcriptional start site of the *LMO1* TF. This single nucleotide alteration gives rise to an APOBEC-like cytidine deaminase mutational signature and generates a new binding site for the MYB transcription factor, leading to the formation of an aberrant transcriptional enhancer complex that drives high levels of expression of the *LMO1* oncogene, similar to the *TAL1* super-enhancer. Sequencing 187 pediatric primary T-ALL samples collected at diagnosis identified four patients (2.14%) with the same heterozygous mutation [37]. As with the *TAL1* indel, the *LMO1* aberrant MYB-dependent super-enhancer was confirmed by the WGS study [36]. However, Shaoyan and colleagues also identified an intrachromosomal inversion event that juxtaposed the active promoter of the *MED17* gene with the coding sequence of *LMO1*, leading to the expression of *LMO1*. This highlights how other structural abnormalities may help explain the abnormal expression of this TF [36]. In the case of *LMO2*, a heterozygous 20-bp duplication in PF-382 cells and a heterozygous 1-bp deletion in DU.528 cells were identified in the same way, both being located closer to a region recently described as an intermediate promoter. These alterations were not limited to T-ALL cell lines, since heterozygous mutations in the *LMO2* intron 1 were detected in diagnostic samples from 6/160 of the pediatric and 9/163 of the adult T-ALL cases sequenced [38]. The confirmatory WGS study, in this case, confirmed the non-coding mutations in regulatory regions of *LMO2*. However, in this case, they were not associated with *LMO2* gene expression [36] (Table 1).

An intronic sequence of 550-kb situated in the neighborhood of the *RNLS* gene and downstream of the *PTEN* gene has very recently been identified and found to interact strongly with the *PTEN* promoter. The presence of enhancer marks in this region, including high levels of H3K27ac and H3K4me1, together with binding of CTCF, BRD4, and ZNF143, defined this region as a *PTEN* enhancer (PE). Screening for genetic lesions in this region in human primary samples identified five cases (5/398, 1.25%) with focal deletions encompassing PE. The deletion was homozygous in two of these samples, and additional simultaneous deletions targeting the coding region of *PTEN* were observed in four of the five cases. Analyses of 1415 BCP-ALL samples failed to identify the same deletion, showing that these alterations are restricted to the T-ALL subtype [39] (Table 1).

Identification of non-coding variants is a burgeoning area of research in which much information is yet to be gathered. The contribution of non-coding sequences to oncogenetics remains largely unknown. In addition to alterations in promoters, regulatory regions and enhancers, as well as other non-coding regions such as intergenic and splicing site sequences, will help refine the immuno-genetic T-ALL classification.

2.2. T-ALL Related Immature Subtypes

Application of WGS and whole transcriptome sequencing has also served to better characterize rare subtypes such as the immature T-ALL leukemias and to provide insight into the cell of origin of these subtypes. This group includes T/Myeloid mixed phenotype acute leukemias (T/M MPALs) and ETP-ALL, which are characterized by different combinations of myeloid and T-lymphoid antigen expression [40]. Other immunophenotypically identified immature T-ALL subtypes include the pro-T [40] and the near-ETP [32,41] forms, but we do not know their genetic basis or clinical implications. Thus, childhood ETP-ALL presents cytokine-activating somatic mutations and mutations in genes involved in the RAS signaling pathway (e.g., *NRAS*, *KRAS*, *FLT3*, *IL7R*, *JAK3*, *JAK1*, *SH2B3*, and *BRAF*), genetic alterations that inactivate genes involved in hematopoietic development (e.g., *GATA3*, *ETV6*, *RUNX1*, *IKZF1*, and *EP300*), and mutations in histone modifier genes (e.g., *EZH2*, *EED*, *SUZ12*, *SETD2*, and *EP300*). It is of note that the mutational spectrum identified in ETP leukemia was similar to that of acute myeloid leukemia (AML) with poor prognosis, in which affected pluripotent genes lend this subtype a myeloid-like profile [29]. In the case of adult ETP-ALL, exclusively genetic alterations have been detected in the *DNMT3A* gene (frequency range from 12 to 16%) [30,31,42,43], in addition to the aforementioned mutations. Specifically, *DNMT3A* mutations are associated with patients aged >60 years with ETP-ALL features [43]. *FAT1* (25%, 17/68) and *FAT3* (20%, 14/68) cadherins are other mutations exclusively found in adult ETP-ALL [30] (Figure 2). In addition to point mutations, structural abnormalities such as rearrangements affecting *KMT2A*, *MLLT10*, *NUP214*, or *NUP98*, which trans activate *HOXA* genes, are often detected in ETP-ALL cases [44,45]. Overexpression of the *BCL11B* gene due to different structural abnormalities including translocations (i.e., t(2;14)(q22.3;q32), t(6;14)(q25.3;q32), hijacking super-enhancers, and other fusion genes has been very recently described as present in one third of ETP-ALL and T/myeloid mixed phenotype acute leukemia (T/M MPAL) cases with a very distinct expression profile [46,47].

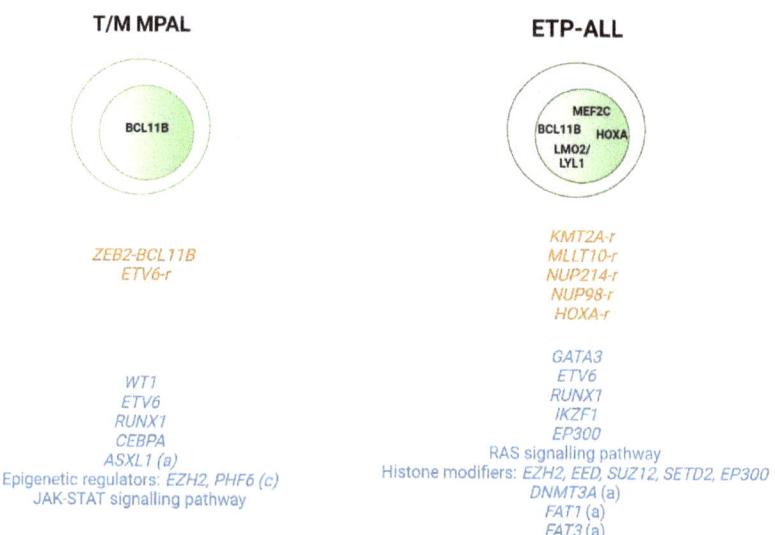

Figure 2. Genomic alterations in T/Myeloid mixed phenotype acute leukemias (T/M MPALs) and ETP-ALL. Active transcription factors in each subtype are represented in the nucleus according to the maturation transition. The rearrangements and fusion genes are written in yellow and most frequently mutations in blue color. (**a**) adult; (**c**) children.

In the case of T/M MPAL leukemias, a study cohort including 49 pediatric cases of this mixed phenotype showed a high number of copy number alterations (CNAs) (average of 4.5 (0–35)) in this subtype compared to KMT2Ar MPAL leukemias. Alterations in genes encoding transcriptional regulators were also detected in the T/M MPAL cases (i.e., *WT1*, *ETV6*, *RUNX1*, and *CEBPA*) [48]. Alterations in JAK–STAT signaling were also common in these leukemias together with mutations in genes encoding epigenetic regulators (69% of cases), including inactivating mutations in *EZH2* (16%) and *PHF6* (16%). Analysis of the transcriptome sequencing identified chimeric in-frame fusions in 15/40 cases, including *ZEB2–BCL11B* (n = 3) and several fusions involving the *ETV6* gene [48].

Comparison of the genetic profiles of ETP-ALL and T/M MPAL with non-immature T-ALL leukemias in pediatric cases has shown that the core TF driving T-ALL (*TAL1*, *TAL2*, *TLX1*, *TLX3*, *LMO1*, *LMO2*, *NKX2-1*, *HOXA10*, and *LYL1*) is less frequently altered in T/M MPAL and ETP-ALL. Other alterations that are common in T-ALL, such as *MYB* amplification, *LEF1* deletion, and *CDKN2A/B* deletions, are also rare in both types of immature leukemia. By contrast, *WT1* alterations are common in T/M MPAL and ETP-ALL, but not in non-immature T-ALL [48]. A similar analysis conducted in adult MPAL leukemias observed that, while myeloid-T/M MPAL and T-ALL shared a number of mutations in common, there were also differences. *PHF6* and *JAK3* mutations, each detected in 21.4% of the adult T-ALL cases analyzed, were not detected in myeloid-T/M MPAL. In contrast, *ASXL1* (11.1%) and *FLT3* (11.1%) mutations were detected in T/M MPAL but not in T-ALL [49]. Collectively, these observations imply that different primary events can drive specific T-ALL subtypes. A summary of these data can be seen in Figure 2.

3. (Epi)genetic Modification

The systematic screening of T-ALL genomes has revealed T-ALL as one of the tumors with the highest frequency of mutations in genes that encode proteins involved in epigenetic regulation [50]. Hence, the field of epigenetics, particularly DNA methylation, is currently being extensively explored in the search for specific methylation patterns that help to explain the oncogenic evolution of pre-leukemic T-cells; to identify specific de-regulated genes to use as a prognosis marker; and to delineate new therapy strategies using DNA methylation inhibitors (iDNMTs) such as 5-azacitidine (vidaza, AZA) and 5-aza-20-deoxycytidine (decitabine, DAC) [51].

Initial epigenetic studies were focused on determining the methylation status of the promoter of specific genes playing a role in the T-ALL oncogenic process such as *CDKN2A/B*. It was observed in T-ALL patients that the percentage of promoter methylation in the *CDKN2B* and *CDKN2A* genes ranged between 46% and 68% and between 0% and 12%, respectively, in pediatric cohorts ([52–54]. In the case of adult T-ALL cohorts, the percentage of *CDKN2B* gene promoter methylation varied from 16% to 49% and was 1% for the *CDKN2A* promoter [55–59]. In T-ALL, the *CDKN2B* methylation status was associated with an immature immunophenotype [58] and with ETP-ALL features [59]. Further investigation of the methylation status in cancer cells using wide genomic approaches (i.e., methylation arrays) have observed that generally malignant cells display a DNA hypermethylation pattern at specific CpG islands; globally, this observation is called a CpG island methylator phenotype (CIMP). CIMP+ in T-ALLs has been associated with a better EF and OS as compared to CIMP− leukemias [60]. Notably, these findings have been confirmed in both pediatric [61] and adult [62] T-ALL cohorts, reinforcing the idea that aberrant DNA methylation might act as a clinically relevant biomarker in human T-ALL. Comparison of the global methylation profile of T-ALL samples with that of normal thymocytes observed that the methylation profile of CIMP− cases was close to normal CD3+ and CD34+ thymocytes [60,61]. That was interpreted as an indication of a shorter proliferation history of the CIMP− blasts as compared to CIMP+ cases [63]. Together, these findings indicate that CIMP− cases are characterized by a hypomethylation pattern that results in a young mitotic age and shorter proliferative history of leukemic cells; at the same time, however, it might be considered as a marker of higher aggressiveness of leukemic cells. In CIMP+ cases, the disease latency is longer, which is reflected by higher methylation acquired during the aging of pre-leukemic cells, [61,63,64]. Altogether, these results indicated that aberrant methylation is likely not a driving force of T-ALL onset and progression but is rather related to the proliferative history of the cells. These concepts have been nicely reviewed by Natalia Mackowska et al. [65] in a recent publication.

4. Germline Variants and Predisposition Alleles

As already mentioned, the incidence of ALL is higher in children between 2 and 5 years than in adults. This, together with the fact that the onset of ALL in children is shorter than in adults, supports the hypothesis of an inherited genetic basis for ALL susceptibility. Here, genetic and non-genetic determinants (i.e., environmental factors) could help explain the etiology of the disease in the very young. A focus on genetic determinants and the investigation and identification of germline variants in "presumably" sporadic cancers such as ALL has rapidly become more common in recent years. It is important to comment, however, that this new area of investigation has some limitations, since predisposition variants are much rarer in hematological cancers such as ALL than in pediatric solid tumors [66], and the incidence of T-ALL in pediatric cases corresponds to 10–15% of the global childhood ALL. Nonetheless, some germline variants have been identified, with possible involvement in disease predisposition. Table 2 summarizes these germline variants. Essentially two types of germline variants can be identified, according to the technical approach used to detect them. Thus, classical genome wide association studies (GWAS) identify predisposition SNPs (alleles) often observed to be altered in T-ALL patients compared with normal (disease-free) cohorts. On the other hand, sequencing of germline DNA using WGS or TDS approximations identifies pathogenic variants in the germline DNA of T-ALL patients with an implication in the disease. The main germline types may be also distinguished by their functional involvement: those contributing to the development of the T-ALL and those affecting the response to specific drugs used during T-ALL treatment (pharmacogenomics). We consider all types below. Nonetheless, germline variants in adults should also be considered in sporadic cancers since common variants can only explain a limited percentage of the genetic burden in cancer [67], and classic tumor suppressor genes (i.e., *TP53*) have been found to harbor rare, predisposing alleles [68]. In this context, a recent publication analyzed the landscape of pathogenic variants in the germline DNA of 10,389 individuals with different types of cancer. Strikingly, 8% of cases were found to carry confirmed or probable pathogenic germline variants, ranging in prevalence from 22.9% in pheochromocytoma and paraganglioma to 2.2% in cholangiocarcinoma [69]. These results dispel the long-held view that germline variants are "non-relevant" in the context of sporadic cancers, even in adult cancers, and will certainly have ramifications in the clinical context.

Table 2. Germline variants and predispositions alleles identified in T-ALL.

Gene	Type of Alteration	SNP ID	Alteration	Association with T-ALL: Odds Ratio (P)	Functional Impact	Reference
			Predisposition alterations contributing to the development of T-ALL			
USP7	allele	rs74010351	wt allele → A Risk allele → G	Discovery cohort → 1.44 (4.51×10^{-8}) Validation cohort → 1.51 (0.04)	Downregulation of *USP7* transcription. Risk allele associated with Higher levels of African ancestry and older age at diagnosis	[70]
ATM	variant		Truncation mutations: R35X 30del215 228delCT	12.9 (0.004)	Aberrant *ATM* protein production → prone to T-ALL	[71]
			Missense mutations: V410A F582L F143C	4.9 (0.03)		
IKZF1	variant		N159S	-	Impaired recognition of the target DNA sequences by IKAROS	[72]
RUNX1	variant	-	36171607G > A 36231773 C > T		Risk to develop T-ALL	[73]
			p.K117* p.A142fs p.S213fs p.R233fs p.Y287* G365R	-	Loss of transcription factor activity	[74]
			Predisposition alterations affecting drug response and treatment			
NT5C2	allele	rs72846714	wt allele → A Risk allele → G	-	Higher level of expression of *NT5C2* and lower level of TGN in erythrocytes.	[75,76]
		rs58700372	wt allele → T Risk allele → C		Activation of *NT5C2* transcription and reduction of 6-MP metabolism	

Abbreviations: *USP7*: ubiquitin-specific peptidase 7; *wt*: wild type; *ATM*: ataxia-telangiectasia-mutated; *IKZF1*: IKAROS family zinc finger 1; *RUNX1*: RUNX family transcription factor 1; *NT5C2*: 5′-nucleotidase cytosolic II; TGN: thioguanine nucleotides.

4.1. Germline Predisposition Alterations Contributing to the Development of T-ALL

USP7

A GWAS of 1191 children with T-ALL and 12,178 control subjects identified eight *USP7* SNPs of genome-wide significance, four of which (rs61426394, rs74010349, rs59591814, and rs74010351) clustered close to the *USP7* transcription start site in a region marked by the strong promoter-active histone modifications H3K4me3 and H3K27ac in two of the T-ALL cell lines analyzed. The region also overlapped with multiple open chromatin segments, suggesting a direct influence of the SNPs on *USP7* transcription. The rs74010351 variant exhibited the most statistically significant difference in a reporter gene transcription assay between the reference and risk alleles. Functional assays suggested that this T-ALL risk allele was located in a putative cis-regulatory DNA element, where it had negative effects on *USP7* transcription. The *USP7* risk allele was specifically restricted to the T-ALL subtype of ALL and was overrepresented in individuals of African descent, thereby contributing to the higher incidence of T-ALL in this ethnic group [70].

ATM

The major feature of ataxia-telangiectasia (A-T) is the increased risk of cancer, particularly of lymphoid malignancies. An interesting risk locus was identified when testing *ATM* (A-T-mutated gene) involvement in leukemia in 39 pediatric T-ALL patients from Israel. Two types of sequence changes —truncating and missense mutations— were identified in eight T-ALL germline samples. It was of particular interest that these eight patients also presented somatic *ATM* mutations. To assess the frequency of A-T heterozygote carriers in childhood T-cell ALL Israeli patients, a control population matched for ethnicity (North African origin (NAJs): $n = 12$, T-ALL vs. 100 non-T-ALL; Arab: $n = 14$, T-ALL vs. 100 non-T-ALL) association study was conducted. This revealed a 12.9-fold higher incidence of A-T carriers in the T-ALL population than in the normal controls, indicating an association between the A-T carrier and T-ALL ($p = 0.004$), and consequently with the susceptibility to develop a T-ALL. The results also support the model of predisposition to cancer in A-T heterozygotes [71].

IKAROS

Exploring the germline DNA of a 10-year-old child with a T-ALL developed 10 years after the diagnosis of a primary combined immunodeficiency, a novel heterozygous *IKZF1* mutation, c.476A > G (p.N159S), was identified in all specimens obtained from the patient. The p.N159S mutation was located within the second N-terminal zinc finger of IKAROS encoded by exon 4, which is essential for its localization to pericentromeric heterochromatin (PC-HC) and its DNA-binding function. The mutant protein displayed diffuse nuclear staining, suggesting that the correct recognition of target DNA sequences by IKAROS was impaired. In vivo experiments performed in immunodeficient mice demonstrated the role of this germline mutation in cooperating with the activation of the *NOTCH1* signaling pathway to develop the disease [72].

RUNX1

Initial studies in the late nineties demonstrated that germline mutations in *RUNX1* define a familial platelet disorder with predisposition to myeloid malignancy (FDP-MM). FDP-MM is an autosomal dominant disorder characterized by variable penetrance of quantitative and/or qualitative platelet defects with a tendency to develop hematological malignancies. The overall lifetime risk of progression to a myeloid disease (or rarely T-ALL) is 44% [77] and most commonly occurs in adulthood [78]. A recent study, that includes the largest series of familial FDP-MM (35 families), has provided a comprehensive overview of all genetic mutations and associated disease phenotypes. Here, two new *RUNX1* germline variants (36171607G > A and 36231773 C > T) were correlated with a high risk of developing T-ALL [73]. The influence of *RUNX1* on predisposing patients to ALL was subsequently assessed by sequencing germline DNA in 4836 children with BCP-ALL and 1354 with T-ALL. Thirty-one and 18 germline *RUNX1* variants were detected, respectively. Of these, *RUNX1* variants in B-ALL consistently showed minimal damaging effects, whereas six T-ALL-related variants (p.K117*, p.A142fs, p.S213fs, p.R233fs, p.Y287*, and p.G365R) caused a significant reduction in *RUNX1* activity as a transcription activator *in vitro*. Further, WGS identified a *JAK3* mutation as being the most frequent somatic genomic abnormality in T-ALL with germline *RUNX1* variants. Co-expression of the *RUNX1* variant and *JAK3* mutation in hematopoietic stem and progenitor cells in mice gave rise to T-ALL with the ETP-ALL phenotype, confirming the highly deleterious role of *RUNX1* germline variants in T-ALL [74].

4.2. Predisposition Alleles Affecting Drug Response

NT5C2

NT5C2 is a ubiquitously expressed cytosolic nucleosidase in charge of maintaining intracellular nucleotide pool homeostasis by promoting the clearance of excess purine nucleotides from cells [79,80]. *NT5C2* preferentially dephosphorylates the 6-hydroxypurine monophosphates inosine monophosphate (IMP), guanosine monophosphate (GMP), and xanthosine monophosphate (XMP), as well as the deoxyribose forms of IMP and GMP (dIMP and dGMP), facilitating the export of purine nucleosides. In the context of ALL therapy, activating mutations in the *NT5C2* gene accelerates the dephosphorylation and inactivation of 6-MP intermediate metabolites and thereby reduces the amount of deoxy thioguanosine triphosphate (TdGTP) available for DNA incorporation during the treatment, which in turn compromises the cytotoxicity of this drug [81].

With the aim of identifying germline DNA variants associated with 6MP pharmacokinetics, a GWAS study of 1009 patients undergoing maintenance therapy for ALL was undertaken. The propensity for DNA-TG incorporation in the discovery cohort (454 patients) was significantly associated with three intronic SNPs in *NT5C2*. Only one of these (rs72846714 at 10q24.3) was significantly associated with DNA-TG incorporation at any treatment step. The association was confirmed in a validation cohort (555 patients). Targeted sequencing of the *NT5C2* gene did not identify any missense variants associated with the SNP. However, the rs72846714 was associated with a more frequent occurrence of relapse-specific *NT5C2* gain-of-function mutations, implying cooperation between gain-of-function *NT5C2* mutations and the germline SNP in relapse [75]. The association between rs72846714 SNP and *NTC5C2* expression was subsequently confirmed [76]. The rs72846714 SNP was not located in a regulatory element of the *NT5C2*. Instead, its association signal was explained by linkage disequilibrium with a proximal functional variant rs12256506, which, in this case, activates *NT5C2* transcription in *cis*. The same study identified another SNP (rs58700372) that directly alters the activity of an intronic enhancer (transactivation), whose variant allele is linked to higher transcription activity of the nucleosidase and therefore to reduced 6-MP metabolism [76].

5. Clonal Hematopoiesis and Aging

Some data suggest that a person typically acquires 10 to 20 non-pathogenic passenger mutations per stem cell by middle age [82], and normal hematopoietic stem cells (HSCs) may acquire approximately 0–1 exonic mutation per decade of life [83]. It is therefore not surprising that HSC populations of elderly humans are somatic mosaics. Some of these mutations (driver mutations*) may confer a survival advantage over non-mutated stem cells, resulting in proliferation of a clonal population or clonal hematopoiesis (CH). A large study of an Icelandic population found that CH was present in 0.5% of those younger than 35 years, but in more than 50% of subjects who were older than 85 years of age [84], arguing in favor of an increased pool of mutational events driving CH in the elderly.

In their review, Silvera and Jaiswal [85] employed two terms to define individuals who showed evidence of CH but lacked signs of a current or previous hematological malignancy. The first is clonal hematopoiesis of indeterminate potential (CHIP) [86]. CHIP defines a state of CH that arises from a somatic mutation affecting a particular set of genes known to be drivers of hematological malignancy: *DNMT3A*, *TET2*, *JAK2*, *SF3B1*, *ASXL1*, *TP53*, *CBL*, *GNB1*, *BCOR*, *U2AF1*, *CREBBP*, *CUX1*, *SRSF2*, *MLL2*, *SETD2*, *SETDB1*, *GNAS*, *PPM1D*, and *BCORL1* [86]. To be categorized as CHIP, a detected somatic variant must be present at a variant allele frequency (VAF) of at least 2% [85]. The second term is age-related clonal hematopoiesis (ARCH) [87]. The difference between this and CHIP is that a recurring alteration is identified as the possible cause of ARCH. Potential copy-number variants, together with mutations in candidate driver genes and epigenetic drift, have to be considered in ARCH development [88]. Despite the name and classification, its relevance is that any form of CH has the potential to transform [85,89] in myeloid [90] or even in lymphoid [89] neoplasms. Therefore, these mutations must be considered in a clinical context.

In this regard, the mutations found in the *DNMT3A* in adult T-ALL are of particular interest. As we have explained, mutations in this gene have been exclusively found in adult T-ALL and are associated with patients aged >60 years [43] as well as with immature subtypes such as the ETP-ALL [30,31,42,43]. Analysis of leukemic and non-leukemic cells of adult T-ALL patients showed that *DNMT3A* mutations were present in the non-leukemic fraction in two of the eight patients analyzed, suggesting that immature T-ALL cases could be derived from a CHIP event [42]. Similar results were obtained in an extended cohort, in which *DNM3TA* mutations were detected in polymorphonuclear cells, as a source of non-leukemic cells, and in leukemic cells [43]. VAFs in the *DNMT3A* gene were lower than or the same as those in the leukemic cells of all seven patients studied, suggesting a role for the *DNMT3A* mutations as a founding event in the development of T-ALL in the elderly and implying that the mutations could arise in an uncommitted myeloid-lymphoid progenitor [43]. In both studies, however, the possible germline origin of *DNMT3A* mutations could not be ruled out. More importantly, adult T-ALL patients with *DNMT3A* mutations have been significantly associated with worse clinical outcomes, a higher cumulative incidence of relapse (HR 2.33, 95% CI: 1.05–5.16, $p = 0.037$), and markedly poorer event-free survival (HR 3.22, 95% CI: 1.81–5.72, $p < 0.001$) and overall survival (HR 2.91, 95% CI: 1.56–5.43, $p = 0.001$) [42].

A driver mutation is an alteration that gives a cancer cell fundamental growth advantage for its neoplastic transformation. It differs from passenger mutations in that these do not necessarily determine the development of the cancer.

6. Relapse

Although intensive chemotherapy treatments have been crucial for improving survival to up to 93% of T-ALL-affected children, the survival rates in adults are still very poor, remaining below 50% [5]. Under both scenarios, T-ALL patients with primary-resistant or relapsed leukemia have a dismal prognosis, mainly due to the rapid progression of the recurrent course of the disease and the lack of therapeutic options. Application of multi-omics techniques in matched-diagnosis (DX), germline, or remission and relapse (RE) DNA samples to identify private and shared variants at DX and RE have helped us understand relapse mechanisms and identify target drugs to apply as new therapies.

The largest cohort studied until now, employing triplets, assessed the mutational profile, including CNVs, of 175 ALL patients ($n = 149$ pediatric and $n = 26$ adult cases; 129 BCP vs. 46 T-ALL) [91]. The WGS revealed that 52% of the relapse samples contained most of the genetic lesions present in the major clone at diagnosis. Overall, there were significantly more relapse-specific mutations than diagnosis-specific variants (chemo-sensitive) and common diagnosis-relapse variants. The most prominent relapse-specific genetic lesions implicated in chemotherapy resistance in ALL were the gain-of-function mutations in *NT5C2* (22/175, 12%), as previously demonstrated [81,92]. *NT5C2* was found exclusively in relapse samples. Other alterations that were more prevalent in relapsed samples were mutations in the *SETD2* (2.3%), *NR3C1* (1%), *WHSC1*9 (4.6%), *WT1* (6.2%), and *CREBBP*9 (9.7%) genes. *TP53* was observed to be more frequent at diagnosis in adult (4/26) than in pediatric (5/149) cases [93]. A similar study, assessing 103 pediatric ALL triplets (87 BCP and 16 T-cell ALL), observed that relapse-specific somatic alterations were enriched in 12 genes (*NR3C1*, *NR3C2*, *TP53*, *NT5C2*, *FPGS*, *CREBBP*, *MSH2*, *MSH6*, *PMS2*, *WHSC1*, *PRPS1*, and *PRPS2*), all of which were involved in the drug response. The mutational relapse signature had a global prevalence of 17% in the very early relapse group (<9 months after DX), 65% in the early relapse group (9–36 months), and 32% in the late relapse (>36 months) group. The authors examined the mechanism/factors by which the leukemic cell can increase the number of mutations at relapse by analyzing mutational signatures based on the trinucleotide context [94]. A novel mutational signature, thought to arise from thiopurine treatment (6-thioguanine and 6-mercaptopurine), was detected in 27% of relapsed ALLs and was responsible for 46% of the acquired resistance mutations in *NT5C2*, *PRPS1*, *NR3C1*, and *TP53*, [95]. Collectively, a summary of the data explained above highlights the role of specific mutations in *NR3C1*, *TP53*, *NT5C2*, and *CREBBP* in ALL relapse (Figure 3).

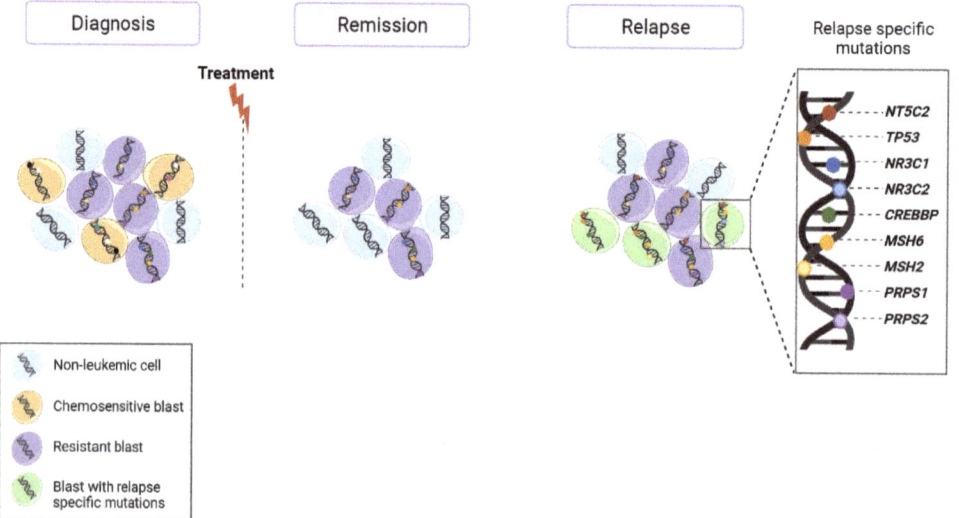

Figure 3. Schematic representation of clonal evolution of leukemic cells from diagnosis to relapse. As described above, relapse blasts contain genetic mutations present at diagnosis and genetic mutations relapse' specific. The most prevalent relapse-specific mutations are shown at the right side of the picture.

As expected, most of the triplets in the two studies mentioned corresponded to BCP-ALL, which limited the possibility of defining relapse mechanisms based on lymphoblastic leukemia type. The work of Oshima et al. is of particular interest for finding no major differences between BCP and T-ALL except for the activating mutations in the *NRAS* and *KRAS* oncogenes, which were primarily early events in T-ALL and more heterogeneously distributed in B-precursor ALL [93]. With the aim of exploring relapse-specific mechanisms in pediatric T-ALL, 313 leukemia-related genes were assessed by targeted deep sequencing (TDS) and multiplex ligation-dependent probe amplification, together with low-coverage WGS, for CNV detections. These techniques detected CNVs in 214 T-ALL patients (67 non-matched relapse and 147 diagnostic cases) and identified activating mutations in *NT5C2* and/or inactivation of *TP53* and/or duplication of chr17 (q11.2; q24.3) in 48% of T-ALL relapse samples. Again, the *NT5C2* was the gene most frequently bearing relapse-specific mutations, although they had no prognostic implications in the pediatric series. Interestingly, *TP53* mutations were very strongly predictive of a second-event relapse [96]. In adult T-ALL cases, data sets analyzing relapse-specific mutations in this subtype of leukemia are very difficult to obtain due to the rarity of the leukemia. However, recently, 19 triplets (DX-remission/germline-RE) from patients treated in two consecutive PETHEMA trials were analyzed by WGS. Data were compared with other open-access genomic data sets of pediatric T-ALL and ALL cases. In this way, clonal mutations in *PHF6* were found to be overrepresented in adult T-ALLs relative to their pediatric counterparts, shared between primary and relapse samples. Alterations in *SMARCA4* (mutations and deletions) were also detected in adult and pediatric T-ALLs, but almost exclusively in relapse malignancies, suggesting a potential role in resistance to treatment [97]. In addition, the authors tried to resolve the outstanding question about relapse mechanisms of whether the treatment (chemotherapy) itself is responsible for genetic variability due to the generation of de novo variants that drive or support relapse. They addressed this by employing computational modeling to estimate the precise divergence time between primary and relapse clonal populations. In the majority of cases, they observed that less than a year passed between the emergence of the relapse clone (single cell) and diagnosis of the primary disease. These findings, and the calculation of the minimum time necessary for the relapse population to reach approximately 7×10^{11} cells, the estimated number for a full-grown leukemia, suggested that in most of the 19 adult T-ALL leukemias analyzed, the relapse population was most probably already present before the treatment began, although it was not possible to detect relapse-specific genetic determinants (mutations) at the time of diagnosis [97]. These results are consistent with the observation of a significantly higher level of branched evolution after diagnosis in pediatric ALL cases compared with adult leukemias, suggesting less divergence between diagnostic and relapsed populations in adults [93]. Data supporting this highly heterogeneous branched clonal structure already present at time of diagnosis have also been validated by modeling relapse in immunodeficient mice [98]. However, another study has suggested that treatment may be responsible for the acquisition of new variants that generate resistance, as the proliferating doubling time model used by the authors is not consistent with the model of a pre-existing clone before diagnosis [95]. This is a very controversial point. The inability to detect resistant mutations at the time of diagnosis due, in part, to the sensitivity of the technique used and to the origin of the sample analyzed, in conjunction with the assumptions required to define a leukemia proliferation model, can dramatically influence the resistance model supported [99].

A very recent technique—variant analysis at single-cell resolution—has proved to be the key to detecting rare variants at diagnosis and during treatment. The technique enables the detection of a limited number of variants in a limited number of cells, the sensitivity being boosted by analyzing a larger number of cells [100,101]. Results obtained using this technique in pediatric T-ALL patients have shown that, at single-cell resolution, *NOTCH1* mutations are also highly heterogeneous [102]. The authors promote the utility of the technique in clinics, based on their success in detecting residual leukemic cells at remission time points (two clones at 0.2% and 0.3%, respectively). However, the sensitivity achieved at the single-cell level is far from that already offered by the high-resolution cytometry currently used in clinics (0.001%) (ALL2019, PETHEMA trial), to track residual leukemic cells. Together with that, the variants specifically observed at relapse could not be detected at the time of diagnosis [102], indicating that sequencing at single-cell resolution is not yet capable of identifying mutations causing relapse in patients at the time of diagnosis, or of increasing the sensitivity of tracking resistant clones in patients following treatment, two key issues to solve to apply the technique in a clinical context.

7. Future Perspectives

The amount of genomic information available has grown rapidly in the last decade as the technology developed to support multi-omics data has become more accessible. From the technical point of view, several private services can currently produce omics data at very reasonable prices, and protocols for generating libraries have been optimized and can be performed in a matter of days with a very high degree of reproducibility. Many of the companies involved in omics have developed easily handled software for analyzing data without the need for a specialized bioinformatician. Sequencing costs have also dropped dramatically. The multi-omic information obtained has helped us better understand the natural history of each T-ALL and reveal the oncogenetic processes operating in non-malignant cells. Genetics is also helping us to understand relapse mechanisms and to design new and more specific therapeutic alternatives. However, it is clear that a large quantity of information is still unavailable to us. In this context, the information provided by the non-coding sequences will help us better define the genetic profile of a T-ALL. Exploration of non-coding sequences needs to be accompanied by the improved assessment of variant functionality. Most of the non-coding variants and a large number of coding variants are classified as being of uncertain significance (many in-dels, small insertions, and deletions), so we cannot predict their impact on the disease. In addition, the contribution of small CNVs in the disease are not well stablished. Functional information is also missing. More importantly, in rare cancers such as T-ALL, especially in adult cases, it is difficult to achieve significant genetic redundancy with which to determine what part of all the genomic information is clinically relevant. To overcome these limitations and advance this area of research, genomic data sets need to be assessed in patients included in standardized treatment protocols in which detailed clinico-biological data at diagnosis, during treatment, and at relapse are registered in detail. More broadly still, groups researching ALL/T-ALL should pool their efforts and collaborate to move definitively towards establishing personalized medicine for these rare types of cancer.

Author Contributions: Study conceptualization and writing of original draft, E.G.; figures and tables, C.G.-G.; review and editing, C.G.-G. and E.G. All authors have read and agreed to the published version of the manuscript.

Funding: This project was supported by the AECC (GC16173697BIGA); ISCIII (PI19/01828), co-funded by ERDF/ESF, "A way to make Europe"/"Investing in your future", CERCA/Generalitat de Catalunya SGR 2017 288 (GRC)/ "La Caixa". C González-Gil was supported by an AGAUR grant (ref: 2020 FI_B2 00210).

Conflicts of Interest: The authors declare no conflict of interest. The funders had no role in writing or publishing the manuscript.

References

1. Yi, M.; Zhou, L.; Li, A.; Luo, S.; Wu, K. Global Burden and Trend of Acute Lymphoblastic Leukemia from 1990 to 2017. *Aging* **2020**, *12*, 22869–22891. [CrossRef] [PubMed]
2. Belver, L.; Ferrando, A. The Genetics and Mechanisms of T Cell Acute Lymphoblastic Leukaemia. *Nat. Rev. Cancer* **2016**, *16*, 494–507. [CrossRef] [PubMed]
3. Guru Murthy, G.S.; Pondaiah, S.K.; Abedin, S.; Atallah, E. Incidence and Survival of T-Cell Acute Lymphoblastic Leukemia in the United States. *Leuk. Lymphoma* **2019**, *60*, 1171–1178. [CrossRef]
4. Bartram, J.; Veys, P.; Vora, A. Improvements in Outcome of Childhood Acute Lymphoblastic Leukaemia (ALL) in the UK—A Success Story of Modern Medicine through Successive UKALL Trials and International Collaboration. *Br. J. Haematol.* **2020**, *191*, 562–567. [CrossRef] [PubMed]
5. Ribera, J.-M.; Morgades, M.; Ciudad, J.; Montesinos, P.; Esteve, J.; Genescà, E.; Barba, P.; Ribera, J.; García-Cadenas, I.; Moreno, M.J.; et al. Chemotherapy or Allogeneic Transplantation in High-Risk Philadelphia Chromosome-Negative Adult Lymphoblastic Leukemia. *Blood* **2021**, *137*, 1879–1894. [CrossRef]
6. Beldjord, K.; Chevret, S.; Asnafi, V.; Huguet, F.; Boulland, M.-L.; Leguay, T.; Thomas, X.; Cayuela, J.-M.; Grardel, N.; Chalandon, Y.; et al. Oncogenetics and Minimal Residual Disease Are Independent Outcome Predictors in Adult Patients with Acute Lymphoblastic Leukemia. *Blood* **2014**, *123*, 3739–3749. [CrossRef]
7. Nguyen, K.; Devidas, M.; Cheng, S.-C.; La, M.; Raetz, E.A.; Carroll, W.L.; Winick, N.J.; Hunger, S.P.; Gaynon, P.S.; Loh, M.L. Factors Influencing Survival After Relapse From Acute Lymphoblastic Leukemia: A Children's Oncology Group Study. *Leukemia* **2008**, *22*, 2142–2150. [CrossRef]
8. Barba, P.; Morgades, M.; Montesinos, P.; Gil, C.; Fox, M.-L.; Ciudad, J.; Moreno, M.-J.; González-Campos, J.; Genescà, E.; Martínez-Carballeira, D.; et al. Increased Survival Due to Lower Toxicity for High-Risk T-Cell Acute Lymphoblastic Leukemia Patients in Two Consecutive Pediatric-Inspired PETHEMA Trials. *Eur. J. Haematol.* **2019**, *102*, 79–86. [CrossRef]
9. Begley, C.G.; Aplan, P.D.; Davey, M.P.; Nakahara, K.; Tchorz, K.; Kurtzberg, J.; Hershfield, M.S.; Haynes, B.F.; Cohen, D.I.; Waldmann, T.A. Chromosomal Translocation in a Human Leukemic Stem-Cell Line Disrupts the T-Cell Antigen Receptor Delta-Chain Diversity Region and Results in a Previously Unreported Fusion Transcript. *Proc. Natl. Acad. Sci. USA* **1989**, *86*, 2031–2035. [CrossRef]
10. Bernard, O.; Guglielmi, P.; Jonveaux, P.; Cherif, D.; Gisselbrecht, S.; Mauchauffe, M.; Berger, R.; Larsen, C.J.; Mathieu-Mahul, D. Two Distinct Mechanisms for the SCL Gene Activation in the t(1;14) Translocation of T-Cell Leukemias. *Genes Chromosom. Cancer* **1990**, *1*, 194–208. [CrossRef]

11. Chen, Q.; Cheng, J.T.; Tasi, L.H.; Schneider, N.; Buchanan, G.; Carroll, A.; Crist, W.; Ozanne, B.; Siciliano, M.J.; Baer, R. The Tal Gene Undergoes Chromosome Translocation in T Cell Leukemia and Potentially Encodes a Helix-Loop-Helix Protein. *EMBO J.* **1990**, *9*, 415–424. [CrossRef]
12. Xia, Y.; Brown, L.; Yang, C.Y.; Tsan, J.T.; Siciliano, M.J.; Espinosa, R.; Le Beau, M.M.; Baer, R.J. TAL2, a Helix-Loop-Helix Gene Activated by the (7;9)(Q34;Q32) Translocation in Human T-Cell Leukemia. *Proc. Natl. Acad. Sci. USA* **1991**, *88*, 11416–11420. [CrossRef]
13. Mellentin, J.D.; Smith, S.D.; Cleary, M.L. Lyl-1, a Novel Gene Altered by Chromosomal Translocation in T Cell Leukemia, Codes for a Protein with a Helix-Loop-Helix DNA Binding Motif. *Cell* **1989**, *58*, 77–83. [CrossRef]
14. McGuire, E.A.; Hockett, R.D.; Pollock, K.M.; Bartholdi, M.F.; O'Brien, S.J.; Korsmeyer, S.J. The t(11;14)(P15;Q11) in a T-Cell Acute Lymphoblastic Leukemia Cell Line Activates Multiple Transcripts, Including Ttg-1, a Gene Encoding a Potential Zinc Finger Protein. *Mol. Cell Biol.* **1989**, *9*, 2124–2132. [PubMed]
15. Boehm, T.; Foroni, L.; Kaneko, Y.; Perutz, M.F.; Rabbitts, T.H. The Rhombotin Family of Cysteine-Rich LIM-Domain Oncogenes: Distinct Members Are Involved in T-Cell Translocations to Human Chromosomes 11p15 and 11p13. *Proc. Natl. Acad. Sci. USA* **1991**, *88*, 4367–4371. [CrossRef] [PubMed]
16. Royer-Pokora, B.; Loos, U.; Ludwig, W.D. TTG-2, a New Gene Encoding a Cysteine-Rich Protein with the LIM Motif, Is Overexpressed in Acute T-Cell Leukaemia with the t(11;14)(P13;Q11). *Oncogene* **1991**, *6*, 1887–1893.
17. Dube, I.; Kamel-Reid, S.; Yuan, C.; Lu, M.; Wu, X.; Corpus, G.; Raimondi, S.; Crist, W.; Carroll, A.; Minowada, J. A Novel Human Homeobox Gene Lies at the Chromosome 10 Breakpoint in Lymphoid Neoplasias with Chromosomal Translocation t(10;14). *Blood* **1991**, *78*, 2996–3003. [CrossRef] [PubMed]
18. Hatano, M.; Roberts, C.W.; Minden, M.; Crist, W.M.; Korsmeyer, S.J. Deregulation of a Homeobox Gene, HOX11, by the t(10;14) in T Cell Leukemia. *Science* **1991**, *253*, 79–82. [CrossRef]
19. Bernard, O.A.; Busson-LeConiat, M.; Ballerini, P.; Mauchauffé, M.; Della Valle, V.; Monni, R.; Nguyen Khac, F.; Mercher, T.; Penard-Lacronique, V.; Pasturaud, P.; et al. A New Recurrent and Specific Cryptic Translocation, t(5;14)(Q35;Q32), Is Associated with Expression of the Hox11L2 Gene in T Acute Lymphoblastic Leukemia. *Leukemia* **2001**, *15*, 1495–1504. [CrossRef]
20. Ferrando, A.A.; Neuberg, D.S.; Staunton, J.; Loh, M.L.; Huard, C.; Raimondi, S.C.; Behm, F.G.; Pui, C.H.; Downing, J.R.; Gilliland, D.G.; et al. Gene Expression Signatures Define Novel Oncogenic Pathways in T Cell Acute Lymphoblastic Leukemia. *Cancer Cell* **2002**, *1*, 75–87. [CrossRef]
21. Soulier, J.; Clappier, E.; Cayuela, J.-M.; Regnault, A.; García-Peydró, M.; Dombret, H.; Baruchel, A.; Toribio, M.-L.; Sigaux, F. HOXA Genes Are Included in Genetic and Biologic Networks Defining Human Acute T-Cell Leukemia (T-ALL). *Blood* **2005**, *106*, 274–286. [CrossRef]
22. Homminga, I.; Pieters, R.; Langerak, A.W.; de Rooi, J.J.; Stubbs, A.; Verstegen, M.; Vuerhard, M.; Buijs-Gladdines, J.; Kooi, C.; Klous, P.; et al. Integrated Transcript and Genome Analyses Reveal NKX2-1 and MEF2C as Potential Oncogenes in T Cell Acute Lymphoblastic Leukemia. *Cancer Cell* **2011**, *19*, 484–497. [CrossRef]
23. Gutierrez, A.; Dahlberg, S.E.; Neuberg, D.S.; Zhang, J.; Grebliunaite, R.; Sanda, T.; Protopopov, A.; Tosello, V.; Kutok, J.; Larson, R.S.; et al. Absence of Biallelic TCRγ Deletion Predicts Early Treatment Failure in Pediatric T-Cell Acute Lymphoblastic Leukemia. *JCO* **2010**, *28*, 3816–3823. [CrossRef]
24. Coustan-Smith, E.; Mullighan, C.G.; Onciu, M.; Behm, F.G.; Raimondi, S.C.; Pei, D.; Cheng, C.; Su, X.; Rubnitz, J.E.; Basso, G.; et al. Early T-Cell Precursor Leukaemia: A Subtype of Very High-Risk Acute Lymphoblastic Leukaemia. *Lancet Oncol.* **2009**, *10*, 147–156. [CrossRef]
25. Van Vlierberghe, P.; Ambesi-Impiombato, A.; De Keersmaecker, K.; Hadler, M.; Paietta, E.; Tallman, M.S.; Rowe, J.M.; Forne, C.; Rue, M.; Ferrando, A.A. Prognostic Relevance of Integrated Genetic Profiling in Adult T-Cell Acute Lymphoblastic Leukemia. *Blood* **2013**, *122*, 74–82. [CrossRef]
26. Vicente, C.; Schwab, C.; Broux, M.; Geerdens, E.; Degryse, S.; Demeyer, S.; Lahortiga, I.; Elliott, A.; Chilton, L.; La Starza, R.; et al. Targeted Sequencing Identifies Associations between IL7R-JAK Mutations and Epigenetic Modulators in T-Cell Acute Lymphoblastic Leukemia. *Haematologica* **2015**, *100*, 1301–1310. [CrossRef]
27. Genescà, E.; Lazarenkov, A.; Morgades, M.; Berbis, G.; Ruíz-Xivillé, N.; Gómez-Marzo, P.; Ribera, J.; Juncà, J.; González-Pérez, A.; Mercadal, S.; et al. Frequency and Clinical Impact of CDKN2A/ARF/CDKN2B Gene Deletions as Assessed by in-Depth Genetic Analyses in Adult T Cell Acute Lymphoblastic Leukemia. *J. Hematol. Oncol.* **2018**, *11*, 96. [CrossRef]
28. Van Vlierberghe, P.; Ambesi-Impiombato, A.; Perez-Garcia, A.; Haydu, J.E.; Rigo, I.; Hadler, M.; Tosello, V.; Della Gatta, G.; Paietta, E.; Racevskis, J.; et al. ETV6 Mutations in Early Immature Human T Cell Leukemias. *J. Exp. Med.* **2011**, *208*, 2571–2579. [CrossRef] [PubMed]
29. Zhang, J.; Ding, L.; Holmfeldt, L.; Wu, G.; Heatley, S.L.; Payne-Turner, D.; Easton, J.; Chen, X.; Wang, J.; Rusch, M.; et al. The Genetic Basis of Early T-Cell Precursor Acute Lymphoblastic Leukaemia. *Nature* **2012**, *481*, 157–163. [CrossRef]
30. Neumann, M.; Heesch, S.; Schlee, C.; Schwartz, S.; Gökbuget, N.; Hoelzer, D.; Konstandin, N.P.; Ksienzyk, B.; Vosberg, S.; Graf, A.; et al. Whole-Exome Sequencing in Adult ETP-ALL Reveals a High Rate of DNMT3A Mutations. *Blood* **2013**, *121*, 4749–4752. [CrossRef] [PubMed]
31. Bond, J.; Graux, C.; Lhermitte, L.; Lara, D.; Cluzeau, T.; Leguay, T.; Cieslak, A.; Trinquand, A.; Pastoret, C.; Belhocine, M.; et al. Early Response-Based Therapy Stratification Improves Survival in Adult Early Thymic Precursor Acute Lymphoblastic Leukemia: A Group for Research on Adult Acute Lymphoblastic Leukemia Study. *J. Clin. Oncol.* **2017**, *35*, 2683–2691. [CrossRef]

32. Liu, Y.; Easton, J.; Shao, Y.; Maciaszek, J.; Wang, Z.; Wilkinson, M.R.; McCastlain, K.; Edmonson, M.; Pounds, S.B.; Shi, L.; et al. The Genomic Landscape of Pediatric and Young Adult T-Lineage Acute Lymphoblastic Leukemia. *Nat. Genet.* **2017**, *49*, 1211–1218. [CrossRef]
33. Gachet, S.; El-Chaar, T.; Avran, D.; Genesca, E.; Catez, F.; Quentin, S.; Delord, M.; Thérizols, G.; Briot, D.; Meunier, G.; et al. Deletion 6q Drives T-Cell Leukemia Progression by Ribosome Modulation. *Cancer Discov.* **2018**, *8*, 1614–1631. [CrossRef] [PubMed]
34. Herranz, D.; Ambesi-Impiombato, A.; Palomero, T.; Schnell, S.A.; Belver, L.; Wendorff, A.A.; Xu, L.; Castillo-Martin, M.; Llobet-Navás, D.; Cordon-Cardo, C.; et al. A NOTCH1-Driven MYC Enhancer Promotes T Cell Development, Transformation and Acute Lymphoblastic Leukemia. *Nat. Med.* **2014**, *20*, 1130–1137. [CrossRef]
35. Mansour, M.R.; Abraham, B.J.; Anders, L.; Berezovskaya, A.; Gutierrez, A.; Durbin, A.D.; Etchin, J.; Lawton, L.; Sallan, S.E.; Silverman, L.B.; et al. Oncogene Regulation. An Oncogenic Super-Enhancer Formed through Somatic Mutation of a Noncoding Intergenic Element. *Science* **2014**, *346*, 1373–1377. [CrossRef] [PubMed]
36. Hu, S.; Qian, M.; Zhang, H.; Guo, Y.; Yang, J.; Zhao, X.; He, H.; Lu, J.; Pan, J.; Chang, M.; et al. Whole-Genome Noncoding Sequence Analysis in T-Cell Acute Lymphoblastic Leukemia Identifies Oncogene Enhancer Mutations. *Blood* **2017**, *129*, 3264–3268. [CrossRef]
37. Li, Z.; Abraham, B.J.; Berezovskaya, A.; Farah, N.; Liu, Y.; Leon, T.; Fielding, A.; Tan, S.H.; Sanda, T.; Weintraub, A.S.; et al. APOBEC Signature Mutation Generates an Oncogenic Enhancer That Drives LMO1 Expression in T-ALL. *Leukemia* **2017**, *31*, 2057–2064. [CrossRef] [PubMed]
38. Rahman, S.; Magnussen, M.; León, T.E.; Farah, N.; Li, Z.; Abraham, B.J.; Alapi, K.Z.; Mitchell, R.J.; Naughton, T.; Fielding, A.K.; et al. Activation of the LMO2 Oncogene through a Somatically Acquired Neomorphic Promoter in T-Cell Acute Lymphoblastic Leukemia. *Blood* **2017**, *129*, 3221–3226. [CrossRef] [PubMed]
39. Tottone, L.; Lancho, O.; Loh, J.-W.; Singh, A.; Kimura, S.; Roels, J.; Kuchmiy, A.; Strubbe, S.; Lawlor, M.A.; da Silva-Diz, V.; et al. A Tumor Suppressor Enhancer of PTEN in T-Cell Development and Leukemia. *Blood Cancer Discov.* **2021**, *2*, 92–109. [CrossRef]
40. Swerdlow, S.H.; Campo, E.; Harris, N.L.; Jaffe, E.S.; Pileri, S.A.; Stein, H.; Thiele, J. *WHO Classification of Tumours of Haematopoietic and Lymphoid Tissues*; IARC Publications: Lyon, France, 2018; ISBN 978-92-832-4494-3.
41. Morita, K.; Jain, N.; Kantarjian, H.; Takahashi, K.; Fang, H.; Konopleva, M.; El Hussein, S.; Wang, F.; Short, N.J.; Maiti, A.; et al. Outcome of T-Cell Acute Lymphoblastic Leukemia/Lymphoma: Focus on near-ETP Phenotype and Differential Impact of Nelarabine. *Am. J. Hematol.* **2021**, *96*, 589–598. [CrossRef]
42. Bond, J.; Touzart, A.; Leprêtre, S.; Graux, C.; Bargetzi, M.; Lhermitte, L.; Hypolite, G.; Leguay, T.; Hicheri, Y.; Guillerm, G.; et al. DNMT3A Mutation Is Associated with Increased Age and Adverse Outcome in Adult T-Cell Acute Lymphoblastic Leukemia. *Haematologica* **2019**, *104*, 1617–1625. [CrossRef]
43. González-Gil, C.; Morgades, M.; Fuster-Tormo, F.; García-Chica, J.; Montesinos, P.; Torrent, A.; Diaz-Beyá, M.; Coll, R.; Ribera, J.; Zhao, R.; et al. Genomic Data Improves Prognostic Stratification in Adult T-Cell Acute Lymphoblastic Leukemia Patients Enrolled in Measurable Residual Disease-Oriented Trials. *Blood* **2021**, *138*, 3486. [CrossRef]
44. Bond, J.; Marchand, T.; Touzart, A.; Cieslak, A.; Trinquand, A.; Sutton, L.; Radford-Weiss, I.; Lhermitte, L.; Spicuglia, S.; Dombret, H.; et al. An Early Thymic Precursor Phenotype Predicts Outcome Exclusively in HOXA-Overexpressing Adult T-Cell Acute Lymphoblastic Leukemia: A Group for Research in Adult Acute Lymphoblastic Leukemia Study. *Haematologica* **2016**, *101*, 732–740. [CrossRef]
45. Ben Abdelali, R.; Asnafi, V.; Petit, A.; Micol, J.-B.; Callens, C.; Villarese, P.; Delabesse, E.; Reman, O.; Lepretre, S.; Cahn, J.-Y.; et al. The Prognosis of CALM-AF10-Positive Adult T-Cell Acute Lymphoblastic Leukemias Depends on the Stage of Maturation Arrest. *Haematologica* **2013**, *98*, 1711–1717. [CrossRef] [PubMed]
46. Montefiori, L.E.; Bendig, S.; Gu, Z.; Chen, X.; Pölönen, P.; Ma, X.; Murison, A.; Zeng, A.; Garcia-Prat, L.; Dickerson, K.; et al. Enhancer Hijacking Drives Oncogenic BCL11B Expression in Lineage-Ambiguous Stem Cell Leukemia. *Cancer Discov.* **2021**, *11*, 2846–2867. [CrossRef] [PubMed]
47. Di Giacomo, D.; La Starza, R.; Gorello, P.; Pellanera, F.; Kalender Atak, Z.; De Keersmaecker, K.; Pierini, V.; Harrison, C.J.; Arniani, S.; Moretti, M.; et al. 14q32 Rearrangements Deregulating BCL11B Mark a Distinct Subgroup of T-Lymphoid and Myeloid Immature Acute Leukemia. *Blood* **2021**, *138*, 773–784. [CrossRef] [PubMed]
48. Alexander, T.B.; Gu, Z.; Iacobucci, I.; Dickerson, K.; Choi, J.K.; Xu, B.; Payne-Turner, D.; Yoshihara, H.; Loh, M.L.; Horan, J.; et al. The Genetic Basis and Cell of Origin of Mixed Phenotype Acute Leukaemia. *Nature* **2018**, *562*, 373–379. [CrossRef] [PubMed]
49. Takahashi, K.; Wang, F.; Morita, K.; Yan, Y.; Hu, P.; Zhao, P.; Zhar, A.A.; Wu, C.J.; Gumbs, C.; Little, L.; et al. Integrative Genomic Analysis of Adult Mixed Phenotype Acute Leukemia Delineates Lineage Associated Molecular Subtypes. *Nat. Commun.* **2018**, *9*, 2670. [CrossRef]
50. Huether, R.; Dong, L.; Chen, X.; Wu, G.; Parker, M.; Wei, L.; Ma, J.; Edmonson, M.N.; Hedlund, E.K.; Rusch, M.C.; et al. The Landscape of Somatic Mutations in Epigenetic Regulators across 1,000 Paediatric Cancer Genomes. *Nat. Commun.* **2014**, *5*, 3630. [CrossRef]
51. Christman, J.K. 5-Azacytidine and 5-Aza-2'-Deoxycytidine as Inhibitors of DNA Methylation: Mechanistic Studies and Their Implications for Cancer Therapy. *Oncogene* **2002**, *21*, 5483–5495. [CrossRef]
52. Batova, A.; Diccianni, M.B.; Yu, J.C.; Nobori, T.; Link, M.P.; Pullen, J.; Yu, A.L. Frequent and Selective Methylation of P15 and Deletion of Both P15 and P16 in T-Cell Acute Lymphoblastic Leukemia. *Cancer Res.* **1997**, *57*, 832–836. [PubMed]

53. Tsellou, E.; Troungos, C.; Moschovi, M.; Athanasiadou-Piperopoulou, F.; Polychronopoulou, S.; Kosmidis, H.; Kalmanti, M.; Hatzakis, A.; Dessypris, N.; Kalofoutis, A.; et al. Hypermethylation of CpG Islands in the Promoter Region of the P15INK4B Gene in Childhood Acute Leukaemia. *Eur. J. Cancer* **2005**, *41*, 584–589. [CrossRef]
54. Takeuchi, S.; Matsushita, M.; Zimmermann, M.; Ikezoe, T.; Komatsu, N.; Seriu, T.; Schrappe, M.; Bartram, C.R.; Koeffler, H.P. Clinical Significance of Aberrant DNA Methylation in Childhood Acute Lymphoblastic Leukemia. *Leuk. Res.* **2011**, *35*, 1345–1349. [CrossRef]
55. Chim, C.S.; Tam, C.Y.; Liang, R.; Kwong, Y.L. Methylation of P15 and P16 Genes in Adult Acute Leukemia: Lack of Prognostic Significance. *Cancer* **2001**, *91*, 2222–2229. [CrossRef]
56. Garcia-Manero, G.; Bueso-Ramos, C.; Daniel, J.; Williamson, J.; Kantarjian, H.M.; Issa, J.-P.J. DNA Methylation Patterns at Relapse in Adult Acute Lymphocytic Leukemia. *Clin. Cancer Res.* **2002**, *8*, 1897–1903.
57. Bueso-Ramos, C.; Xu, Y.; McDonnell, T.J.; Brisbay, S.; Pierce, S.; Kantarjian, H.; Rosner, G.; Garcia-Manero, G. Protein Expression of a Triad of Frequently Methylated Genes, P73, P57Kip2, and P15, Has Prognostic Value in Adult Acute Lymphocytic Leukemia Independently of Its Methylation Status. *J. Clin. Oncol.* **2005**, *23*, 3932–3939. [CrossRef]
58. Grossmann, V.; Haferlach, C.; Weissmann, S.; Roller, A.; Schindela, S.; Poetzinger, F.; Stadler, K.; Bellos, F.; Kern, W.; Haferlach, T.; et al. The Molecular Profile of Adult T-Cell Acute Lymphoblastic Leukemia: Mutations in RUNX1 and DNMT3A Are Associated with Poor Prognosis in T-ALL. *Genes Chromosom. Cancer* **2013**, *52*, 410–422. [CrossRef] [PubMed]
59. Jang, W.; Park, J.; Kwon, A.; Choi, H.; Kim, J.; Lee, G.D.; Han, E.; Jekarl, D.W.; Chae, H.; Han, K.; et al. CDKN2B Downregulation and Other Genetic Characteristics in T-Acute Lymphoblastic Leukemia. *Exp. Mol. Med.* **2019**, *51*, 1–15. [CrossRef] [PubMed]
60. Borssén, M.; Palmqvist, L.; Karrman, K.; Abrahamsson, J.; Behrendtz, M.; Heldrup, J.; Forestier, E.; Roos, G.; Degerman, S. Promoter DNA Methylation Pattern Identifies Prognostic Subgroups in Childhood T-Cell Acute Lymphoblastic Leukemia. *PLoS ONE* **2013**, *8*, e65373. [CrossRef] [PubMed]
61. Kimura, S.; Seki, M.; Kawai, T.; Goto, H.; Yoshida, K.; Isobe, T.; Sekiguchi, M.; Watanabe, K.; Kubota, Y.; Nannya, Y.; et al. DNA Methylation-Based Classification Reveals Difference between Pediatric T-Cell Acute Lymphoblastic Leukemia and Normal Thymocytes. *Leukemia* **2020**, *34*, 1163–1168. [CrossRef]
62. Touzart, A.; Boissel, N.; Belhocine, M.; Smith, C.; Graux, C.; Latiri, M.; Lhermitte, L.; Mathieu, E.-L.; Huguet, F.; Lamant, L.; et al. Low Level CpG Island Promoter Methylation Predicts a Poor Outcome in Adult T-Cell Acute Lymphoblastic Leukemia. *Haematologica* **2020**, *105*, 1575–1581. [CrossRef]
63. Roels, J.; Thénoz, M.; Szarzyńska, B.; Landfors, M.; De Coninck, S.; Demoen, L.; Provez, L.; Kuchmiy, A.; Strubbe, S.; Reunes, L.; et al. Aging of Preleukemic Thymocytes Drives CpG Island Hypermethylation in T-Cell Acute Lymphoblastic Leukemia. *Blood Cancer Discov.* **2020**, *1*, 274–289. [CrossRef] [PubMed]
64. Haider, Z.; Larsson, P.; Landfors, M.; Köhn, L.; Schmiegelow, K.; Flægstad, T.; Kanerva, J.; Heyman, M.; Hultdin, M.; Degerman, S. An Integrated Transcriptome Analysis in T-cell Acute Lymphoblastic Leukemia Links DNA Methylation Subgroups to Dysregulated *TAL1* and ANTP Homeobox Gene Expression. *Cancer Med.* **2018**, *8*, 311–324. [CrossRef] [PubMed]
65. Maćkowska, N.; Drobna-Śledzińska, M.; Witt, M.; Dawidowska, M. DNA Methylation in T-Cell Acute Lymphoblastic Leukemia: In Search for Clinical and Biological Meaning. *Int. J. Mol. Sci.* **2021**, *22*, 1388. [CrossRef]
66. Newman, S.; Nakitandwe, J.; Kesserwan, C.A.; Azzato, E.M.; Wheeler, D.A.; Rusch, M.; Shurtleff, S.; Hedges, D.J.; Hamilton, K.V.; Foy, S.G.; et al. Genomes for Kids: The Scope of Pathogenic Mutations in Pediatric Cancer Revealed by Comprehensive DNA and RNA Sequencing. *Cancer Discov.* **2021**, *11*, 3008–3027. [CrossRef]
67. Bodmer, W.; Tomlinson, I. Rare Genetic Variants and the Risk of Cancer. *Curr. Opin. Genet. Dev.* **2010**, *20*, 262–267. [CrossRef] [PubMed]
68. Rahman, N. Realizing the Promise of Cancer Predisposition Genes. *Nature* **2014**, *505*, 302–308. [CrossRef]
69. Huang, K.-L.; Mashl, R.J.; Wu, Y.; Ritter, D.I.; Wang, J.; Oh, C.; Paczkowska, M.; Reynolds, S.; Wyczalkowski, M.A.; Oak, N.; et al. Pathogenic Germline Variants in 10,389 Adult Cancers. *Cell* **2018**, *173*, 355–370.e14. [CrossRef]
70. Qian, M.; Zhao, X.; Devidas, M.; Yang, W.; Gocho, Y.; Smith, C.; Gastier-Foster, J.M.; Li, Y.; Xu, H.; Zhang, S.; et al. Genome-Wide Association Study of Susceptibility Loci for T-Cell Acute Lymphoblastic Leukemia in Children. *J. Natl. Cancer Inst.* **2019**, *111*, 1350–1357. [CrossRef]
71. Liberzon, E.; Avigad, S.; Stark, B.; Zilberstein, J.; Freedman, L.; Gorfine, M.; Gavriel, H.; Cohen, I.J.; Goshen, Y.; Yaniv, I.; et al. Germ-Line ATM Gene Alterations Are Associated with Susceptibility to Sporadic T-Cell Acute Lymphoblastic Leukemia in Children. *Genes Chromosom. Cancer* **2004**, *39*, 161–166. [CrossRef]
72. Yoshida, N.; Sakaguchi, H.; Muramatsu, H.; Okuno, Y.; Song, C.; Dovat, S.; Shimada, A.; Ozeki, M.; Ohnishi, H.; Teramoto, T.; et al. Germline IKAROS Mutation Associated with Primary Immunodeficiency That Progressed to T-Cell Acute Lymphoblastic Leukemia. *Leukemia* **2017**, *31*, 1221–1223. [CrossRef] [PubMed]
73. Brown, A.L.; Arts, P.; Carmichael, C.L.; Babic, M.; Dobbins, J.; Chong, C.-E.; Schreiber, A.W.; Feng, J.; Phillips, K.; Wang, P.P.S.; et al. RUNX1-Mutated Families Show Phenotype Heterogeneity and a Somatic Mutation Profile Unique to Germline Predisposed AML. *Blood Adv.* **2020**, *4*, 1131–1144. [CrossRef]
74. Li, Y.; Yang, W.; Devidas, M.; Winter, S.S.; Kesserwan, C.; Yang, W.; Dunsmore, K.P.; Smith, C.; Qian, M.; Zhao, X.; et al. Germline *RUNX1* Variation and Predisposition to Childhood Acute Lymphoblastic Leukemia. *J. Clin. Invest.* **2021**, *131*, e147898. [CrossRef]

75. Tulstrup, M.; Grosjean, M.; Nielsen, S.N.; Grell, K.; Wolthers, B.O.; Wegener, P.S.; Jonsson, O.G.; Lund, B.; Harila-Saari, A.; Abrahamsson, J.; et al. NT5C2 Germline Variants Alter Thiopurine Metabolism and Are Associated with Acquired NT5C2 Relapse Mutations in Childhood Acute Lymphoblastic Leukaemia. *Leukemia* **2018**, *32*, 2527–2535. [CrossRef] [PubMed]
76. Jiang, C.; Yang, W.; Moriyama, T.; Liu, C.; Smith, C.; Yang, W.; Qian, M.; Li, Z.; Tulstrup, M.; Schmiegelow, K.; et al. Effects of NT5C2 Germline Variants on 6-Mecaptopurine Metabolism in Children With Acute Lymphoblastic Leukemia. *Clin. Pharmacol. Ther.* **2021**, *109*, 1538–1545. [CrossRef] [PubMed]
77. Godley, L.A. Inherited Predisposition to Acute Myeloid Leukemia. *Semin. Hematol.* **2014**, *51*, 306–321. [CrossRef]
78. Antony-Debré, I.; Duployez, N.; Bucci, M.; Geffroy, S.; Micol, J.-B.; Renneville, A.; Boissel, N.; Dhédin, N.; Réa, D.; Nelken, B.; et al. Somatic Mutations Associated with Leukemic Progression of Familial Platelet Disorder with Predisposition to Acute Myeloid Leukemia. *Leukemia* **2016**, *30*, 999–1002. [CrossRef]
79. Spychała, J.; Madrid-Marina, V.; Fox, I.H. High Km Soluble 5′-Nucleotidase from Human Placenta. Properties and Allosteric Regulation by IMP and ATP. *J. Biol. Chem.* **1988**, *263*, 18759–18765. [CrossRef]
80. Gazziola, C.; Ferraro, P.; Moras, M.; Reichard, P.; Bianchi, V. Cytosolic High K(m) 5′-Nucleotidase and 5′(3′)-Deoxyribonucleotidase in Substrate Cycles Involved in Nucleotide Metabolism. *J. Biol. Chem.* **2001**, *276*, 6185–6190. [CrossRef]
81. Moriyama, T.; Liu, S.; Li, J.; Meyer, J.; Zhao, X.; Yang, W.; Shao, Y.; Heath, R.; Hnízda, A.; Carroll, W.L.; et al. Mechanisms of NT5C2-Mediated Thiopurine Resistance in Acute Lymphoblastic Leukemia. *Mol. Cancer Ther.* **2019**, *18*, 1887–1895. [CrossRef]
82. Cooper, J.N.; Young, N.S. Clonality in Context: Hematopoietic Clones in Their Marrow Environment. *Blood* **2017**, *130*, 2363–2372. [CrossRef] [PubMed]
83. Welch, J.S.; Ley, T.J.; Link, D.C.; Miller, C.A.; Larson, D.E.; Koboldt, D.C.; Wartman, L.D.; Lamprecht, T.L.; Liu, F.; Xia, J.; et al. The Origin and Evolution of Mutations in Acute Myeloid Leukemia. *Cell* **2012**, *150*, 264–278. [CrossRef] [PubMed]
84. Zink, F.; Stacey, S.N.; Norddahl, G.L.; Frigge, M.L.; Magnusson, O.T.; Jonsdottir, I.; Thorgeirsson, T.E.; Sigurdsson, A.; Gudjonsson, S.A.; Gudmundsson, J.; et al. Clonal Hematopoiesis, with and without Candidate Driver Mutations, Is Common in the Elderly. *Blood* **2017**, *130*, 742–752. [CrossRef] [PubMed]
85. Silver, A.J.; Jaiswal, S. Clonal Hematopoiesis: Pre-Cancer PLUS. *Adv. Cancer Res.* **2019**, *141*, 85–128. [CrossRef]
86. Steensma, D.P.; Bejar, R.; Jaiswal, S.; Lindsley, R.C.; Sekeres, M.A.; Hasserjian, R.P.; Ebert, B.L. Clonal Hematopoiesis of Indeterminate Potential and Its Distinction from Myelodysplastic Syndromes. *Blood* **2015**, *126*, 9–16. [CrossRef]
87. Busque, L.; Buscarlet, M.; Mollica, L.; Levine, R.L. Age-Related Clonal Hematopoiesis: Stem Cells Tempting the Devil. *Stem Cells* **2018**, *36*, 1287–1294. [CrossRef]
88. Abelson, S.; Collord, G.; Ng, S.W.K.; Weissbrod, O.; Mendelson Cohen, N.; Niemeyer, E.; Barda, N.; Zuzarte, P.C.; Heisler, L.; Sundaravadanam, Y.; et al. Prediction of Acute Myeloid Leukaemia Risk in Healthy Individuals. *Nature* **2018**, *559*, 400–404. [CrossRef]
89. Jaiswal, S.; Fontanillas, P.; Flannick, J.; Manning, A.; Grauman, P.V.; Mar, B.G.; Lindsley, R.C.; Mermel, C.H.; Burtt, N.; Chavez, A.; et al. Age-Related Clonal Hematopoiesis Associated with Adverse Outcomes. *N. Engl. J. Med.* **2014**, *371*, 2488–2498. [CrossRef]
90. Desai, P.; Mencia-Trinchant, N.; Savenkov, O.; Simon, M.S.; Cheang, G.; Lee, S.; Samuel, M.; Ritchie, E.K.; Guzman, M.L.; Ballman, K.V.; et al. Somatic Mutations Precede Acute Myeloid Leukemia Years before Diagnosis. *Nat. Med.* **2018**, *24*, 1015–1023. [CrossRef]
91. Oshima, K.; Khiabanian, H.; da Silva-Almeida, A.C.; Tzoneva, G.; Abate, F.; Ambesi-Impiombato, A.; Sanchez-Martin, M.; Carpenter, Z.; Penson, A.; Perez-Garcia, A.; et al. Mutational Landscape, Clonal Evolution Patterns, and Role of RAS Mutations in Relapsed Acute Lymphoblastic Leukemia. *Proc. Natl. Acad. Sci. USA* **2016**, *113*, 11306–11311. [CrossRef]
92. Tzoneva, G.; Perez-Garcia, A.; Carpenter, Z.; Khiabanian, H.; Tosello, V.; Allegretta, M.; Paietta, E.; Racevskis, J.; Rowe, J.M.; Tallman, M.S.; et al. Activating Mutations in the NT5C2 Nucleotidase Gene Drive Chemotherapy Resistance in Relapsed ALL. *Nat. Med.* **2013**, *19*, 368–371. [CrossRef]
93. Oshima, K.; Zhao, J.; Pérez-Durán, P.; Brown, J.A.; Patiño-Galindo, J.A.; Chu, T.; Quinn, A.; Gunning, T.; Belver, L.; Ambesi-Impiombato, A.; et al. Mutational and Functional Genetics Mapping of Chemotherapy Resistance Mechanisms in Relapsed Acute Lymphoblastic Leukemia. *Nat. Cancer* **2020**, *1*, 1113–1127. [CrossRef] [PubMed]
94. Alexandrov, L.B.; Nik-Zainal, S.; Wedge, D.C.; Aparicio, S.A.J.R.; Behjati, S.; Biankin, A.V.; Bignell, G.R.; Bolli, N.; Borg, A.; Børresen-Dale, A.-L.; et al. Signatures of Mutational Processes in Human Cancer. *Nature* **2013**, *500*, 415–421. [CrossRef] [PubMed]
95. Li, B.; Brady, S.W.; Ma, X.; Shen, S.; Zhang, Y.; Li, Y.; Szlachta, K.; Dong, L.; Liu, Y.; Yang, F.; et al. Therapy-Induced Mutations Drive the Genomic Landscape of Relapsed Acute Lymphoblastic Leukemia. *Blood* **2020**, *135*, 41–55. [CrossRef] [PubMed]
96. Richter-Pechańska, P.; Kunz, J.B.; Hof, J.; Zimmermann, M.; Rausch, T.; Bandapalli, O.R.; Orlova, E.; Scapinello, G.; Sagi, J.C.; Stanulla, M.; et al. Identification of a Genetically Defined Ultra-High-Risk Group in Relapsed Pediatric T-Lymphoblastic Leukemia. *Blood Cancer J.* **2017**, *7*, e523. [CrossRef]
97. Sentís, I.; Gonzalez, S.; Genescà, E.; García-Hernández, V.; Muiños, F.; Gonzalez, C.; López-Arribillaga, E.; Gonzalez, J.; Fernandez-Ibarrondo, L.; Mularoni, L.; et al. The Evolution of Relapse of Adult T Cell Acute Lymphoblastic Leukemia. *Genome Biol.* **2020**, *21*, 1–24. [CrossRef]
98. Waanders, E.; Gu, Z.; Dobson, S.M.; Antić, Ž.; Crawford, J.C.; Ma, X.; Edmonson, M.N.; Payne-Turner, D.; van de Vorst, M.; Jongmans, M.C.J.; et al. Mutational Landscape and Patterns of Clonal Evolution in Relapsed Pediatric Acute Lymphoblastic Leukemia. *Blood Cancer Discov.* **2020**, *1*, 96–111. [CrossRef]

99. Gaynon, P.S.; Orgel, E.; Ji, L. Preexisting or Therapy-Induced Mutations in Relapsed Acute Lymphoblastic Leukemia? *Blood* **2020**, *136*, 2233–2235. [CrossRef]
100. Pellegrino, M.; Sciambi, A.; Yates, J.L.; Mast, J.D.; Silver, C.; Eastburn, D.J. RNA-Seq Following PCR-Based Sorting Reveals Rare Cell Transcriptional Signatures. *BMC Genom.* **2016**, *17*, 361. [CrossRef]
101. Pellegrino, M.; Sciambi, A.; Treusch, S.; Durruthy-Durruthy, R.; Gokhale, K.; Jacob, J.; Chen, T.X.; Geis, J.A.; Oldham, W.; Matthews, J.; et al. High-Throughput Single-Cell DNA Sequencing of Acute Myeloid Leukemia Tumors with Droplet Microfluidics. *Genome Res.* **2018**, *28*, 1345–1352. [CrossRef]
102. Albertí-Servera, L.; Demeyer, S.; Govaerts, I.; Swings, T.; De Bie, J.; Gielen, O.; Brociner, M.; Michaux, L.; Maertens, J.; Uyttebroeck, A.; et al. Single-Cell DNA Amplicon Sequencing Reveals Clonal Heterogeneity and Evolution in T-Cell Acute Lymphoblastic Leukemia. *Blood* **2021**, *137*, 801–811. [CrossRef] [PubMed]

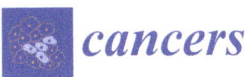

Review

Genomics of Plasma Cell Leukemia

Elizabeta A. Rojas [1,2] and Norma C. Gutiérrez [1,2,3,4,*]

1. Hematology Department, University Hospital of Salamanca, Institute of Biomedical Research of Salamanca (IBSAL), 37007 Salamanca, Spain; elirr@usal.es
2. Cancer Research Center-Institute of Cancer Molecular and Cellular Biology (CIC-IBMCC) (USAL-CSIC), 37007 Salamanca, Spain
3. Centro de Investigación Biomédica en Red de Cáncer (CIBERONC), CB16/12/00233, 28029 Madrid, Spain
4. Grupo Español de Mieloma (GEM), 28040 Madrid, Spain
* Correspondence: normagu@usal.es; Tel.: +34-923-291-200 (ext. 56617)

Simple Summary: Plasma cell leukemia (PCL) is a very aggressive plasma cell disorder with a dismal prognosis, despite the therapeutic progress made in the last few years. The implementation of genomic high-throughput technologies in the clinical setting has revealed new insights into the genomic landscape of PCL, some of which may have an impact on the development of novel therapeutic approaches. The purpose of this review is to provide a comprehensive overview and update of the genomic studies carried out in PCL.

Abstract: Plasma cell leukemia (PCL) is a rare and highly aggressive plasma cell dyscrasia characterized by the presence of clonal circulating plasma cells in peripheral blood. PCL accounts for approximately 2–4% of all multiple myeloma (MM) cases. PCL can be classified in primary PCL (pPCL) when it appears de novo and in secondary PCL (sPCL) when it arises from a pre-existing relapsed/refractory MM. Despite the improvement in treatment modalities, the prognosis remains very poor. There is growing evidence that pPCL is a different clinicopathological entity as compared to MM, although the mechanisms underlying its pathogenesis are not fully elucidated. The development of new high-throughput technologies, such as microarrays and new generation sequencing (NGS), has contributed to a better understanding of the peculiar biological and clinical features of this disease. Relevant information is now available on cytogenetic alterations, genetic variants, transcriptome, methylation patterns, and non-coding RNA profiles. Additionally, attempts have been made to integrate genomic alterations with gene expression data. However, given the low frequency of PCL, most of the genetic information comes from retrospective studies with a small number of patients, sometimes leading to inconsistent results.

Keywords: plasma cell leukemia; PCL; genetics; primary and secondary PCL; multiple myeloma; mutations; transcriptome

1. Introduction

Plasma cell leukemia (PCL) is an uncommon plasma cell dyscrasia with an aggressive course and poor prognosis. PCL represents less than 3% of all plasma cells neoplasms, and its incidence has been estimated at 0.04 cases per 100,000 persons/year [1,2].

Historically, PCL has been defined by the presence of more than 20% of circulating plasma cells (PCs) and an absolute number of $\geq 2 \times 10^9$/L of PCs in peripheral blood [3]. However, in some studies, only the presence of one of these criteria had been considered to define PCL. Moreover, recent studies have shown that much lower levels of circulating PC have the same adverse prognostic impact. Accordingly, the consensus recently published by the International Myeloma Working Group (IMWG) states that PCL is defined by the presence of 5% or more circulating plasma cells in peripheral blood [4].

PCL is classified as primary PCL (pPCL) when it occurs de novo so that the patient has no evidence of previous multiple myeloma (MM), and as secondary PCL (sPCL) when

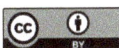

leukemic progression occurs in the context of pre-existing refractory or relapsing MM [5,6]. pPCL is more frequent than sPCL, representing about 60–70% of patients, [7] and occurs in patients significantly younger than sPCL. Nevertheless, the number of sPCL cases has been increasing in recent years, which is probably related to the increased survival of MM patients.

The clinical presentation of PCL is more aggressive than that observed in MM, including more severe cytopenias, hypercalcemia, and renal insufficiency. Higher tumor burden and proliferation activity of PCL are manifested by greater levels of B2-microglobulin and lactate dehydrogenase (LDH). Extramedullary involvement (lymph nodes, liver, spleen, pleura, and central nervous system) at diagnosis is more common in pPCL and sPCL than in MM, but osteolytic lesions are more frequent in sPCL and MM than in pPCL [8–13].

Various studies have analyzed the immunophenotype of PCL. The two common PCs markers, CD38 and CD138 antigens, are similarly expressed in MM and PCL. However, PCL displays a more immature phenotype than MM, expressing more frequently CD20, CD23, CD28, CD44, and CD45, and less frequently CD9, CD56, CD71, CD117, and HLA-DR antigens [14–16].

PCL patients are characterized by short remissions and early relapses. The 5-year survival rate from the diagnosis of PCL does not exceed 10%. Survival of sPCL patients is consistently shorter than pPCL [8]. The incorporation of new therapeutic agents has not achieved significant improvements in the survival of PCL, unlike what has been attained in MM. The low incidence of PCL makes it difficult to conduct studies aimed at exploring the efficacy of new drugs that would eventually help to establish an optimal therapeutic option. Thus, therapeutic recommendations are supported by small prospective and retrospective studies and sometimes by data extrapolated from clinical trials with MM patients. The therapeutic strategy usually followed in transplant-candidate patients generally includes an intensive induction with bortezomib-based regimens also containing lenalidomide and chemotherapeutic agents. After autologous stem cell transplantation (ASCT), there is increasing consensus on continuing a consolidation and maintenance therapy, although the therapeutic agents that should be included are not well established. A tandem transplant with an ASCT followed by reduced-intensity allogenic transplantation can also be considered. However, even using the most intensive therapeutic arsenal, the prognosis of PCL remains ominous. There is, therefore, a compelling need to advance in the search for new drugs with different mechanisms of action and more closely related to the genetic features of tumor PC. In this regard, the development of *BCL2* inhibitors and the new immunotherapeutic approaches, such as chimeric antigen receptor T-cells (CAR-T cells) and monoclonal and bispecific antibodies, opens up new opportunities in the treatment of PCL patients.

Early cytogenetic studies performed in PCL had already revealed some differences between this entity and MM. Later on, the widespread use of fluorescence in situ hybridization (FISH) has increased our knowledge of genetic alterations. In recent years, the development of high-throughput genomic analysis tools has helped to better understand the genetic particularities of PCL. However, the robustness of the results is undermined by the limited number of patients included in the studies because of the low incidence of this disease. In this review, we mainly focus on the genomic characteristics of pPCL, although some data concerning sPCL are provided when considered of interest. A summary of the most relevant results provided by the main genomic studies carried out in PCL is shown in Table 1.

Table 1. Summary of the most relevant genomic studies carried out in PCL.

Study/Reference	Number of Patients	Methodologies	Summary of Results *
Avet-Loiseau et al., 1998 [17]	14 pPCL/127 MM	FISH	*IGH* translocations in 71% pPCL.
García-Sanz et al., 1999 [14]	26 pPCL/664 MM	Cell DNA content, immunophenotypic studies, FISH	Numeric abnormalities in 92% pPCL. DNA content: diploid in 85% pPCL.
Avet-Loiseau et al., 2001 [18]	40 pPCL/247 MM	FISH, conventional karyotyping	Higher proportion of t(11;14), t(14;16), and hypodiploid karyotype in pPCL.
Gutiérrez et al., 2001 [19]	5 pPCL/25 MM	CGH	Losses of chromosomal material significantly more frequent in pPCL.
Bezieau et al., 2001 [20]	10 pPCL/3 sPCL/33 MM/6 MGUS/2 SMM/11 MM at relapse	Allele-specific PCR amplification and *K/NRAS* direct sequencing	*K/NRAS* mutations in 55% MM at diagnosis, 81% MM at relapse, and 50% pPCL. *KRAS* mutations were always more frequent than *NRAS*.
Avet-Loiseau et al., 2002 [21]	46 pPCL/147 MGUS/39 SMM/669 MM	FISH	Higher proportion of t(11;14), t(14;16), and 13q deletions in pPCL.
Tiedemann et al., 2008 [8]	41 pPCL/39 sPCL/439 MM	FISH, conventional karyotyping, methylation-sensitive PCR, *TP53*, and *N/K-RAS* DNA sequencing	t(11;14) significantly more frequent in pPCL than in sPCL. High proportion of del(17p), *TP53* mutation, and biallelic inactivation in pPCL and sPCL.
Chang et al., 2009 [22]	15 pPCL/26 sPCL/220 MM	cIg-FISH, FISH	del(13q), del(17p), t(4;14), 1q21 amplification and del(1p21) significantly more common in PCL than in MM. t(4;14) and del(1p21) associated with shorter OS. In multivariant analysis, t(4;14) remained a significant predictor for adverse OS in PCL.
Chiecchio et al., 2009 [23]	10 pPCL/2 sPCL/861 MM	FISH, conventional karyotyping, aCGH, qRT-PCR	t(11;14) and t(14;16) significantly more frequent in PCL. Structural and numerical abnormalities frequently involve 8q24. *MYC* upregulation in PCL.
Pagano et al., 2011 [24]	73 pPCL (41 FISH), 53 sPCL	Conventional karyotyping ($n = 28$), FISH ($n = 23$)	Unfavorable cytogenetics: 56%.
Usmani et al., 2012 [25]	13 pPCL/19 sPCL/1018 MM	GEP, FISH	GEP analyses distinguished pPCL from MM based on 203 gene probes.

Table 1. Cont.

Study/Reference	Number of Patients	Methodologies	Summary of Results *
Lionetti et al., 2013 [26]	18 pPCL	FISH, GEP, SNP arrays, miRNA microarrays	83 deregulated miRNAs in pPCL compared to MM. Expression levels of miR-497, miR-106b, miR-181a, and miR-181b correlated with treatment response, and of miR-92a, miR-330-3p, miR-22, and miR-146a correlated with clinical outcome.
Mosca et al., 2013 [27]	23 pPCL	FISH, SNP array, and GEP	Predominance of t(11;14) (40%) and t(14;16) (30%) Absence of activating mutations of N/KRAS in pPCL. GEP analysis revealed deregulated genes involved in metabolic processes.
Todoerti et al., 2013 [28]	21 pPCL/55 MM	GEP	503-gene transcriptional signature distinguishes pPCL from MM. Underexpression of YIPF6, EDEM3, and CYB5D2 associated with nonresponder pPCL. 27-gene model identifies pPCL patients with shorter OS.
Cifola et al., 2015 [29]	12 pPCL	WES	First study of mutational pattern in pPCL patients using WES. Identification of 14 candidate cancer driver genes, mainly involved in cell cycle, genome stability, RNA metabolism, and protein folding.
Lionetti et al., 2015 [30]	24 pPCL/11 sPCL/132 MM	Targeted NGS for BRAF (exons 11 and 15), NRAS (exons 2 and 3) and KRAS (exons 2–4)	MAPK pathway affected in 42% pPCL, 64% sPCL, and 60% MM. BRAF mutations in 21% pPCL, 9% sPCL and 11% MM.
Ronchetti et al., 2016 [31]	24 pPCL/12 sPCL/170 MM/33 SMM/20 MGUS/9 NPC	lncRNA expression profiling by arrays	15 lncRNAs progressively increased, and six decreased from normal PCs to MGUS, SMM, MM, and PCL samples.
Lionetti et al., 2016 [32]	12 pPCL/10 sPCL/129 MM	Targeted NGS for TP53 (exons 4–9)	TP53 mutations in 25% pPCL, 20% sPCL and 3% MM. del(17p) in 29% pPCL, 44% sPCL, and 5% MM. TP53 mutations and del(17p) are markers of progression.
Todoerti et al., 2018 [33]	14 pPCL/60 MM/5 MGUS	Global methylation patterns by high-density arrays	Global hypomethylation profile in pPCL. Decreasing methylation levels from MGUS to MM and pPCL.

Table 1. Cont.

Study/Reference	Number of Patients	Methodologies	Summary of Results *
Rojas et al., 2019 [34]	9 pPCL/ 10 MM	Transcriptome arrays	Different transcriptome profiles between pPCL and MM carrying del(17p). RNA splicing machinery was one of the most deregulated processes in pPCL.
Yu et al., 2020 [35]	46 pPCL	Conventional karyotyping (n = 34) and FISH (n = 37)	Predominance of del(13q) (38%), 1q gains (30%), del(17p) (27%), and t(11;14) (24%). t(4;14): not found.
Schinke et al., 2020 [36]	23 pPCL/1273 MM	FISH, WES, and GEP	Predominance of complex structural changes and high-risk mutational patterns in pPCL. Driver genes with more mutations in pPCL than in MM: KRAS, TP53, EGR1, LTB, PRDM1, EP300, NF1, PIK3CA, and ZFP36L1.
Nandakumar et al., 2021 [37]	68 pPCL (defined by ≥5% of clonal circulating PC)	FISH (n = 58)	Predominance of t(11;14) (47%), del(17p) (28%) and t(14;16) (12%).
Todoerti et al., 2021 [38]	15 pPCL/50 MM	GEP, FISH	Different transcriptome profiles between pPCL and MM carrying t(11;14).
Bútová et al., 2021 [39]	12 pPCL/11 sPCL/34 MM	lncRNA expression profile by NGS. Validation with qRT-PCR	13 deregulated lncRNAs between PCL and MM. Downregulation of LY86-AS1 and VIM-AS1 in PCL compared to MM.
Papadhimitriou et al., 2022 [40]	25 pPCL/19 sPCL/965 MM	FISH and NGF	Distinct cytogenetic profile between pPCL and sPCL, predominantly more del(13q) (95%) and del(17p) (68%) in sPCL than in pPCL, but t(11;14) only detected in pPCL and MM cases, and significantly higher incidence of 8q24 rearrangements in pPCL (40%) compared to sPCL (26%) and MM (9%).
Cazaubiel et al., 2020 [41] and Cazaubiel et al., 2022 [42]	96 pPCL/907 MM	Targeted NGS, RNA-seq, and FISH	TP53 and IRF4 mutations significantly more frequent in pPCL. Increased proportion of double hit profiles in pPCL. Different transcriptome profiles between pPCL with and without t(11;14).

FISH—fluorescence in situ hybridization; CGH—comparative genomic hybridization; aCGH—comparative genome hybridization arrays; NGS—next-generation sequencing; WES—whole-exome sequencing; SNP—single nucleotide polymorphism; GEP—gene expression profiling by microarrays; cIg-FISH—Cytoplasm light chain immunofluorescence with simultaneous interphase fluorescence in situ hybridization; qRT-PCR—quantitative real-time PCR; OS—overall survival; NGF—next-generation flow cytometry. * Only results related to genetic/genomic alterations are summarized.

2. Cytogenetic Abnormalities

Early cytogenetic and DNA content studies carried out in PCL revealed that there was a predominance of non-hyperdiploid cases (more than 50% of pPCL) compared to that observed in MM [8,14,18]. These results were confirmed in subsequent studies using not only conventional karyotyping but also molecular cytogenetic techniques such as comparative genomic hybridization (CGH) and single nucleotide polymorphism (SNP)-arrays, which showed that pPCL had more DNA copy number changes with a predominance of chromosomal losses in contrast to MM [19,27]. As in MM, FISH has been routinely carried out to identify cytogenetic alterations present in pPCL at the time of diagnosis. Virtually all the studies reporting data provided by FISH analysis, sometimes in combination with other cytogenetic techniques, point out that the chromosomal abnormalities observed in pPCL are mostly the same recurrently found in MM, although many of them are present with greater frequency (Figure 1).

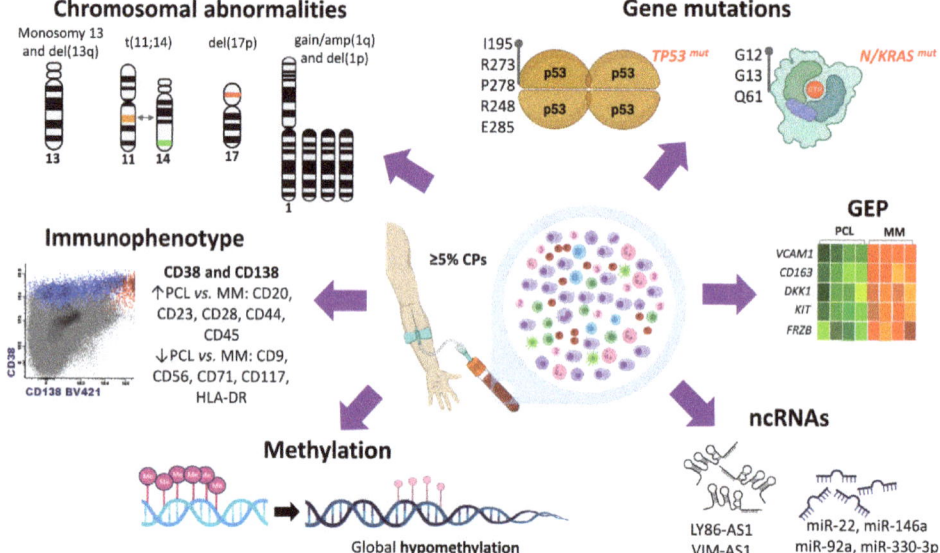

Figure 1. Genomic abnormalities of primary plasma cell leukemia (pPCL). The updated consensus of the IMWG defines pPCL by the presence of 5% or more circulating plasma cells in peripheral blood. Cytogenetic studies by FISH show predominance of monosomy and deletions of chromosome 13, t(11;14), del(17p), gain/amp(1q) and del(1p). Mutation studies by conventional DNA sequencing, WES, and targeted NGS detect a high frequency of mutations in *TP53* and *K/NRAS* genes. The amino acids most frequently mutated in *TP53* are I195, R273, P278, R248, and E285. Activating mutations of *K/NRAS* most frequently found in pPCL patients affect codons 12, 13, and 61 (G12, G13, and Q61). Immunophenotyping of plasma cells reveals expression of CD38 and CD138 in both pPCL and MM, although higher expression of CD20, CD23, CD28, CD44, and CD45 and lower expression of CD9, CD56, CD71, CD117, and HLA-DR may be found in pPCL compared to MM. Gene expression profiling in pPCL has shown downregulation of genes associated with bone marrow microenvironment and bone diseases in MM, such as *DKK1*, *KIT*, and *NCAM1* genes. A global hypomethylation profile has been found in pPCL samples. Non-coding RNAs (miRNAs and lncRNAs) are dysregulated in pPCL, and some of them are associated with survival of patients (as shown in the figure).

Monosomy and deletions of chromosome 13 (del(13q)) have been observed in approximately 85% of pPCL [8,22,35]. Abnormalities of chromosome 1 are also frequent in pPCL patients. Gain (3 copies) and amplification (≥4 copies) of chromosome arm 1q21 (gain/amp(1q)) have been reported in around 70% of pPCL cases [35,36]. Although the frequency of gain/amp(1q) does not reach such a high percentage in newly diagnosed MM patients, the incidence of this abnormality increases in relapsed/refractory MM up to 50–80% [22,43,44]. Likewise, most of the studies have shown greater frequency of deletion of 1p (del(1p)) in pPCL than in MM patients (24–33% vs. 9–18%, respectively) [22,41]. While the impact of abnormalities in chromosome 1, both gain/amp(1q) and del(1p), on the survival of patients with MM is well established [45,46], their effect on the prognosis of pPCL is still poorly substantiated. Only one study has reported that del(1p), but not gain/amp(1q), is associated with shorter survival of PCL patients, although the set of sPCL included in the study may be biasing the influence that this chromosomal alteration might have on pPCL considered as a separate entity [22]. Deletion of 17p (del(17p)), although uncommon in MM at the time of diagnosis, reaches frequencies of 50% in pPCL [8,22,27,32,37]. However, it seems to have no impact on the prognosis of pPCL, unlike in MM [8,22].

Taken together, all these results showing the increasing frequency of the aforementioned chromosome imbalances from MM to PCL support the multistep transformation model from monoclonal gammopathy of undetermined significance (MGUS) through smoldering multiple myeloma (SMM) and MM to PCL that leads to progressive accumulation of secondary genetic alterations.

The incidence of *IGH* translocations is significantly higher in pPCL than in MM. Several studies show that t(11;14) leading to *CCND1* dysregulation are significantly more frequent in pPCL than in MM, reaching percentages as high as 45–70% in some series [8,17,18,21–24,27,40,41]; also noteworthy is the high proportion of t(14;16) detected in pPCL compared with MM (13–25% vs. 1–5%, respectively), which is supported by five studies [18,21,23,36,41]. Conversely, in most of the studies, t(4;14) has been found to be less frequent in pPCL than in MM [23,36,38].

The t(11;14) has largely been demonstrated to be a neutral prognostic factor for MM survival [47]. Although no influence of t(11;14) in the survival of pPCL patients was initially observed [8,22], it has recently been reported that pPCL patients bearing t(11;14) had a significantly longer OS than those without this abnormality [42]. On the contrary, t(4;14) has been associated with poor prognosis [22].

MYC rearrangements have also been found in PCL, although the reported incidence varies between 13% and 40% [8,40,48]. Moreover, an association between *MYC* rearrangement and shorter overall survival of pPCL patients has been shown [8].

Other chromosomal abnormalities have been identified in pPCL, especially the loss of chromosome 16 (80%) [19,23,49], 7 (11%) [50] and X (25%) [14], and the trisomy of chromosome 8 (43%) [14].

3. Gene Mutations

Before the availability of next-generation sequencing (NGS) technologies, the mutational status of *RAS* oncogenes (*NRAS* and *KRAS*), the two most prevalent mutated genes in MM, and of the tumor suppressor *TP53*, had been explored in pPCL using traditional DNA sequencing methodologies. Two studies demonstrated a high incidence of *NRAS* and *KRAS* activating mutations: one of them reported these mutations at codons 12, 13, or 61 in 27% of pPCL and 15% of sPCL cases [8], and in the other study *NRAS* and/or *KRAS* mutations were found in 50% of pPCL cases and in 55% of MM [20]. Strikingly, these findings were not confirmed in a subsequent study [27]. *TP53* is one of the most frequently mutated genes in pPCL in all the published series, reaching frequencies of 25% [8,23,27]. The proportion of cases with biallelic inactivation of *TP53* is also greater in pPCL than in MM (17–35% vs. 3–4%) [8,27]. *TP53* coding mutations involving 5–8 exons were found, predicting all of them a non-functional p53 protein [8,27] (Figure 1).

The first whole-exome sequencing (WES) analysis of pPCL revealed a highly heterogeneous mutational profile [29]. Almost 2000 coding somatic non-silent variants on 1643 genes were described, with more than 160 variants per sample, although with hardly any recurrent mutations in two or more samples. Fourteen mutated genes mainly involved in cell cycle and apoptosis (*CIDEC*), RNA binding and degradation (*DIS3, RPL17*), and cell-matrix adhesion and membrane organization (*SPTB*, *CELA1*) were considered as potential cancer driver genes in pPCL. Other studies have confirmed that the number of nonsynonymous mutations per sample is higher in pPCL than in MM [36].

As in MM, activating *N/KRAS* mutations have been identified in pPCL using WES methodologies, although the proportions were significantly unequal between the two of the studies. The first study reported mutations of *KRAS* and *NRAS* only in two distinct samples (<10% of the pPCL). This study highlighted that *KRAS* and *NRAS* were three-fold less frequently mutated in pPCL compared to that observed in MM [29]. On the contrary, the second study also using WES methodology found that *KRAS* was the most frequently mutated gene in pPCL samples (around 39%), and mutations of *NRAS* were present in 13% of pPCL [36]. Using targeted NGS approaches, *KRAS* mutations were detected in 17% of pPCL, 18% of sPCL, and 33% of MM, and *NRAS* mutations in 4% of pPCL, 36% of sPCL, and 27% of MM [30]. Apparently, the *MEK/ERK* signaling pathway was less affected by mutation events in pPCL than in sPCL and MM [30].

Mutations of the *BRAF* gene have also been detected in pPCL samples. A low frequency and even absence of *BRAF* mutations in pPCL patients have been described using WES [29,36]. However, when targeted NGS was applied, the frequency of *BRAF* mutations detected in pPCL was higher (21% in pPCL and 9% in sPCL). It is worth highlighting the role that the different coverage levels among NGS studies and the small number of patients analyzed may be playing in the conflicting results.

TP53 gene has also been analyzed by NGS in pPCL [32,36,41], confirming the results previously observed using traditional DNA sequencing methodologies, namely, the high proportion of *TP53* mutations in pPCL. Interestingly, the presence of *TP53* mutations has been associated with significantly shorter survival in the study, including the largest number of patients with pPCL to date [41]. *IRF4* mutations have recently been shown to be significantly more frequent in pPCL than in MM patients (11% vs. 4%) [41]. Other gene mutations commonly observed in MM have also been reported in pPCL but with different frequencies. Schinke et al. detected *DIS3* and *PRMD1* mutations in 5% and 13% of patients with pPCL, respectively, while Cifola et al. identified *DIS3* mutations in 25% of cases and no variants in the *PRMD1* gene. Both studies have described a similar incidence of *FAM46C* mutation (10–12%) in pPCL patients [29,36].

4. Transcriptome Characterization

Several studies have explored the gene expression profile (GEP) analyzed by microarrays in pPCL. All of them have identified a transcriptome signature characteristic of pPCL and different from that of MM. The first two reports identified a gene-specific signature that distinguished pPCL from MM cases, although the number of overlapped genes between both datasets containing the differentially expressed genes was only around 15%. The functional annotation analysis identified dysregulation of lipid metabolism, glucocorticoid receptor, and *IL6* pathways in one study [25], and alterations of *NF-kB* pathway, *FAS* signaling, structural organization of the cell and migration processes in the other study [28]. A transcriptional signature including 27 genes has been associated with the overall survival of pPCL, despite the cytogenetic alterations. Interestingly, none of these genes had been selected in MM-high risk signatures [28].

More recently, the GEP of 41 pPCL patients has been compared to that of more than 700 newly diagnosed MM [36]. In pPCL, the analysis showed overexpression of genes previously related to MM biology or prognosis, such as *PHF19* and *TAGLN2*, and underexpression of the adhesion molecules *VCAM1* and *CD163*, which are highly expressed in MM and have been correlated with poor survival [51,52].

RNA-seq analysis of pPCL has also shown a specific transcriptional landscape of pPCL, as previously demonstrated by GEP using microarrays. Compared to MM, pPCL showed significantly higher expression of genes involved in G2M checkpoint and *MYC* target genes and lower expression of genes involved in p53 pathway, hypoxia, and *TNF alpha* signaling via *NF-κB* [41]. In this regard, significant overexpression of *CDKN2A*, *CCND3*, and *CCND1* genes, using quantitative RT-PCR, has been reported in PCL compared to MM samples, indicating a marked cell cycle dysregulation in the transition from MM to PCL [53].

A comprehensive molecular analysis of pPCL integrating data from FISH, SNP-arrays, and GEP has revealed a strong correlation between chromosomal imbalances and transcriptional modulation. The gene dosage effect was particularly observed in those genes mapping 1q chromosome [27]. In addition, the analysis of upregulated and downregulated transcripts in the gained and lost chromosomal regions, respectively, found that protein transport, translation, and biosynthesis functional categories were upregulated in pPCL cases with gained chromosomal regions, whereas RNA splicing, protein catabolic process, and regulation of apoptosis were downregulated in pPCL cases with deleted regions.

Differences between the gene expression signature of pPCL and MM could be partly attributed to the dissimilar distribution of genetic abnormalities between the two diseases. This fact prompted us to compare the transcriptome of pPCL and MM patients using samples with del(17p) and a similar cytogenetic background [34]. This approach revealed that pPCL and MM were separated into two differentiated clusters despite the equivalent cytogenetic profile shared by both entities. Differentially expressed genes were mostly downregulated in pPCL, among which were genes associated with bone marrow microenvironment and bone diseases in MM, such as *DKK1*, *KIT*, *NCAM1*, and *FRZB* (Figure 1). Interestingly, the analysis focused on isoform expression showed that dysregulation of RNA splicing machinery may be a relevant molecular mechanism underlying the biological differences between the pPCL and MM.

A similar approach has been used to ascertain the differences in the transcriptome between pPCL and MM samples harboring t(11;14) [38]. In line with our results, this study shows that both plasma cell dyscrasias are clearly distinguishable based on the transcriptome profile despite sharing a uniform genetic background. pPCL with t(11;14) were positively associated with genes involved in *IL2-STAT5* signaling but negatively associated with the regulation of cell and cell adhesion pathways. In any case, the most relevant finding of this study was that pPCL showed a different expression pattern of the *BCL2* family genes and of the B-cell-associated genes, despite the presence of t(11;14) in both PCL and MM samples. These results suggest that the efficacy of venetoclax in pPCL and MM patients with t(11;14) may be associated with different molecular programs.

5. Non-Coding RNA Profile

Non-coding RNAs (ncRNAs) are classified as short (<200 nucleotides) and long (>200 nucleotides). The miRNAs are short ncRNAs of 19–22 nucleotides that regulate gene expression at the post-transcriptional level. Since their discovery, numerous studies have attributed a wide variety of functions for ncRNAs in the pathogenic mechanisms of MM [54–56].

There is only one study analyzing the expression pattern of miRNAs in pPCL [26]. The analysis of 18 pPCL identified 42 upregulated and 41 downregulated miRNAs in pPCL when compared with MM samples. Moreover, seven miRNAs were found to be differentially expressed depending on the type of *IGH* translocation. Three miRNAs (let-7e, miR-135a, and miR-148a) were overexpressed in PCL patients with t(4;14); three (miR-7, miR-7-1, and miR-454) underexpressed in PCL with t(14;16); and the miR-342-3p was underexpressed in PCL with t(11;14). Notably, four miRNAs, miR-22, miR-146a, miR-92a, and miR-330-3p, were found to have an impact on the survival of pPCL patients. The overexpression of miR-146a, which was associated with shorter progression-free survival (PFS) in pPCL cases, and miR-22, which was associated with longer PFS, showed a pro- and anti-survival effect, respectively, in myeloma cell lines [26]. Accordingly, one study has demonstrated that MM cells stimulate the overexpression of miR-146a in mesenchymal stromal cells, resulting in more cytokine secretion and enhancing cell viability of MM cells [57] (Figure 1).

Long non-coding RNAs (lncRNAs) are a group of very heterogeneous non-coding RNAs with a length of more than 200 nucleotides. They have a similar structure to mR-

NAs but are not translated to functional proteins. LncRNAs represent more than 50% of the non-coding RNAs, and their functions are related to the regulation of transcription, genome integrity, cell differentiation, X-chromosome inactivation, and development, among others [58].

LncRNAs expression profile has also been investigated in a large cohort of PC dyscrasias, including samples from MGUS, SMM, MM, and PCL together with NPC [31]. Differential expression of 160 lncRNAs between NPC and the four premalignant and malignant entities was detected. In particular, expression levels of 15 lncRNAs were progressively increased from NPC to PCL patients, while six lncRNAs showed a significant decrease in the transition from NPC and premalignant entities to more aggressive forms. LncRNAs involved in the progression from MM to PCL have recently been explored [39]. A total of 13 dysregulated lncRNAs was detected. A significant underexpression of lymphocyte antigen antisense RNA 1 (*LY86-AS1*) and VIM antisense RNA 1 (*VIM-AS1*) was observed in PCL compared to MM and further validated by qRT-PCR. However, their functions in MM to PCL progression remain unknown.

Differential expression of lncRNAs has also been detected between pPCL and MM samples with t(11;14) [38]. In particular, the lncRNA *SNHG6*, whose overexpression was associated with significantly inferior overall survival in MM patients from the CoMMpass dataset, was found to be upregulated in the pPCL patients.

6. Methylation Patterns

The analysis of global methylation patterns in pPCL using high-density arrays has identified a global hypomethylation profile in pPCL samples [33] (Figure 1). The comparison of methylation levels between pPCL, MM, MGUS, and NPC samples revealed that genes highly methylated in NPC underwent a progressive decrease in the levels of methylation as the aggressiveness of the disease increased from MGUS to MM and pPCL. Curiously, pPCL patients showed distinct methylation profiles depending on the presence of *DIS3* gene mutations, t(11;14), and t(14;16). On the contrary, Walker et al. [59] had previously found gene-specific hypermethylation of almost 2000 genes in the transition from MM to PCL, although the number of PCL cases was quite small.

7. Concluding Remarks

Chromosomal, genetic, and genomic alterations found in pPCL are sufficiently different from those observed in MM to consider it a distinct clinicopathological entity and not merely a more aggressive form of MM. However, the low incidence of this disease makes it extremely difficult to gather enough pPCL cases to carry out genomic studies that provide consistent results. On the other hand, the paucity of clinical trials specifically designed for this disease precludes prospective studies. In this regard, proposals aimed at collecting hundreds of pPCL samples involving numerous centers in order to conduct biological studies could represent a breakthrough in identifying dysregulations of signaling pathways that could be therapeutically targeted.

Author Contributions: Conceptualization, N.C.G.; writing original draft, preparation, review, and editing, E.A.R. and N.C.G. All authors have read and agreed to the published version of the manuscript.

Funding: E.A.R. was supported by a fellowship from the Consejería de Educación de Castilla y León and FEDER funds. This study was funded by the Instituto de Salud Carlos III and co-financed by FEDER (PI16/01074 and PI19/00674); by the Asociación Española Contra el Cáncer (AECC) (Proyectos Estratégicos: PROYE20047GUTI); and by the Gerencia Regional de Salud, Junta de Castilla y León grants (GRS 2058/A/19 and GRS 2331/A/21).

Acknowledgments: The authors would like to thank Luzalba Sanoja-Flores for providing the image of flow cytometry.

Conflicts of Interest: E.A.R. declares no conflict of interest. N.C.G.: honoraria from Janssen.

References

1. Gundesen, M.T.; Lund, T.; Moeller, H.E.H.; Abildgaard, N. Plasma Cell Leukemia: Definition, Presentation, and Treatment. *Curr. Oncol. Rep.* **2019**, *21*, 8. [CrossRef] [PubMed]
2. Gonsalves, W.I.; Rajkumar, S.V.; Go, R.S.; Dispenzieri, A.; Gupta, V.; Singh, P.P.; Buadi, F.K.; Lacy, M.Q.; Kapoor, P.; Dingli, D.; et al. Trends in Survival of Patients with Primary Plasma Cell Leukemia: A Population-Based Analysis. *Blood* **2014**, *124*, 907–912. [CrossRef] [PubMed]
3. Fernández de Larrea, C.; Kyle, R.A.; Durie, B.G.M.; Ludwig, H.; Usmani, S.; Vesole, D.H.; Hajek, R.; San Miguel, J.F.; Sezer, O.; Sonneveld, P.; et al. Plasma Cell Leukemia: Consensus Statement on Diagnostic Requirements, Response Criteria and Treatment Recommendations by the International Myeloma Working Group. *Leukemia* **2013**, *27*, 780–791. [CrossRef] [PubMed]
4. Fernández de Larrea, C.; Kyle, R.; Rosiñol, L.; Paiva, B.; Engelhardt, M.; Usmani, S.; Caers, J.; Gonsalves, W.; Schjesvold, F.; Merlini, G.; et al. Primary Plasma Cell Leukemia: Consensus Definition by the International Myeloma Working Group According to Peripheral Blood Plasma Cell Percentage. *Blood Cancer J.* **2021**, *11*, 192. [CrossRef]
5. Noel, P.; Kyle, R.A. Plasma Cell Leukemia: An Evaluation of Response to Therapy. *Am. J. Med.* **1987**, *83*, 1062–1068. [CrossRef]
6. Albarracin, F.; Fonseca, R. Plasma Cell Leukemia. *Blood Rev.* **2011**, *25*, 107–112. [CrossRef]
7. International Myeloma Working Group. Criteria for the Classification of Monoclonal Gammopathies, Multiple Myeloma and Related Disorders: A Report of the International Myeloma Working Group. *Br. J. Haematol.* **2003**, *121*, 749–757. [CrossRef]
8. Tiedemann, R.E.; Gonzalez-Paz, N.; Kyle, R.A.; Santana-Davila, R.; Price-Troska, T.; Van Wier, S.A.; Chng, W.J.; Ketterling, R.P.; Gertz, M.A.; Henderson, K.; et al. Genetic Aberrations and Survival in Plasma Cell Leukemia. *Leukemia* **2008**, *22*, 1044–1052. [CrossRef]
9. Chaulagain, C.P.; Diacovo, M.-J.; Van, A.; Martinez, F.; Fu, C.-L.; Jimenez Jimenez, A.M.; Ahmed, W.; Anwer, F. Management of Primary Plasma Cell Leukemia Remains Challenging Even in the Era of Novel Agents. *Clin. Med. Insights Blood Disord.* **2021**, *14*. [CrossRef]
10. Mina, R.; D'Agostino, M.; Cerrato, C.; Gay, F.; Palumbo, A. Plasma Cell Leukemia: Update on Biology and Therapy. *Leuk. Lymphoma* **2017**, *58*, 1538–1547. [CrossRef]
11. Jimenez-Zepeda, V.H.; Dominguez-Martinez, V.J. Plasma Cell Leukemia: A Highly Aggressive Monoclonal Gammopathy with a Very Poor Prognosis. *Int. J. Hematol.* **2009**, *89*, 259–268. [CrossRef] [PubMed]
12. Jurczyszyn, A.; Radocha, J.; Davila, J.; Fiala, M.A.; Gozzetti, A.; Grząśko, N.; Robak, P.; Hus, I.; Waszczuk-Gajda, A.; Guzicka-Kazimierczak, R.; et al. Prognostic Indicators in Primary Plasma Cell Leukaemia: A Multicentre Retrospective Study of 117 Patients. *Br. J. Haematol.* **2018**, *180*, 831–839. [CrossRef] [PubMed]
13. Ramsingh, G.; Mehan, P.; Luo, J.; Vij, R.; Morgensztern, D. Primary Plasma Cell Leukemia: A Surveillance, Epidemiology, and End Results Database Analysis between 1973 and 2004. *Cancer* **2009**, *115*, 5734–5739. [CrossRef]
14. García-Sanz, R.; Orfão, A.; González, M.; Tabernero, M.D.; Bladé, J.; Moro, M.J.; Fernández-Calvo, J.; Sanz, M.A.; Pérez-Simón, J.A.; Rasillo, A.; et al. Primary Plasma Cell Leukemia: Clinical, Immunophenotypic, DNA Ploidy, and Cytogenetic Characteristics. *Blood* **1999**, *93*, 1032–1037. [CrossRef]
15. Kraj, M.; Pogłód, R.; Kopeć-Szlęzak, J.; Sokołowska, U.; Woźniak, J.; Kruk, B. C-Kit Receptor (CD117) Expression on Plasma Cells in Monoclonal Gammopathies. *Leuk. Lymphoma* **2004**, *45*, 2281–2289. [CrossRef]
16. Kraj, M.; Kopeć-Szlęzak, J.; Pogłód, R.; Kruk, B. Flow Cytometric Immunophenotypic Characteristics of 36 Cases of Plasma Cell Leukemia. *Leuk. Res.* **2011**, *35*, 169–176. [CrossRef] [PubMed]
17. Avet-Loiseau, H.; Li, J.Y.; Facon, T.; Brigaudeau, C.; Morineau, N.; Maloisel, F.; Rapp, M.J.; Talmant, P.; Trimoreau, F.; Jaccard, A.; et al. High Incidence of Translocations t(11;14)(Q13;Q32) and t(4;14)(P16;Q32) in Patients with Plasma Cell Malignancies. *Cancer Res.* **1998**, *58*, 5640–5645. [PubMed]
18. Avet-Loiseau, H.; Daviet, A.; Brigaudeau, C.; Callet-Bauchu, E.; Terré, C.; Lafage-Pochitaloff, M.; Désangles, F.; Ramond, S.; Talmant, P.; Bataille, R. Cytogenetic, Interphase, and Multicolor Fluorescence in Situ Hybridization Analyses in Primary Plasma Cell Leukemia: A Study of 40 Patients at Diagnosis, on Behalf of the Intergroupe Francophone Du Myélome and the Groupe Français de Cytogénétique Hématologique. *Blood* **2001**, *97*, 822–825. [CrossRef] [PubMed]
19. Gutiérrez, N.C.; Hernández, J.M.; García, J.L.; Cañizo, M.C.; González, M.; Hernández, J.; González, M.B.; García-Marcos, M.A.; San Miguel, J.F. Differences in Genetic Changes between Multiple Myeloma and Plasma Cell Leukemia Demonstrated by Comparative Genomic Hybridization. *Leukemia* **2001**, *15*, 840–845. [CrossRef]
20. Bezieau, S.; Devilder, M.C.; Avet-Loiseau, H.; Mellerin, M.P.; Puthier, D.; Pennarun, E.; Rapp, M.J.; Harousseau, J.L.; Moisan, J.P.; Bataille, R. High Incidence of N and K-Ras Activating Mutations in Multiple Myeloma and Primary Plasma Cell Leukemia at Diagnosis. *Hum. Mutat.* **2001**, *18*, 212–224. [CrossRef]
21. Avet-Loiseau, H.; Facon, T.; Grosbois, B.; Magrangeas, F.; Rapp, M.-J.; Harousseau, J.-L.; Minvielle, S.; Bataille, R. Intergroupe Francophone du Myélome Oncogenesis of Multiple Myeloma: 14q32 and 13q Chromosomal Abnormalities Are Not Randomly Distributed, but Correlate with Natural History, Immunological Features, and Clinical Presentation. *Blood* **2002**, *99*, 2185–2191. [CrossRef] [PubMed]
22. Chang, H.; Qi, X.; Yeung, J.; Reece, D.; Xu, W.; Patterson, B. Genetic Aberrations Including Chromosome 1 Abnormalities and Clinical Features of Plasma Cell Leukemia. *Leuk. Res.* **2009**, *33*, 259–262. [CrossRef] [PubMed]

23. Chiecchio, L.; Dagrada, G.P.; White, H.E.; Towsend, M.R.; Protheroe, R.K.M.; Cheung, K.L.; Stockley, D.M.; Orchard, K.H.; Cross, N.C.P.; Harrison, C.J.; et al. Frequent Upregulation of MYC in Plasma Cell Leukemia. *Genes Chromosomes Cancer* **2009**, *48*, 624–636. [CrossRef]
24. Pagano, L.; Valentini, C.G.; De Stefano, V.; Venditti, A.; Visani, G.; Petrucci, M.T.; Candoni, A.; Specchia, G.; Visco, C.; Pogliani, E.M.; et al. Primary Plasma Cell Leukemia: A Retrospective Multicenter Study of 73 Patients. *Ann. Oncol.* **2011**, *22*, 1628–1635. [CrossRef] [PubMed]
25. Usmani, S.Z.; Nair, B.; Qu, P.; Hansen, E.; Zhang, Q.; Petty, N.; Waheed, S.; Shaughnessy, J.D.; Alsayed, Y.; Heuck, C.J.; et al. Primary Plasma Cell Leukemia: Clinical and Laboratory Presentation, Gene-Expression Profiling and Clinical Outcome with Total Therapy Protocols. *Leukemia* **2012**, *26*, 2398–2405. [CrossRef] [PubMed]
26. Lionetti, M.; Musto, P.; Di Martino, M.T.; Fabris, S.; Agnelli, L.; Todoerti, K.; Tuana, G.; Mosca, L.; Gallo Cantafio, M.E.; Grieco, V.; et al. Biological and Clinical Relevance of MiRNA Expression Signatures in Primary Plasma Cell Leukemia. *Clin. Cancer Res.* **2013**, *19*, 3130–3142. [CrossRef] [PubMed]
27. Mosca, L.; Musto, P.; Todoerti, K.; Barbieri, M.; Agnelli, L.; Fabris, S.; Tuana, G.; Lionetti, M.; Bonaparte, E.; Sirchia, S.M.; et al. Genome-Wide Analysis of Primary Plasma Cell Leukemia Identifies Recurrent Imbalances Associated with Changes in Transcriptional Profiles. *Am. J. Hematol.* **2013**, *88*, 16–23. [CrossRef]
28. Todoerti, K.; Agnelli, L.; Fabris, S.; Lionetti, M.; Tuana, G.; Mosca, L.; Lombardi, L.; Grieco, V.; Bianchino, G.; D'Auria, F.; et al. Transcriptional Characterization of a Prospective Series of Primary Plasma Cell Leukemia Revealed Signatures Associated with Tumor Progression and Poorer Outcome. *Clin. Cancer Res.* **2013**, *19*, 3247–3258. [CrossRef]
29. Cifola, I.; Lionetti, M.; Pinatel, E.; Todoerti, K.; Mangano, E.; Pietrelli, A.; Fabris, S.; Mosca, L.; Simeon, V.; Petrucci, M.T.; et al. Whole-Exome Sequencing of Primary Plasma Cell Leukemia Discloses Heterogeneous Mutational Patterns. *Oncotarget* **2015**, *6*, 17543–17558. [CrossRef]
30. Lionetti, M.; Barbieri, M.; Todoerti, K.; Agnelli, L.; Marzorati, S.; Fabris, S.; Ciceri, G.; Galletti, S.; Milesi, G.; Manzoni, M.; et al. Molecular Spectrum of BRAF, NRAS and KRAS Gene Mutations in Plasma Cell Dyscrasias: Implication for MEK-ERK Pathway Activation. *Oncotarget* **2015**, *6*, 24205–24217. [CrossRef]
31. Ronchetti, D.; Agnelli, L.; Taiana, E.; Galletti, S.; Manzoni, M.; Todoerti, K.; Musto, P.; Strozzi, F.; Neri, A. Distinct LncRNA Transcriptional Fingerprints Characterize Progressive Stages of Multiple Myeloma. *Oncotarget* **2016**, *7*, 14814–14830. [CrossRef] [PubMed]
32. Lionetti, M.; Barbieri, M.; Manzoni, M.; Fabris, S.; Bandini, C.; Todoerti, K.; Nozza, F.; Rossi, D.; Musto, P.; Baldini, L.; et al. Molecular Spectrum of TP53 Mutations in Plasma Cell Dyscrasias by next Generation Sequencing: An Italian Cohort Study and Overview of the Literature. *Oncotarget* **2016**, *7*, 21353–21361. [CrossRef] [PubMed]
33. Todoerti, K.; Calice, G.; Trino, S.; Simeon, V.; Lionetti, M.; Manzoni, M.; Fabris, S.; Barbieri, M.; Pompa, A.; Baldini, L.; et al. Global Methylation Patterns in Primary Plasma Cell Leukemia. *Leuk. Res.* **2018**, *73*, 95–102. [CrossRef]
34. Rojas, E.A.; Corchete, L.A.; Mateos, M.V.; García-Sanz, R.; Misiewicz-Krzeminska, I.; Gutiérrez, N.C. Transcriptome Analysis Reveals Significant Differences between Primary Plasma Cell Leukemia and Multiple Myeloma Even When Sharing a Similar Genetic Background. *Blood Cancer J.* **2019**, *9*, 90. [CrossRef] [PubMed]
35. Yu, T.; Xu, Y.; An, G.; Tai, Y.-T.; Ho, M.; Li, Z.; Deng, S.; Zou, D.; Yu, Z.; Hao, M.; et al. Primary Plasma Cell Leukemia: Real-World Retrospective Study of 46 Patients From a Single-Center Study in China. *Clin. Lymphoma Myeloma Leuk.* **2020**, *20*, e652–e659. [CrossRef] [PubMed]
36. Schinke, C.; Boyle, E.M.; Ashby, C.; Wang, Y.; Lyzogubov, V.; Wardell, C.; Qu, P.; Hoering, A.; Deshpande, S.; Ryan, K.; et al. Genomic Analysis of Primary Plasma Cell Leukemia Reveals Complex Structural Alterations and High-Risk Mutational Patterns. *Blood Cancer J.* **2020**, *10*, 70. [CrossRef] [PubMed]
37. Nandakumar, B.; Kumar, S.K.; Dispenzieri, A.; Buadi, F.K.; Dingli, D.; Lacy, M.Q.; Hayman, S.R.; Kapoor, P.; Leung, N.; Fonder, A.; et al. Clinical Characteristics and Outcomes of Patients With Primary Plasma Cell Leukemia in the Era of Novel Agent Therapy. *Mayo Clin. Proc.* **2021**, *96*, 677–687. [CrossRef]
38. Todoerti, K.; Taiana, E.; Puccio, N.; Favasuli, V.; Lionetti, M.; Silvestris, I.; Gentile, M.; Musto, P.; Morabito, F.; Gianelli, U.; et al. Transcriptomic Analysis in Multiple Myeloma and Primary Plasma Cell Leukemia with t(11;14) Reveals Different Expression Patterns with Biological Implications in Venetoclax Sensitivity. *Cancers (Basel)* **2021**, *13*, 4898. [CrossRef]
39. Bútová, R.; Vychytilová-Faltejsková, P.; Gregorová, J.; Radová, L.; Almáši, M.; Bezděková, R.; Brožová, L.; Jarkovský, J.; Knechtová, Z.; Štork, M.; et al. LncRNAs LY86-AS1 and VIM-AS1 Distinguish Plasma Cell Leukemia Patients from Multiple Myeloma Patients. *Biomedicines* **2021**, *9*, 1637. [CrossRef]
40. Papadhimitriou, S.I.; Terpos, E.; Liapis, K.; Pavlidis, D.; Marinakis, T.; Kastritis, E.; Dimopoulos, M.-A.; Tsitsilonis, O.E.; Kostopoulos, I.V. The Cytogenetic Profile of Primary and Secondary Plasma Cell Leukemia: Etiopathogenetic Perspectives, Prognostic Impact and Clinical Relevance to Newly Diagnosed Multiple Myeloma with Differential Circulating Clonal Plasma Cells. *Biomedicines* **2022**, *10*, 209. [CrossRef]
41. Cazaubiel, T.; Buisson, L.; Maheo, S.; Do Souto Ferreira, L.; Lannes, R.; Perrot, A.; Hulin, C.; Avet-Loiseau, H.; Corre, J. The Genomic and Transcriptomic Landscape of Plasma Cell Leukemia. *Blood* **2020**, *136*, 48–49. [CrossRef]
42. Cazaubiel, T.; Leleu, X.; Perrot, A.; Manier, S.; Buisson, L.; Mahéo, S.; Do Souto Ferreira, L.; Lannes, R.; Pavageau, L.; Hulin, C.; et al. Primary Plasma Cell Leukemia Displaying t(11;14) Have Specific Genomic, Transcriptional and Clinical Feature. *Blood* **2021**, *in press.* [CrossRef] [PubMed]

43. Hanamura, I.; Stewart, J.P.; Huang, Y.; Zhan, F.; Santra, M.; Sawyer, J.R.; Hollmig, K.; Zangarri, M.; Pineda-Roman, M.; van Rhee, F.; et al. Frequent Gain of Chromosome Band 1q21 in Plasma-Cell Dyscrasias Detected by Fluorescence in Situ Hybridization: Incidence Increases from MGUS to Relapsed Myeloma and Is Related to Prognosis and Disease Progression Following Tandem Stem-Cell Transplantation. *Blood* **2006**, *108*, 1724–1732. [CrossRef]
44. Hanamura, I. Gain/Amplification of Chromosome Arm 1q21 in Multiple Myeloma. *Cancers (Basel)* **2021**, *13*, 256. [CrossRef]
45. Chang, H.; Qi, X.; Jiang, A.; Xu, W.; Young, T.; Reece, D. 1p21 Deletions Are Strongly Associated with 1q21 Gains and Are an Independent Adverse Prognostic Factor for the Outcome of High-Dose Chemotherapy in Patients with Multiple Myeloma. *Bone Marrow Transpl.* **2010**, *45*, 117–121. [CrossRef] [PubMed]
46. Chang, H.; Qi, C.; Jiang, A.; Xu, W.; Trieu, Y.; Reece, D.E. Loss of Chromosome 1p21 Band Is Associated with Disease Progression and Poor Survival in Multiple Myeloma Patients Undergoing Autologous Stem Cell Transplantation. *Blood* **2008**, *112*, 1702. [CrossRef]
47. Rajkumar, S.V.; Dimopoulos, M.A.; Palumbo, A.; Blade, J.; Merlini, G.; Mateos, M.-V.; Kumar, S.; Hillengass, J.; Kastritis, E.; Richardson, P.; et al. International Myeloma Working Group Updated Criteria for the Diagnosis of Multiple Myeloma. *Lancet Oncol.* **2014**, *15*, e538–e548. [CrossRef]
48. Avet-Loiseau, H.; Gerson, F.; Magrangeas, F.; Minvielle, S.; Harousseau, J.L.; Bataille, R. Intergroupe Francophone du Myélome Rearrangements of the C-Myc Oncogene Are Present in 15% of Primary Human Multiple Myeloma Tumors. *Blood* **2001**, *98*, 3082–3086. [CrossRef]
49. Jonveaux, P.; Berger, R. Chromosome Studies in Plasma Cell Leukemia and Multiple Myeloma in Transformation. *Genes Chromosomes Cancer* **1992**, *4*, 321–325. [CrossRef]
50. Dimopoulos, M.A.; Palumbo, A.; Delasalle, K.B.; Alexanian, R. Primary Plasma Cell Leukaemia. *Br. J. Haematol.* **1994**, *88*, 754–759. [CrossRef]
51. Andersen, M.N.; Abildgaard, N.; Maniecki, M.B.; Møller, H.J.; Andersen, N.F. Monocyte/Macrophage-Derived Soluble CD163: A Novel Biomarker in Multiple Myeloma. *Eur. J. Haematol.* **2014**, *93*, 41–47. [CrossRef] [PubMed]
52. Terpos, E.; Migkou, M.; Christoulas, D.; Gavriatopoulou, M.; Eleutherakis-Papaiakovou, E.; Kanellias, N.; Iakovaki, M.; Panagiotidis, I.; Ziogas, D.C.; Fotiou, D.; et al. Increased Circulating VCAM-1 Correlates with Advanced Disease and Poor Survival in Patients with Multiple Myeloma: Reduction by Post-Bortezomib and Lenalidomide Treatment. *Blood Cancer J.* **2016**, *6*, e428. [CrossRef] [PubMed]
53. Kryukov, F.; Dementyeva, E.; Kubiczkova, L.; Jarkovsky, J.; Brozova, L.; Petrik, J.; Nemec, P.; Sevcikova, S.; Minarik, J.; Stefanikova, Z.; et al. Cell Cycle Genes Co-Expression in Multiple Myeloma and Plasma Cell Leukemia. *Genomics* **2013**, *102*, 243–249. [CrossRef] [PubMed]
54. Chen, D.; Yang, X.; Liu, M.; Zhang, Z.; Xing, E. Roles of MiRNA Dysregulation in the Pathogenesis of Multiple Myeloma. *Cancer Gene Ther.* **2021**, *28*, 1256–1268. [CrossRef] [PubMed]
55. Carrasco-Leon, A.; Ezponda, T.; Meydan, C.; Valcárcel, L.V.; Ordoñez, R.; Kulis, M.; Garate, L.; Miranda, E.; Segura, V.; Guruceaga, E.; et al. Characterization of Complete LncRNAs Transcriptome Reveals the Functional and Clinical Impact of LncRNAs in Multiple Myeloma. *Leukemia* **2021**, *35*, 1438–1450. [CrossRef]
56. Misiewicz-Krzeminska, I.; Krzeminski, P.; Corchete, L.A.; Quwaider, D.; Rojas, E.A.; Herrero, A.B.; Gutiérrez, N.C. Factors Regulating MicroRNA Expression and Function in Multiple Myeloma. *Noncoding RNA* **2019**, *5*, 9. [CrossRef]
57. De Veirman, K.; Wang, J.; Xu, S.; Leleu, X.; Himpe, E.; Maes, K.; De Bruyne, E.; Van Valckenborgh, E.; Vanderkerken, K.; Menu, E.; et al. Induction of MiR-146a by Multiple Myeloma Cells in Mesenchymal Stromal Cells Stimulates Their pro-Tumoral Activity. *Cancer Lett.* **2016**, *377*, 17–24. [CrossRef]
58. Statello, L.; Guo, C.-J.; Chen, L.-L.; Huarte, M. Gene Regulation by Long Non-Coding RNAs and Its Biological Functions. *Nat. Rev. Mol. Cell Biol.* **2021**, *22*, 96–118. [CrossRef]
59. Walker, B.A.; Wardell, C.P.; Chiecchio, L.; Smith, E.M.; Boyd, K.D.; Neri, A.; Davies, F.E.; Ross, F.M.; Morgan, G.J. Aberrant Global Methylation Patterns Affect the Molecular Pathogenesis and Prognosis of Multiple Myeloma. *Blood* **2011**, *117*, 553–562. [CrossRef]

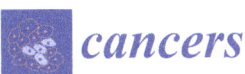

Review

Genomic and Epigenomic Landscape of Juvenile Myelomonocytic Leukemia

Claudia Fiñana [1,2,†], Noel Gómez-Molina [1,2,†], Sandra Alonso-Moreno [1,2] and Laura Belver [1,2,*]

[1] Cancer and Leukemia Epigenetics and Biology Program, Josep Carreras Leukemia Research Institute (IJC), 08916 Badalona, Barcelona, Spain; cfinana@carrerasresearch.org (C.F.); ngomez@carrerasresearch.org (N.G.-M.); salonso@carrerasresearch.org (S.A.-M.)
[2] Immuno Procure, Catalan Institute of Oncology (ICO), 08916 Badalona, Barcelona, Spain
* Correspondence: lbelver@carrerasresearch.org
† These authors contributed equally to this work.

Simple Summary: Juvenile myelomonocytic leukemia (JMML) is a rare pediatric myelodysplastic/myeloproliferative neoplasm characterized by the constitutive activation of the RAS pathway. In spite of the recent progresses in the molecular characterization of JMML, this disease is still a clinical challenge due to its heterogeneity, difficult diagnosis, poor prognosis, and the lack of curative treatment options other than hematopoietic stem cell transplantation (HSCT). In this review, we will provide a detailed overview of the genetic and epigenetic alterations occurring in JMML, and discuss their clinical relevance in terms of disease prognosis and risk of relapse after HSCT. We will also present the most recent advances on novel preclinical and clinical therapeutic approaches directed against JMML molecular targets. Finally, we will outline future research perspectives to further explore the oncogenic mechanism driving JMML leukemogenesis and progression, with special attention to the application of single-cell next-generation sequencing technologies.

Abstract: Juvenile myelomonocytic leukemia (JMML) is a rare myelodysplastic/myeloproliferative neoplasm of early childhood. Most of JMML patients experience an aggressive clinical course of the disease and require hematopoietic stem cell transplantation, which is currently the only curative treatment. JMML is characterized by RAS signaling hyperactivation, which is mainly driven by mutations in one of five genes of the RAS pathway, including *PTPN11*, *KRAS*, *NRAS*, *NF1*, and *CBL*. These driving mutations define different disease subtypes with specific clinico-biological features. Secondary mutations affecting other genes inside and outside the RAS pathway contribute to JMML pathogenesis and are associated with a poorer prognosis. In addition to these genetic alterations, JMML commonly presents aberrant epigenetic profiles that strongly correlate with the clinical outcome of the patients. This observation led to the recent publication of an international JMML stratification consensus, which defines three JMML clinical groups based on DNA methylation status. Although the characterization of the genomic and epigenomic landscapes in JMML has significantly contributed to better understand the molecular mechanisms driving the disease, our knowledge on JMML origin, cell identity, and intratumor and interpatient heterogeneity is still scarce. The application of new single-cell sequencing technologies will be critical to address these questions in the future.

Keywords: juvenile myelomonocytic leukemia; RAS pathway; DNA methylation; experimental therapeutics

Citation: Fiñana, C.; Gómez-Molina, N.; Alonso-Moreno, S.; Belver, L. Genomic and Epigenomic Landscape of Juvenile Myelomonocytic Leukemia. *Cancers* **2022**, *14*, 1335. https://doi.org/10.3390/cancers14051335

Academic Editors: Ferenc Gallyas, Jr., Enrico Garattini and Paula Ludovico

Received: 6 January 2022
Accepted: 2 March 2022
Published: 4 March 2022

Publisher's Note: MDPI stays neutral with regard to jurisdictional claims in published maps and institutional affiliations.

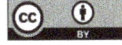

Copyright: © 2022 by the authors. Licensee MDPI, Basel, Switzerland. This article is an open access article distributed under the terms and conditions of the Creative Commons Attribution (CC BY) license (https://creativecommons.org/licenses/by/4.0/).

1. Introduction

Juvenile myelomonocytic leukemia (JMML) is a rare and very heterogeneous myelodysplastic/myeloproliferative neoplasm of early childhood resulting from the malignant transformation of hematopoietic stem/progenitor cells (HSPCs) and characterized by the hyperactivation of the RAS signaling pathway. Children with JMML typically show symptoms related to the infiltration of the bone marrow (BM) and other organs by malignant mature and immature myeloid cells. Formal diagnosis of JMML requires the presence of prominent monocytosis ($\geq 1 \times 10^9$/L), a low proportion of blasts in the BM (<20%), splenomegaly, absence of BCR-ABL fusions, and mutations in genes encoding for proteins of the RAS signaling pathway [1]. Granulocyte–macrophage colony-stimulating factor (GM-CSF) in vitro hypersensitivity is a common hallmark in JMML and can be used as a diagnostic criterion in patients in which RAS pathway mutations are not identified [2,3]. Although JMML karyotype is predominantly normal, recurrent cases of monosomy 7 are observed in approximately 25% of the patients, as well as other karyotype abnormalities involving 10% of cases [4]. JMML therapeutic options are scarce, with early allogeneic hematopoietic stem cell transplantation (HSCT) being the only effective therapy for achieving long-term disease control. However, this treatment entails a significant risk of transplant-related mortality and the overall survival at five years in treated patients remains at 64%, largely due to unsuccessful HSCT [3,5,6].

Despite the major advances in the study of the underlying molecular defects in JMML, this disease is still a puzzling disorder with a wide variety of phenotypes and outcomes, ranging from rare self-limiting forms that spontaneously resolve, to aggressive cases prone to relapse and with dismal prognosis. In this context, the characterization of the genomic and epigenomic landscapes in JMML has not only contributed to identify novel oncogenic mechanisms involved in the pathogenesis of the disease, but also provided critical insights in predicting patient prognosis and making clinical decisions.

2. Genetic Alterations in JMML

The RAS signaling pathway is one of the most studied pathways in cell biology and its deregulation is widely observed in approximately 40% of cancer patients [7]. Under normal conditions, RAS pathway activation triggers a phosphorylation signaling cascade that ultimately boosts cell proliferation, survival, differentiation, and migration, among other functions (Figure 1) [8].

Around 90% of JMML patients carry mutations in one of five genes of the RAS pathway, including *PTPN11*, *NRAS*, *KRAS*, *CBL*, and *NF1*. Concomitantly, some other secondary mutations affecting either additional RAS pathway components or external elements have been described in JMML patients [9].

2.1. PTPN11

Activating *PTPN11* somatic mutations are the most common genetic drivers of JMML, accounting for approximately 35–40% of the patients (Figure 2), and are associated with an aggressive clinical course and poor disease outcome [10–12]. The *PTPN11* gene encodes for the protein tyrosine phosphatase SHP2, which acts downstream of various receptor and cytoplasmic tyrosine kinases, and promotes RAS signaling activation (Figure 1) [13].

SHP2 structure consists in two tandem Src homology 2 recognition domains (N-SH2 and C-SH2), followed by a catalytic protein tyrosine phosphatase (PTP) domain, and a C-terminal hydrophilic tail containing phosphorylation sites [14]. In the inactive state, the N-SH2 domain engages the PTP domain, keeping the phosphatase in a close autoinhibited conformation [15]. Under physiological conditions, the binding of tyrosine-phosphorylated ligands to the tandem SH2 domains stabilizes an open SHP2 conformation that renders the active site accessible and allows the dephosphorylation of target substrates [16].

JMML *PTPN11* mutations occur mainly in the N-SH2 domain of SHP2, particularly in the residues G60, D61, A72, and E76, which account for more than 70% of *PTPN11*-mutated patients [12]. These mutations result in ligand-independent forms of the enzyme that constitutively activate downstream effectors of the RAS pathway [17].

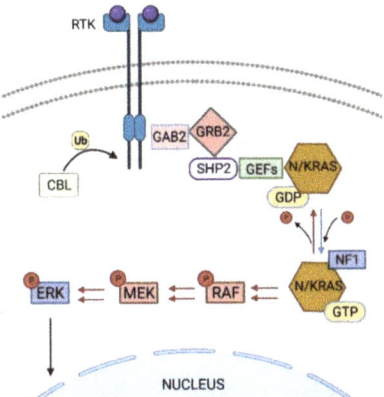

Figure 1. The RAS signaling pathway. NRAS and KRAS are small GTPase switch proteins that act downstream receptor and non-receptor tyrosine kinases (RTKs and TKs). RAS activation status is regulated by a two-stage molecular system directed by phosphorylation and dephosphorylation changes in RAS, which are regulated by the opposing activities of guanine nucleotide-exchange factors (GEFs) and GTPase activating proteins (GAPs). RTK/TK stimulation promotes the recruitment of adaptor proteins (such as GAB2, GRB2, and SHP2) and GEFs to mediate RAS-GDP phosphorylation to a RAS-GTP active status. Active RAS then triggers a signaling cascade that sequentially activates RAF, and phosphorylates MEK and ERK proteins, which ultimately signal to the nucleus to control specific cell functions such as proliferation, survival, and differentiation, among others. RAS pathway is inactivated by the activity of GAPs, such as NF1, which promote RAS-GTP dephosphorylation to a RAS-GDP inactive form. In addition, the ubiquitin ligase CBL can also act as a negative regulator of the RAS pathway by targeting active RTKs for proteasomal degradation. Figure was created with BioRender.com.

Interestingly, germline mutations in *PTPN11* are highly prevalent in Noonan Syndrome (NS), a developmental disorder characterized by unusual facial features, a restricted growth, and cardiovascular defects [18]. Approximately 5% of NS patients are affected by a mild myeloproliferative disorder, which is hematologically indistinguishable from JMML, but usually resolves spontaneously without intervention [12,19]. However, a small subset of NS patients (approximately 3%) progress into bona fide JMML and half of them die within the first month of life [19]. The distribution of NS-associated *PTPN11* germline mutations differs from the one observed in *PTPN11*-mutated JMML patients and results in weaker SHP2 forms [12,19].

2.2. NRAS and KRAS

Approximately 25–30% of JMML patients present heterozygous somatic-activating mutations in the *RAS* paralogs *NRAS* and *KRAS* (Figure 2) [20]. The NRAS and KRAS proteins are small GTPases that act as binary molecular switches of the RAS signaling pathway. NRAS and KRAS are active when bound to guanosine triphosphate (GTP) and inactive when bound to guanosine diphosphate (GDP) [20]. This phosphorylation exchange is regulated by the opposing activity of guanine nucleotide-exchange factors (GEFs) and GTPase-activating proteins (GAPs) (Figure 1) and results in allosteric conformational changes at the RAS protein G domain, which is critical for RAS activation [21].

JMML mutations occur mostly in the residues G12, G13, and Q61, which are located at the G domain both in KRAS and NRAS, and render the proteins insensitive to GAP inactivation, stabilize their GTP-bound conformation, and/or affect nucleotide-exchange rate [22–26]. Duplication of *NRAS* and *KRAS* oncogenic alleles through acquired uniparental disomy (UPD) by mitotic recombination is observed in some JMML patients and is associated with higher aggressiveness and worst outcomes [27,28]. Interestingly, there is a strong association between *KRAS* mutations and monosomy 7, being the latter present in approximately 50% of *KRAS*-mutated JMML patients [29]. This observation suggests an interaction between the oncogenic mechanisms driven by these two genetic alterations.

Germline mutations in RAS proteins have been described in different RASopathies, including NS. However, the distribution of these mutations is different to the one observed in JMML patients harboring *NRAS*/*KRAS* somatic mutations, and the evidence pointing to a driver role in JMML leukemogenesis is scarce [30–33]. A *NRAS* germline mutation at G13D was found as a possible driver event in a JMML patient, and somatic mosaicism of *NRAS* mutations, acquired at early developmental stages, has been reported in two JMML patients, who developed a mild clinical form of the disease [34,35]. In addition, a *KRAS* germline mutation at T58I was identified in a NS patient who presented a JMML-like disorder [36].

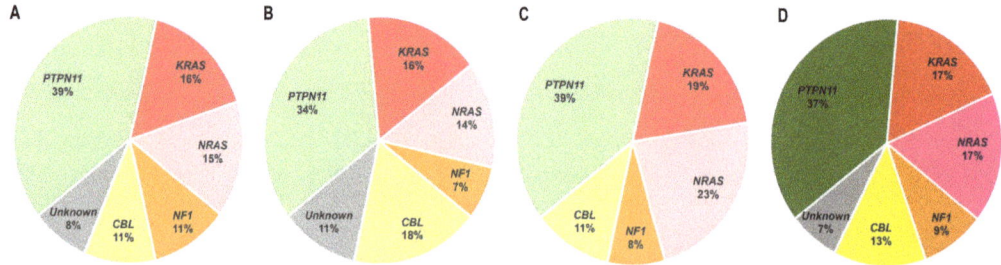

Figure 2. Distribution of RAS pathway mutations in children with JMML. Data reported by Lipka et al. [25] (**A**), Murakami et al. [37] (**B**), and Caye et al. [29] (**C**). Panel (**D**) summarizes the three studies. NS cases were excluded from the analysis.

2.3. CBL

Germline and somatic *CBL* loss-of-function mutations account for 10–15% of JMML patients [38,39]. Germline *CBL* mutations are associated to Noonan-like CBL syndrome, a constitutional disease that is presented as a mild form of NS with a heterogeneous set of clinical features with a variable penetrance (developmental delay, reduced growth, facial dysmorphism, among others) and an increased risk to develop JMML [38,40,41]. Disease progression to JMML normally occurs after loss of heterozygosity of the *CBL* wild type allele, typically through UPD encompassing the *CBL* locus [42–44]. *CBL*-mutant JMML patients usually develop indolent forms of the disease that resolve spontaneously, and only a subset of them require HSCT treatment [38,45].

The *CBL* gene encodes for the RING E3 ubiquitin ligase CBL that acts as negative regulator of activated protein tyrosine kinases by promoting their targeting for degradation by the proteasome (Figure 1) [46]. The CBL protein comprises a highly conserved N-terminal tyrosine kinase-binding (TKB) domain, followed by a central region containing a helical linker and a RING finger domain, which are critical for CBL ubiquitin ligase activity, and a C-terminal proline-rich sequence, that mediates interactions of CBL with SH3 domain-containing proteins [46,47].

Most JMML somatic mutations in CBL occur in the linker region, especially in Y371, or in different residues at the RING finger domain, and lead to the loss of E3 ubiquitin ligase activity against tyrosine kinase substrates [9,38,42]. CBL linker mutants have been shown to enhance LYN- and JAK2-mediated GM-CSF signaling by activating the PI3K/AKT/mTOR and JAK/STAT pathways, respectively [48,49]. Moreover, CBL can also regulate the RAS pathway through an indirect mechanism involving the adaptor protein GRB2 [50]. CBL interaction with GRB2 prevents the binding of this protein to SOS, a GEF that promotes the formation of active RAS-GTP complexes (Figure 1) [51]. *CBL* loss-of-function mutations impair the binding of CBL to GRB2, indirectly promoting RAS pathway activation by allowing GRB2-SOS interaction and SOS-mediated GDP/GTP nucleotide exchange in RAS proteins [52,53]. Interestingly, GRB2 is a core component of a multiprotein complex that includes SHP2, among other factors (Figure 1) [13,54]. The interaction of this complex with SOS allows SHP2 to dephosphorylate the RAS residue Y32, which increases the binding of RAS to RAF, thus contributing to RAS activation [55]. This adaptor activity of SHP2 and the inhibitory role of CBL in the regulation of GRB2-SOS complex function illustrate how *CBL* loss-of-function mutations and *PTPN11* gain-of-function mutations (through the adaptor activity of SHP2) functionally converge through a similar molecular mechanism to induce RAS activation, which could explain why these two genetic alterations are mutually exclusive in JMML [42].

2.4. NF1

Germline and somatic loss-of-function mutations at the *NF1* tumor suppressor gene are found in 10% to 15% of JMML patients (Figure 2) [4]. Germline *NF1* mutations are associated to neurofibromatosis type 1, a common autosomal congenital disorder characterized by the presence of café-au-lait macules, skinfold freckling, development of tumors of the nervous system, and overlapping features with other RASopathies, such as NS and Legius syndrome [56]. Although it is not a common complication, *NF1*-mutated neurofibromatosis type 1 patients have an increased predisposition to develop JMML, with a 200- to 350-fold increased risk compared to their wild type *NF1* counterparts [4]. In *NF1*-mutant patients, JMML progression is triggered by loss of heterozygosity of the wild type *NF1* allele, typically by UPD or compound-heterozygous mutations [57].

NF1 encodes for neurofibromin, a GAP that functions as negative regulator of the RAS signaling pathway. Neurofibromin binds to RAS family proteins and stimulates the hydrolysis of active RAS-GTP to RAS-GDP inactive forms (Figure 1) [58–60].

Most of JMML reported alterations in *NF1* are nonsense or frameshift mutations resulting in a truncated protein due to a premature termination codon [61,62]. NF1 loss-of-function mutations result in a reduced dephosphorylation of RAS-GTP activated proteins and confer sustained activation of the RAS signaling pathway [63].

2.5. Other Driver Genetic Alterations in the RAS Pathway

Although *PTPN11*, *NRAS*, *KRAS*, *CBL*, and *NF1* mutations account for approximately 90% of JMML cases, around 10% of the patients that are clinically diagnosed with JMML do not present mutations in any of these five RAS pathway genes [37]. However, several studies have reported other genetic alterations that can possibly act as molecular drivers of the disease in cases of unknown origin.

Gain-of-function somatic mutations affecting known oncogenic hotspots of the *RAS* genes were identified in *RRAS* (Q87L) and *RRAS2* (Q72L) in two independent patients that lacked any of the canonical JMML mutations at diagnosis, supporting a driver role of these alterations [64]. In addition, the analysis of a cohort of 16 patients presenting a JMML-like phenotype without mutations in any of the five canonical JMML genes revealed three patients that harbored gain-of-function *ALK* and *ROS1* tyrosine kinase fusions, including *RANBP2-ALK*, *DCTN1-ALK*, and *TBL1XR1-ROS1* [37]. Fusions involving the tyrosine kinase genes *PDGFRB* (*SPECC1-PDGFRB* and *NDEL1-PDGFRB*) and *FLT3* (*CCDC88C-FLT3*) were also identified in case reports of JMML-diagnosed patients lacking mutations in the classical JMML drivers [65–67]. Similar rearrangements involving these tyrosine kinases have been also described in other hematologic malignancies [68–72], supporting the role for these alterations as an alternative oncogenic mechanism of RAS pathway hyperactivation in leukemia transformation. However, although these patients harboring tyrosine kinase fusions recapitulate the clinical features of JMML, it is still a matter of controversy whether they should be diagnosed as JMML or instead represent an as yet undefined category of myelodysplastic/myeloproliferative neoplasms. Further research must be carried out to shed light on this debate.

2.6. Secondary Genetic Alterations in JMML

JMML is characterized by a low mutational rate, suggesting that a limited number of genetic alterations is required to support JMML leukemogenesis [29]. However, secondary mutational events that contribute to the pathogenesis of the disease have been recurrently identified in different cohorts of JMML patients.

Although the mutations in the five canonical JMML genes are in general mutually exclusive, around 10% of JMML patients harbor co-existing alterations in these genes, being the association of *PTPN11* and *NF1* mutations the most common co-mutational event [37]. In addition, approximately 50% of the cases present secondary somatic mutations in other genes, which are specifically associated with particular RAS pathway initiating lesions and expand clonally, indicating a cooperative role with the driver event in JMML maintenance (Table 1; Figure 3) [29]. Within the RAS pathway, heterozygous mutations in signaling components (*RRAS*, *RAC2*, and *SOS1*) or RAS regulators (*PLXNB2*, *ABI1*, and *PDE8A*) have been described in JMML in combination with some of the classical driver events and contribute to JMML pathogenesis by enhancing RAS pathway activation (Table 1) [29,37,64]. In addition, other genetic events outside the RAS pathway have been reported as major secondary mutations in some JMML subsets. Among them, *SETBP1* activating mutations are the most prevalent genetic events, being present in around 30% of JMML patients and correlating with poorer disease outcomes [73,74]. SETBP1 directly binds to SET, which functions as an inhibitor of the protein phosphatase PP2A, a well-known tumor suppressor in hematopoietic malignancies [75,76]. This interaction protects SET from degradation, potentiating its inhibitory activity over PP2A [77]. *SETBP1* mutations disrupt the degron motif of the protein, resulting in an impaired proteasome cleavage and subsequent SETBP1 protein accumulation, which further enhances the inhibitory effects of SET over PP2A and support leukemia cell proliferation [77,78]. In addition to this function, SETBP1 has been shown to directly bind AT-rich promoter regions and contribute to the transcriptional activation a set of target genes that include the hematopoietic master regulators *HOXA9* and *HOXA10* [79,80]. This effect correlates with an increase in myeloid progenitor self-renewal capacity in Setbp1-overexpressing mouse bone marrow, supporting the existence of additional PP2A-independent oncogenic mechanisms driven by SETBP1 aberrant expression [79]. In JMML, *SETBP1* mutations associate with *PTPN11* or *NRAS* somatic mutations [74]. Interestingly, a recently published mouse model combining *SETBP1* and *NRAS* mutations has shed some light on the mechanism of interaction between these two factors by showing that the aberrant expression of SETBP1 enhances both NRAS gene expression signature and NRAS-driven MAPK protein phosphorylation [81].

Table 1. Recurrent genetic alterations in JMML.

Pathway		Affected Gene	Alteration	%	References
RAS pathway	Tyrosine phosphatases	*PTPN11*	GoF-M	39%	[12,25,37,82]
	Tyrosine kinases	*ALK*	GoF-F	<3%	[37]
		PDGFRB	GoF-F	<3%	[65,66]
	RAS signaling components	*KRAS*	GoF-M	16%	[37,82]
		NRAS	GoF-M	15%	[37,82]
		RRAS	GoF-M	<3%	[29,64,83,84]
		RRAS2	GoF-M	<3%	[37,64]
	RAS regulators	*NF1*	LoF-M	11%	[37,57,82]
		CBL	LoF-M	11%	[38]
		SOS1	MS	<3%	[37]

Table 1. Cont.

Pathway		Affected Gene	Alteration	%	References
JAK/STAT pathway		SETBP1	GoF-M	30%	[37,73,81,84,85]
		JAK3	GoF-M	8%	[29,73,74]
		SH2B3	LoF-M	7%	[64]
Hematopoietic commitment transcription factors		RUNX1	LoF-M	<3%	[64,84]
		GATA2	MS	<3%	[64]
Spliceosome components		ZRSR2	LoF-M	<3%	[29,64]
Epigenetic machinery	Histone modifiers	DNMT3A	LoF-M	3%	[64]
	PRC2 complex components and associated factors	ASXL1	LoF-M	8%	[64,84]
		EZH2	LoF-M	4%	[64]
		SUZ12	LOH	<3%	[29]
		CDYL	LOH	<3%	[29]

Abbreviations: GoF-M, gain-of-function mutations; GoF-F, gain-of-function gene fusions; LoF-M, loss-of-function mutations; MS, missense mutations (undetermined effect); LOH, loss of heterozygosity.

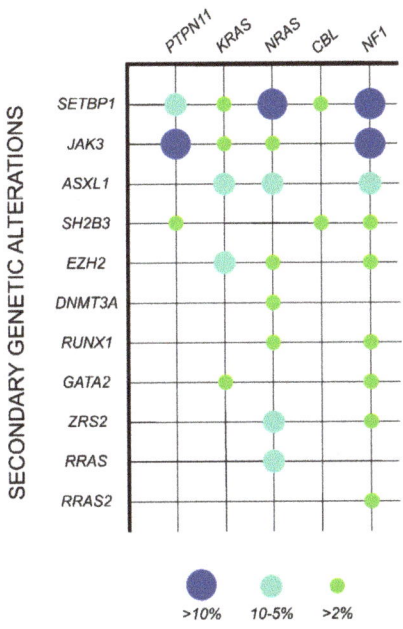

Figure 3. Association of secondary mutations with specific genetic drivers in JMML. Data reported by Murakami et al. [37], Caye et al. [29], and Stieglitz et al. [64,85]. Colored circles represent the relative frequency of a secondary mutation in patients with each of the five JMML canonical drivers (green > 2%; light blue 5–10%; dark blue > 10%).

Along with the mutations in *SETBP1*, other secondary genetic alterations are also observed as clonal events in JMML patients, including mutations in hematopoietic commitment transcription factors (*RUNX1*, *GATA2*, *RARA*, and *HOXA11*), spliceosome components (*ZRSR2*), cAMP pathway components (*PDE8A*), structural protein components and regulators (*WASP*, *DYNC1H1*, *TNS3*, *COL22A1*, *KRT1*, and *SMC1A*), or JAK/STAT pathway components (*JAK3* and *SH2B3*), among others (Table 1) [29,37,64,73,74,81,84,86–89]. These secondary mutations are associated with an aggressive clinical course of the disease and an increased risk of relapse after HSCT [64].

Of special relevance are the genetic alterations that affect components of the epigenetic machinery, which are observed in approximately 15% of JMML patients [29,64]. These genetic alterations include mostly mutations at the genes encoding for the polycomb repressive complex 2 (PRC2) core component EZH2 and the PRC2-associated factor ASXL1. Of note, the *EZH2* gene is located at chromosome 7 and all JMML-associated *EZH2* mutations are hemizygous due to co-occurring monosomy 7 [29,64]. In addition to these mutations, copy number variations (CVN) in genes encoding for other PRC2 complex components and associated factors, such as *SUZ12, AEBP2, CDYL*, or *JARID*, have been found in some subsets of JMML patients [29]. Mutations at the *DNMT3A* gene, encoding for the DNA methyltransferase 3 alpha, have been also described; however, the recurrence of this genetic alterations in JMML is lower than in other hematologic malignancies [64,90].

The PRC2 complex directs the transcriptional repression of target genes by catalyzing histone H3 trimethylation at lysine 27 (H3K27me3) [91]. Interestingly, a recent study demonstrated that JMML patients that present an impaired PRC2 activity show a global decrease in H3K27me3 and a concomitant increase in H3K27 acetylation, suggesting a critical role of PRC2-associated mutations in regulating the JMML transcriptional program at the epigenetic level [29]. These findings illustrate the crosstalk between genetics and epigenetics in JMML and highlight the importance of a better understanding of the oncogenic mechanisms driven by epigenetic dysregulation during JMML leukemogenesis.

3. Epigenetic Alterations in JMML

Although genetic mutational events are generally considered the main drivers of cancer transformation, alterations in the epigenetic landscape of tumor cells have a critical role in cancer pathogenesis, providing additional mechanisms to consolidate specific oncogenic transcriptional programs [92]. Over the last decade, several research groups have explored the epigenetic landscape in JMML and identified important alterations in the methylome of JMML cells that correlate with the severity and prognosis of the disease. This fact highlights the urgent need of a better understanding of the oncogenic mechanisms driven by JMML epigenetic aberrations and postulates the use of epigenetic modifiers as a potential therapeutic strategy for the treatment of this disease.

3.1. Early Studies on DNA Methylation in JMML

CpG island methylation at gene promoters is an important repressive mechanism of gene expression, which has been shown to play a relevant oncogenic role in different cancers, including myeloid malignancies [93]. In JMML, methylation in CpG islands was first analyzed in a European cohort of 86 patients, in which 14 candidate genes were selected based on their hypermethylation status in other cancer types (*CALCA, CDKN1C, CDKN2B, DAPK1, MGMT, MLH1, RARB, RASSF1, SOCS1*, and *TP73*) or their involvement in RAS signaling (*BMP4, PAWR, RASA1*, and *RECK*). Among the selected candidates, four genes were found recurrently hypermethylated, including *BMP4, CALCA, CDKN2B*, and *RARB* (Table 2; Figure 4). Interestingly, this hypermethylation phenotype correlated with poorer prognosis and a high risk of treatment failure due to relapse after HSCT [94].

These results were further validated in a Japanese cohort of 92 JMML patients, in which the CpG methylation status of 16 genes was analyzed, including nine genes that were common to the European study (*CALCA, CDKN2B, DAPK1, MGMT, MLH1, RARB, RASSF1, TP73*, and *BMP4*) and seven new candidate genes (*APC, CDH13, CDKN1A, CHFR, ESR1, H19*, and *IGF2AS*). This study not only confirmed the hypermethylation of *BMP4, CALCA, CDKN2B*, and *RARB*, but also provided a novel prognostic tool based on the "aberrant methylation score" (AMS). AMS stratifies the patients in three groups based on the number of hypermethylated genes (0, 1–2, or 3–4) and predicts their 5-year overall survival and transplant-free survival, with high AMS patients presenting a dismal prognosis [95].

Table 2. Recurrent epigenetic alterations in JMML.

	Affected Gene	Alteration	%	References
Polypeptide from TGF-β superfamily of proteins	BMP4	Hypermethylation	36%	[94]
Family of G-protein-coupled receptors	CALCA	Hypermethylation	54%	[94]
Cyclin-dependent kinase inhibitor	CDKN2B	Hypermethylation	22%	[94]
Retinoic acid receptor	RARB	Hypermethylation	13%	[94]
RAS Regulator	RASA4	Hypermethylation	51%	[96]
Histone acetylation	CREBBP	Hypermethylation	77%	[97]
Scaffold protein in signal transduction	AKAP12	Hypermethylation	42%	[98]

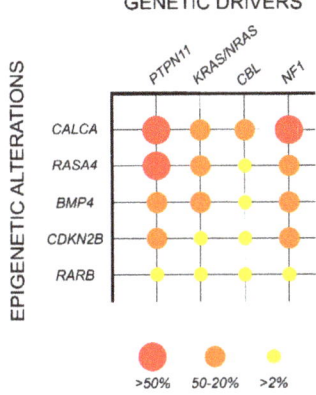

Figure 4. Association of epigenetic alterations with specific genetic drivers in JMML. Data reported by Olk-Batz et al. [94] and Poetsch et al. [96]. Colored circles represent the relative frequency of a specific epigenetic alteration in patients with each of the five JMML canonical drivers (yellow > 2%; orange 20–50%; red > 50%).

In addition to the genes identified in these studies, hypermethylation in other genes such as *RASA4*, *CREBBP*, and *AKAP12* was also observed in JMML patients in correlation with a poor survival and high risk of relapse after HSCT, further supporting the significance of DNA methylation in aggressive JMML phenotypes (Table 2; Figure 4) [96–98].

3.2. The JMML Methylation Landscape

Early methylation studies in JMML focused on the analysis of specific gene subsets. However, a global view on the DNA methylation landscape in JMML was not obtained until the first genome-wide CpG methylation analyses were performed [25,37,99]. Based on these studies, patients were clustered according to their global methylation status in three groups: low methylation (LM), intermediate methylation (IM), and high methylation (HM). These groups were not only associated with particular outcomes [99], but also to specific molecular profiles [25,37]. Thus, LM patients showed enrichment of somatic *NRAS* and *CBL* mutations and presented high survival rates, the IM group was associated to somatic *KRAS* mutations and monosomy 7, and the HM patients showed an enrichment in *PTPN11* mutations and were characterized by a poor clinical outcome [25]. Interestingly, the analysis of HM samples showed an upregulation in the expression of the genes encoding for the DNA methyltransferases *DNMT1* and *DNMT3B*, suggesting an association between activation of DNA methylation mechanisms and specific JMML mutational profiles [25]. Overall, these data further supported the diagnostic value of DNA methylation in JMML patients.

3.3. DNA Methylation as a Prognostic Tool in JMML

The accumulating evidences on the role of DNA methylation in the pathogenesis of JMML has led to the recent publication of an international JMML stratification consensus, which has defined the parameters and characteristics of the different DNA methylation subgroups in JMML [100]. In here, the Illumina Infinium 450 k/EPIC array technology was applied to develop and validate a machine learning classifier for prospective patient classification.

To complement this novel prognostic tool, a new technique called Digital Restriction Enzyme Analysis of Methylation (DREAM) was developed to provide an easy and robust method to evaluate DNA methylation in JMML clinical samples [101]. In this method, DNA is sequentially digested with a methylation-sensitive restriction enzyme (SmaI), followed by a restriction enzyme that is tolerant to DNA methylation (XmaI). This digestion results in the generation of two DNA fragment types, carrying either a CCGGG tag in their 5′ end in methylated DNA sites, or a GGG tag in unmethylated DNA sites. These fragments are then analyzed by Next-Generation Sequencing (NGS), allowing a quantitative whole-genome evaluation of DNA methylation [102]. DREAM represents a promising and cost-efficient technology for the evaluation of DNA methylation in clinical settings; however, further research will be required to address its implementation and determine the robustness of the approach in different laboratories.

The standardized use of DNA methylation as a biomarker in JMML and the incorporation of techniques such as Illumina Infinium 450 k/EPIC arrays or new techniques such as DREAM as prognostic methods represent a unique breakthrough for the stratification and management of JMML patients. These tools will not only improve clinical decision-making, but also contribute to optimize the inclusion criteria of specific JMML subsets in future clinical trials.

4. Genetic and Epigenetic Therapeutic Targets for the Treatment of JMML

JMML has historically represented a clinical challenge mainly due to the limited number of therapeutic options for its treatment and the inevitable fatal outcome in children with the most aggressive forms of the disease [103,104]. HSCT is currently the only effective therapy for achieving long-term disease control in JMML [103]. However, the advances in the characterization of the molecular mechanisms driving and supporting the progression of JMML have provided new potential genetic and epigenetic therapeutic targets that are currently being explored in different preclinical assays and clinical trials as alternative treatments for JMML (Table 3). These studies hold promise for an improvement in the pre- and post-HSCT management of the disease, and might have a direct impact on the prognosis and survival of JMML patients in the future.

4.1. JMML Therapeutic Targets on Signaling Pathways

4.1.1. RAS Pathway Targeting

Although RAS hyperactivation is a hallmark in JMML, the therapeutic targeting of factors involved in RAS signaling has been shown to provide limited benefits due to the frequent treatment-associated toxicities, and the functional redundancy and complexity of the pathway [105–107]. However, some studies have explored the use of different tyrosine kinase (TK) and mitogen-activated protein kinase (MEK) inhibitors to target RAS signaling, as a therapeutic alternative for JMML treatment.

A small subset of clinically-diagnosed JMML patients harbor fusions involving diverse RAS components, which result in the abnormal activation of specific TKs, such as *ALK*, *ROS1*, or *FLT3* [37,67]. Some examples illustrate how drug repurposing of TK inhibitors (TKIs) that are approved for the treatment of other pathologies could have a potential therapeutic benefit on this atypical subset of JMML patients. Such is the case of crizotinib, a potent inhibitor of ALK and ROS1 that is approved for the treatment of non-small cell lung cancer [108]. Current evidences on the benefits of crizotinib treatment on JMML are limited to the case of a patient carrying *RANBP2-ALK* fusion that was refractory to conventional cytotoxic chemotherapy. The addition of crizotinib to the treatment resulted in complete molecular remission and allowed successful HSCT in this patient [37]. In the same study, another two patients who harbored *ALK* or *ROS1* fusions were not treated with crizotinib and succumbed due to tumor progression [37].

Similar to this case, the use of another TKI, sorafenib, has been also explored in the context of JMML [67]. Sorafenib, is currently approved for the treatment of different types of cancer, including acute myeloid leukemia patients that carry an activating internal tandem duplication mutation on FLT3 (FLT3-ITD) [109]. A JMML patient harboring a *CCDC88C-FLT3* fusion who was refractory to conventional chemotherapy, was treated with sorafenib, resulting in FLT3 inhibition and cytogenetic remission, which also in this case allowed successful HSCT [67].

In the case of *PTPN11*-mutant JMML, a recent study has identified the non-receptor tyrosine kinase ACK1 (encoded by the *TNK2* gene) as a potential therapeutic target for these patients [110]. In vitro assays showed that the ACK1-specific inhibitors AIM-100 and XMD8-87 can reduce the transforming potential of JMML-associated *PTPN11* mutations [110]. Clinically, the use of dasatinib, a TKI that is approved for the treatment of different types of leukemia and can target ACK1 (among other TKs), was shown to reduce disease burden and provide extended survival in a *PTPN11*-mutant JMML patient [110].

Together, these data postulate the use of TKIs as a potential therapeutic approach to achieve disease remission and facilitate HSCT in some JMML patient subsets; however, further research is required to validate these observations.

In addition to TKIs, the use of MEK inhibitors (MEKi) in JMML has also been explored. Especially remarkable is the case of trametinib, a MAP2K1/MAP2K2 inhibitor that is currently approved for the treatment of metastatic melanoma [111]. The first evidences on the potential therapeutic effect of trametinib in JMML were obtained in in vitro assays using induced pluripotent stem cells (iPSCs) derived from *PTPN11*- and *CBL*-mutant JMML cells [112]. In this experimental setting, trametinib treatment resulted in efficient RAS signaling and cell growth inhibition in *PTPN11*-mutant iPSCs [112]. More recently, trametinib has also been shown to provide a survival benefit in a mouse model in which leukemogenesis is driven by the combined expression of JMML-associated *NRAS* and *SETBP1* mutations [81]. The application of trametinib for the treatment of JMML is currently being explored in a phase II clinical trial, which aims to determine the safety and efficacy of this drug in refractory or relapsed JMML patients (ClinicalTrials.gov Identifier: NCT03190915).

4.1.2. Targeting of Other Signaling Pathways

The PI3K/AKT/mTOR pathway is one of the main downstream effectors of the RAS pathway and it is also affected by RAS hyperactivation [106]. In JMML, some studies have provided evidence of the beneficial effects of PI3K/AKT/mTOR inhibition. The use of rapamycin, a specific and potent mTOR inhibitor, has been shown to reduce signaling and proliferation of JMML-derived *PTPN11*-mutant iPSCs in vitro [112]. Similar results were obtained in the same experimental setting upon treatment with idelalisib, a PI3Kδ inhibitor [112]. Moreover, the use of idelalisib on primary JMML cells resulted in a dose-dependent reduction in GM-CSF hypersensitivity in two of the three samples analyzed [113]. Finally, both rapamycin and idelalisib have also shown a therapeutic effect in in vivo leukemia mouse models driven by the expression of JMML-associated *PTPN11* mutations [114,115].

Secondary mutations affecting components of the JAK/STAT pathway, such as *JAK3* or *SH2B3*, are recurrently found in JMML patients, indicating a relevant role of this signaling pathway in the pathogenesis of JMML [29,64,73,74]. Therefore, targeting the JAK/STAT pathway could potentially report beneficial effects in some JMML patient subsets. In this context, a recent in vitro study revealed that JMML-derived *CBL*-mutant iPSCs are sensitive to the JAK inhibitors momelotinib and ruxolitinib, reducing both cell proliferation and aberrant signaling [112].

Although clinical data on the use of these inhibitors in JMML are not available, the promising results obtained in in vitro and in vivo preclinical models support a potential therapeutic benefit of these treatments in JMML patients. However, further research will be required to explore this possibility in a clinical setting.

4.2. Epigenetic Therapeutic Targets in JMML

DNA hypermethylation has been showed to be a hallmark in the most aggressive cases of JMML [25,37,99]. For that reason, the use of the DNA methyltransferase inhibitor azacitidine has been explored as a potential therapeutic agent for the treatment of this disease, alone or in combination with conventional cytotoxic chemotherapy [116]. Azacitidine use in JMML was first reported on a patient that achieved complete clinical and genetic remission of the disease after eight cycles of treatment prior to HSCT [117]. Later on, a retrospective study showed that low-dose azacitidine was effective and tolerable in JMML, and documented another three JMML cases in which this drug induced complete remission before HSCT [118]. Finally, the beneficial effects of pre-HSCT azacitidine treatment were formally validated in a phase II clinical trial (NCT02447666) that demonstrated that the use of this drug as a single agent is a suitable option for newly diagnosed JMML patients, independent of their methylation status [116]. In addition, the histone deacetylase inhibitor vorinostat, is currently being explored in a phase I clinical trial (NCT03843528) in combination with low dose azacitidine for the treatment of pediatric myeloid malignancies, including JMML. Further clinical studies will be required to determine long-term safety and efficacy of these treatments in JMML.

Table 3. Experimental therapeutic strategies for JMML treatment.

	Pathway	Target	Inhibitor	Status	References
Signaling pathway inhibitors	RAS	ACK1	Dasatinib	In vitro	[110]
		ALK/ROS1/MET	Crizotinib	In vitro	[37]
		MEK	Trametinib	Phase II clinical trial	[81,112,119,120]
		FLT3	Sorafenib	Clinical use	[67]
	PI3K	mTOR	Rapamycin	Preclinical in vivo	[112,114,115]
		PI3Kδ	Idelalisib	Preclinical in vivo	[112–115]
	JAK/STAT	JAK1/JAK2	Momelotinib	In vitro	[112]
		JAK1/JAK2	Ruxolitinib	In vitro	[112]
Epigenetic inhibitors	Methylation	DNMTs	Azacitidine	Clinical use	[37,116–118,121,122]
	Acetylation	HDACs	Vorinostat	Phase I clinical trial	

5. Current Challenges and Future Perspectives in JMML Research

Despite of the advances in the genetic and epigenetic characterization of JMML, there are still several experimental challenges and clinically relevant open questions that remain to be addressed.

5.1. JMML Experimental Models

JMML research has been traditionally hindered due to its low incidence (1.2 cases per million children under 14 years of age), and the impossibility of maintaining primary JMML cells in vitro for extended periods of time or establishing immortalized JMML cells lines [123,124]. In this context, the development of methods to generate JMML patient-derived xenografts (PDX) and iPSCs has been instrumental to overcome low sample number difficulties and provide an unlimited source of JMML cells for experimental purposes.

JMML PDXs have been established in immunodeficient NSG (NOD/SCID/IL2rγ$^{-/-}$) and NSG-S (NOD/SCID/IL2rγ$^{-/-}$/IL-3/GM/SF) mice, and in both cases these models present not only the immunophenotypical features of the primary sample, but also maintain the clonal diversity of the original tumor [84,125]. On the other hand, different reprogramming techniques have been successfully applied towards the generation of JMML-derived iPSCs, providing a unique experimental tool to perform high-throughput analysis, such as drug or CRISPR screens [112,126–128]. However, the lack of a physiological bone marrow microenvironment in iPSC models gives rise to important concerns regarding whether these systems can faithfully recapitulate the molecular and functional features of the tumor. Future JMML modeling efforts should focus on the establishment of biomimetic 3D culture systems that replicate the molecular and cellular complexity of the bone marrow microenvironment [129–131]. The development of these approaches might help to overcome the limitations of primary JMML cultures and provide new physiologically relevant in vitro models to study the oncogenic mechanism driving JMML pathogenesis and resistance to therapy.

5.2. State-of-the-Art Methods to Explore JMML Tumor Origin, Heterogeneity and Evolution

Although the phenotype of JMML patients is dominated by the expansion of myeloid cells, there is evidence that also indicates the involvement of other hematopoietic lineages [4,20,132]. For this reason, JMML is considered a disease of the HSPC compartment [1,84,133]. However, very little is known about the cell hierarchies involved in leukemia progression, the intratumor heterogeneity, the specific identity of the leukemia initiating cells, or the clonal evolution of the disease. However, all these features might have an important impact in the prognosis of the disease and risk of relapse after HSCT.

Over the last years, the rapid development of new technologies based on the use of next generation sequencing has changed the paradigms of cancer research. More specifically, the analysis of genomic, epigenomic, and/or transcriptomic information at single-cell resolution, and the comprehensive integration of these data can provide critical information on tumor origin, progression, and cellular heterogeneity.

In JMML, these approaches have only been applied to the transcriptomic analysis of HSPCs from two JMML patient samples by single-cell RNA sequencing (scRNA-seq) [134]. In this study, different JMML-specific HSPC clusters were identified, each of them showing upregulation of particular sets of genes, including myeloid genes, stem cell, and fetal genes, or genes associated to proliferation, leukemia, and erythroid differentiation [134]. These results demonstrated a broad heterogeneity within the JMML HSPC compartment, with the expression of aberrant transcriptional signatures that are not found in control cord blood HSPCs [134]. However, the collection of only transcriptional data and the low number of samples analyzed, limited the conclusions that could be extracted regarding the role of each of these clusters in tumor progression or maintenance.

Although not yet applied to JMML research, single-cell DNA-sequencing (scDNA-seq) combined with scRNA-seq has been successfully applied to the analysis of different types of cancers [135,136]. In these analyses, scRNA-seq data are used to identify specific cell clusters based on their transcriptomic profile. Then, this information is integrated with the scDNA-seq results to correlate different cell subpopulations with a specific mutational status and assess tumor clonal evolution during the differentiation process. In addition, transcriptomic data can be used to infer cell lineage differentiation between the annotated cell subpopulations by trajectory-based differential expression analysis using pseudotime analytical tools [137–139]. These bioinformatic approaches could be applied to the study of JMML tumoral heterogeneity and clonal evolution by tracking "first hit" mutations to a cell of origin, and studying their differentiation trajectories and acquisition of mutations.

Similarly, JMML epigenomic intratumoral heterogeneity could be studied using methods that allow the analysis of DNA methylation at single-cell level. Simultaneous profiling of the transcriptome and DNA methylome from individual cells (scMT-seq) provides both a functional annotation of different cell subsets and a methylation profile [140]. A similar approach integrating scRNA-seq with methylome microarray data has been recently used to track the cell of origin in chronic lymphocytic leukemia [141]. The application of these technologies to the study of JMML could be critical to decipher the molecular mechanisms driving JMML leukemogenesis and progression.

6. Conclusions

The characterization of the genetic and epigenetic landscapes of JMML has significantly improved our understanding of the oncogenic pathways controlling the pathogenesis of this disease. Moreover, these analyses have turned the spotlight on DNA hypermethylation and secondary mutations as critical alterations that cooperate with canonical RAS pathway mutations and have an important prognostic value in the clinic. However, key questions regarding JMML origin, tumor cell identity, and intratumor and interpatient heterogeneity, remain open and must be addressed in the future. The use of new technologies allowing single-cell molecular profiling will be instrumental to achieve this aim and provide new relevant information on JMML pathobiology. This will in turn improve JMML diagnostic and prognostic criteria and contribute to identify potential therapeutic targets for the treatment of this disease.

Author Contributions: Conceptualization: L.B. Literature review: C.F. and N.G.-M. Manuscript preparation: C.F., N.G.-M. and L.B. Figure preparation: C.F., N.G.-M. and S.A.-M. Supervision: L.B. All authors have read and agreed to the published version of the manuscript.

Funding: This work was supported by Spanish Ministry of Science and Innovation (PID2020-117645RB-I00/AEI/10.13039/501100011033 and RYC2020-029400-I/AEI/10.13039/501100011033), the FERO Foundation (BFero2020.03), and the Government of Andorra (ATC025-AND-2020).

Acknowledgments: We thank the CERCA Program (Generalitat de Catalunya), the Josep Carreras Leukemia Research Institute and the Catalan Institute of Oncology for their institutional support. LB is supported by the Spanish Ministry of Science and Innovation (MCI) (PID2020-117645RB-I00/AEI/10.13039/501100011033 and RYC2020-029400-I/AEI/10.13039/501100011033), and the FERO Foundation (BFero2020.03). CF is supported by a PhD grant from the Government of Andorra (ATC025-AND-2020).

Conflicts of Interest: The authors declare no conflict of interest.

References

1. Arber, D.A.; Orazi, A.; Hasserjian, R.; Thiele, J.; Borowitz, M.J.; Le Beau, M.M.; Bloomfield, C.D.; Cazzola, M.; Vardiman, J.W. The 2016 revision to the World Health Organization classification of myeloid neoplasms and acute leukemia. *Blood* **2016**, *127*, 2391–2405. [CrossRef] [PubMed]
2. Emanuel, P.; Bates, L.; Castleberry, R.; Gualtieri, R.; Zuckerman, K. Selective Hypersensitivity to Granulocyte-Macrophage Colony-Stimulating Factor by Juvenile Chronic Myeloid Leukemia Hematopoietic Progenitors. *Blood* **1991**, *77*, 925–929. [CrossRef] [PubMed]
3. Locatelli, F.; Niemeyer, C.M. How I treat juvenile myelomonocytic leukemia. *Blood* **2015**, *125*, 1083–1090. [CrossRef] [PubMed]
4. Niemeyer, C.M.; Aricó, M.; Basso, G.; Biondi, A.; Cantú Rajnoldi, A.; Creutzig, U.; Haas, O.; Harbott, J.; Hasle, H.; Kerndrup, G.; et al. Chronic Myelomonocytic Leukemia in Childhood: A Retrospective Analysis of 110 Cases. *Blood* **1997**, *89*, 3534–3543. [CrossRef]
5. Yabe, M.; Ohtsuka, Y.; Watanabe, K.; Inagaki, J.; Yoshida, N.; Sakashita, K.; Kakuda, H.; Yabe, H.; Kurosawa, H.; Kudo, K.; et al. Transplantation for juvenile myelomonocytic leukemia: A retrospective study of 30 children treated with a regimen of busulfan, fludarabine, and melphalan. *Int. J. Hematol.* **2014**, *101*, 184–190. [CrossRef]
6. Dvorak, C.C.; Satwani, P.; Stieglitz, E.; Cairo, M.S.; Dang, H.; Pei, Q.; Gao, Y.; Wall, D.; Mazor, T.; Olshen, A.B.; et al. Disease Burden and Conditioning Regimens in ASCT1221, A Randomized Phase II Trial in Children with Juvenile Myelomonocytic Leukemia: A Children's Oncology Group Study. *Pediatr. Blood Cancer* **2018**, *65*, e27034. [CrossRef]
7. Sanchez-Vega, F.; Mina, M.; Armenia, J.; Chatila, W.K.; Luna, A.; La, K.C.; Dimitriadoy, S.; Liu, D.L.; Kantheti, H.S.; Saghafinia, S.; et al. Oncogenic Signaling Pathways in The Cancer Genome Atlas. *Cell* **2018**, *173*, 321–337. [CrossRef]
8. Chung, E.; Kondo, M. Role of Ras/Raf/MEK/ERK signaling in physiological hematopoiesis and leukemia development. *Immunol. Res.* **2011**, *49*, 248–268. [CrossRef]
9. Niemeyer, C.M. RAS diseases in children. *Haematologica* **2014**, *99*, 1653–1662. [CrossRef]
10. Tartaglia, M.; Niemeyer, C.M.; Fragale, A.; Song, X.; Buechner, J.; Jung, A.; Hählen, K.; Hasle, H.; Licht, J.D.; Gelb, B.D.; et al. Somatic mutations in PTPN11 in juvenile myelomonocytic leukemia, myelodysplastic syndromes and acute myeloid leukemia. *Nat. Genet.* **2003**, *34*, 148–150. [CrossRef]

11. Loh, M.L.; Vattikuti, S.; Schubbert, S.; Reynolds, M.G.; Carlson, E.; Lleuw, K.H.; Cheng, J.W.; Lee, C.M.; Stokoe, D.; Bonifas, J.M.; et al. Mutations in PTPN11 implicate the SHP-2 phosphatase in leukemogenesis. *Blood* **2004**, *103*, 2325–2331. [CrossRef]
12. Kratz, C.P.; Niemeyer, C.M.; Castleberry, R.P.; Cetin, M.; Bergsträsser, E.; Emanuel, P.D.; Hasle, H.; Kardos, G.; Klein, C.; Kojima, S.; et al. The mutational spectrum of PTPN11 in juvenile myelomonocytic leukemia and Noonan syndrome/myeloproliferative disease. *Blood* **2005**, *106*, 2183–2185. [CrossRef]
13. Dance, M.; Montagner, A.; Salles, J.P.; Yart, A.; Raynal, P. The molecular functions of Shp2 in the Ras/Mitogen-activated protein kinase (ERK1/2) pathway. *Cell. Signal.* **2008**, *20*, 453–459. [CrossRef]
14. Neel, B.G.; Gu, H.; Pao, L. The 'Shp'ing news: SH2 domain-containing tyrosine phosphatases in cell signaling. *Trends Biochem. Sci.* **2003**, *28*, 284–293. [CrossRef]
15. Hof, P.; Pluskey, S.; Dhe-Paganon, S.; Eck, M.J.; Shoelson, S.E. Crystal Structure of the Tyrosine Phosphatase SHP-2. *Cell* **1998**, *92*, 441–450. [CrossRef]
16. Pluskey, S.; Wandless, T.J.; Walsh, C.T.; Shoelson, S.E. Potent stimulation of SH-PTP2 phosphatase activity by simultaneous occupancy of both SH2 domains. *J. Biol. Chem.* **1995**, *270*, 2897–2900. [CrossRef]
17. LaRochelle, J.R.; Fodor, M.; Xu, X.; Durzynska, I.; Fan, L.; Stams, T.; Chan, H.M.; LaMarche, M.J.; Chopra, R.; Wang, P.; et al. Structural and Functional Consequences of Three Cancer-Associated Mutations of the Oncogenic Phosphatase SHP2. *Biochemistry* **2016**, *55*, 2269–2277. [CrossRef]
18. Tartaglia, M.; Kalidas, K.; Shaw, A.; Song, X.; Musat, D.L.; van der Burgt, I.; Brunner, H.G.; Bertola, D.R.; Crosby, A.; Ion, A.; et al. PTPN11 Mutations in Noonan Syndrome: Molecular Spectrum, Genotype-Phenotype Correlation, and Phenotypic Heterogeneity. *Am. J. Hum. Genet.* **2002**, *70*, 1555. [CrossRef]
19. Strullu, M.; Caye, A.; Lachenaud, J.; Cassinat, B.; Gazal, S.; Fenneteau, O.; Pouvreau, N.; Pereira, S.; Baumann, C.; Contet, A.; et al. Juvenile myelomonocytic leukaemia and Noonan syndrome. *J. Med. Genet.* **2014**, *51*, 689–697. [CrossRef]
20. Flotho, C.; Valcamonica, S.; Mach-Pascual, S.; Schmahl, G.; Corral, L.; Ritterbach, J.; Hasle, H.; Aricò, M.; Biondi, A.; Niemeyer, C.; et al. RAS mutations and clonality analysis in children with juvenile myelomonocytic leukemia (JMML). *Leukemia* **1999**, *13*, 32–37. [CrossRef]
21. Shima, F.; Ijiri, Y.; Muraoka, S.; Liao, J.; Ye, M.; Araki, M.; Matsumoto, K.; Yamamoto, N.; Sugimoto, T.; Yoshikawa, Y.; et al. Structural Basis for Conformational Dynamics of GTP-bound Ras Protein. *J. Biol. Chem.* **2010**, *285*, 22696. [CrossRef] [PubMed]
22. Matsuda, K.; Shimada, A.; Yoshida, N.; Ogawa, A.; Watanabe, A.; Yajima, S.; Iizuka, S.; Koike, K.K.; Yanai, F.; Kawasaki, K.; et al. Spontaneous improvement of hematologic abnormalities in patients having juvenile myelomonocytic leukemia with specific RAS mutations. *Blood* **2007**, *109*, 5477–5480. [CrossRef] [PubMed]
23. Kraoua, L.; Journel, H.; Bonnet, P.; Amiel, J.; Pouvreau, N.; Baumann, C.; Verloes, A.; Cavé, H. Constitutional NRAS mutations are rare among patients with Noonan syndrome or juvenile myelomonocytic leukemia. *Am. J. Med. Genet. Part A* **2012**, *158A*, 2407–2411. [CrossRef] [PubMed]
24. Hobbs, G.A.; Der, C.J.; Rossman, K.L. RAS isoforms and mutations in cancer at a glance. *J. Cell Sci.* **2016**, *129*, 1287. [CrossRef]
25. Lipka, D.B.; Witte, T.; Toth, R.; Yang, J.; Wiesenfarth, M.; Nöllke, P.; Fischer, A.; Brocks, D.; Gu, Z.; Park, J.; et al. RAS-pathway mutation patterns define epigenetic subclasses in juvenile myelomonocytic leukemia. *Nat. Commun.* **2017**, *8*, 2126. [CrossRef]
26. Simanshu, D.K.; Nissley, D.V.; Mccormick, F. Leading Edge Review RAS Proteins and Their Regulators in Human Disease. *Cell* **2017**, *170*, 17–33. [CrossRef]
27. Matsuda, K.; Nakazawa, Y.; Sakashita, K.; Shiohara, M.; Yamauchi, K.; Koike, K. Acquisition of loss of the wild-type NRAS locus with aggressive disease progression in a patient with juvenile myelomonocytic leukemia and a heterozygous NRAS mutation. *Haematologica* **2007**, *92*, 1576–1578. [CrossRef]
28. Kato, M.; Yasui, N.; Seki, M.; Kishimoto, H.; Sato-Otsubo, A.; Hasegawa, D.; Kiyokawa, N.; Hanada, R.; Ogawa, S.; Manabe, A.; et al. Aggressive Transformation of Juvenile Myelomonocytic Leukemia Associated with Duplication of Oncogenic KRAS due to Acquired Uniparental Disomy. *J. Pediatr.* **2013**, *162*, 1285–1288.e1. [CrossRef]
29. Caye, A.; Strullu, M.; Guidez, F.; Cassinat, B.; Gazal, S.; Fenneteau, O.; Lainey, E.; Nouri, K.; Nakhaei-Rad, S.; Dvorsky, R.; et al. Juvenile myelomonocytic leukemia displays mutations in components of the RAS pathway and the PRC2 network. *Nat. Genet.* **2015**, *47*, 1334–1340. [CrossRef]
30. Schubbert, S.; Zenker, M.; Rowe, S.L.; Böll, S.; Klein, C.; Bollag, G.; van der Burgt, I.; Musante, L.; Kalscheuer, V.; Wehner, L.-E.E.; et al. Germline KRAS mutations cause Noonan syndrome. *Nat. Genet.* **2006**, *38*, 331–336. [CrossRef]
31. Zenker, M.; Lehmann, K.; Schulz, A.L.; Barth, H.; Hansmann, D.; Koenig, R.; Korinthenberg, R.; Kreiss-Nachtsheim, M.; Meinecke, P.; Morlot, S.; et al. Expansion of the genotypic and phenotypic spectrum in patients with KRAS germline mutations. *J. Med. Genet.* **2007**, *44*, 131–135. [CrossRef]
32. Ekvall, S.; Wilbe, M.; Dahlgren, J.; Legius, E.; van Haeringen, A.; Westphal, O.; Annerén, G.; Bondeson, M.L. Mutation in NRAS in familial Noonan syndrome-case report and review of the literature. *BMC Med. Genet.* **2015**, *16*, 95. [CrossRef]
33. Altmüller, F.; Lissewski, C.; Bertola, D.; Flex, E.; Stark, Z.; Spranger, S.; Baynam, G.; Buscarilli, M.; Dyack, S.; Gillis, J.; et al. Genotype and phenotype spectrum of NRAS germline variants. *Eur. J. Hum. Genet.* **2017**, *25*, 823–831. [CrossRef]
34. De Filippi, P.; Zecca, M.; Lisini, D.; Rosti, V.; Cagioni, C.; Carlo-Stella, C.; Radi, D.; Veggiotti, P.; Mastronuzzi, A.; Acquaviva, A.; et al. Germ-line mutation of the NRAS gene may be responsible for the development of juvenile myelomonocytic leukaemia. *Br. J. Haematol.* **2009**, *147*, 706–709. [CrossRef]

35. Doisaki, S.; Muramatsu, H.; Shimada, A.; Takahashi, Y.; Mori-Ezaki, M.; Sato, M.; Kawaguchi, H.; Kinoshita, A.; Sotomatsu, M.; Hayashi, Y.; et al. Somatic mosaicism for oncogenic NRAS mutations in juvenile myelomonocytic leukemia. *Blood* **2012**, *120*, 1485–1488. [CrossRef]
36. Kratz, C.P.; Schubert, S.; Bollag, G.; Niemeyer, C.M.; Shannon, K.M.; Zenker, M. Germline Mutations in Components of the Ras Signaling Pathway in Noonan Syndrome and Related Disorders. *Cell Cycle* **2006**, *5*, 1607–1611. [CrossRef]
37. Murakami, N.; Okuno, Y.; Yoshida, K.; Shiraishi, Y.; Nagae, G.; Suzuki, K.; Narita, A.; Sakaguchi, H.; Kawashima, N.; Wang, X.; et al. Integrated molecular profiling of juvenile myelomonocytic leukemia. *Blood* **2018**, *131*, 1576–1586. [CrossRef]
38. Niemeyer, C.M.; Kang, M.W.; Shin, D.H.; Furlan, I.; Erlacher, M.; Bunin, N.J.; Bunda, S.; Finklestein, J.Z.; Gorr, T.A.; Mehta, P.; et al. Germline CBL mutations cause developmental abnormalities and predispose to juvenile myelomonocytic leukemia. *Nat. Genet.* **2010**, *42*, 794. [CrossRef]
39. Hecht, A.; Meyer, J.A.; Behnert, A.; Wong, E.; Chehab, F.; Olshen, A.; Hechmer, A.; Aftandilian, C.; Bhat, R.; Choi, S.W.; et al. Molecular and phenotypic diversity of CBL-mutated juvenile myelomonocytic leukemia. *Haematologica* **2022**, *107*, 178–186. [CrossRef]
40. Pérez, B.; Mechinaud, F.; Galambrun, C.; Ben Romdhane, N.; Isidor, B.; Philip, N.; Derain-Court, J.; Cassinat, B.; Lachenaud, J.; Kaltenbach, S.; et al. Germline mutations of the CBL gene define a new genetic syndrome with predisposition to juvenile myelomonocytic leukaemia. *J. Med. Genet.* **2010**, *47*, 686–691. [CrossRef]
41. Martinelli, S.; De Luca, A.; Stellacci, E.; Rossi, C.; Checquolo, S.; Lepri, F.; Caputo, V.; Silvano, M.; Buscherini, F.; Consoli, F.; et al. Heterozygous germline mutations in the CBL tumor-suppressor gene cause a Noonan syndrome-like phenotype. *Am. J. Hum. Genet.* **2010**, *87*, 250–257. [CrossRef]
42. Loh, M.L.; Sakai, D.S.; Flotho, C.; Kang, M.; Fliegauf, M.; Archambeault, S.; Mullighan, C.G.; Chen, L.; Bergstraesser, E.; Bueso-Ramos, C.E.; et al. Mutations in CBL occur frequently in juvenile myelomonocytic leukemia. *Blood* **2009**, *114*, 1859–1863. [CrossRef]
43. Muramatsu, H.; Makishima, H.; Jankowska, A.M.; Cazzolli, H.; O'Keefe, C.; Yoshida, N.; Xu, Y.; Nishio, N.; Hama, A.; Yagasaki, H.; et al. Mutations of an E3 ubiquitin ligase c-Cbl but not TET2 mutations are pathogenic in juvenile myelomonocytic leukemia. *Blood* **2010**, *115*, 1969–1975. [CrossRef]
44. Pérez, B.; Kosmider, O.; Cassinat, B.; Renneville, A.; Lachenaud, J.; Kaltenbach, S.; Bertrand, Y.; Baruchel, A.; Chomienne, C.; Fontenay, M.; et al. Genetic typing of CBL, ASXL1, RUNX1, TET2 and JAK2 in juvenile myelomonocytic leukaemia reveals a genetic profile distinct from chronic myelomonocytic leukaemia. *Br. J. Haematol.* **2010**, *151*, 460–468. [CrossRef]
45. Matsuda, K.; Taira, C.; Sakashita, K.; Saito, S.; Tanaka-Yanagisawa, M.; Yanagisawa, R.; Nakazawa, Y.; Shiohara, M.; Fukushima, K.; Oda, M.; et al. Long-term survival after nonintensive chemotherapy in some juvenile myelomonocytic leukemia patients with CBL mutations, and the possible presence of healthy persons with the mutations. *Blood* **2010**, *115*, 5429–5431. [CrossRef]
46. Mohapatra, B.; Ahmad, G.; Nadeau, S.; Zutshi, N.; An, W.; Scheffe, S.; Dong, L.; Feng, D.; Goetz, B.; Arya, P.; et al. Protein tyrosine kinase regulation by ubiquitination: Critical roles of Cbl-family ubiquitin ligases. *Biochim. Biophys. Acta* **2013**, *1833*, 122–139. [CrossRef]
47. Zheng, N.; Wang, P.; Jeffrey, P.D.; Pavletich, N.P. Structure of a c-Cbl–UbcH7 Complex: RING Domain Function in Ubiquitin-Protein Ligases. *Cell* **2000**, *102*, 533–539. [CrossRef]
48. Javadi, M.; Richmond, T.D.; Huang, K.; Barber, D.L. CBL Linker Region and RING Finger Mutations Lead to Enhanced Granulocyte-Macrophage Colony-stimulating Factor (GM-CSF) Signaling via Elevated Levels of JAK2 and LYN. *J. Biol. Chem.* **2013**, *288*, 19459. [CrossRef] [PubMed]
49. Belizaire, R.; Koochaki, S.H.J.; Udeshi, N.D.; Vedder, A.; Sun, L.; Svinkina, T.; Hartigan, C.; McConkey, M.; Kovalcik, V.; Bizuayehu, A.; et al. CBL mutations drive PI3K/AKT signaling via increased interaction with LYN and PIK3R1. *Blood* **2021**, *137*, 2209–2220. [CrossRef] [PubMed]
50. Park, R.K.; Kyono, W.T.; Liu, Y.; Durden, D.L. CBL-GRB2 Interaction in Myeloid Immunoreceptor Tyrosine Activation Motif Signaling. *J. Immunol.* **1998**, *160*, 5018–5027. [PubMed]
51. Schmidt, M.H.H.; Dikic, I. The Cbl interactome and its functions. *Nat. Rev. Mol. Cell Biol.* **2005**, *6*, 907–919. [CrossRef]
52. Budays, L.; Egan, S.E.; Rodriguez Viciana, P.; Cantrello, D.A.; Downward, J. A Complex of Grb2 Adaptor Protein, Sos Exchange Factor, and a 36-kDa Membrane-bound Tyrosine Phosphoprotein Is Implicated in Ras Activation in T Cells. *J. Biol. Chem.* **1994**, *269*, 9019–9023. [CrossRef]
53. Buday, L.; Khwaja, A.; Sipeki, S.; Faragó, A.; Downward, J. Interactions of Cbl with two adapter proteins, Grb2 and Crk, upon T cell activation. *J. Biol. Chem.* **1996**, *271*, 6159–6163. [CrossRef]
54. Grossmann, K.S.; Rosário, M.; Birchmeier, C.; Birchmeier, W. The Tyrosine Phosphatase Shp2 in Development and Cancer. *Adv. Cancer Res.* **2010**, *106*, 53–89. [CrossRef]
55. Bunda, S.; Heir, P.; Srikumar, T.; Cook, J.D.; Burrell, K.; Kano, Y.; Lee, J.E.; Zadeh, G.; Raught, B.; Ohh, M. Src promotes GTPase activity of Ras via tyrosine 32 phosphorylation. *Proc. Natl. Acad. Sci. USA* **2014**, *111*, E3785–E3794. [CrossRef]
56. Rauen, K.A. The RASopathies. *Annu. Rev. Genomics Hum. Genet.* **2013**, *14*, 355. [CrossRef]
57. Steinemann, D.; Arning, L.; Praulich, I.; Stuhrmann, M.; Hasle, H.; Starý, J.; Schlegelberger, B.; Niemeyer, C.M.; Flotho, C. Mitotic recombination and compound-heterozygous mutations are predominant NF1-inactivating mechanisms in children with juvenile myelomonocytic leukemia and neurofibromatosis type 1. *Haematologica* **2010**, *95*, 320–323. [CrossRef]

58. Martin, G.A.; Viskoohil, D.; Bollag, G.; McCabe, P.C.; Crosier, W.J.; Haubruck, H.; Conroy, L.; Clark, R.; O'Connell, P.; Cawthon, R.M.; et al. The GAP-related domain of the neurofibromatosis type 1 gene product interacts with ras p21. *Cell* **1990**, *63*, 843–849. [CrossRef]
59. Xu, G.; Lin, B.; Tanaka, K.; Dunn, D.; Wood, D.; Gesteland, R.; White, R.; Weiss, R.; Tamanoi, F.; GF, X.; et al. The catalytic domain of the neurofibromatosis type 1 gene product stimulates ras GTPase and complements ira mutants of S. cerevisiae. *Cell* **1990**, *63*, 835–841. [CrossRef]
60. Scheffzek, K.; Ahmadian, M.R.; Wiesmüller, L.; Kabsch, W.; Stege, P.; Schmitz, F.; Wittinghofer, A. Structural analysis of the GAP-related domain from neurofibromin and its implications. *EMBO J.* **1998**, *17*, 4313. [CrossRef]
61. Flotho, C.; Steinemann, D.; Mullighan, C.G.; Neale, G.; Mayer, K.; Kratz, C.P.; Schlegelberger, B.; Downing, J.R.; Niemeyer, C.M. Genome-wide single-nucleotide polymorphism analysis in juvenile myelomonocytic leukemia identifies uniparental disomy surrounding the NF1 locus in cases associated with neurofibromatosis but not in cases with mutant RAS or PTPN11. *Oncogene* **2007**, *26*, 5816–5821. [CrossRef] [PubMed]
62. Side, L.E.; Emanuel, P.D.; Taylor, B.; Franklin, J.; Thompson, P.; Castleberry, R.P.; Shannon, K.M. Mutations of the NF1 Gene in Children with Juvenile Myelomonocytic Leukemia Without Clinical Evidence of Neurofibromatosis, Type 1. *Blood* **1998**, *92*, 267–272. [CrossRef] [PubMed]
63. Cichowski, K.; Santiago, S.; Jardim, M.; Johnson, B.W.; Jacks, T. Dynamic regulation of the Ras pathway via proteolysis of the NF1 tumor suppressor. *Genes Dev.* **2003**, *17*, 449. [CrossRef] [PubMed]
64. Stieglitz, E.; Taylor-Weiner, A.N.; Chang, T.Y.; Gelston, L.C.; Wang, Y.-D.D.; Mazor, T.; Esquivel, E.; Yu, A.; Seepo, S.; Olsen, S.R.; et al. The genomic landscape of juvenile myelomonocytic leukemia. *Nat. Genet.* **2015**, *47*, 1326–1333. [CrossRef] [PubMed]
65. Morerio, C.; Acquila, M.; Rosanda, C.; Rapella, A.; Dufour, C.; Locatelli, F.; Maserati, E.; Pasquali, F.; Panarello, C. HCMOGT-1 Is a Novel Fusion Partner to PDGFRB in Juvenile Myelomonocytic Leukemia with t(5;17)(q33;p11.2). *Cancer Res.* **2004**, *64*, 2649–2651. [CrossRef] [PubMed]
66. Byrgazov, K.; Kastner, R.; Dworzak, M.; Hoermann, G.; Haas, O.A.; Ulreich, R.; Urban, C.E.; Hantschel, O.D.; Valent, P.; Lion, T. A Novel Fusion Gene NDEL1-Pdgfrb in a Patient with JMML with a New Variant of TKI-Resistant Mutation in the Kinase Domain of PDGFRβ. *Blood* **2014**, *124*, 613. [CrossRef]
67. Chao, A.K.; Meyer, J.A.; Lee, A.G.; Hecht, A.; Tarver, T.; Van Ziffle, J.; Koegel, A.K.; Golden, C.; Braun, B.S.; Sweet-Cordero, E.A.; et al. Fusion driven JMML: A novel CCDC88C–FLT3 fusion responsive to sorafenib identified by RNA sequencing. *Leukemia* **2020**, *34*, 662–666. [CrossRef] [PubMed]
68. Morris, S.W.; Kirstein, M.N.; Valentine, M.B.; Dittmer, K.G.; Shapiro, D.N.; Saltman, D.L.; Look, A.T. Fusion of a kinase gene, ALK, to a nucleolar protein gene, NPM, in non-Hodgkin's lymphoma. *Science* **1994**, *263*, 1281–1284. [CrossRef] [PubMed]
69. Maesako, Y.; Izumi, K.; Okamori, S.; Takeoka, K.; Kishimori, C.; Okumura, A.; Honjo, G.; Akasaka, T.; Ohno, H. inv(2)(p23q13)/RAN-binding protein 2 (RANBP2)-ALK fusion gene in myeloid leukemia that developed in an elderly woman. *Int. J. Hematol.* **2014**, *99*, 202–207. [CrossRef]
70. Ma, Z.; Hill, D.A.; Collins, M.H.; Morris, S.W.; Sumegi, J.; Zhou, M.; Zuppan, C.; Bridge, J.A. Fusion of ALK to the Ran-binding protein 2 (RANBP2) gene in inflammatory myofibroblastic tumor. *Genes Chromosomes Cancer* **2003**, *37*, 98–105. [CrossRef]
71. Heilmann, A.M.; Schrock, A.B.; He, J.; Nahas, M.; Curran, K.; Shukla, N.; Cramer, S.; Draper, L.; Verma, A.; Erlich, R.; et al. Novel PDGFRB fusions in childhood B- and T-acute lymphoblastic leukemia. *Leukemia* **2017**, *31*, 1989–1992. [CrossRef]
72. Zhang, H.; Paliga, A.; Hobbs, E.; Moore, S.; Olson, S.; Long, N.; Dao, K.H.T.; Tyner, J.W. Two myeloid leukemia cases with rare FLT3 fusions. *Cold Spring Harb. Mol. Case Stud.* **2018**, *4*, a003079. [CrossRef]
73. Sakaguchi, H.; Okuno, Y.; Muramatsu, H.; Yoshida, K.; Shiraishi, Y.; Takahashi, M.; Kon, A.; Sanada, M.; Chiba, K.; Tanaka, H.; et al. Exome sequencing identifies secondary mutations of SETBP1 and JAK3 in juvenile myelomonocytic leukemia. *Nat. Genet.* **2013**, *45*, 937–941. [CrossRef]
74. Bresolin, S.; De Filippi, P.; Vendemini, F.; D'Alia, M.; Zecca, M.; Meyer, L.H.; Danesino, C.; Locatelli, F.; Masetti, R.; Basso, G.; et al. Mutations of SETBP1 and JAK3 in juvenile myelomonocytic leukemia: A report from the Italian AIEOP study group. *Oncotarget* **2016**, *7*, 28914. [CrossRef]
75. Cristóbal, I.; Blanco, F.J.; Garcia-Orti, L.; Marcotegui, N.; Vicente, C.; Rifon, J.; Novo, F.J.; Bandres, E.; Calasanz, M.J.; Bernabeu, C.; et al. SETBP1 overexpression is a novel leukemogenic mechanism that predicts adverse outcome in elderly patients with acute myeloid leukemia. *Blood* **2010**, *115*, 615–625. [CrossRef]
76. Piazza, R.; Valletta, S.; Winkelmann, N.; Redaelli, S.; Spinelli, R.; Pirola, A.; Antolini, L.; Mologni, L.; Donadoni, C.; Papaemmanuil, E.; et al. Recurrent SETBP1 mutations in atypical chronic myeloid leukemia. *Nat. Genet.* **2013**, *45*, 18. [CrossRef]
77. Bayarkhangai, B.; Noureldin, S.; Yu, L.; Zhao, N.; Gu, Y.; Xu, H.; Guo, C. A comprehensive and perspective view of oncoprotein SET in cancer. *Cancer Med.* **2018**, *7*, 3084–3094. [CrossRef]
78. Acuna-Hidalgo, R.; Deriziotis, P.; Steehouwer, M.; Gilissen, C.; Graham, S.A.; van Dam, S.; Hoover-Fong, J.; Telegrafi, A.B.; Destree, A.; Smigiel, R.; et al. Overlapping SETBP1 gain-of-function mutations in Schinzel-Giedion syndrome and hematologic malignancies. *PLoS Genet.* **2017**, *13*, e1006683. [CrossRef]
79. Oakley, K.; Han, Y.; Vishwakarma, B.A.; Chu, S.; Bhatia, R.; Gudmundsson, K.O.; Keller, J.; Chen, X.; Vasko, V.; Jenkins, N.A.; et al. Setbp1 promotes the self-renewal of murine myeloid progenitors via activation of Hoxa9 and Hoxa10. *Blood* **2012**, *119*, 6099–6108. [CrossRef]

80. Piazza, R.; Magistroni, V.; Redaelli, S.; Mauri, M.; Massimino, L.; Sessa, A.; Peronaci, M.; Lalowski, M.; Soliymani, R.; Mezzatesta, C.; et al. SETBP1 induces transcription of a network of development genes by acting as an epigenetic hub. *Nat. Commun.* **2018**, *9*. [CrossRef]
81. Carratt, S.A.; Braun, T.P.; Coblentz, C.; Schonrock, Z.; Callahan, R.; Smith, B.M.; Maloney, L.; Foley, A.C.; Maxson, J.E.; SA, C.; et al. Mutant SETBP1 enhances NRAS-driven MAPK pathway activation to promote aggressive leukemia. *Leukemia* **2021**, *35*, 3594–3599. [CrossRef] [PubMed]
82. Niemeyer, C.M. JMML genomics and decisions. *Hematol. Am. Soc. Hematol. Educ. Progr.* **2018**, *2018*, 307–312. [CrossRef] [PubMed]
83. Flex, E.; Jaiswal, M.; Pantaleoni, F.; Martinelli, S.; Strullu, M.; Fansa, E.K.; Caye, A.; De Luca, A.; Lepri, F.; Dvorsky, R.; et al. Activating mutations in RRAS underlie a phenotype within the RASopathy spectrum and contribute to leukaemogenesis. *Hum. Mol. Genet.* **2014**, *23*, 4315–4327. [CrossRef] [PubMed]
84. Caye, A.; Rouault-Pierre, K.; Strullu, M.; Lainey, E.; Abarrategi, A.; Fenneteau, O.; Arfeuille, C.; Osman, J.; Cassinat, B.; Pereira, S.; et al. Despite mutation acquisition in hematopoietic stem cells, JMML-propagating cells are not always restricted to this compartment. *Leukemia* **2020**, *34*, 1658–1668. [CrossRef]
85. Stieglitz, E.; Troup, C.B.; Gelston, L.C.; Haliburton, J.; Chow, E.D.; Yu, K.B.; Akutagawa, J.; Taylor-Weiner, A.N.; Liu, Y.L.; Wang, Y.D.; et al. Subclonal mutations in SETBP1 confer a poor prognosis in juvenile myelomonocytic leukemia. *Blood* **2015**, *125*, 516–524. [CrossRef]
86. Huang, H.; Bauer, D.E.; Loh, M.L.; Bhagat, G.; Cantor, A.B.; Kung, A.L. Potential Role of RUNX1 In the Pathogenesis of Juvenile Myelomonocytic Leukemia (JMML). *Blood* **2013**, *122*, 45. [CrossRef]
87. Buijs, A.; Bruin, M. Fusion of FIP1L1 and RARA as a result of a novel t(4;17)(q12;q21) in a case of juvenile myelomonocytic leukemia. *Leukemia* **2007**, *21*, 1104–1108. [CrossRef]
88. Mizoguchi, Y.; Fujita, N.; Taki, T.; Hayashi, Y.; Hamamoto, K. Juvenile myelomonocytic leukemia with t(7;11)(p15;p15) and NUP98-HOXA11 fusion. *Am. J. Hematol.* **2009**, *84*, 295–297. [CrossRef]
89. Coppe, A.; Nogara, L.; Pizzuto, M.S.; Cani, A.; Cesaro, S.; Masetti, R.; Locatelli, F.; Kronnie, G.; Basso, G.; Bortoluzzi, S.; et al. Somatic mutations activating Wiskott–Aldrich syndrome protein concomitant with RAS pathway mutations in juvenile myelomonocytic leukemia patients. *Hum. Mutat.* **2018**, *39*, 579–587. [CrossRef]
90. Yang, L.; Rau, R.; Goodell, M.A. DNMT3A in haematological malignancies. *Nat. Rev. Cancer* **2015**, *15*, 152. [CrossRef]
91. Laugesen, A.; Højfeldt, J.W.; Helin, K. Role of the Polycomb Repressive Complex 2 (PRC2) in Transcriptional Regulation and Cancer. *Cold Spring Harb. Perspect. Med.* **2016**, *6*, a026575. [CrossRef]
92. Shen, H.; Laird, P.W. Interplay between the cancer genome and epigenome. *Cell* **2013**, *153*, 38–55. [CrossRef]
93. Galm, O.; Herman, J.G.; Baylin, S.B. The fundamental role of epigenetics in hematopoietic malignancies. *Blood Rev.* **2006**, *20*, 1–13. [CrossRef]
94. Olk-Batz, C.; Poetsch, A.R.; Nöllke, P.; Claus, R.; Zucknick, M.; Sandrock, I.; Witte, T.; Strahm, B.; Hasle, H.; Zecca, M.; et al. Aberrant DNA methylation characterizes juvenile myelomonocytic leukemia with poor outcome. *Blood* **2011**, *117*, 4871–4880. [CrossRef]
95. Sakaguchi, H.; Muramatsu, H.; Okuno, Y.; Makishima, H.; Xu, Y.; Furukawa-Hibi, Y.; Wang, X.; Narita, A.; Yoshida, K.; Shiraishi, Y.; et al. Aberrant DNA Methylation Is Associated with a Poor Outcome in Juvenile Myelomonocytic Leukemia. *PLoS ONE* **2015**, *10*, e0145394. [CrossRef]
96. Poetsch, A.R.; Lipka, D.B.; Witte, T.; Claus, R.; Nöllke, P.; Zucknick, M.; Olk-Batz, C.; Fluhr, S.; Dworzak, M.; De Moerloose, B.; et al. RASA4 undergoes DNA hypermethylation in resistant juvenile myelomonocytic leukemia. *Epigenetics* **2014**, *9*, 1252–1260. [CrossRef]
97. Fluhr, S.; Boerries, M.; Busch, H.; Symeonidi, A.; Witte, T.; Lipka, D.B.; Mücke, O.; Nöllke, P.; Krombholz, C.F.; Niemeyer, C.M.; et al. CREBBP is a target of epigenetic, but not genetic, modification in juvenile myelomonocytic leukemia. *Clin. Epigenet.* **2016**, *8*, 50. [CrossRef]
98. Wilhelm, T.; Lipka, D.B.; Witte, T.; Wierzbinska, J.A.; Fluhr, S.; Helf, M.; Mücke, O.; Claus, R.; Konermann, C.; Nöllke, P.; et al. Epigenetic silencing of AKAP12 in juvenile myelomonocytic leukemia. *Epigenetics* **2016**, *11*, 110–119. [CrossRef]
99. Stieglitz, E.; Mazor, T.; Olshen, A.B.; Geng, H.; Gelston, L.C.; Akutagawa, J.; Lipka, D.B.; Plass, C.; Flotho, C.; Chehab, F.F.; et al. Genome-wide DNA methylation is predictive of outcome in juvenile myelomonocytic leukemia. *Nat. Commun.* **2017**, *8*, 2127. [CrossRef]
100. Schönung, M.; Meyer, J.; Nöllke, P.; Olshen, A.; Hartmann, M.; Murakami, N.; Wakamatsu, M.; Okuno, Y.; Plass, C.; Loh, M.L.; et al. International consensus definition of DNA methylation subgroups in juvenile myelomonocytic leukemia. *Clin. Cancer Res.* **2021**, *27*, 158. [CrossRef]
101. Kitazawa, H.; Okuno, Y.; Muramatsu, H.; Aoki, K.; Murakami, N.; Wakamatsu, M.; Suzuki, K.; Narita, K.; Kataoka, S.; Ichikawa, D.; et al. A simple and robust methylation test for risk stratification of patients with juvenile myelomonocytic leukemia. *Blood Adv.* **2021**, *5*, 5507–5518. [CrossRef]
102. Jelinek, J.; Lee, J.T.; Cesaroni, M.; Madzo, J.; Liang, S.; Lu, Y.; Issa, J.P.J. Digital Restriction Enzyme Analysis of Methylation (DREAM). *Methods Mol. Biol.* **2018**, *1708*, 247–265. [CrossRef] [PubMed]
103. Niemeyer, C.M.; Flotho, C. Juvenile myelomonocytic leukemia: Who's the driver at the wheel? *Blood* **2019**, *133*, 1060–1070. [CrossRef] [PubMed]

104. Yoshida, N.; Yagasaki, H.; Xu, Y.; Matsuda, K.; Yoshimi, A.; Takahashi, Y.; Hama, A.; Nishio, N.; Muramatsu, H.; Watanabe, N.; et al. Correlation of clinical features with the mutational status of GM-CSF signaling pathway-related genes in juvenile myelomonocytic leukemia. *Pediatr. Res.* **2009**, *65*, 334–340. [CrossRef]
105. Stephen, A.G.; Esposito, D.; Bagni, R.G.; McCormick, F. Dragging ras back in the ring. *Cancer Cell* **2014**, *25*, 272–281. [CrossRef] [PubMed]
106. Ward, A.F.; Braun, B.S.; Shannon, K.M. Targeting oncogenic Ras signaling in hematologic malignancies. *Blood* **2012**, *120*, 3397–3406. [CrossRef] [PubMed]
107. Stieglitz, E.; Ward, A.F.; Gerbing, R.B.; Alonzo, T.A.; Arceci, R.J.; Liu, Y.L.; Emanuel, P.D.; Widemann, B.C.; Cheng, J.W.; Jayaprakash, N.; et al. Phase II/III trial of a pre-transplant farnesyl transferase inhibitor in juvenile myelomonocytic leukemia: A report from the Children's Oncology Group. *Pediatr. Blood Cancer* **2015**, *62*, 629. [CrossRef]
108. Kazandjian, D.; Blumenthal, G.M.; Chen, H.-Y.; He, K.; Patel, M.; Justice, R.; Keegan, P.; Pazdur, R. FDA approval summary: Crizotinib for the treatment of metastatic non-small cell lung cancer with anaplastic lymphoma kinase rearrangements. *Oncologist* **2014**, *19*, e5–e11. [CrossRef]
109. Kennedy, V.E.; Smith, C.C. FLT3 Mutations in Acute Myeloid Leukemia: Key Concepts and Emerging Controversies. *Front. Oncol.* **2020**, *10*, 612880. [CrossRef]
110. Jenkins, C.; Luty, S.B.; Maxson, J.E.; Eide, C.A.; Abel, M.L.; Togiai, C.; Nemecek, E.R.; Bottomly, D.; McWeeney, S.K.; Wilmot, B.; et al. Synthetic lethality of TNK2 inhibition in PTPN11-mutant leukemia. *Sci. Signal.* **2018**, *11*, eaao5617. [CrossRef]
111. Wright, C.J.M.; McCormack, P.L. Trametinib: First global approval. *Drugs* **2013**, *73*, 1245–1254. [CrossRef]
112. Tasian, S.K.; Casas, J.A.; Posocco, D.; Gandre-Babbe, S.; Gagne, A.L.; Liang, G.; Loh, M.L.; Weiss, M.J.; French, D.L.; Chou, S.T.; et al. Mutation-specific signaling profiles and kinase inhibitor sensitivities of juvenile myelomonocytic leukemia revealed by induced pluripotent stem cells. *Leukemia* **2019**, *33*, 181–190. [CrossRef]
113. Goodwin, C.B.; Li, X.J.; Mali, R.S.; Chan, G.; Kang, M.; Liu, Z.; Vanhaesebroeck, B.; Neel, B.G.; Loh, M.L.; Lannutti, B.J.; et al. PI3K p110δ uniquely promotes gain-of-function Shp2-induced GM-CSF hypersensitivity in a model of JMML. *Blood* **2014**, *123*, 2838–2842. [CrossRef]
114. Deng, L.; Virts, E.L.; Kapur, R.; Chan, R.J. Pharmacologic inhibition of PI3K p110δ in mutant Shp2E76K-expressing mice. *Oncotarget* **2017**, *8*, 84776–84781. [CrossRef]
115. Liu, W.; Yu, W.-M.M.; Zhang, J.; Chan, R.J.; Loh, M.L.; Zhang, Z.; Bunting, K.D. Inhibition of the Gab2/PI3K/mTOR signaling ameliorates myeloid malignancy caused by Ptpn11 (Shp2) gain-of-function mutations. *Leukemia* **2017**, *31*, 1415–1422. [CrossRef]
116. Niemeyer, C.M.; Flotho, C.; Lipka, D.B.; Stary, J.; Rössig, C.; Baruchel, A.; Klingebiel, T.; Micalizzi, C.; Michel, G.; Nysom, K.; et al. Response to upfront azacitidine in juvenile myelomonocytic leukemia in the AZA-JMML-001 trial. *Blood Adv.* **2021**, *5*, 2901–2908. [CrossRef]
117. Furlan, I.; Niemeyer, C.M.; Batz, C.; Flotho, C.; Mohr, B.; Lübbert, M.; Suttorp, M. Intriguing response to azacitidine in a patient with juvenile myelomonocytic leukemia and monosomy 7. *Blood* **2009**, *113*, 2867–2868. [CrossRef]
118. Cseh, A.; Niemeyer, C.M.; Yoshimi, A.; Dworzak, M.; Hasle, H.; Van Den Heuvel-Eibrink, M.M.; Locatelli, F.; Masetti, R.; Schmugge, M.; Groß-Wieltsch, U.; et al. Bridging to transplant with azacitidine in juvenile myelomonocytic leukemia: A retrospective analysis of the EWOG-MDS study group. *Blood* **2015**, *125*, 2311–2313. [CrossRef]
119. Chang, T.; Krisman, K.; Theobald, E.H.; Xu, J.; Akutagawa, J.; Lauchle, J.O.; Kogan, S.; Braun, B.S.; Shannon, K. Sustained MEK inhibition abrogates myeloproliferative disease in Nf1 mutant mice. *J. Clin. Invest.* **2013**, *123*, 335–339. [CrossRef]
120. Lyubynska, N.; Gorman, M.F.; Lauchle, J.O.; Hong, W.X.; Akutagawa, J.K.; Shannon, K.; Braun, B.S. A MEK Inhibitor Abrogates Myeloproliferative Disease in Kras Mutant Mice. *Sci. Transl. Med.* **2011**, *3*, 76ra27. [CrossRef]
121. Fabri, O.; Horakova, J.; Bodova, I.; Svec, P.; Striezencova, Z.L.; Bubanska, E.; Cermak, M.; Galisova, V.; Skalicka, K.; Vaska, A.; et al. Diagnosis and treatment of juvenile myelomonocytic leukemia in Slovak Republic: Novel approaches. *Neoplasma* **2019**, *66*, 818–824. [CrossRef]
122. Hashmi, S.K.; Punia, J.N.; Marcogliese, A.N.; Gaikwad, A.S.; Fisher, K.E.; Roy, A.; Rao, P.; Lopez-Terrada, D.H.; Ringrose, J.; Loh, M.L.; et al. Sustained remission with azacitidine monotherapy and an aberrantprecursor B-lymphoblast population in juvenile myelomonocyticleukemia. *Pediatr. Blood Cancer* **2019**, *66*, e27905. [CrossRef]
123. Chan, R.J.; Cooper, T.; Kratz, C.P.; Weiss, B.; Loh, M.L. Juvenile Myelomonocytic Leukemia: A Report from the 2nd International JMML Symposium. *Leuk. Res.* **2009**, *33*, 355. [CrossRef]
124. Wehbe, Z.; Ghanjati, F.; Flotho, C. Induced Pluripotent Stem Cells to Model Juvenile Myelomonocytic Leukemia: New Perspectives for Preclinical Research. *Cells* **2021**, *10*, 2335. [CrossRef]
125. Yoshimi, A.; Balasis, M.E.; Vedder, A.; Feldman, K.; Ma, Y.; Zhang, H.; Lee, S.C.W.; Letson, C.; Niyongere, S.; Lu, S.X.; et al. Robust patient-derived xenografts of MDS/MPN overlap syndromes capture the unique characteristics of CMML and JMML. *Blood* **2017**, *130*, 397–407. [CrossRef]
126. Gandre-Babbe, S.; Paluru, P.; Aribeana, C.; Chou, S.T.; Bresolin, S.; Lu, L.; Sullivan, S.K.; Tasian, S.K.; Weng, J.; Favre, H.; et al. Patient-derived induced pluripotent stem cells recapitulate hematopoietic abnormalities of juvenile myelomonocytic leukemia. *Blood* **2013**, *121*, 4925–4929. [CrossRef]
127. Mulero-Navarro, S.; Sevilla, A.; Roman, A.C.; Lee, D.F.; D'Souza, S.L.; Pardo, S.; Riess, I.; Su, J.; Cohen, N.; Schaniel, C.; et al. Myeloid dysregulation in a human induced pluripotent stem cell model of PTPN11-associated juvenile myelomonocytic leukemia. *Cell Rep.* **2015**, *13*, 504. [CrossRef]

128. Shigemura, T.; Matsuda, K.; Kurata, T.; Sakashita, K.; Okuno, Y.; Muramatsu, H.; Yue, F.; Ebihara, Y.; Tsuji, K.; Sasaki, K.; et al. Essential role of PTPN11 mutation in enhanced haematopoietic differentiation potential of induced pluripotent stem cells of juvenile myelomonocytic leukaemia. *Br. J. Haematol.* **2019**, *187*, 163–173. [CrossRef] [PubMed]
129. Sbrana, F.V.; Pinos, R.; Barbaglio, F.; Ribezzi, D.; Scagnoli, F.; Scarfò, L.; Redwan, I.N.; Martinez, H.; Farè, S.; Ghia, P.; et al. 3D Bioprinting Allows the Establishment of Long-Term 3D Culture Model for Chronic Lymphocytic Leukemia Cells. *Front. Immunol.* **2021**, *12*. [CrossRef] [PubMed]
130. Janagama, D.; Hui, S.K. 3-D Cell Culture Systems in Bone Marrow Tissue and Organoid Engineering, and BM Phantoms as In Vitro Models of Hematological Cancer Therapeutics-A Review. *Materials* **2020**, *13*, 5609. [CrossRef] [PubMed]
131. Wolf, D.M.C.; Langhans, S.A. Moving Myeloid Leukemia Drug Discovery into the Third Dimension. *Front. Pediatr.* **2019**, *7*, 314. [CrossRef]
132. Lau, R.C.; Squire, J.; Brisson, L.; Kamel-Reid, S.; Grunberger, T.; Dubé, I.; Letarte, M.; Shannon, K.; Freedman, M.H. Lymphoid blast crisis of B-lineage phenotype with monosomy 7 in a patient with juvenile chronic myelogenous leukemia (JCML). *Leukemia* **1994**, *8*, 903–908.
133. Roy, A.; Wang, G.; Iskander, D.; O'Byrne, S.; Elliott, N.; O'Sullivan, J.; Buck, G.; Heuston, E.F.; Wen, W.X.; Meira, A.R.; et al. Transitions in lineage specification and gene regulatory networks in hematopoietic stem/progenitor cells over human development. *Cell Rep.* **2021**, *36*, 109698. [CrossRef]
134. Louka, E.; Povinelli, B.; Rodriguez-Meira, A.; Buck, G.; Wen, W.X.; Wang, G.; Sousos, N.; Ashley, N.; Hamblin, A.; Booth, C.A.G.; et al. Heterogeneous disease-propagating stem cells in juvenile myelomonocytic leukemia. *J. Exp. Med.* **2021**, *218*, e20180853. [CrossRef] [PubMed]
135. Kim, C.; Gao, R.; Sei, E.; Brandt, R.; Hartman, J.; Hatschek, T.; Crosetto, N.; Foukakis, T.; Navin, N.E. Chemoresistance Evolution in Triple-Negative Breast Cancer Delineated by Single Cell Sequencing. *Cell* **2018**, *173*, 879. [CrossRef]
136. Andor, N.; Lau, B.T.; Catalanotti, C.; Sathe, A.; Kubit, M.; Chen, J.; Blaj, C.; Cherry, A.; Bangs, C.D.; Grimes, S.M.; et al. Joint single cell DNA-seq and RNA-seq of gastric cancer cell lines reveals rules of in vitro evolution. *NAR Genom. Bioinform.* **2020**, *2*. [CrossRef]
137. Van den Berge, K.; Roux de Bézieux, H.; Street, K.; Saelens, W.; Cannoodt, R.; Saeys, Y.; Dudoit, S.; Clement, L. Trajectory-based differential expression analysis for single-cell sequencing data. *Nat. Commun.* **2020**, *11*, 1–13. [CrossRef]
138. Qiu, X.; Mao, Q.; Tang, Y.; Wang, L.; Chawla, R.; Pliner, H.A.; Trapnell, C. Reversed graph embedding resolves complex single-cell trajectories. *Nat. Methods.* **2017**, *14*, 979. [CrossRef]
139. Lönnberg, T.; Svensson, V.; James, K.R.; Fernandez-Ruiz, D.; Sebina, I.; Montandon, R.; Soon, M.S.F.; Fogg, L.G.; Nair, A.S.; Liligeto, U.N.; et al. Single-cell RNA-seq and computational analysis using temporal mixture modelling resolves Th1/Tfh fate bifurcation in malaria. *Sci. Immunol.* **2017**, *2*, eaal2192. [CrossRef]
140. Hu, Y.; Huang, K.; An, Q.; Du, G.; Hu, G.; Xue, J.; Zhu, X.; Wang, C.Y.; Xue, Z.; Fan, G. Simultaneous profiling of transcriptome and DNA methylome from a single cell. *Genome Biol.* **2016**, *17*, 1–11. [CrossRef]
141. Wierzbinska, J.A.; Toth, R.; Ishaque, N.; Rippe, K.; Mallm, J.P.; Klett, L.C.; Mertens, D.; Zenz, T.; Hielscher, T.; Seifert, M.; et al. Methylome-based cell-of-origin modeling (Methyl-COOM) identifies aberrant expression of immune regulatory molecules in CLL. *Genome Med.* **2020**, *12*, 1–19. [CrossRef] [PubMed]

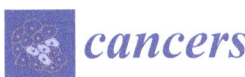

Review

The Genomics of Hairy Cell Leukaemia and Splenic Diffuse Red Pulp Lymphoma

David Oscier [1,*], Kostas Stamatopoulos [2], Amatta Mirandari [3] and Jonathan Strefford [3]

1. Department of Haematology, Royal Bournemouth and Christchurch NHS Trust, Bournemouth BH7 7DW, UK
2. Institute of Applied Biosciences, Centre for Research and Technology-Hellas, 57001 Thessaloniki, Greece; kostas.stamatopoulos@certh.gr
3. Cancer Genomics Group, Southampton General Hospital, Tremona Road, Southampton SO16 6YD, UK; a.mirandari@soton.ac.uk (A.M.); jcs@soton.ac.uk (J.S.)
* Correspondence: david.oscier@uhd.nhs.uk

Simple Summary: Hairy cell leukaemia is a rare chronic lymphoid malignancy with distinctive clinical and laboratory features which include an enlarged spleen, low blood counts, and infiltration of the spleen and bone marrow, with lymphocytes that have a villous or hairy cytoplasmic border. Historically it has been responsive to a range of treatment modalities including splenectomy, alpha interferon, and more recently chemotherapy, but none are curative. This review describes the chromosome abnormalities, genomic mutations, DNA methylation patterns, and immunoglobulin gene usage in this disease. We then discuss how the discovery of a specific mutation in a single gene (*BRAF*), present in almost all cases but not in hairy cell variant or splenic lymphoma with villous lymphocytes, two other splenic lymphomas with similar features, has provided new insights into its biology, a new diagnostic test, and a new therapeutic target.

Abstract: Classical hairy cell leukaemia (HCLc), its variant form (HCLv), and splenic diffuse red pulp lymphoma (SDRPL) constitute a subset of relatively indolent B cell tumours, with low incidence rates of high-grade transformations, which primarily involve the spleen and bone marrow and are usually associated with circulating tumour cells characterised by villous or irregular cytoplasmic borders. The primary aim of this review is to summarise their cytogenetic, genomic, immunogenetic, and epigenetic features, with a particular focus on the clonal *BRAFV600E* mutation, present in most cases currently diagnosed with HCLc. We then reflect on their cell of origin and pathogenesis as well as present the clinical implications of improved biological understanding, extending from diagnosis to prognosis assessment and therapy response.

Keywords: hairy cell leukaemia; HCLc; HCLv; SDRPL; *BRAFV600E*; Tbet

Citation: Oscier, D.; Stamatopoulos, K.; Mirandari, A.; Strefford, J. The Genomics of Hairy Cell Leukaemia and Splenic Diffuse Red Pulp Lymphoma. *Cancers* 2022, 14, 697. https://doi.org/10.3390/cancers14030697

Academic Editor: Gianpietro Semenzato

Received: 29 December 2021
Accepted: 25 January 2022
Published: 29 January 2022

Publisher's Note: MDPI stays neutral with regard to jurisdictional claims in published maps and institutional affiliations.

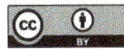

Copyright: © 2022 by the authors. Licensee MDPI, Basel, Switzerland. This article is an open access article distributed under the terms and conditions of the Creative Commons Attribution (CC BY) license (https://creativecommons.org/licenses/by/4.0/).

1. Introduction

The 2017 WHO classification of haematological malignancies recognises classical hairy cell leukaemia (HCLc) as a discrete entity and its variant form (HCLv) and splenic diffuse red pulp lymphoma (SDRPL) as provisional entities [1]. HCLc is a rare chronic lymphoproliferative disorder, with an incidence of 0.4/100,000. It is approximately four times more common in men than women and typically presents in middle age, with fatigue, infections, and abdominal discomfort due to splenomegaly. A complete blood count frequently shows cytopenia with almost universal monocytopenia, and a blood film usually reveals small numbers of medium-sized lymphoid cells with a 'kidney-shaped nucleus', infrequent nucleoli, weakly basophilic cytoplasm, and hairy projections. A modest lymphocytosis is seen in 5–10% of cases. Splenic histology shows diffuse infiltration of the red pulp with atrophy of the white pulp, a pattern also seen in HCLv and SDRPL, in contrast to the predominant white pulp involvement found in Splenic Marginal Zone Lymphoma (SMZL), which is the subject of a separate review in this series. Although originally believed to represent a tumour of haemopoietic progenitor reticuloendothelial cells [2], immunophenotyping identified HCLc as a tumour of mature B cells, typically expressing CD19, CD20, CD200, Tbet, PD1, and four markers of diagnostic value: CD11c and CD103, components of integrin receptors, and CD25 and CD123, components of interleukin receptors, of which at least three are expressed in all cases. Hairy cells do not express CD5 or CD27. Immunohistochemistry of bone marrow trephines additionally shows the expression of cyclin D1, CD72 (DBA-44), and Annexin A1, a specific marker for HCLc among B-cell malignancies, while bone marrow aspiration is usually unsuccessful due to the presence of reticulin fibrosis [3,4].

HCLv has an incidence of 0.04/100,000, a median age at presentation of 70 years, and a male-to-female ratio of 1.5–2. It was first described in 1980 in two patients with bulky splenomegaly, a marked leucocytosis with villous lymphocytes, and splenic histology showing red pulp involvement similar to that seen in HCLc, together with a number of distinctive features not found in HCLc. These include the absence of monocytopenia, larger tumour cells with prominent nucleoli, and bone marrow that is easy to aspirate due to absence or minimal marrow reticulin. Immunophenotyping shows the expression of CD19, CD20, and of the four archetypal HCLc markers, only CD11c and CD103 are commonly expressed, while CD25, CD123, and CD200 are negative or only weakly expressed. Immunohistochemistry shows the expression of CD72 but not annexin A1, and cyclin D1 is negative or weak [5,6].

In 2008, the term SDRPL was introduced to describe a further type of splenic lymphoma with circulating villous lymphocytes [7]. The frequency of SDRPL has not been established in the general population but represented 9% of splenic B-cell lymphomas seen in a 12-year period reviewed at the Spanish National Cancer Research Centre [8]. The clinical and laboratory features overlap those seen in HCLv, but the tumour cells generally lack a prominent nucleolus, and patients pursue a more indolent clinical course. Key demographic, morphological, phenotypic, and clinical differences between the three disorders are shown in Table 1.

Table 1. Key Differences between HCLc, HCLv, and SDRPL.

		HCLc	HCLv	SDRPL
Demographics	Incidence	0.4/100,000	0.03/100,000	?
	Median age	55–63	70	70
	M:F ratio	3–4: 1	1–2: 1	1.6–2.4: 1
Haematology	Monocytopenia	Yes	No	No
	Nucleolus	Inconspicuous	Single prominent	Inconspicuous
Immunophenotype	Surface IgH	Usually, multiple isotypes	Usually IgG +/− other isotypes	M+/−D, M+G, G
	CD11c	Strong	Strong	Moderate
	CD25	Strong	Negative	Negative (weak in 3%)
	CD103	Strong	Moderate	Negative (weak in 33%)
	CD123	Strong	Negative	Negative (weak in 15%)
	CD27	Negative	?	Negative (positive in 20%)
	CD200	Strong	Weak or negative	Weak
Immunohistochemistry	Annexin A1	Positive	Negative	Negative
	Cyclin D1	Positive	Negative	Negative
Outcome	Need for treatment	Yes	Yes	Approx. 50%

2. Hairy Cell Leukaemia

2.1. BRAF V600E Mutations

The whole-exome sequencing of a single case of HCLc led to the discovery of a single somatic, point mutation in the DNA sequence of v-Raf murine sarcoma viral oncogene homolog B (*BRAF*), a kinase-encoding proto-oncogene. The same mutation was subsequently found in all 47 additional cases studied. The mutation replaces thymine (T) with adenine (A) in exon 15 of *BRAF* at position 1799 of the gene-coding sequence located in chromosome 7q34. In turn, this produces an amino acid change from valine (V) to glutamate (E) at position 600 (V600E) of the protein sequence, ultimately leading to aberrant activation of the *BRAF* oncogenic kinase and, thus, of the downstream MEK–ERK signalling pathway, such that ERK phosphorylation (pERK), detectable by immunohistochemistry, is a ubiquitous finding in *BRAF-V600E* positive HCLc [9,10]. The *BRAF-V600E* mutation in HCL is clonal and heterozygous, except in a minority of patients who lose the wild-type allele as a result of a concomitant 7q deletion [11]. Details of the RAS–RAF–MEK–ERK pathway and the *BRAF* protein with the site of the *BRAFV600E* mutation are shown in Figures 1 and 2, respectively, and described in the accompanying legends.

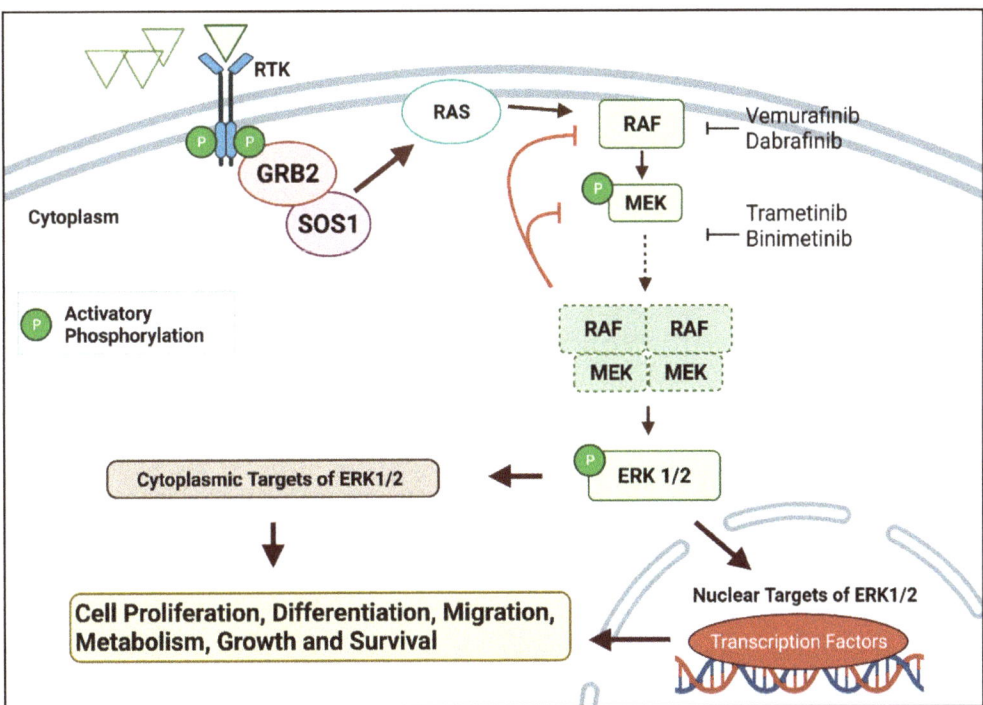

Figure 1. The RAS–RAF–MEK–ERK signal transduction cascade is one of four mitogen-activated protein kinase (MAPK) cascades which are activated in response to extracellular signals. RAS activation occurs within biomolecular condensates at the inner part of the cell membrane and recruits members of the RAF kinase family (A-RAF, B-RAF, and C-RAF/RAF-1) to the plasma membrane for activation. Active RAF kinases phosphorylate downstream mitogen-activated protein kinase/extracellular signal-regulated kinase ERK kinase (MEK). A transient tetramer, consisting of two RAF-MEK dimers, is formed to facilitate MEK activation by RAF. Active MEK then dually phosphorylates its only downstream targets, extracellular signal-related kinases 1 and 2 (ERK1/2). In contrast, ERK1/2 has extremely broad substrate specificity and is capable of activating both nuclear and cytosolic targets, many of which are transcription factors essential for the regulation of cell proliferation, survival, growth, metabolism, migration, and differentiation. In addition, ERKs also phosphorylate RAFs themselves at specific inhibitory amino acid residues, which releases RAF from RAS and extinguishes the signal via a negative feedback mechanism [12,13]. Created with Biorender.com (accessed on 28 December 2021).

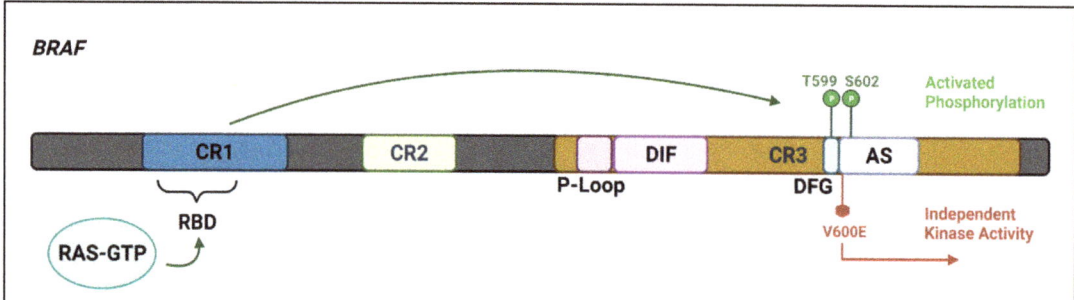

Figure 2. The *BRAF* protein includes three highly conserved regions—CR1 which functions as an auto-inhibitor of the *BRAF* kinase domain and contains a RAS-GTP binding domain (RBD), CR2 which acts as a flexible hinge between CR1 and CR3, and CR3, the kinase domain, which comprises multiple subregions including the P loop, the dimerisation interface (DIF), the DFG motif, and the activation segment. In the wild-type protein, inactive RAF exists in an auto-inhibited state. Under activating conditions, RAS-GTP binds to the RBD, disrupting auto-inhibition. *BRAF* is then phosphorylated at T599 and S602 within the DFG motif and activation segments, destabilising interactions with the P loop and allowing the activation segment to flip into its active conformation. The majority of *BRAF* mutants are located within either the P loop or the activation segment and adjacent DFG motif. The *BRAF-V600E* mutation occurs in the kinase activation segment, thereby inducing a change to the active conformation independently from upstream RAS activation. This results in constitutive kinase activity and aberrant signalling through the RAF–MEK–ERK pathway [14,15]. Created with Biorender.com (accessed on 28 December 2021).

BRAF mutations are found in a wide range of both solid and haematopoietic tumours, with a particularly high incidence in benign melanocytic nevi, malignant melanoma, papillary carcinoma of the thyroid [16], and the primary histiocytic disorders, Langerhans cell histiocytosis (LCH) and Erdheim–Chester disease (ECD) [17,18]. The clinical and biological consequences of *BRAF* mutations are highly variable and include the induction of a senescent phenotype, oncogenic transformation, and the emergence of secondary histiocytic sarcomas in a variety of acute or chronic, B or T cell, leukaemia, or lymphomas [19–21]. This variability may reflect the acquisition of additional genomic abnormalities such as the inactivation of cell cycle inhibitors, and the differentiation stage, transcriptomic and epigenetic features of the cell type in which the *BRAF* mutation arises [22,23].

2.1.1. Haematopoietic Stem Cell Origin of *BRAFV600E* Mutation in HCLc

To identify the cell population from which the *BRAFV600E* mutation arises, immunophenotypically distinct CD34+, CD38− lineage-negative cells which encompass haemopoietic stem cells (HSCs) and their immediate multipotent progenitors [24,25], CD34+, CD38+ pro-B cells, myeloid progenitor cells, and HCLc cells were isolated with >97% purity from the bone marrow of 14 HCLc patients and age-matched controls [26].

HCLc patients were characterised by an expansion of HSCs and a marked decrease in the frequency of granulocyte-macrophage progenitor cells, consistent with the neutropenia and monocytopenia characteristics of HCLc. The *BRAFV600E* mutation was identified in the HSC, pro-B cell, and HCL cell populations, and quantitative sequencing analysis revealed a mean *BRAFV600E*-mutant allele frequency of 4.97% in the HSCs. Furthermore, in one patient who also had chronic lymphocytic leukaemia (CLL), the *BRAFV600E* mutation was present in both tumour cell populations, consistent with the mutation arising in a common precursor. To identify additional co-occurring genetic lesions that might cooperate with the *BRAFV600E* mutation to promote haematopoietic transformation, targeted mutational analysis was performed on HCL cells from three patients in whom the *BRAFV600E* mutation had been detected in HSCs. An additional *ARID1A* or *KMT2C* mutation was present in the leukemic cells but not the HSCs of 2/3 cases. HCLc patients treated with vemurafenib showed restoration of normal myelopoiesis, demonstrating that the impaired myeloid differentiation in HCL is dependent on mutant *BRAFV600E* signalling. This raises the question as to whether the clinical response to *BRAF* inhibitors may be mediated through their effects on mature leukemic cells, as well as through targeted inhibition of signalling and survival in mutant HSPCs.

Although both arise from HSCs, the co-existence of HCLc and LCH in the same patient has rarely been reported [27], possibly reflecting the different skewing of *BRAFV600E* mutant HPC differentiation in mouse models along lymphoid or myeloid pathways in HCLc and LCH, respectively. [26,28,29].

2.1.2. Biological Consequences of the *BRAFV600E* Mutation in HCLc

The biology of HCLc reflects both cell-intrinsic factors as well as interactions with antigen(s), the extracellular matrix, the multiple cell types, and their secreted products present in the tissue microenvironment (TME) [30,31]. To ascertain the contribution of mutant *BRAF* to the HCLc phenotype, hairy cells from 26 patients were exposed in vitro to the specific *BRAF* inhibitors, vemurafenib or dabrafenib, or the MEK inhibitor trametinib. This resulted in the silencing of a gene expression signature which is specific to HCLc among B-cell tumours, with downregulation of genes including *CCND1*, *CD25*, and feedback inhibitors of ERK signalling such as members of the dual-specificity phosphatase (DSP) gene family. Additionally, *BRAF* or MEK inhibition caused loss of the hairy morphology and induced apoptosis which could be partially abrogated by co-culture with a bone marrow stromal cell line. *BRAF* and MEK inhibitors did not elicit any of the above-described biological effects in leukemic cells from four cases with HCLv, although the *MAP2K1* mutation status of these cases was not documented [32–34].

2.1.3. Incidence of *BRAFV600E* in HCLc

The initial description of the *BRAFV600E* mutation in HCLc identified the mutation in all 48 patients tested [9], and several subsequent studies also found an incidence of 100% [11,35–37]. In contrast, other studies of patients reported having the typical clinical, morphological, and immunophenotypic features of HCLc have included a varying percentage of cases lacking the *BRAFV600E* mutation, with by far the highest incidence (21–25%) found among cases with relapsed/refractory disease [38,39]. Alternate methods of MAPK pathway activation have been discovered in some of these cases, including rare *BRAF* exon 11 mutations [40] and a single case with a t(7;14) (q34;q32) translocation resulting in an *IGH-BRAF* fusion [41]. The translocation juxtaposes the IGM switch region with exons 10–18 of BRAF, including the protein kinase domain, while removing the N-terminal auto-inhibitory Ras binding domain which spans exons 3–5. This results in ERK phosphorylation of tumour cells, indicating upregulation of MAPK signalling. Of potential clinical relevance, this patient would be expected to respond to MEK, but not *BRAFV600E*, mutation-specific inhibitors.

In a study of targeted gene sequencing in 20 HCLc cases, 2 lacked a *BRAF* mutation, of which 1 had a *MAP2K1* mutation, while no genomic abnormality was detected in the other case [42]. Among 53 cases with relapsed/refractory disease, *BRAF* was wild type in 11 (21%), including all 5 cases with clonotypic B-cell receptor immunoglobulin (BcR IG) utilising the *IGHV4-34* gene [38]. In a follow-up study of 27 HCLc cases, 7 were *IGHV4-34* positive, and activating *MAP2K1* mutations were identified in 5 *IGHV4-34*-positive but only 1 *IGHV4-34*-negative case [43].

2.2. Other Genomic Abnormalities

The most frequent cytogenetic and genomic abnormalities and immunogenetic features found in *BRAFV600E* mutated HCLc, *BRAF* WT HCLc, HCLv, and SDRPL are summarised in Table 2.

Table 2. Most frequent features of HCLc, HCLv, and SDRPL.

			HCLc		HCLv	SDRPL
			HCLc *BRAF* WT	HCLc *BRAF* Mutated or Upregulated		
Recurring CNAs *		7q Loss		Y	Y	Y
		8q Loss (MAPK15)		Y	N	N
		17p Loss		Rare	Y	Rare
		X or Xp Loss (BCOR)		N	N	Y
		5q Gain		Y	Y	N
Genomic Mutations	MAPK Pathway	*BRAFV600E*	0%	>99%	0%	0%
		MAP2K1	22%	0%	22–41%	7–13%
	Cell Cycle	*CDKN1B*		16%		
		CCND3		0%	13%	21–24%
	Epigenetic Regulators **	*KMT2C*		15%	25%	
		KDM6A		0%	50%	
		CREBBP		5%	12–25%	
		ARID1A		4%	4%	9%
	Transcriptional Repressors	*BCOR*		0%	0%	16%
	NFKβ Pathway	*KLF2*		13%	0%	2%
	Spliceosome	*U2AF1*		0%	2/7	0%
		TP53		2%		
IGHV Genes	Homology	100%		<5%	18–22%	11%
		98–100%		17–20%	27–53%	14%
		<98%		80%	47–73%	86%
	Gene Usage	IGHV3-23		7–10%		14%
		IGHV3-30		7–10%		6%
		IGHV4-34	50%	7–10%	17–36%	22%

* % incidence of CNAs is not provided due to wide variations among studies. ** % incidence of mutations in epigenetic regulators is based on small samples.

2.2.1. Cytogenetic and DNA Copy Number Aberrations in HCL

Chromosome banding analysis (CBA) using a variety of B-cell mitogens identified clonal abnormalities in 70–80% of evaluable metaphases, but the nature and frequency of recurring abnormalities differed among studies. Abnormalities of chromosome 5, most commonly trisomy 5, or pericentric inversions and interstitial deletions involving band 5q13 were the most frequent abnormality in one study, detected in 12/30 cases [44]. Subsequent studies employing comparative genomic hybridisation also showed a varying incidence of copy number abnormalities (CNAs) but confirmed recurrent gains of 5q13-q31 and loss of 7q [45–48].

Two deep-targeted sequencing studies have enabled copy number analysis of regions sequenced by the panels. Among 53 *BRAFV600E* mutated cases of whom 22 were treatment naïve, recurrent abnormalities included deletions of 7q and of 13q14.3, encompassing *RB1* and the miR-15a and miR-16-1 microRNA cluster at 13q [11]. A second study of 20 cases sampled at diagnosis found loss of *MAPK15* in 7 (35%) of patients. The *MAPK15* gene, located on chromosome 8, encodes extracellular regulated kinase 8 (ERK8), a member of the MAPK family. The presence of a *MAPK15* CNA had no impact on treatment-free survival (TFS) and overall survival (OS), but progression-free survival (PFS) was significantly longer in cases with a *MAPK15* deletion [42].

2.2.2. Somatic Genomic Mutations

Current information on the nature and incidence of somatic mutations other than *BRAF* in HCLc is based on limited data—namely, whole-exome sequencing (WES) of 9 cases [9,49,50] and targeted sequencing using a large panel of cancer-related genes in 73 cases [11,26,42], together with targeted sequencing of specific genes: *CDKN1B*, *MAP2K1*, and *KLF2*. Mutations in these genes are described in more detail below. Recurring low-frequency mutations also involve chromatin modifiers, discussed in the next section on epigenetic abnormalities and genes involved in Notch signalling (*NOTCH1* and *NOTCH2*), and DNA repair (*RAD50*).

- CDKN1B

CDKN1B maps to 12p13 and encodes p27Kip1(p27), an intrinsically unstructured protein which regulates the transition from the G1 to the S phase of the cell cycle (Figure 3) and also has CDK-independent functions [51].

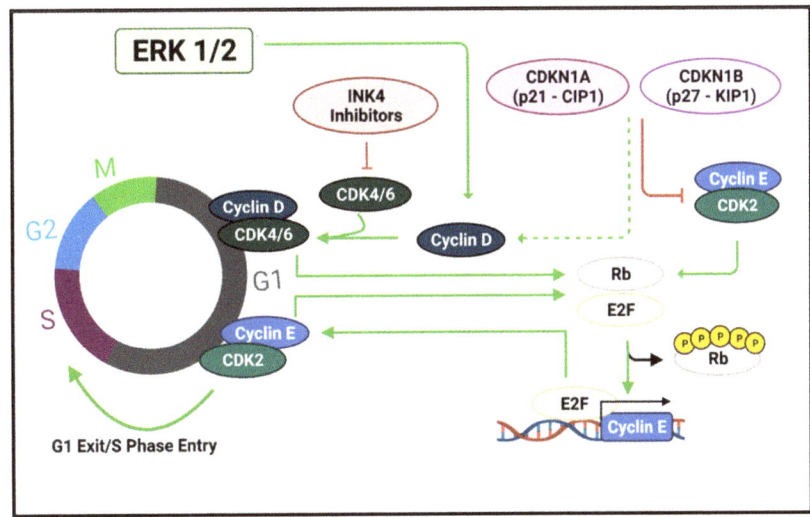

Figure 3. Mitogenic signals received during the G1 phase of the cell cycle, partially mediated through RAS-induced ERK signalling, upregulate the D-type cyclins D1, D2, D3, encoded by *CCND1*, *CCND2*, and *CCND3*, respectively. These bind and activate their catalytic partners, CDK4 or CDK6, whose activity is, in turn, negatively regulated by the INK4 family of inhibitors which include p16INK4A and p15INKB encoded by *CDKN2A* and *CDKN2B*, respectively. The formation of stable cyclin D-CDK4/6 complexes also requires the KIP/CIP proteins p21CIP1, p27KIP1, and p57KIP2, encoded by *CDKN1A*, *CDKN1B*, and *CDKN1C*, respectively, which serve as assembly factors for cyclin D-CDK4/6 but also act as inhibitors of Cdk2–cyclin E complexes required for transition into S phase [52]. Created with Biorender.com (accessed on 28 December 2021).

Low expression of p27 was demonstrated in all 58 cases of HCL studied and was associated with post-transcriptional downregulation, although the precise cause was not ascertained [53]. Subsequent studies in melanoma revealed a direct role for the *BRAFV600E* mutation: Expression of mutant *BRAF* was sufficient to upregulate cyclin D1 and down-regulate p27 in human melanocytes [54], while in melanoma cells, mutant B-RAF controls p27Kip1 expression via mRNA abundance and proteasomal degradation [55]. A further potential mechanism for low p27 in HCLc emerged from microarray expression profiling of HCLc, compared with normal and other malignant B cells, which identified overexpression of miR-221/miR-222c which negatively regulates the expression of p27 [56,57].

More recently mutations of *CDKN1B* were identified in 13 of 81 (16%) patients with HCLc. All harboured at least one *CDKN1B* nonsense or splice site variant, except for one case in which a missense mutation was identified. Three patients had more than one mutation. implying selective pressure to inactivate *CDKN1B*. Overall, 11/13 *CDKN1B* mutations had allele frequencies very similar to those of the *BRAF* mutant clone, suggesting that *CDKN1B* mutations are early lesions that may contribute to HCLc pathogenesis by impairing cell cycle control and/or circumventing oncogene-induced senescence. *CDKN1B* mutations did not impact treatment response to PNAs [49].

- KLF2

The Krüppel-like factor 2 (*KLF2*) zinc-finger gene, located at chromosome 19p13.1, encodes a transcription factor widely expressed in haemopoietic, endothelial, and lung cells. In B cells, *KLF2* regulates the expression of genes involved in cell homing, NF-κB signalling, and cell cycle control. B-cell-specific Klf2-deficient mice show a dramatic increase in cells with a marginal zone-like phenotype [58,59]. The KLF2 protein comprises activating and inhibitory domains, two nuclear localisation sequences (NLSs), and three zinc finger motifs (ZnFs). *KLF2* mutations are present in 20–40% of SMZL cases [60,61] and in three studies were also found in 9/74 (12%) cases of HCLc cases [42,62,63]. Mutations may occur in the activation, inhibitory, zinc finger or nuclear localisation domains, are predominantly truncating or missense, and reduce the transcriptional activity of *KLF2*, partly by displacement from the nucleus if mutations involve the NLS (Figure 4).

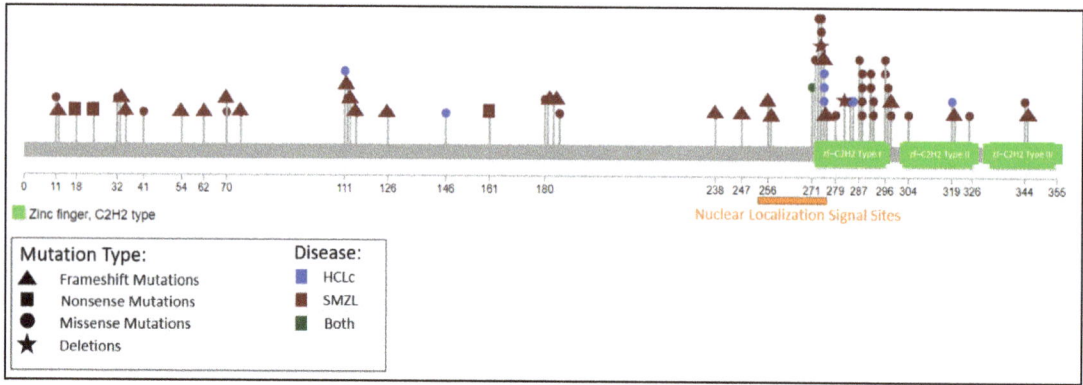

Figure 4. Distribution of *KLF2* mutations in HCLc and SMZL. Mutations were compiled from [42,62,64]. Diagram produced using Lollipops [65].

2.3. Germline Variants

Familial HCLc exhibits similar clinical features to sporadic HCLc but is rare, with fewer than 20 families reported in the literature. Four multiplex HCLc pedigrees were recently screened for shared germline variants, conferring HCLc susceptibility. Although there was only limited overlap between the pedigrees on a variant or gene level, several functional pathways such as neutrophil-mediated immunity and G-protein-coupled receptor signalling were shared in 3/4 and MAPK and RAS signalling in 2/4 pedigrees, respectively [66].

2.4. Epigenetic Abnormalities

The epigenome comprises chemical modifications to DNA and DNA-associated proteins which modify gene expression mediated through DNA methylation, histone tail modifications, chromatin accessibility, and DNA architecture and are critical for cellular differentiation and response to environmental stimuli. Post-translational modifications (PTM) of histone proteins regulate the accessibility of DNA to transcription factors and

DNA repair enzymes by a variety of mechanisms which include recruiting additional chromatin-modifying factors, reducing the positive charge of histones, and altering the positioning of nucleosomes [67]. Mutations of genes that encode chromatin modifiers may also target nonhistone proteins.

2.4.1. Mutations in Chromatin Modifiers

Mutations in genes involved in transcriptional regulation were found in 26/74 (35%) of HCLc cases [11,26,42]. The most frequently mutated gene was the histone methyltransferase *KMT2C* (MLL3) in which loss-of-function mutations throughout the coding region were identified in 15% (8 of 53) of cases [11]. *KMT2C* is a member of the KMT2 gene family which promotes methylation of H3K4 at enhancers and super-enhancers and transcription of genes related to cell differentiation or tumour suppression [68]. Other recurring mutations involve *CREBBP* and *EP300*, two interacting histone acetylation genes, and *BRD4*, *CEBPA*, *RUNX1*, and *MED12*. The transcriptional and phenotypic consequences of these mutations are highly context dependent, and their functional consequences in HCLc are unknown.

2.4.2. DNA Methylation Profile

DNA methylation profiling was analysed with the low-resolution Infinium Human-Methylation27 array in 11 cases of *BRAFV600E* mutated HCLc, together with cases of CLL, SMZL, and normal B-cell subsets. HCLc had a distinct global methylation profile which, nevertheless, was more closely related to SMZL than to CLL and to normal post germinal centre (GC) memory B cells and marginal zone B cells than to pre-GC and GC B cells. When probes inside or outside cytosine guanine dinucleotide islands (CGIs) were analysed separately, the CGI-only methylation profile clustered all HCLc samples in an independent branch, separately from post-GC B cells but together with two of seven SMZL cases.

An integrated analysis of the HCL methylation profile and the previously published gene expression profile showed an inverse correlation between gene expression and methylation, alluding to a role for DNA promoter methylation in the regulation of specific gene expression. Independent supervised analyses were then performed to compare HCL methylation with that of post-GC B cells, SMZL, and CLL. Differential methylation changes observed in HCLc that were also reflected in gene expression patterns were consistent with constitutive activation of the RAS–RAF–MEK–ERK pathway and also affected pathways involved in the homing, migration, and survival of HCL cells [69].

2.5. Immunogenetic Features

The analysis of immunoglobulin gene repertoires in B-cell malignancies has provided key insights into their ontogeny, including their cell(s) of origin, the role and nature of antigenic stimulation in tumour development and evolution; moreover, in some diseases, especially CLL, *IGHV* gene SHM status has prognostic and predictive value [70].

While the majority of cases of HCLc have mutated *IGHV* genes, 17–20% are unmutated using a 98% cut-off and <5% have completely unmutated *IGHV* genes, with 100% identity to the germline. Compared with the normal B-cell repertoire [71], there is biased usage of the *IGHV3-21*, *IGHV3-30*, *IGHV3-33*, and *IGHV4-34* genes, each found in 7–10% of cases, with preferential use of *IGHV3-30* and *IGHV4-34*, especially among the unmutated cases. Biased usage of *IGHD* genes has also been documented [72–75].

While kappa is the most frequently used immunoglobulin light chain in the normal B-cell repertoire and in other B-cell tumours, HCLc is associated with preferential use of lambda light chains, resulting in an inverted Igκ:Igλ ratio (0.7:1). The explanation for this is unclear but may derive from secondary IG light chain gene rearrangements as part of receptor editing, a physiological process leading to the pairing of the authentic heavy chain with a novel light chain as a means to alleviate intense autoreactivity.

While there is much less diversity within the light chain, compared with the heavy chain repertoire, there is evidence of biased usage in HCLc, as virtually all cases that express lambda light chains utilise the IGLJ3 gene. In addition, the variable lambda complementarity determining region 3 (VL CDR3) of lambda-expressing cases frequently share structural features, while restricted pairings exist between certain conserved lambda light chains and heavy chains encoded by the *IGHV3-21/30/33* genes [72].

All of the above features support a role for antigen selective pressure in tumour ontogeny. Moreover, the presence of intra-clonal diversification within the clonotypic IG genes indicates that ongoing SHM occurs post-transformation likely in a context of continuous interactions with antigen(s).

An unusual feature of HCLc is the expression of multiple *IGH* isotypes on the cell surface, documented in 40% to over 80% of cases. Single-cell analysis has confirmed that this phenomenon is attributable to the expression of multiple isotypes in individual cells rather than to clonal heterogeneity [76]. Heavy-chain isotype switching is mediated through class-switch DNA recombination (CSR) which occurs between two switch (S) regions located 5' of each *IGHC* gene. The intervening DNA segments are extruded via a cohesion-driven process and form extrachromosomal DNA switch circles. Deleted circle transcripts are not seen in HCLc cases expressing multiple isotypes, suggesting an arrest of CSR prior to deletional switching but where multiple isotypes can still be generated. CSR requires the upregulation of AID, enhanced chromatin accessibility mediated by histone modifications, and upregulation of factors such as IL-4, TGFβ, or IFNγ whose transcription is dependent on microenvironmental stimuli which determine the choice of specific isotypes. No genomic differences have been reported between cases that express either a single or multiple H chain isotypes, and the cause of the aberrant CSR remains uncertain [77,78].

The expression of multiple CH isotypes, including IgM with IgG or IgA, has also been reported in HCLv and SDRPL, although it has not been demonstrated if they are expressed in single cells. If so, this might point to a microenvironmental factor.

A further anomalous immunogenetic feature of HCLc is an increased incidence of cells expressing both IG kappa and lambda light chains. Dual expression of IG K and L light chains is rare in health, documented in only 0.2–0.5% of B cells from five normal controls [79]. Immunophenotypic analysis of 105 HCLc cases identified 3 (2.86%) that co-expressed surface kappa/lambda in virtually all cells. The immunogenetic analysis identified an additional case with a functional IGK/IGL transcript that also expressed multiple *IGH* isotypes and a RAG1 transcript. An increased incidence of dual light chain expressing cells is also seen in SLE [80] and in mouse models of autoimmunity [81–83]. The functional consequences of dual kappa and lambda light-chain expression are still unknown. That notwithstanding, evidence exists that compromised allelic exclusion leading to dual kappa/lambda expression might allow autoreactive cells to avoid clonal deletion, a mechanism described by the term receptor dilution [81].

2.6. Biological Implications: Cell of Origin

The identity and behaviour of tumour cells are largely controlled by the activity of transcriptional programs which reflect the programs active in, or available to, their cell(s) of origin, and/or their dysregulation by either cell-intrinsic genomic/epigenetic factors or cell-extrinsic interactions with the TME [84,85]. The biological and clinical significance of these variables has been well documented among mature B-cell tumours such as diffuse large B-cell lymphoma (DLBCL), mantle cell lymphoma (MCL), and SMZL [86–88].

The stem cell origin of the clonal *BRAFV600E* mutation in HCLc, together with the induction of a lethal haematopoietic disorder with features of HCLc in *BRAFV600E* mice [26], are consistent with the role of *BRAFV600E* as an early/initiating event in hairy cell leukemogenesis. However, there remains uncertainty about the nature of the mature B-cell population(s) expanded in HCLc and whether additional genetic and/or epigenetic alterations or a suitable TME are required to give rise to mature HCL cells. Dysregulation of the G1 phase of the cell cycle is a common finding in HCLc, but as yet, no subsequent genomic final transforming event has been discovered.

Data relevant to determining the COO in HCLc include the following:

1. The presence of mutated *IGHV* genes, with evidence for antigen selection, in the majority of cases and preferential use of the *IGHV4-34* gene in the minority of cases with low or no SHM;
2. A gene expression profile and methylome more similar to that of CD27 positive memory and marginal zone B cells than to naïve or germinal centre B cells [32,69];
3. A phenotype which includes expression of CD11c+, Tbet+, and PD1+ but not CD27 [89–92].

This phenotype also delineates a subset of normal B cells present in blood and splenic red pulp but rarely in lymph nodes. These cells also lack expression of CD21 and the chemokine receptors CD185 (CXCR5) and CD184 (CXCR4), reflecting their distribution within lymphoid organs. They frequently express sIgG, consistent with the role of Tbet in regulating antibody class switching to IgG1 or IgG3. Cells with a CD11c+ Tbet+ phenotype are found within B-cell populations variously described as age-associated B cells, atypical B cells, and double-negative B cells. CD11c+, Tbet+ B cell numbers increase with age and are expanded in conditions associated with chronic antigenic stimulation such as infections with human immunodeficiency virus and malaria, and in autoimmune diseases such as SLE. However, the CD11c+ Tbet+ phenotype does not, by itself, identify a distinct B-cell population, nor a specific B-cell lineage, and can be found in activated naïve B cells and in memory B cells believed to be generated through follicular or extra-follicular maturation pathways [93–99].

Immunogenetic, transcriptomic, and epigenetic analysis of B cells based either on the expression of CD11chi, Tbet, or a double-negative phenotype (CD19+ IgD- CD27- CXCR5-) shows significant differences from canonical CD11-ve Tbet -memory B cells [96,100,101]. Interestingly, the CD11c+ cohort is associated with enrichment of *IGHV4-34* gene usage [100]. Immunoglobulins encoded by the *IGHV4-34* gene display autoreactivity to the I/i antigens present on erythrocytes by virtue of a germline motif within the VH FR1 and additionally show cross-reactivity with other self and microbial antigens. Naïve B cells expressing *IGHV4-34* are often anergic, while this gene is largely excluded from switched memory and plasma cells. The persistence of this gene in a spleen-resident Tbet+ memory B-cell subset has been postulated to reflect either positive selection of B cells that may facilitate clearing of self-antigens or neutralisation of microbial antigens [102] or a defect in negative selection during GC transit [100].

It would be interesting to review the transcriptomic and methylation data in HCLc using normal splenic CD11c+ Tbet+ CD27- cells rather than CD27+ memory B cells as the comparator. However, currently, and as in CLL despite extensive studies [103], the COO of HCLc remains enigmatic.

2.7. Clinical Implications of Genetic Features

2.7.1. Diagnosis

The initial description of *BRAFV600E* in HCLc failed to find the same mutation in 195 cases of other mature B-cell tumours including CLL, follicular lymphoma, DLBCL, and other splenic lymphomas [9]. However, subsequent screening of larger cohorts of CLL and myeloma for both *BRAFV600E* and other *BRAF* hotspot mutations has identified a low incidence of predominantly subclonal V600E and non V600E *BRAF* mutations, usually associated with a poorer outcome [104–108].

Whilst a confident diagnosis of HCLc can be made without knowledge of the *BRAF* mutation status, the specificity of the *BRAFV600E* mutation for HCLc among splenic lymphomas is valuable when there is diagnostic uncertainty, and its presence underpins the use of targeted inhibitors. If it emerges that widely available diagnostic criteria are unable to distinguish *BRAFV600E* HCLc from *BRAFWT* HCLc, this would provide an additional rationale for *BRAFV600E* mutation screening. Allele-specific PCR performed on blood or marrow aspirate samples has superseded less sensitive molecular techniques such as Sanger sequencing, pyrosequencing, or melting curve analysis [109]. Digital, droplet PCR has comparable specificity and superior sensitivity to QT–PCR and is a potential method for MRD analysis [110]. Immunohistochemistry (IHC) using a *BRAFV600E*-specific antibody is an alternative method suitable for bone marrow trephine or other tissue sections, with comparable sensitivity and specificity to allele-specific PCR. Next-generation sequencing (NGS) also has high sensitivity but, currently, also has higher costs and longer turnaround time, compared with allele-specific tests [111].

2.7.2. Prognostic Significance of *IGHV* Gene Somatic Hypermutation Status

The clinical significance of *IGHV* gene SHM status in HCLc has been evaluated in two studies with discordant results. In a trial of single-agent cladribine in 58 previously untreated patients, all expressing annexin A1, failure to respond was observed in 5/6 patients with unmutated *IGHV* genes using a 98% cut-off value, only one of whom used *IGHV4-34*. Bulky splenomegaly, leucocytosis, and *TP53* abnormalities were present in four, three, and two of the five cases, respectively [73].

In a cohort of 62 patients with HCLc and 20 with HCLv diagnosed according to the WHO 2008 criteria [112], *IGHV4-34* was used in 6 (10%) of HCLc and 8 (40%) of HCLv cases, respectively, and was unmutated in all but 1 case, using a 98% cut-off value. A suboptimal response to first-line treatment with cladribine was seen in 4/6 *IGHV4-34* HCLc positive cases, compared with 4/56 *IGHV4-34* negative cases. A worse response was also seen in *IGHV4-34* positive HCLv cases, suggesting that outcome was more closely related to *IGHV4-34* status than to whether or not patients had HCL or HCLv. However, many of the HCLc cases were *BRAFV600E* negative [113].

2.7.3. *BRAFV600E* as a Therapeutic Target

The purine nucleoside analogues (PNAs), pentostatin, and cladribine remain the current treatment of choice for first-line therapy of HCLc. However, PNAs may cause short-term myelosuppression, with an increased risk of infection and an increased risk of secondary malignancies, and approximately 50% of patients eventually relapse. Single-agent vemurafenib or dabrafenib resulted in high overall response rates without minimal/measurable residual disease (MRD) negativity in relapsed/refractory HCL, but the median relapse-free survival in responders was less than 1 year [114,115]. In contrast, a phase II study of vemurafenib plus rituximab achieved a CR rate of 87%, of whom 65% were MRD negative and with relapse-free survival of 85% at a median follow-up of 34 months [116].

2.7.4. Genomic Abnormalities as Predictors of Drug Resistance

- To PNAs

Targeted mutational and copy number analysis showed no difference in the pattern of genomic abnormalities between treatment naïve cases and those refractory to a PNA [11]. Serial samples from two HCL-c cases tested both at diagnosis and relapse post-PNA therapy, revealed two additional subclonal mutations of *BCOR* (BCORE1430X) and *XPO1* (XPO1E571K) in one case, while the second case remained genomically stable [42]. However, there is no clear evidence to suggest that genomic mutations confer resistance to PNAs in HCLc.

- To BRAF Inhibitors

Of 13 evaluable HCLc cases treated with vemurafenib, 6 showed persistence of ERK phosphorylation in bone marrow cells, suggesting that, in at least some patients, the growth of HCL cells remains dependent on MEK–ERK signalling, likely reactivated through mechanisms bypassing *BRAF* inhibition by vemurafenib. In support, targeted sequencing of 300 genes performed in one patient who was refractory to vemurafenib showed two separate activating subclonal *KRAS* mutations at relapse [116].

A further case with vemurafenib resistance had heterozygous deletions of *BRAF*, *NF1*, *NF2*, and *TP53* and subclonal mutations in *CREBBP* and *IRS1* in a pretreatment sample. *NF1* and *NF2* encode tumour suppressors that have been experimentally implicated in RAF inhibitor resistance in epithelial cancer cells [117] and downregulation of either or both

Nf1 or Nf2 in Ba/F3 cells stably expressing *BRAFV600E* conferred vemurafenib resistance in vitro [11].

Seven distinct activating mutations in *KRAS* and two mutations in *MAP2K1* were detected in the relapse sample of a patient resistant to a PNA and vemurafenib plus rituximab. Allele frequencies were consistent with the parallel, convergent evolution of multiple clones with *KRAS* mutations appearing before *MAP2K1* mutations. Treatment with MEK inhibitor cobimetinib in combination with vemurafenib resulted in significant clinical and haematological improvement, associated with suppression of mutant allele frequencies for *BRAF*, *KRAS*, and *MAP2K1* mutations and of ERK activity [118].

Elucidating the mechanisms of resistance to *BRAF* inhibitors in solid tumours, especially melanoma, is an area of intensive investigation. In addition to the selection of genomic mutations such as mutations of *RAS* or *MAP2K1/MEK1* or of drug-tolerant persister cells, it is increasingly recognised that tumour cells may undergo non-genetic adaptive changes such as metabolic reprograming or reversion to a progenitor cell phenotype which result in drug resistance. It remains to be seen whether such adaptive changes will emerge in HCLc, a tumour with significantly less genomic complexity and instability [119–123].

3. Hairy Cell Variant

3.1. Cytogenetic and Copy Number Abnormalities

CBA showed an abnormal karyotype in 12/17 (71%) of cases, of which 5 (29%) were complex, defined as three or more chromosomal abnormalities. Recurrent aberrations included 17p abnormalities and del(18q) each in three cases. FISH analysis showed TP53 deletion or monosomy 17 in 5 of 12 (42%) cases and *ATM* deletion or monosomy 11 was detected in 2 of 9 (22.2%) cases. One case showed del(7q) by both conventional karyotype and FISH analysis [124]. Using single-nucleotide polymorphism (SNP) arrays in 15 previously untreated cases, CNAs were identified in 14 (93%) cases, with a mean of 7.9 abnormalities per case. Although the data are limited, combined CBA and SNP results suggest a greater degree of genomic complexity in HCLv than HCLc. Gains on chromosome 5 were identified in 5 cases and deletions of 17p and 7q in five and three cases, respectively [47]. Copy number analysis of regions covered in a targeted sequencing study identified 7q deletions and also recurrent 3p deletions which included a critical tumour suppressor locus encoding *VHL*, *SETD2*, *BAP1*, and *PBRM1* [11].

3.1.1. Recurring Mutations

Information on the genomic landscape of HCLv is also based on limited data—namely, WGS in 7 cases published in abstract from only [125], WES in 7 cases [43] targeted sequencing using a cancer gene panel in 12 cases [11,42], and targeted sequencing of *MAP2K1* in 25 cases [42,124,126] and of *TP53* in 30 cases [127]. No case had the *BRAF-V600E* mutation. Recurring mutations have been found in *TP53*, among cases with a 17p deletion [47], in *MAP2K1*, *U2AF1*, and *KDM6A*, as discussed below, and in *ARID1A* and *CREBBP*, while single mutations were identified in *CCND3*, in genes involved in transcriptional regulation (*CEBPA*, *DDX3X*, and *PBRM1*) and chromatin remodelling (*KMT2C* and *KDM5C*).

- MAP2K1

Waterfall first identified *MAP2K1* mutations in HCLv in 10/24 (41%) cases. The mutations mapped predominantly to the regions encoding the negative regulatory region and catalytic core (Figure 5) and are functionally active, increasing the basal enzymatic activity of MEK, encoded by *MAP2K1* [128]. The only non-missense mutation was a 48 bp in-frame deletion (amino acids 42 through 57) that almost entirely removed the autoinhibitory helix A13. Subsequent studies have confirmed the finding of recurring *MAP2K1* mutations but at a varying and predominantly lower incidence, with 2/4, 3/8, 2/11, and 1/14 cases and an overall incidence of 8/37 (22%) [11,42,124,126].

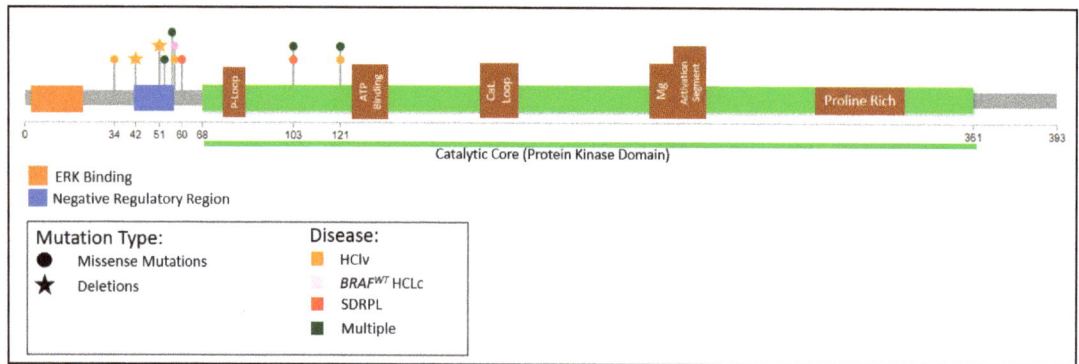

Figure 5. Distribution of *MAP2K1* mutations in *BRAF*^{WT} HCLc, HCLv, and SDRPL. Mutations compiled from [11,42,43,62]. Diagram produced using Lollipops [65].

- U2AF1

U2AF1 encodes the U2AF1 protein which heterodimerises with U2AF2, to form a key component of the splicesome. Among haematological malignancies, *U2AF1* and *U2AF2* mutations are largely restricted to myeloid neoplasms, especially high-risk myelodysplastic syndromes and acute myeloid leukaemia in which *U2AF1* mutants may alter the differential splicing of many genes that affect various biological pathways, including DNA damage response (*ATR* and *FANCA*) and epigenetic regulation (*H2AFY*, *ASXL1*, *BCOR*, and *DNMT3B*). Subclonal hotspot p.Ser34Phe *U2AF1* mutations were identified in 2/7 cases of HCLv [43] and in one case which underwent a high-grade transformation in a lymph node 7 years after presentation, the mutation was found in both pre- and post-transformation samples [129]. The biological significance of *U2AF1* mutations in HCLv is unknown, but they are potential targets for splicing inhibitors.

- KDM6A

KDM6A encodes a lysine demethylase protein that removes di- and tri-methyl groups from lysine 27 of Histone 3 (H3K27). Potentially deleterious mutations resulting in the loss of the highly conserved C-terminal region of *KDM6A*, essential for its demethylase activity, were identified in 2/4 cases, one of which was unresponsive to first- and second-line therapies [42]. Their biological and clinical significance in HCLv is unknown but the loss of *KDM6A* activity may sensitise tumour cells to demethylating agents such as EZH2 inhibitors [130].

3.1.2. Immunogenetic Features

Immunogenetic profiling in HCLv shows distinct differences in the incidence of somatic hypermutation and *IGHV* gene usage, compared with HCLc. A study of 41 patients revealed that 22% had truly unmutated *IGHV* genes, with 100% germline identity, and 5% were borderline mutated, with 97–99.9% germline identity. The most commonly used gene was *IGHV4-34*, in 17% of cases, of which 67% were truly unmutated [74]. Similar findings were reported in 26 patients, with 5/28 (18%) of rearrangements truly unmutated and 10/28 (36%) borderline mutated. *IGHV4-34* was used in 10 (36%) cases, and all were unmutated, using a 98% cut-off [75].

3.2. Clinical Implications

3.2.1. Prognostic Significance of TP53 Aberrations

A significant association was found between 17p deletion and shorter overall survival [127]. In a recently reported phase II study of CDA plus rituximab in 20 patients, the overall CR rate was 95%, and 80% achieved bone marrow MRD negativity at 6 months.

The five patients with a *TP53* mutation had a significantly shorter PFS and OS than those with wild-type *TP53* [131].

3.2.2. Targeted Therapy

In contrast to HCLc, current treatments for HCLv are suboptimal, with chemoimmunotherapy remaining the preferred initial therapy [6,132]. A patient with *IGHV4-34* expressing HCLv who had relapsed with skin nodules following multiple previous treatments, including chemoimmunotherapy and allogeneic transplantation, was found to have a somatic *MAP2K1* p.K57N mutation, with a VAF of 43.26% in skin and 20.08% in blood. He received the MEK inhibitor trametinib and achieved a partial response [133]. Based on partial or complete remissions following compassionate use of MEK inhibitors in patients with either HCLc with wild-type *BRAF* or HCLv, use of the MEK inhibitor binimetinib is currently being explored in a phase II trial of both patient groups who have relapsed or refractory disease, have received at least one course of a purine analogue, and who require further treatment. Trial inclusion criteria do not include a requirement to show evidence for dysregulation of the MAPK pathway such as a *MAP2K1* mutation or increased pERK expression [134].

4. Splenic Diffuse Red Pulp Lymphoma

4.1. Cytogenetic and Copy Number Abnormalities

The largest studies in SDRPL employing CBA identified cytogenetic abnormalities in 35–57% of cases, of which 13% had a complex karyotype. The most frequent abnormality was 7q deletion in 18–25%, while recurring trisomies of chromosomes 3, 12, or 18 were also seen [7,64,135]. In contrast, copy number analysis in 16 cases using array-comparative genomic hybridisation identified aberrations in 69% of samples, including recurrent losses of 10q23, 14q31–q32, and 17p13 in three, and 9p21 in two cases. Deletion of 7q31.3–q32.3 was present in only one case, and trisomy 3 or 18 were not detected [136].

4.2. Genomic Mutations

As with HCLc, the data are limited and based on WES in 33 cases, targeted sequencing using a panel of 109 genes relevant to lymphomagenesis in 42 cases, and targeted sequencing of *CCND3* in 34 cases and of *BRAF*, *MAP2K1*, *MYD88*, *NOTCH1*, *NOTCH2*, *SF3B1* and *TP53* in 23–36 cases. The most frequent recurring abnormalities involved *CCND3* and *BCOR*, as described below, while single- or low-frequency recurrent mutations were found in genes encoding proteins involved in cell cycle regulation, epigenetic regulation, the RAS–MAPK pathway, NF-κB and NOTCH signalling, cytoskeleton, and cell–matrix interactions [64,135,136]. No *BRAFV600E* mutations were found, but a single *BRAF* mutation (p.G469A) was identified in a case with a non-HCLc (CD103+, CD25-, CD123-) immunophenotype, expression of an unmutated *IGHV4-34*-encoded BcR IG and a *MAP2K1* mutation, highlighting the overlap of genomic and immunogenetic features in some cases diagnosed as HCLv or SDRPL.

4.2.1. CCND3 Mutations

CCND3 located at 12p13 encodes cyclin D3, required in normal B cells for the proliferative expansion of pre-B cells and of B cells within the dark zone of germinal centres [137,138]. In addition, cyclin D3 has several non-canonical functions which include the activation or repression of transcription either directly or via the recruitment of chromatin modifiers to gene promotors [139].

CCND3 mutations have been identified in 20–24% cases of SDRPL and almost invariably comprise missense variants in the negative regulatory proline, glutamic acid, serine, and threonine (PEST) domain, involving the amino acids T283, P284, and I290 which are part of a phosphorylation motif that regulates cyclin D3 phosphorylation and stability [64,140].

Cyclin D3 was shown to be overexpressed in >50% of tumour cells from splenectomy samples in all cases with a *CCND3* mutation and also in 19/24 cases without a *CCND3* mutation. *CCND3/IGH* translocations resulting in cyclin D3 overexpression have previously been documented in other B-cell lymphomas, but no *CCND3* translocations were detected using a *CCND3* Break Apart FISH Probe Kit [140]. Currently, neither the functional consequences of cyclin D3 overexpression in SDRPL nor the explanation for cyclin D3 overexpression in *CCND3* WT cases is understood. However, a subsequent study in cyclin D1 negative MCL expressing cyclin D3 revealed cryptic insertion of the IGK/L enhancer upstream of the *CCND3* gene that was undetectable by standard FISH probes and was associated with *CCND3* overexpression [141].

4.2.2. BCOR Abnormalities

The BCL6 co-repressor (*BCOR*) gene, located at Xp11.4., encodes the widely expressed BCOR protein whose function is highly tissue specific. In germinal centres (GC), BCOR interacts with polycomb repressive complex 1 (PCR1) and BCL6, facilitating the transient repression of genes associated with DNA damage response, cell cycle checkpoint control, GC exit, and plasma cell differentiation [142].

BCOR mutations, found in 16% of SDRPL cases, are characterised by splicing site (1/6), nonsense (2/6), and frameshift (3/6) alterations across the coding sequence, consistent with loss of function, as seen in other lymphoid and myeloid malignancies. Overall, 4/6 mutations exhibited a high variant allele frequency. Additionally, loss of the *BCOR* locus due either to a microdeletion or loss of a whole X chromosome was found in four SDRPL female patients, with no *BCOR* mutation within the remaining allele, resulting in an overall incidence of *BCOR* abnormalities in 11/42 cases.

BCOR mutations have also been identified in other non-GC-derived B-cell tumours such as SMZL, MCL, prolymphocytic leukaemia, and CLL. The functional consequences of mutations in these tumours and in SDRPL are unknown [64,143].

4.3. Immunogenetic Features

The great majority (79–89%) of cases have been found to carry hypermutated *IGHV* genes (<100% identity), with overrepresentation of the *IGHV3-23* and *IGHV4-34* genes. Of 10 cases using *IGHV4-34*, 6 were borderline unmutated, and 4 were truly unmutated, comparable to the findings in HCLv. *IGHV1-2* usage was confined to a single case [64,135]. Broadly similar findings were reported in another study of 13 patients [136].

5. Conclusions and Future Studies

A major focus of this review was the key role that the discovery of the almost ubiquitous clonal *BRAFV600E* mutation has played in understanding the biology of HCLc and its importance both in differential diagnosis and as a therapeutic target. However, there remain many unanswered questions regarding the diagnosis and biology of both HCLc and, particularly, HCLv and SDRPL. Of greater clinical importance is an unmet need for potentially curative non-chemotherapeutic regimens for HCLc and more effective treatments for HCLv which additional genetic data may help to resolve.

While the finding of a *BRAFV600E* mutation in HCLc unequivocally identifies a disorder with largely uniform laboratory and clinical features, methylome and clinical course, the pathogenesis of less frequent features such as skeletal involvement, found in 3% of cases [144], and a propensity to autoimmune disease [145] remain unexplained. Additionally, there is still much to learn about the incidence, biology, and optimal management of cases with a typical HCLc phenotype that lacks the *BRAFV600E* mutation or another mechanism for *BRAF* upregulation.

It is also unlikely to be coincidental that *BRAF* WT HCLc cases display enrichment for *IGHV4-34* gene usage, frequently accompanied by activating *MAP2K1* mutations, and that these two features are also found in a subset of cases with HCLv, raising questions about the inter-relationship between these two patient groups. If *IGHV4-34*-positive, *MAP2K1*-

mutated cases of HCLc and HCLv do exhibit the typical phenotypes of HCLc and HCLv, respectively, what might account for the differences between the two phenotypes?

There is also uncertainty about the relationship between HCLv and SDRPL, given their many overlapping features and the current absence of disease-defining genetic abnormalities. The absence of reports of the rare cases of SDRPL with progressive disease acquiring typical features of HCLv such as *TP53* abnormalities or prominent nucleoli would suggest they are not simply different stages of a single disease.

These uncertainties are, in large part, a consequence of the rarity of these disorders, the lack of cell lines and animal models, and the difficulty in obtaining tumour cells, especially in HCLc, where the circulating tumour cell count is usually low, bone marrow aspiration is unsuccessful, and splenectomy rarely performed [146,147]. This is reflected in the lack of genomic data on HCLc and especially HCLv and SDRPL, compared with that available in the more common B-cell tumours, such that the published genomic landscapes are unlikely to reflect the full range or true incidence of CNAs and mutations present in all three disorders.

New biological insights are likely to require studies in larger multi-institution patient cohorts, together with the application of newer technologies such as WGS, and transcriptomic and epigenetic analyses, both at the bulk and single-cell levels, comparing data from tumour cells with that from normal splenic B-cell subsets.

It is conceivable that these studies, in conjunction with a more detailed analysis of the TME, may lead to the identification of new disease subsets within or spanning the current diagnoses of *BRAF WT* HCLc, HCLv, and SDRPL, offer new insights into their cells of origin, and give rise to a more genetically based classification, offering more precise diagnostic and prognostic features and targeted therapies.

Author Contributions: Conceptualisation, D.O. and K.S.; data curation, A.M.; writing—original draft preparation, D.O.; writing—review and editing, D.O., K.S., A.M. and J.S. All authors have read and agreed to the published version of the manuscript.

Funding: A.M. is funded by the University of Southampton Centre for Cancer Immunology Talent Fund; J.S. is supported by the Cancer Research UK (CRUK) ECRIN-M3 program (grant C42023/A29370); the CRUK B-cell malignancy program (C2750/A23669); and CRUK Southampton Centre core funding (C36811/A29101).

Conflicts of Interest: The authors declare no conflict of interest.

References

1. Swerdlow, S.H.; Campo, E.; Pileri, S.A.; Harris, N.L.; Stein, H.; Siebert, R.; Advani, R.; Ghielmini, M.; Salles, G.A.; Zelenetz, A.D.; et al. The 2016 revision of the World Health Organization classification of lymphoid neoplasms. *Blood* **2016**, *127*, 2375–2390. [CrossRef] [PubMed]
2. Bouroncle, B.A.; Wiseman, B.K.; Doan, C.A. Leukemic reticuloendotheliosis. *Blood* **1958**, *13*, 609–630. [CrossRef] [PubMed]
3. Cross, M.; Dearden, C. Hairy Cell Leukaemia. *Curr. Oncol. Rep.* **2020**, *22*, 42. [CrossRef] [PubMed]
4. Maitre, E.; Cornet, E.; Troussard, X. Hairy cell leukemia: 2020 update on diagnosis, risk stratification, and treatment. *Am. J. Hematol.* **2019**, *94*, 1413–1422. [CrossRef]
5. Cawley, J.C.; Burns, G.F.; Hayhoe, F.G. A chronic lymphoproliferative disorder with distinctive features: A distinct variant of hairy-cell leukaemia. *Leuk. Res.* **1980**, *4*, 547–559. [CrossRef]
6. Matutes, E. Diagnostic and therapeutic challenges in hairy cell leukemia-variant: Where are we in 2021? *Expert Rev. Hematol.* **2021**, *14*, 355–363. [CrossRef]
7. Traverse-Glehen, A.; Baseggio, L.; Bauchu, E.C.; Morel, D.; Gazzo, S.; Ffrench, M.; Verney, A.; Rolland, D.; Thieblemont, C.; Magaud, J.P.; et al. Splenic red pulp lymphoma with numerous basophilic villous lymphocytes: A distinct clinicopathologic and molecular entity? *Blood* **2008**, *111*, 2253–2260. [CrossRef]
8. Kanellis, G.; Mollejo, M.; Montes-Moreno, S.; Rodriguez-Pinilla, S.M.; Cigudosa, J.C.; Algara, P.; Montalban, C.; Matutes, E.; Wotherspoon, A.; Piris, M.A. Splenic diffuse red pulp small B-cell lymphoma: Revision of a series of cases reveals characteristic clinico-pathological features. *Haematologica* **2010**, *95*, 1122–1129. [CrossRef]
9. Tiacci, E.; Trifonov, V.; Schiavoni, G.; Holmes, A.; Kern, W.; Martelli, M.P.; Pucciarini, A.; Bigerna, B.; Pacini, R.; Wells, V.A.; et al. BRAF mutations in hairy-cell leukemia. *N. Engl. J. Med.* **2011**, *364*, 2305–2315. [CrossRef]

10. Tiacci, E.; Schiavoni, G.; Martelli, M.P.; Boveri, E.; Pacini, R.; Tabarrini, A.; Zibellini, S.; Santi, A.; Pettirossi, V.; Fortini, E.; et al. Constant activation of the RAF-MEK-ERK pathway as a diagnostic and therapeutic target in hairy cell leukemia. *Haematologica* **2013**, *98*, 635–639. [CrossRef]
11. Durham, B.H.; Getta, B.; Dietrich, S.; Taylor, J.; Won, H.; Bogenberger, J.M.; Scott, S.; Kim, E.; Chung, Y.R.; Chung, S.S.; et al. Genomic analysis of hairy cell leukemia identifies novel recurrent genetic alterations. *Blood* **2017**, *130*, 1644–1648. [CrossRef] [PubMed]
12. Lavoie, H.; Therrien, M. Regulation of RAF protein kinases in ERK signalling. *Nat. Rev. Mol. Cell Biol.* **2015**, *16*, 281–298. [CrossRef] [PubMed]
13. Lavoie, H.; Gagnon, J.; Therrien, M. ERK signalling: A master regulator of cell behaviour, life and fate. *Nat. Rev. Mol. Cell Biol.* **2020**, *21*, 607–632. [CrossRef] [PubMed]
14. Wan, P.T.; Garnett, M.J.; Roe, S.M.; Lee, S.; Niculescu-Duvaz, D.; Good, V.M.; Jones, C.M.; Marshall, C.J.; Springer, C.J.; Barford, D.; et al. Mechanism of activation of the RAF-ERK signaling pathway by oncogenic mutations of B-RAF. *Cell* **2004**, *116*, 855–867. [CrossRef]
15. Dankner, M.; Rose, A.A.N.; Rajkumar, S.; Siegel, P.M.; Watson, I.R. Classifying BRAF alterations in cancer: New rational therapeutic strategies for actionable mutations. *Oncogene* **2018**, *37*, 3183–3199. [CrossRef]
16. Michaloglou, C.; Vredeveld, L.C.; Mooi, W.J.; Peeper, D.S. BRAF(E600) in benign and malignant human tumours. *Oncogene* **2008**, *27*, 877–895. [CrossRef]
17. Allen, C.E.; Merad, M.; McClain, K.L. Langerhans-Cell Histiocytosis. *N. Engl. J. Med.* **2018**, *379*, 856–868. [CrossRef]
18. Gulati, N.; Allen, C.E. Langerhans cell histiocytosis: Version 2021. *Hematol. Oncol.* **2021**, *39* (Suppl. S1), 15–23. [CrossRef] [PubMed]
19. Feldman, A.L.; Arber, D.A.; Pittaluga, S.; Martinez, A.; Burke, J.S.; Raffeld, M.; Camos, M.; Warnke, R.; Jaffe, E.S. Clonally related follicular lymphomas and histiocytic/dendritic cell sarcomas: Evidence for transdifferentiation of the follicular lymphoma clone. *Blood* **2008**, *111*, 5433–5439. [CrossRef]
20. Tsai, Y.T.; Lakshmanan, A.; Lehman, A.; Harrington, B.K.; Lucas, F.M.; Tran, M.; Sass, E.J.; Long, M.; Flechtner, A.D.; Jaynes, F.; et al. BRAF(V600E) accelerates disease progression and enhances immune suppression in a mouse model of B-cell leukemia. *Blood Adv.* **2017**, *1*, 2147–2160. [CrossRef] [PubMed]
21. Egan, C.; Lack, J.; Skarshaug, S.; Pham, T.A.; Abdullaev, Z.; Xi, L.; Pack, S.; Pittaluga, S.; Jaffe, E.S.; Raffeld, M. The mutational landscape of histiocytic sarcoma associated with lymphoid malignancy. *Mod. Pathol.* **2021**, *34*, 336–347. [CrossRef] [PubMed]
22. Tao, Y.; Kang, B.; Petkovich, D.A.; Bhandari, Y.R.; In, J.; Stein-O'Brien, G.; Kong, X.; Xie, W.; Zachos, N.; Maegawa, S.; et al. Aging-like Spontaneous Epigenetic Silencing Facilitates Wnt Activation, Stemness, and Braf(V600E)-Induced Tumorigenesis. *Cancer Cell* **2019**, *35*, 315–328. [CrossRef]
23. Baggiolini, A.; Callahan, S.J.; Montal, E.; Weiss, J.M.; Trieu, T.; Tagore, M.M.; Tischfield, S.E.; Walsh, R.M.; Suresh, S.; Fan, Y.; et al. Developmental chromatin programs determine oncogenic competence in melanoma. *Science* **2021**, *373*, eabc1048. [CrossRef] [PubMed]
24. Velten, L.; Haas, S.F.; Raffel, S.; Blaszkiewicz, S.; Islam, S.; Hennig, B.P.; Hirche, C.; Lutz, C.; Buss, E.C.; Nowak, D.; et al. Human haematopoietic stem cell lineage commitment is a continuous process. *Nat. Cell Biol.* **2017**, *19*, 271–281. [CrossRef] [PubMed]
25. Triana, S.; Vonficht, D.; Jopp-Saile, L.; Raffel, S.; Lutz, R.; Leonce, D.; Antes, M.; Hernandez-Malmierca, P.; Ordonez-Rueda, D.; Ramasz, B.; et al. Single-cell proteo-genomic reference maps of the hematopoietic system enable the purification and massive profiling of precisely defined cell states. *Nat. Immunol.* **2021**, *22*, 1577–1589. [CrossRef] [PubMed]
26. Chung, S.S.; Kim, E.; Park, J.H.; Chung, Y.R.; Lito, P.; Teruya-Feldstein, J.; Hu, W.; Beguelin, W.; Monette, S.; Duy, C.; et al. Hematopoietic stem cell origin of BRAFV600E mutations in hairy cell leukemia. *Sci. Transl. Med.* **2014**, *6*, 238ra271. [CrossRef] [PubMed]
27. Loghavi, S.; Khoury, J.D. Langerhans cell histiocytosis in a patient with hairy cell leukemia: A tale of divergence. *Blood* **2017**, *129*, 1563. [CrossRef]
28. Bigenwald, C.; Le Berichel, J.; Wilk, C.M.; Chakraborty, R.; Chen, S.T.; Tabachnikova, A.; Mancusi, R.; Abhyankar, H.; Casanova-Acebes, M.; Laface, I.; et al. BRAF(V600E)-induced senescence drives Langerhans cell histiocytosis pathophysiology. *Nat. Med.* **2021**, *27*, 851–861. [CrossRef]
29. Biavasco, R.; Lettera, E.; Giannetti, K.; Gilioli, D.; Beretta, S.; Conti, A.; Scala, S.; Cesana, D.; Gallina, P.; Norelli, M.; et al. Oncogene-induced senescence in hematopoietic progenitors features myeloid restricted hematopoiesis, chronic inflammation and histiocytosis. *Nat. Commun.* **2021**, *12*, 4559. [CrossRef]
30. Sivina, M.; Burger, J.A. The importance of the tissue microenvironment in hairy cell leukemia. *Best Pract. Res. Clin. Haematol.* **2015**, *28*, 208–216. [CrossRef]
31. Bohn, J.P.; Salcher, S.; Pircher, A.; Untergasser, G.; Wolf, D. The Biology of Classic Hairy Cell Leukemia. *Int. J. Mol. Sci.* **2021**, *22*, 7780. [CrossRef] [PubMed]
32. Basso, K.; Liso, A.; Tiacci, E.; Benedetti, R.; Pulsoni, A.; Foa, R.; Di Raimondo, F.; Ambrosetti, A.; Califano, A.; Klein, U.; et al. Gene expression profiling of hairy cell leukemia reveals a phenotype related to memory B cells with altered expression of chemokine and adhesion receptors. *J. Exp. Med.* **2004**, *199*, 59–68. [CrossRef] [PubMed]

33. Pratilas, C.A.; Taylor, B.S.; Ye, Q.; Viale, A.; Sander, C.; Solit, D.B.; Rosen, N. (V600E)BRAF is associated with disabled feedback inhibition of RAF-MEK signaling and elevated transcriptional output of the pathway. *Proc. Natl. Acad. Sci. USA* **2009**, *106*, 4519–4524. [CrossRef] [PubMed]
34. Pettirossi, V.; Santi, A.; Imperi, E.; Russo, G.; Pucciarini, A.; Bigerna, B.; Schiavoni, G.; Fortini, E.; Spanhol-Rosseto, A.; Sportoletti, P.; et al. BRAF inhibitors reverse the unique molecular signature and phenotype of hairy cell leukemia and exert potent antileukemic activity. *Blood* **2015**, *125*, 1207–1216. [CrossRef] [PubMed]
35. Boyd, E.M.; Bench, A.J.; van't Veer, M.B.; Wright, P.; Bloxham, D.M.; Follows, G.A.; Scott, M.A. High resolution melting analysis for detection of BRAF exon 15 mutations in hairy cell leukaemia and other lymphoid malignancies. *Br. J. Haematol.* **2011**, *155*, 609–612. [CrossRef] [PubMed]
36. Arcaini, L.; Zibellini, S.; Boveri, E.; Riboni, R.; Rattotti, S.; Varettoni, M.; Guerrera, M.L.; Lucioni, M.; Tenore, A.; Merli, M.; et al. The BRAF V600E mutation in hairy cell leukemia and other mature B-cell neoplasms. *Blood* **2012**, *119*, 188–191. [CrossRef]
37. Blombery, P.A.; Wong, S.Q.; Hewitt, C.A.; Dobrovic, A.; Maxwell, E.L.; Juneja, S.; Grigoriadis, G.; Westerman, D.A. Detection of BRAF mutations in patients with hairy cell leukemia and related lymphoproliferative disorders. *Haematologica* **2012**, *97*, 780–783. [CrossRef]
38. Xi, L.; Arons, E.; Navarro, W.; Calvo, K.R.; Stetler-Stevenson, M.; Raffeld, M.; Kreitman, R.J. Both variant and *IGHV4-34*-expressing hairy cell leukemia lack the BRAF V600E mutation. *Blood* **2012**, *119*, 3330–3332. [CrossRef]
39. Rogers, K.A.; Andritsos, L.A.; Wei, L.; McLaughlin, E.M.; Ruppert, A.S.; Anghelina, M.; Blachly, J.S.; Call, T.; Chihara, D.; Dauki, A.; et al. Phase 2 study of ibrutinib in classic and variant hairy cell leukemia. *Blood* **2021**, *137*, 3473–3483. [CrossRef]
40. Tschernitz, S.; Flossbach, L.; Bonengel, M.; Roth, S.; Rosenwald, A.; Geissinger, E. Alternative BRAF mutations in BRAF V600E-negative hairy cell leukaemias. *Br. J. Haematol.* **2014**, *165*, 529–533. [CrossRef]
41. Thompson, E.R.; Lim, K.J.C.; Kuzich, J.A.; McBean, M.; Westerman, D.; Tam, C.S.; Blombery, P. Detection of an IGH-BRAF fusion in a patient with BRAF Val600Glu negative hairy cell leukemia. *Leuk. Lymphoma* **2020**, *61*, 2024–2026. [CrossRef] [PubMed]
42. Maitre, E.; Bertrand, P.; Maingonnat, C.; Viailly, P.J.; Wiber, M.; Naguib, D.; Salaun, V.; Cornet, E.; Damaj, G.; Sola, B.; et al. New generation sequencing of targeted genes in the classical and the variant form of hairy cell leukemia highlights mutations in epigenetic regulation genes. *Oncotarget* **2018**, *9*, 28866–28876. [CrossRef] [PubMed]
43. Waterfall, J.J.; Arons, E.; Walker, R.L.; Pineda, M.; Roth, L.; Killian, J.K.; Abaan, O.D.; Davis, S.R.; Kreitman, R.J.; Meltzer, P.S. High prevalence of MAP2K1 mutations in variant and *IGHV4-34*-expressing hairy-cell leukemias. *Nat. Genet.* **2014**, *46*, 8–10. [CrossRef] [PubMed]
44. Haglund, U.; Juliusson, G.; Stellan, B.; Gahrton, G. Hairy cell leukemia is characterized by clonal chromosome abnormalities clustered to specific regions. *Blood* **1994**, *83*, 2637–2645. [CrossRef] [PubMed]
45. Dierlamm, J.; Stefanova, M.; Wlodarska, I.; Michaux, L.; Hinz, K.; Penas, E.M.; Maes, B.; Hagemeijer, A.; De Wolf-Peeters, C.; Hossfeld, D.K. Chromosomal gains and losses are uncommon in hairy cell leukemia: A study based on comparative genomic hybridization and interphase fluorescence in situ hybridization. *Cancer Genet. Cytogenet.* **2001**, *128*, 164–167. [CrossRef]
46. Andersen, C.L.; Gruszka-Westwood, A.; Ostergaard, M.; Koch, J.; Jacobsen, E.; Kjeldsen, E.; Nielsen, B. A narrow deletion of 7q is common to HCL, and SMZL, but not CLL. *Eur. J. Haematol.* **2004**, *72*, 390–402. [CrossRef]
47. Hockley, S.L.; Morgan, G.J.; Leone, P.E.; Walker, B.A.; Morilla, A.; Else, M.; Wotherspoon, A.; Dearden, C.; Catovsky, D.; Gonzalez, D.; et al. High-resolution genomic profiling in hairy cell leukemia-variant compared with typical hairy cell leukemia. *Leukemia* **2011**, *25*, 1189–1192. [CrossRef] [PubMed]
48. Rinaldi, A.; Kwee, I.; Young, K.H.; Zucca, E.; Gaidano, G.; Forconi, F.; Bertoni, F. Genome-wide high resolution DNA profiling of hairy cell leukaemia. *Br. J. Haematol.* **2013**, *162*, 566–569. [CrossRef]
49. Dietrich, S.; Hullein, J.; Lee, S.C.; Hutter, B.; Gonzalez, D.; Jayne, S.; Dyer, M.J.; Oles, M.; Else, M.; Liu, X.; et al. Recurrent CDKN1B (p27) mutations in hairy cell leukemia. *Blood* **2015**, *126*, 1005–1008. [CrossRef] [PubMed]
50. Weston-Bell, N.J.; Tapper, W.; Gibson, J.; Bryant, D.; Moreno, Y.; John, M.; Ennis, S.; Kluin-Nelemans, H.C.; Collins, A.R.; Sahota, S.S. Exome Sequencing in Classic Hairy Cell Leukaemia Reveals Widespread Variation in Acquired Somatic Mutations between Individual Tumours Apart from the Signature BRAF V(600)E Lesion. *PLoS ONE* **2016**, *11*, e0149162. [CrossRef]
51. Bencivenga, D.; Caldarelli, I.; Stampone, E.; Mancini, F.P.; Balestrieri, M.L.; Della Ragione, F.; Borriello, A. p27(Kip1) and human cancers: A reappraisal of a still enigmatic protein. *Cancer Lett.* **2017**, *403*, 354–365. [CrossRef] [PubMed]
52. Suski, J.M.; Braun, M.; Strmiska, V.; Sicinski, P. Targeting cell-cycle machinery in cancer. *Cancer Cell* **2021**, *39*, 759–778. [CrossRef] [PubMed]
53. Chilosi, M.; Chiarle, R.; Lestani, M.; Menestrina, F.; Montagna, L.; Ambrosetti, A.; Prolla, G.; Pizzolo, G.; Doglioni, C.; Piva, R.; et al. Low expression of p27 and low proliferation index do not correlate in hairy cell leukaemia. *Br. J. Haematol.* **2000**, *111*, 263–271. [CrossRef]
54. Bhatt, K.V.; Spofford, L.S.; Aram, G.; McMullen, M.; Pumiglia, K.; Aplin, A.E. Adhesion control of cyclin D1 and p27Kip1 levels is deregulated in melanoma cells through BRAF-MEK-ERK signaling. *Oncogene* **2005**, *24*, 3459–3471. [CrossRef] [PubMed]
55. Bhatt, K.V.; Hu, R.; Spofford, L.S.; Aplin, A.E. Mutant B-RAF signaling and cyclin D1 regulate Cks1/S-phase kinase-associated protein 2-mediated degradation of p27Kip1 in human melanoma cells. *Oncogene* **2007**, *26*, 1056–1066. [CrossRef]
56. le Sage, C.; Nagel, R.; Egan, D.A.; Schrier, M.; Mesman, E.; Mangiola, A.; Anile, C.; Maira, G.; Mercatelli, N.; Ciafre, S.A.; et al. Regulation of the p27(Kip1) tumor suppressor by miR-221 and miR-222 promotes cancer cell proliferation. *EMBO J.* **2007**, *26*, 3699–3708. [CrossRef]

57. Kitagawa, Y.; Brahmachary, M.; Tiacci, E.; Dalla-Favera, R.; Falini, B.; Basso, K. A microRNA signature specific for hairy cell leukemia and associated with modulation of the MAPK-JNK pathways. *Leukemia* **2012**, *26*, 2564–2567. [CrossRef]
58. Hoek, K.L.; Gordy, L.E.; Collins, P.L.; Parekh, V.V.; Aune, T.M.; Joyce, S.; Thomas, J.W.; Van Kaer, L.; Sebzda, E. Follicular B cell trafficking within the spleen actively restricts humoral immune responses. *Immunity* **2010**, *33*, 254–265. [CrossRef]
59. Hart, G.T.; Wang, X.; Hogquist, K.A.; Jameson, S.C. Kruppel-like factor 2 (KLF2) regulates B-cell reactivity, subset differentiation, and trafficking molecule expression. *Proc. Natl. Acad. Sci. USA* **2011**, *108*, 716–721. [CrossRef]
60. Campos-Martin, Y.; Martinez, N.; Martinez-Lopez, A.; Cereceda, L.; Casado, F.; Algara, P.; Oscier, D.; Menarguez, F.J.; Garcia, J.F.; Piris, M.A.; et al. Clinical and diagnostic relevance of NOTCH2-and KLF2-mutations in splenic marginal zone lymphoma. *Haematologica* **2017**, *102*, e310–e312. [CrossRef]
61. Oquendo, C.J.; Parker, H.; Oscier, D.; Ennis, S.; Gibson, J.; Strefford, J.C. The (epi)genomic landscape of splenic marginal zone lymphoma, biological implications, clinical utility, and future questions. *J. Transl. Genet. Genom.* **2021**, *5*, 89–111. [CrossRef]
62. Piva, R.; Deaglio, S.; Famà, R.; Buonincontri, R.; Scarfò, I.; Bruscaggin, A.; Mereu, E.; Serra, S.; Spina, V.; Brusa, D.; et al. The Krüppel-like factor 2 transcription factor gene is recurrently mutated in splenic marginal zone lymphoma. *Leukemia* **2015**, *29*, 503–507. [CrossRef] [PubMed]
63. Clipson, A.; Wang, M.; de Leval, L.; Ashton-Key, M.; Wotherspoon, A.; Vassiliou, G.; Bolli, N.; Grove, C.; Moody, S.; Escudero-Ibarz, L.; et al. KLF2 mutation is the most frequent somatic change in splenic marginal zone lymphoma and identifies a subset with distinct genotype. *Leukemia* **2015**, *29*, 1177–1185. [CrossRef] [PubMed]
64. Jallades, L.; Baseggio, L.; Sujobert, P.; Huet, S.; Chabane, K.; Callet-Bauchu, E.; Verney, A.; Hayette, S.; Desvignes, J.P.; Salgado, D.; et al. Exome sequencing identifies recurrent BCOR alterations and the absence of KLF2, TNFAIP3 and MYD88 mutations in splenic diffuse red pulp small B-cell lymphoma. *Haematologica* **2017**, *102*, 1758–1766. [CrossRef] [PubMed]
65. Jay, J.J.; Brouwer, C. Lollipops in the Clinic: Information Dense Mutation Plots for Precision Medicine. *PLoS ONE* **2016**, *11*, e0160519. [CrossRef] [PubMed]
66. Pemov, A.; Pathak, A.; Jones, S.J.; Dewan, R.; Merberg, J.; Karra, S.; Kim, J.; Arons, E.; Ravichandran, S.; Luke, B.T.; et al. In search of genetic factors predisposing to familial hairy cell leukemia (HCL): Exome-sequencing of four multiplex HCL pedigrees. *Leukemia* **2020**, *34*, 1934–1938. [CrossRef] [PubMed]
67. Zhao, S.; Allis, C.D.; Wang, G.G. The language of chromatin modification in human cancers. *Nat. Rev. Cancer* **2021**, *21*, 413–430. [CrossRef] [PubMed]
68. Fagan, R.J.; Dingwall, A.K. COMPASS Ascending: Emerging clues regarding the roles of MLL3/KMT2C and MLL2/KMT2D proteins in cancer. *Cancer Lett.* **2019**, *458*, 56–65. [CrossRef] [PubMed]
69. Arribas, A.J.; Rinaldi, A.; Chiodin, G.; Kwee, I.; Mensah, A.A.; Cascione, L.; Rossi, D.; Kanduri, M.; Rosenquist, R.; Zucca, E.; et al. Genome-wide promoter methylation of hairy cell leukemia. *Blood Adv.* **2019**, *3*, 384–396. [CrossRef]
70. Gemenetzi, K.; Agathangelidis, A.; Zaragoza-Infante, L.; Sofou, E.; Papaioannou, M.; Chatzidimitriou, A.; Stamatopoulos, K. B Cell Receptor Immunogenetics in B Cell Lymphomas: Immunoglobulin Genes as Key to Ontogeny and Clinical Decision Making. *Front. Oncol.* **2020**, *10*, 67. [CrossRef]
71. Brezinschek, H.P.; Foster, S.J.; Brezinschek, R.I.; Dorner, T.; Domiati-Saad, R.; Lipsky, P.E. Analysis of the human VH gene repertoire. Differential effects of selection and somatic hypermutation on human peripheral CD5(+)/IgM+ and CD5(−)/IgM+ B cells. *J. Clin. Investig.* **1997**, *99*, 2488–2501. [CrossRef] [PubMed]
72. Forconi, F.; Sozzi, E.; Rossi, D.; Sahota, S.S.; Amato, T.; Raspadori, D.; Trentin, L.; Leoncini, L.; Gaidano, G.; Lauria, F. Selective influences in the expressed immunoglobulin heavy and light chain gene repertoire in hairy cell leukemia. *Haematologica* **2008**, *93*, 697–705. [CrossRef] [PubMed]
73. Forconi, F.; Sozzi, E.; Cencini, E.; Zaja, F.; Intermesoli, T.; Stelitano, C.; Rigacci, L.; Gherlinzoni, F.; Cantaffa, R.; Baraldi, A.; et al. Hairy cell leukemias with unmutated IGHV genes define the minor subset refractory to single-agent cladribine and with more aggressive behavior. *Blood* **2009**, *114*, 4696–4702. [CrossRef] [PubMed]
74. Hockley, S.L.; Giannouli, S.; Morilla, A.; Wotherspoon, A.; Morgan, G.J.; Matutes, E.; Gonzalez, D. Insight into the molecular pathogenesis of hairy cell leukaemia, hairy cell leukaemia variant and splenic marginal zone lymphoma, provided by the analysis of their IGH rearrangements and somatic hypermutation patterns. *Br. J. Haematol.* **2010**, *148*, 666–669. [CrossRef] [PubMed]
75. Arons, E.; Roth, L.; Sapolsky, J.; Suntum, T.; Stetler-Stevenson, M.; Kreitman, R.J. Evidence of canonical somatic hypermutation in hairy cell leukemia. *Blood* **2011**, *117*, 4844–4851. [CrossRef] [PubMed]
76. Forconi, F.; Sahota, S.S.; Raspadori, D.; Ippoliti, M.; Babbage, G.; Lauria, F.; Stevenson, F.K. Hairy cell leukemia: At the crossroad of somatic mutation and isotype switch. *Blood* **2004**, *104*, 3312–3317. [CrossRef] [PubMed]
77. Xu, Z.; Zan, H.; Pone, E.J.; Mai, T.; Casali, P. Immunoglobulin class-switch DNA recombination: Induction, targeting and beyond. *Nat. Rev. Immunol.* **2012**, *12*, 517–531. [CrossRef]
78. Zhang, Y.; Zhang, X.; Ba, Z.; Liang, Z.; Dring, E.W.; Hu, H.; Lou, J.; Kyritsis, N.; Zurita, J.; Shamim, M.S.; et al. The fundamental role of chromatin loop extrusion in physiological V(D)J recombination. *Nature* **2019**, *573*, 600–604. [CrossRef]
79. Giachino, C.; Padovan, E.; Lanzavecchia, A. $\kappa^+\lambda^+$ dual receptor B cells are present in the human peripheral repertoire. *J. Exp. Med.* **1995**, *181*, 1245–1250. [CrossRef] [PubMed]
80. Fraser, L.D.; Zhao, Y.; Lutalo, P.M.; D'Cruz, D.P.; Cason, J.; Silva, J.S.; Dunn-Walters, D.K.; Nayar, S.; Cope, A.P.; Spencer, J. Immunoglobulin light chain allelic inclusion in systemic lupus erythematosus. *Eur. J. Immunol.* **2015**, *45*, 2409–2419. [CrossRef] [PubMed]

81. Kenny, J.J.; Rezanka, L.J.; Lustig, A.; Fischer, R.T.; Yoder, J.; Marshall, S.; Longo, D.L. Autoreactive B cells escape clonal deletion by expressing multiple antigen receptors. *J. Immunol.* **2000**, *164*, 4111–4119. [CrossRef] [PubMed]
82. Li, Y.; Li, H.; Weigert, M. Autoreactive B cells in the marginal zone that express dual receptors. *J. Exp. Med.* **2002**, *195*, 181–188. [CrossRef] [PubMed]
83. Fournier, E.M.; Velez, M.G.; Leahy, K.; Swanson, C.L.; Rubtsov, A.V.; Torres, R.M.; Pelanda, R. Dual-reactive B cells are autoreactive and highly enriched in the plasmablast and memory B cell subsets of autoimmune mice. *J. Exp. Med.* **2012**, *209*, 1797–1812. [CrossRef] [PubMed]
84. Visvader, J.E. Cells of origin in cancer. *Nature* **2011**, *469*, 314–322. [CrossRef] [PubMed]
85. Bradner, J.E.; Hnisz, D.; Young, R.A. Transcriptional Addiction in Cancer. *Cell* **2017**, *168*, 629–643. [CrossRef]
86. Holmes, A.B.; Corinaldesi, C.; Shen, Q.; Kumar, R.; Compagno, N.; Wang, Z.; Nitzan, M.; Grunstein, E.; Pasqualucci, L.; Dalla-Favera, R.; et al. Single-cell analysis of germinal-center B cells informs on lymphoma cell of origin and outcome. *J. Exp. Med.* **2020**, *217*, e20200483. [CrossRef]
87. Nadeu, F.; Martin-Garcia, D.; Clot, G.; Diaz-Navarro, A.; Duran-Ferrer, M.; Navarro, A.; Vilarrasa-Blasi, R.; Kulis, M.; Royo, R.; Gutierrez-Abril, J.; et al. Genomic and epigenomic insights into the origin, pathogenesis, and clinical behavior of mantle cell lymphoma subtypes. *Blood* **2020**, *136*, 1419–1432. [CrossRef]
88. Bonfiglio, F.; Bruscaggin, A.; Guidetti, F.; Terzi di Bergamo, L.; Faderl, M.R.; Spina, V.; Condoluci, A.; Bonomini, L.; Forestieri, G.; Koch, R.; et al. Genetic and Phenotypic Attributes of Splenic Marginal Zone Lymphoma. *Blood* **2021**. [CrossRef]
89. Dorfman, D.M.; Hwang, E.S.; Shahsafaei, A.; Glimcher, L.H. T-bet, a T-cell-associated transcription factor, is expressed in a subset of B-cell lymphoproliferative disorders. *Am. J. Clin. Pathol.* **2004**, *122*, 292–297. [CrossRef]
90. Toth-Liptak, J.; Piukovics, K.; Borbenyi, Z.; Demeter, J.; Bagdi, E.; Krenacs, L. A comprehensive immunophenotypic marker analysis of hairy cell leukemia in paraffin-embedded bone marrow trephine biopsies—A tissue microarray study. *Pathol. Oncol. Res.* **2015**, *21*, 203–211. [CrossRef]
91. Johrens, K.; Moos, V.; Schneider, T.; Anagnostopoulos, I. T-box-expressed-in-T-cells (T-bet) expression by the tumor cells of hairy-cell leukemia correlates with interferon-gamma production. *Leuk. Lymphoma* **2009**, *50*, 1687–1692. [CrossRef] [PubMed]
92. Kumar, P.; Gao, Q.; Chan, A.; Lewis, N.; Sigler, A.; Pichardo, J.; Xiao, W.; Roshal, M.; Dogan, A. Hairy cell leukemia expresses programmed death-1. *Blood Cancer J.* **2020**, *10*, 115. [CrossRef] [PubMed]
93. Cancro, M.P. Age-Associated B Cells. *Annu. Rev. Immunol.* **2020**, *38*, 315–340. [CrossRef] [PubMed]
94. Elsner, R.A.; Shlomchik, M.J. Germinal Center and Extrafollicular B Cell Responses in Vaccination, Immunity, and Autoimmunity. *Immunity* **2020**, *53*, 1136–1150. [CrossRef] [PubMed]
95. Glass, D.R.; Tsai, A.G.; Oliveria, J.P.; Hartmann, F.J.; Kimmey, S.C.; Calderon, A.A.; Borges, L.; Glass, M.C.; Wagar, L.E.; Davis, M.M.; et al. An Integrated Multi-omic Single-Cell Atlas of Human B Cell Identity. *Immunity* **2020**, *53*, 217–232.e215. [CrossRef]
96. Johnson, J.L.; Rosenthal, R.L.; Knox, J.J.; Myles, A.; Naradikian, M.S.; Madej, J.; Kostiv, M.; Rosenfeld, A.M.; Meng, W.; Christensen, S.R.; et al. The Transcription Factor T-bet Resolves Memory B Cell Subsets with Distinct Tissue Distributions and Antibody Specificities in Mice and Humans. *Immunity* **2020**, *52*, 842–855.e846. [CrossRef]
97. Sutton, H.J.; Aye, R.; Idris, A.H.; Vistein, R.; Nduati, E.; Kai, O.; Mwacharo, J.; Li, X.; Gao, X.; Andrews, T.D.; et al. Atypical B cells are part of an alternative lineage of B cells that participates in responses to vaccination and infection in humans. *Cell Rep.* **2021**, *34*, 108684. [CrossRef]
98. Sanz, I.; Wei, C.; Jenks, S.A.; Cashman, K.S.; Tipton, C.; Woodruff, M.C.; Hom, J.; Lee, F.E. Challenges and Opportunities for Consistent Classification of Human B Cell and Plasma Cell Populations. *Front. Immunol.* **2019**, *10*, 2458. [CrossRef]
99. Stewart, A.; Ng, J.C.; Wallis, G.; Tsioligka, V.; Fraternali, F.; Dunn-Walters, D.K. Single-Cell Transcriptomic Analyses Define Distinct Peripheral B Cell Subsets and Discrete Development Pathways. *Front. Immunol.* **2021**, *12*, 602539. [CrossRef]
100. Maul, R.W.; Catalina, M.D.; Kumar, V.; Bachali, P.; Grammer, A.C.; Wang, S.; Yang, W.; Hasni, S.; Ettinger, R.; Lipsky, P.E.; et al. Transcriptome and IgH Repertoire Analyses Show That CD11c(hi) B Cells Are a Distinct Population With Similarity to B Cells Arising in Autoimmunity and Infection. *Front. Immunol.* **2021**, *12*, 649458. [CrossRef]
101. Scharer, C.D.; Blalock, E.L.; Mi, T.; Barwick, B.G.; Jenks, S.A.; Deguchi, T.; Cashman, K.S.; Neary, B.E.; Patterson, D.G.; Hicks, S.L.; et al. Epigenetic programming underpins B cell dysfunction in human SLE. *Nat. Immunol.* **2019**, *20*, 1071–1082. [CrossRef] [PubMed]
102. Pugh-Bernard, A.E.; Silverman, G.J.; Cappione, A.J.; Villano, M.E.; Ryan, D.H.; Insel, R.A.; Sanz, I. Regulation of inherently autoreactive VH4-34 B cells in the maintenance of human B cell tolerance. *J. Clin. Investig.* **2001**, *108*, 1061–1070. [CrossRef]
103. Ng, A.; Chiorazzi, N. Potential Relevance of B-cell Maturation Pathways in Defining the Cell(s) of Origin for Chronic Lymphocytic Leukemia. *Hematol. Oncol. Clin. N. Am.* **2021**, *35*, 665–685. [CrossRef]
104. Gimenez, N.; Martinez-Trillos, A.; Montraveta, A.; Lopez-Guerra, M.; Rosich, L.; Nadeu, F.; Valero, J.G.; Aymerich, M.; Magnano, L.; Rozman, M.; et al. Mutations in the RAS-BRAF-MAPK-ERK pathway define a specific subgroup of patients with adverse clinical features and provide new therapeutic options in chronic lymphocytic leukemia. *Haematologica* **2019**, *104*, 576–586. [CrossRef]
105. Vendramini, E.; Bomben, R.; Pozzo, F.; Benedetti, D.; Bittolo, T.; Rossi, F.M.; Dal Bo, M.; Rabe, K.G.; Pozzato, G.; Zaja, F.; et al. KRAS, NRAS, and BRAF mutations are highly enriched in trisomy 12 chronic lymphocytic leukemia and are associated with shorter treatment-free survival. *Leukemia* **2019**, *33*, 2111–2115. [CrossRef]

106. Blakemore, S.J.; Clifford, R.; Parker, H.; Antoniou, P.; Stec-Dziedzic, E.; Larrayoz, M.; Davis, Z.; Kadalyayil, L.; Colins, A.; Robbe, P.; et al. Clinical significance of TP53, BIRC3, ATM and MAPK-ERK genes in chronic lymphocytic leukaemia: Data from the randomised UK LRF CLL4 trial. *Leukemia* **2020**, *34*, 1760–1774. [CrossRef]
107. Andrulis, M.; Lehners, N.; Capper, D.; Penzel, R.; Heining, C.; Huellein, J.; Zenz, T.; von Deimling, A.; Schirmacher, P.; Ho, A.D.; et al. Targeting the BRAF V600E mutation in multiple myeloma. *Cancer Discov.* **2013**, *3*, 862–869. [CrossRef] [PubMed]
108. Rustad, E.H.; Dai, H.Y.; Hov, H.; Coward, E.; Beisvag, V.; Myklebost, O.; Hovig, E.; Nakken, S.; Vodak, D.; Meza-Zepeda, L.A.; et al. BRAF V600E mutation in early-stage multiple myeloma: Good response to broad acting drugs and no relation to prognosis. *Blood Cancer J.* **2015**, *5*, e299. [CrossRef] [PubMed]
109. Tiacci, E.; Schiavoni, G.; Forconi, F.; Santi, A.; Trentin, L.; Ambrosetti, A.; Cecchini, D.; Sozzi, E.; Francia di Celle, P.; Di Bello, C.; et al. Simple genetic diagnosis of hairy cell leukemia by sensitive detection of the BRAF-V600E mutation. *Blood* **2012**, *119*, 192–195. [CrossRef]
110. Guerrini, F.; Paolicchi, M.; Ghio, F.; Ciabatti, E.; Grassi, S.; Salehzadeh, S.; Ercolano, G.; Metelli, M.R.; Del Re, M.; Iovino, L.; et al. The Droplet Digital PCR: A New Valid Molecular Approach for the Assessment of B-RAF V600E Mutation in Hairy Cell Leukemia. *Front. Pharmacol.* **2016**, *7*, 363. [CrossRef]
111. Cardus, B.; Colling, R.; Hamblin, A.; Soilleux, E. Comparison of methodologies for the detection of BRAF mutations in bone marrow trephine specimens. *J. Clin. Pathol.* **2019**, *72*, 406–411. [CrossRef] [PubMed]
112. WHO. *WHO Classification of Tumours of Haematopoietic and Lymphoid Tissues*; Swerdlow, S.H., Campo, E., Harris, N.L., Jaffe, E.S., Pileri, S.A., Stein, H., Thiele, J., Vardiman, J.W., Eds.; WHO Press: Geneva, Switzerland, 2008.
113. Arons, E.; Suntum, T.; Stetler-Stevenson, M.; Kreitman, R.J. VH4-34+ hairy cell leukemia, a new variant with poor prognosis despite standard therapy. *Blood* **2009**, *114*, 4687–4695. [CrossRef] [PubMed]
114. Tiacci, E.; Park, J.H.; De Carolis, L.; Chung, S.S.; Broccoli, A.; Scott, S.; Zaja, F.; Devlin, S.; Pulsoni, A.; Chung, Y.R.; et al. Targeting Mutant BRAF in Relapsed or Refractory Hairy-Cell Leukemia. *N. Engl. J. Med.* **2015**, *373*, 1733–1747. [CrossRef] [PubMed]
115. Tiacci, E.; De Carolis, L.; Simonetti, E.; Merluzzi, M.; Bennati, A.; Perriello, V.M.; Pucciarini, A.; Santi, A.; Venanzi, A.; Pettirossi, V.; et al. Safety and efficacy of the BRAF inhibitor dabrafenib in relapsed or refractory hairy cell leukemia: A pilot phase-2 clinical trial. *Leukemia* **2021**, *35*, 3314–3318. [CrossRef]
116. Tiacci, E.; De Carolis, L.; Simonetti, E.; Capponi, M.; Ambrosetti, A.; Lucia, E.; Antolino, A.; Pulsoni, A.; Ferrari, S.; Zinzani, P.L.; et al. Vemurafenib plus Rituximab in Refractory or Relapsed Hairy-Cell Leukemia. *N. Engl. J. Med.* **2021**, *384*, 1810–1823. [CrossRef]
117. Whittaker, S.R.; Theurillat, J.P.; Van Allen, E.; Wagle, N.; Hsiao, J.; Cowley, G.S.; Schadendorf, D.; Root, D.E.; Garraway, L.A. A genome-scale RNA interference screen implicates NF1 loss in resistance to RAF inhibition. *Cancer Discov.* **2013**, *3*, 350–362. [CrossRef]
118. Caeser, R.; Collord, G.; Yao, W.Q.; Chen, Z.; Vassiliou, G.S.; Beer, P.A.; Du, M.Q.; Scott, M.A.; Follows, G.A.; Hodson, D.J. Targeting MEK in vemurafenib-resistant hairy cell leukemia. *Leukemia* **2019**, *33*, 541–545. [CrossRef]
119. Marine, J.C.; Dawson, S.J.; Dawson, M.A. Non-genetic mechanisms of therapeutic resistance in cancer. *Nat. Rev. Cancer* **2020**, *20*, 743–756. [CrossRef]
120. Ciriello, G.; Magnani, L. The many faces of cancer evolution. *iScience* **2021**, *24*, 102403. [CrossRef]
121. Emert, B.L.; Cote, C.J.; Torre, E.A.; Dardani, I.P.; Jiang, C.L.; Jain, N.; Shaffer, S.M.; Raj, A. Variability within rare cell states enables multiple paths toward drug resistance. *Nat. Biotechnol.* **2021**, *39*, 865–876. [CrossRef]
122. Sadras, T.; Chan, L.N.; Xiao, G.; Muschen, M. Metabolic Gatekeepers of Pathological B Cell Activation. *Annu. Rev. Pathol.* **2021**, *16*, 323–349. [CrossRef] [PubMed]
123. Waldschmidt, J.M.; Kloeber, J.A.; Anand, P.; Frede, J.; Kokkalis, A.; Dimitrova, V.; Potdar, S.; Nair, M.S.; Vijaykumar, T.; Im, N.G.; et al. Single-Cell Profiling Reveals Metabolic Reprogramming as a Resistance Mechanism in BRAF-Mutated Multiple Myeloma. *Clin. Cancer Res.* **2021**, *27*, 6432–6444. [CrossRef] [PubMed]
124. Angelova, E.A.; Medeiros, L.J.; Wang, W.; Muzzafar, T.; Lu, X.; Khoury, J.D.; Ravandi, F.; Patel, K.P.; Hu, Z.; Kanagal-Shamanna, R. Clinicopathologic and molecular features in hairy cell leukemia-variant: Single institutional experience. *Mod. Pathol.* **2018**, *31*, 1717–1732. [CrossRef]
125. Haferlach, T.; Nadarajah, N.; Meggendorfer, M.; Haferlach, C.; Kern, W. Whole Genome Sequencing in Hairy Cell Leukemia-Variant (HCL-v) and Splenic Marginal Zone Lymphoma (SMZL). *Blood* **2017**, *130*, 4003. [CrossRef]
126. Mason, E.F.; Brown, R.D.; Szeto, D.P.; Gibson, C.J.; Jia, Y.; Garcia, E.P.; Jacobson, C.A.; Dal Cin, P.; Kuo, F.C.; Pinkus, G.S.; et al. Detection of activating MAP2K1 mutations in atypical hairy cell leukemia and hairy cell leukemia variant. *Leuk. Lymphoma* **2017**, *58*, 233–236. [CrossRef] [PubMed]
127. Hockley, S.L.; Else, M.; Morilla, A.; Wotherspoon, A.; Dearden, C.; Catovsky, D.; Gonzalez, D.; Matutes, E. The prognostic impact of clinical and molecular features in hairy cell leukaemia variant and splenic marginal zone lymphoma. *Br. J. Haematol.* **2012**, *158*, 347–354. [CrossRef]
128. Hanrahan, A.J.; Sylvester, B.E.; Chang, M.T.; Elzein, A.; Gao, J.; Han, W.; Liu, Y.; Xu, D.; Gao, S.P.; Gorelick, A.N.; et al. Leveraging Systematic Functional Analysis to Benchmark an In Silico Framework Distinguishes Driver from Passenger MEK Mutants in Cancer. *Cancer Res.* **2020**, *80*, 4233–4243. [CrossRef]

129. Zanelli, M.; Ragazzi, M.; Valli, R.; Piattoni, S.; Alvarez De Celis, M.I.; Farnetti, E.; Orcioni, G.F.; Longo, R.; Ascani, S.; Falini, B.; et al. Transformation of *IGHV4-34+* hairy cell leukaemia-variant with U2AF1 mutation into a clonally-related high grade B-cell lymphoma responding to immunochemotherapy. *Br. J. Haematol.* **2016**, *173*, 491–495. [CrossRef]
130. Ler, L.D.; Ghosh, S.; Chai, X.; Thike, A.A.; Heng, H.L.; Siew, E.Y.; Dey, S.; Koh, L.K.; Lim, J.Q.; Lim, W.K.; et al. Loss of tumor suppressor KDM6A amplifies PRC2-regulated transcriptional repression in bladder cancer and can be targeted through inhibition of EZH2. *Sci. Transl. Med.* **2017**, *9*, eaai8312. [CrossRef]
131. Chihara, D.; Arons, E.; Stetler-Stevenson, M.; Yuan, C.; Wang, H.W.; Zhou, H.; Raffeld, M.; Xi, L.; Steinberg, S.M.; Feurtado, J.; et al. Long term follow-up of a phase II study of cladribine with concurrent rituximab with hairy cell leukemia variant. *Blood Adv.* **2021**, *5*, 4807–4816. [CrossRef]
132. Liu, Q.; Harris, N.; Epperla, N.; Andritsos, L.A. Current and Emerging Therapeutic Options for Hairy Cell Leukemia Variant. *OncoTargets Ther.* **2021**, *14*, 1797–1805. [CrossRef] [PubMed]
133. Andritsos, L.A.; Grieselhuber, N.R.; Anghelina, M.; Rogers, K.A.; Roychowdhury, S.; Reeser, J.W.; Timmers, C.D.; Freud, A.G.; Blachly, J.S.; Lucas, D.M.; et al. Trametinib for the treatment of *IGHV4-34*, MAP2K1-mutant variant hairy cell leukemia. *Leuk. Lymphoma* **2018**, *59*, 1008–1011. [CrossRef] [PubMed]
134. Binimetinib for People with Relapsed/Refractory BRAF Wild Type Hairy Cell Leukemia and Variant. Available online: https://clinicaltrials.gov/ct2/show/NCT04322383 (accessed on 20 December 2021).
135. Traverse-Glehen, A.; Verney, A.; Gazzo, S.; Jallades, L.; Chabane, K.; Hayette, S.; Coiffier, B.; Callet-Bauchu, E.; Ffrench, M.; Felman, P.; et al. Splenic diffuse red pulp lymphoma has a distinct pattern of somatic mutations amongst B-cell malignancies. *Leuk. Lymphoma* **2017**, *58*, 666–675. [CrossRef] [PubMed]
136. Martinez, D.; Navarro, A.; Martinez-Trillos, A.; Molina-Urra, R.; Gonzalez-Farre, B.; Salaverria, I.; Nadeu, F.; Enjuanes, A.; Clot, G.; Costa, D.; et al. NOTCH1, TP53, and MAP2K1 Mutations in Splenic Diffuse Red Pulp Small B-cell Lymphoma Are Associated With Progressive Disease. *Am. J. Surg. Pathol.* **2016**, *40*, 192–201. [CrossRef]
137. Ramezani-Rad, P.; Chen, C.; Zhu, Z.; Rickert, R.C. Cyclin D3 Governs Clonal Expansion of Dark Zone Germinal Center B Cells. *Cell Rep.* **2020**, *33*, 108403. [CrossRef] [PubMed]
138. Pae, J.; Ersching, J.; Castro, T.B.R.; Schips, M.; Mesin, L.; Allon, S.J.; Ordovas-Montanes, J.; Mlynarczyk, C.; Melnick, A.; Efeyan, A.; et al. Cyclin D3 drives inertial cell cycling in dark zone germinal center B cells. *J. Exp. Med.* **2021**, *218*, e20201699. [CrossRef] [PubMed]
139. Hydbring, P.; Malumbres, M.; Sicinski, P. Non-canonical functions of cell cycle cyclins and cyclin-dependent kinases. *Nat. Rev. Mol. Cell Biol.* **2016**, *17*, 280–292. [CrossRef] [PubMed]
140. Curiel-Olmo, S.; Mondejar, R.; Almaraz, C.; Mollejo, M.; Cereceda, L.; Mares, R.; Derdak, S.; Campos-Martin, Y.; Batlle, A.; Gonzalez de Villambrosia, S.; et al. Splenic diffuse red pulp small B-cell lymphoma displays increased expression of cyclin D3 and recurrent CCND3 mutations. *Blood* **2017**, *129*, 1042–1045. [CrossRef]
141. Martin-Garcia, D.; Navarro, A.; Valdes-Mas, R.; Clot, G.; Gutierrez-Abril, J.; Prieto, M.; Ribera-Cortada, I.; Woroniecka, R.; Rymkiewicz, G.; Bens, S.; et al. CCND2 and CCND3 hijack immunoglobulin light-chain enhancers in cyclin D1(-) mantle cell lymphoma. *Blood* **2019**, *133*, 940–951. [CrossRef] [PubMed]
142. Mlynarczyk, C.; Fontan, L.; Melnick, A. Germinal center-derived lymphomas: The darkest side of humoral immunity. *Immunol. Rev.* **2019**, *288*, 214–239. [CrossRef]
143. Sportoletti, P.; Sorcini, D.; Falini, B. BCOR gene alterations in hematologic diseases. *Blood* **2021**, *138*, 2455–2468. [CrossRef] [PubMed]
144. Robak, P.; Jesionek-Kupnicka, D.; Kupnicki, P.; Polliack, A.; Robak, T. Bone lesions in hairy cell leukemia: Diagnosis and treatment. *Eur. J. Haematol.* **2020**, *105*, 682–691. [CrossRef] [PubMed]
145. Dasanu, C.A.; Van den Bergh, M.; Pepito, D.; Alvarez Argote, J. Autoimmune disorders in patients with hairy cell leukemia: Are they more common than previously thought? *Curr. Med. Res. Opin.* **2015**, *31*, 17–23. [CrossRef] [PubMed]
146. Weston-Bell, N.J.; Hendriks, D.; Sugiyarto, G.; Bos, N.A.; Kluin-Nelemans, H.C.; Forconi, F.; Sahota, S.S. Hairy cell leukemia cell lines expressing annexin A1 and displaying B-cell receptor signals characteristic of primary tumor cells lack the signature BRAF mutation to reveal unrepresentative origins. *Leukemia* **2013**, *27*, 241–245. [CrossRef]
147. Falini, B.; Martelli, M.P.; Tiacci, E. BRAF V600E mutation in hairy cell leukemia: From bench to bedside. *Blood* **2016**, *128*, 1918–1927. [CrossRef]

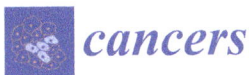

Review

Recent Advances in the Genetic of MALT Lymphomas

Juan José Rodríguez-Sevilla [1,2] and Antonio Salar [1,2,3,*]

1. Department of Hematology, Hospital del Mar-IMIM, 08003 Barcelona, Spain; 63639@parcdesalutmar.cat
2. Group of Applied Clinical Research in Hematology, Cancer Research Program-IMIM (Hospital del Mar Medical Research Institute), 08003 Barcelona, Spain
3. Life and Health Sciences Department, Pompeu Fabra University, 08003 Barcelona, Spain
* Correspondence: asalar@parcdesalutmar.cat; Tel.: +34-93-248-3341

Simple Summary: Mucosa-associated lymphoid tissue (MALT) lymphoma is the most common subtype of marginal zone lymphomas. These B-cell neoplasms may arise from many organs and usually have an indolent behavior. Recurrent chromosomal translocations and cytogenetic alterations are well characterized, some of them being associated to specific sites. Through next-generation sequencing technologies, the mutational landscape of MALT lymphomas has been explored and available data to date show that there are considerable variations in the incidence and spectrum of mutations among MALT lymphoma of different sites. Interestingly, most of these mutations affect several common pathways and some of them are potentially targetable. Gene expression profile and epigenetic studies have also added new information, potentially useful for diagnosis and treatment. This article provides a comprehensive review of the genetic landscape in MALT lymphomas.

Abstract: Mucosa-associated lymphoid tissue (MALT) lymphomas are a diverse group of lymphoid neoplasms with B-cell origin, occurring in adult patients and usually having an indolent clinical behavior. These lymphomas may arise in different anatomic locations, sharing many clinicopathological characteristics, but also having substantial variances in the aetiology and genetic alterations. Chromosomal translocations are recurrent in MALT lymphomas with different prevalence among different sites, being the 4 most common: t(11;18)(q21;q21), t(1;14)(p22;q32), t(14;18)(q32;q21), and t(3;14)(p14.1;q32). Several chromosomal numerical abnormalities have also been described, but probably represent secondary genetic events. The mutational landscape of MALT lymphomas is wide, and the most frequent mutations are: *TNFAIP3, CREBBP, KMT2C, TET2, SPEN, KMT2D, LRP1B, PRDM1, EP300, TNFRSF14, NOTCH1/NOTCH2,* and *B2M*, but many other genes may be involved. Similar to chromosomal translocations, certain mutations are enriched in specific lymphoma types. In the same line, variation in immunoglobulin gene usage is recognized among MALT lymphoma of different anatomic locations. In the last decade, several studies have analyzed the role of microRNA, transcriptomics and epigenetic alterations, further improving our knowledge about the pathogenic mechanisms in MALT lymphoma development. All these advances open the possibility of targeted directed treatment and push forward the concept of precision medicine in MALT lymphomas.

Keywords: MALT lymphoma; marginal zone; *Helicobacter pylori*; extranodal lymphoma; gastric lymphoma

Citation: Rodríguez-Sevilla, J.J.; Salar, A. Recent Advances in the Genetic of MALT Lymphomas. *Cancers* 2022, 14, 176. https://doi.org/10.3390/cancers14010176

Academic Editor: Francesco Bertoni

Received: 28 November 2021
Accepted: 29 December 2021
Published: 30 December 2021

Publisher's Note: MDPI stays neutral with regard to jurisdictional claims in published maps and institutional affiliations.

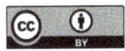

Copyright: © 2021 by the authors. Licensee MDPI, Basel, Switzerland. This article is an open access article distributed under the terms and conditions of the Creative Commons Attribution (CC BY) license (https://creativecommons.org/licenses/by/4.0/).

1. Introduction

Mucosa-associated lymphoid tissue (MALT) lymphoma was first described in 1983 by Isaacson and Wright in the stomach but may arise from other mucosal tissues [1]. According to the WHO classification [2], MALT lymphomas are one of the three recognized subtypes of marginal zone lymphomas (MZL), a group of indolent lymphoid neoplasms which represents 7% of all mature non-Hodgkin lymphomas (NHL) [3]. Based on data from SEER-18 program, MALT lymphomas represent 60.8% of MZLs, followed by nodal MZL (NMZL) (30.3%) and splenic MZL (SMZL) (8.9%) [4]. According to this program, the incidence of

MALT lymphomas in the US from 2001–2017 has increased +1.1% per year [4], despite the decrease in the incidence of gastric MALT lymphomas associated with *Helicobacter pylori* (*H. pylori*) recently described in several studies [5].

MALT lymphomas mainly occur in adults, with a median age about 60 years. Men and women are affected equally, although there is site specific female predominance in the parotid gland and breast [6]. MALT lymphomas can occur at any extranodal site. In health, these tissues are usually almost devoid of lymphoid tissue; however, they accumulate B lymphocytes in response to persistent antigenic stimulation due to chronic infections or autoimmune disorders [7,8]. The most common anatomic sites are the stomach (30%), followed by eye/adnexa (12%), skin (10%), lung (9%) and salivary gland (7%) [4]. However, these lymphomas have been described at many other mucosal organs, such as thyroid, liver, small intestine, large intestine, bladder, dura, and many other sites [7,9].

Gastric MALT lymphoma is linked with chronic *H. pylori* infection, satisfying Koch's postulates for an etiologic agent [10]. Albeit not with the same clear evidence, other infectious agents have been associated with MALT lymphomas: *Helicobacter heilmannii* in the stomach [11], *Chlamydia psittaci* (*C. psittaci*) in the ocular adnexa [12,13], *Borrelia burgdorferi* in the skin [14,15], *Campylobacter jejuni* in immunoproliferative small intestine disease [16] and, *Achromobacter xylosoxidans* in the lung [17]. Autoimmune conditions have been further associated with MALT lymphoma, including Sjogren's disease, lymphoepithelial sialadenitis and Hashimoto's thyroiditis [18]. There are also promising leads related to other infections (hepatitis B and C viruses and human immunodeficiency virus), other B-cell activating autoimmune conditions (systemic lupus erythematosus), trichloroethylene exposure, certain occupations, hair dye, recreational sun exposure, smoking, and alcohol use, but these require further research [4].

MALT lymphomas are considered indolent neoplasms with 5-year relative survival rate of 93.8%, higher than that observed in SMZL (85.3%) and NMZL (82.8%) [4]. Among MALT lymphoma sites, 5-year survival is highest for skin (100%) and lowest for small intestine (87.9%). However, occasionally, MALT lymphomas can progress and transform into aggressive high-grade (diffuse large B cell lymphoma (DLBCL)) and in those cases the survival rate drops sharply.

High throughput genome-wide methodologies, the complete sequencing of the human genome and recent developments in next generation sequencing (NGS) have allowed for unprecedented insights into the genomic alterations that underlie oncogenesis, tumor biology, and survival. Since more than 95% of patients with hematologic malignancies have adequate tissue for genomic profiling, this represents an excellent opportunity to improve diagnosis and classification, to look for prognostic markers and also for detection of pharmacologically tractable targets [19]. This review will summarize the latest advances in the genetics and molecular insights of MALT lymphomas.

2. IGHV Usage

A functional B-cell receptor (BCR) is essential for the biology of B-cells. MALT lymphoma cells almost always express surface immunoglobulin (Ig) M and its BCR signalling is functional. This is supported by their proliferative responses to mitogens [20] and the responses achieved with treatment with Bruton Tyrosine Kinase (BTK) inhibitors [21].

MALT lymphomas have highly altered variable heavy chain immunoglobulin (IGHV) and variable light chain immunoglobulin (IGLV) genes, which are consistent with germinal center (GC) or post-GC origin [22–24]. A role for antigen-driven clonal expansion of the lymphoma cells is shown through the evidence of ongoing somatic hypermutation in the IGHV [25]. The involvement of antigens is also supported by evidence of clonal evolution within the tumor, suggesting selective pressure to increase affinity of the Ig for antigens [26–28]. Despite large mutation loads, the overall structure of the Ig is typically retained in these lymphomas [25].

The variation in Ig gene usage among MALT lymphoma of different anatomic locations is presumably the result of adaptive response and clonal selection induced by their varied aetiologies, resulting in different antigen exposures [29]. The Ig from MALT lymphoma of various anatomic sites is autoreactive rather than recognizing antigens from infectious agents. The auto-reactivity may range from polyreactive to various self-antigens to a high-affinity binding to IgG-Fc, a characteristic of rheumatoid factors (RF) [25,30]. In fact, many of these MALT lymphoma derived immunoglobulins share the fundamental features of known autoantibodies [31].

In MALT lymphomas of the salivary gland (SGMZL), there is a clear skewed usage of IGHV1-69/J4 (55%) or IGHV3-7/J3 (15%) rearrangements, and this together with other less frequent (IGHV4-59/J2(J5) and IGHV3-30/JH4) rearrangements indicates that most salivary gland MALT lymphomas express BCR that potentially bears RF activities [32,33].

IGHV4-34 (18%) is the most often usage in ocular adnexal MALT lymphoma (OAMZL), followed by IGHV3-23 (12–17%), IGHV3-30 (10–14%), and IGHV3–7 (9%) [34–39]. OAMZL carry no or very rare mutation at the conserved VH FR1 Q6W7A24V25Y26 residues, and in contrast, IGVH4-34 mutations are common at the CDR2 N-link glycosylation site and FR3 K90L91S92 residues [40]. In addition, IGHV gene usage in OAMZL is biased by the presence of *C. psittaci* infection. *C. psittaci*-negative cases have a much greater prevalence of IGHV4-34 usage than those *C. psittaci*-positive [41], raising the possibility that other yet unknown pathogens may be involved in their pathogenesis, boosting the formation of an inflammatory environment in which autoantigen exposure could promote the malignant proliferation of autoreactive cells. Moreover, *TNFAIP3* inactivation by deletion or mutation was significantly higher in MALT lymphomas with IGHV4-34 rearrangement (54%), particularly in those of OAMZL (70%), than in those using other IGHV genes (20%). The concurrence of IGHV4-34 rearrangement and *TNFAIP3* inactivation points toward a cooperative relationship of between these two events in OAMZL lymphomagenesis [37].

MALT lymphomas from other sites have also biased usage of IG genes, albeit those coding for autoantibodies are still overrepresented. Gastric MALT lymphomas (GMZL) have a biased use of IGHV4-34, IGHV3-7 and IGHV1-69 genes [25,30,37,42–46] and those responsive to *H. pylori* antibiotic treatment and without the t(11;18)(q21;q21) of IGHV3-30 or IGHV3-23. MALT lymphomas of the lung and skin have also found to have biased usage of IGHV3 or IGHV4 and IGHVH1-69 or IGHVH4-59, respectively [47]. Moreover, the usage of IGHV4-34 and IGHV1-69 in MALT lymphoma is frequently associated with a biased usage of IGLV (IGKV3-20), suggesting recognition of certain antigenic determinants [25,48]. However, the prognostic impact of both the biased usage of Ig genes or their mutational status (unmutated vs. mutated) remains to be determined in MALT lymphomas.

3. Cytogenetics

The identification of cytogenetic abnormalities constitutes an important tool for establishing the diagnosis, monitoring the clinical course, and assessing the prognosis of patients with B-cell lymphomas. Cytogenetic analysis in MALT lymphomas was initially hampered by the facts that biopsies are usually small (most taken by endoscopic procedures) and then rarely subjected to conventional cytogenetic analysis and also, because its proliferation in vitro is often poor. Then, during several years, data were limited in comparison with other types of indolent B-cell lymphomas. However, the application of FISH (fluorescence in-situ hybridization), SKY (spectral karyotyping) and high-resolution technologies such as array based comparative genomic hybridization (array-CGH) have improved our knowledge of chromosomal abnormalities in MALT lymphomas.

In the last two decades, a variety of chromosomal structural and numerical alterations have been described in MALT lymphomas (Table 1). Chromosomal translocations are recurrent in MALT lymphomas, but not in NMZL or SMZL, and their prevalence differs according to disease sites [49,50]. Many translocations have been reported in MALT lymphomas, but the 4 most common are t(1;14) (p22;q32), t(11;18)(q21;q21), t(14;18)(q32;q21), and t(3;14)(p14.1;q32). All these translocations and their products target the activation of nuclear factor k-light-chain-enhancer of activated B-cells (NF-kB) pathway [51–53].

Table 1. Most common genetic aberrations detected in MALT lymphomas at different sites.

Location	Antigen Exposure Association	IGHV Usage	Abnormality	Involved Genes	Copy Number Variations	Other Imbalances
GASTRIC	Helicobacter pylori Helicobacter heilmannii Campylobacter jejuni (small intestine)	IGHV4-34 IGHV3-7 IGHV1-69 IGHV1-2 IGHV3-23	t(11;18)(q21;q21) 20–25% (intestinal 33%) t(1;14)(p22;q32) 4%	BIRC3-MALT1 IGHV-BCL10	Trisomy 3 Trisomy 18	TNFAIP3 deletion
OCULAR ADNEXA	Chlamydia psittaci	IGHV4-34: 18% IGHV3-23: 12–17% IGHV3-30: 10–14% IGHV3-7: 9%	t(11;18)(q21;q21) 10% t(14;18)(q32;q21) 7% t(3;14)(p14.1;q32)	BIRC3-MALT1 IGHV-MALT1 IGHV-FOXP1	Trisomy 18 6q gain 30% 3q gain 18q gain	TNFAIP3 deletion 19%
THRYOID	Hashimoto thyroiditis	IGHV3-30	t(3;14)(p14.1;q32) 7–56% t(14;18)(q32;q21)	IGHV-FOXP1 IGHV-MALT1	Trisomy 3	TNFAIP3 deletion 11% PD-L1 deletion 53%
SALIVAL GLAND	Lymphoepithelial sialadenitis Sjögren syndrome	IGHV1-69/J4: 55% IGHV3-7/J3 15% IGHV4-59/J2(J5) IGHV3-30/JH4	t(X;14)(p11.4;q32)	IGHV-GPR34		TNFAIP3 deletion 8%
SKIN	Borrelia burgdorferi	IGHV1-69 IGHV4-59 IGHV3-30	t(14;18)(q32;q21) 10% t(3;14)(p14.1;q32),	IGHV-MALT1		
LUNG	Achromobacter xylosoxidans	IGHV3 IGHV4-34	t(11;18)(q21;q21) 40% t(11;12;18)(q21;q13;q21) t(11;14;18)(q21;q32;q21) t(1;14)(p22;q32) 9% t(14;18)(q32;q21) 6–9%	BIRC3-MALT1 IGHV-BCL10 IGHV-MALT1	3q gain 18q gain	

The most common recurrent translocation is t(11;18)(q21;q21) which juxtaposes the N-terminal region API2 gene, containing 3 BIR domains with inhibitor caspase activity, and the C-terminal region of MALT1 gene, containing an intact caspase p20-like domain [54–59]. The resulting fusion product undergo oligomerization, generating a chimeric protein that induces aberrant nuclear expression of BCL-10 and activation of both canonical and non-canonical NF-κB pathways, promoting cell survival and proliferation [55,60–64]. A recent molecular mechanism described for the API2/MALT1 fusion protein shows that the tumor suppressor gene LIMA1 binds BIRC2 and is proteolytically cleaved by MALT1 through its paracaspase activity. This cleavage originates a LIM domain-only-containing fragment with oncogenic properties in vitro and in vivo [65].

t(11;18)(q21;q21) is most frequent in MALT lymphomas of the lung (40%) and stomach (20–25%). This translocation is also found in the intestinal (33%; with different frequencies between primary (12.5%) and secondary forms (57%), but rare in colorectal cases), the ocular adnexa (10%), and it is uncommon or not present in MALT lymphomas of the thyroid, salivary gland, and skin [49,50,56,59,63,66–72]. Aneuploidy is rarely observed. Variant translocations of the t(11;18)(q21;q21) have been described, the three-way translocation t(11;12;18)(q21;q13;q21) in the lung [73,74], t(6;18;11)(q24;q21;q21) in the stomach [75] and t(11;14;18)(q21;q32;q21) in the lung [75].

In the MALT lymphomas of the stomach, t(11;18)(q21;q21) is found in 47% and 68% of cases with stage IE and stage IIE or above, respectively, which do not respond to *H. pylori* antibiotic treatment, but only in 3% of those that respond to *H. pylori* eradication [76–87]. Additionally, these t(11;18)(q21;q21) positive cases often show residual disease and have a higher risk of lymphoma relapse after antibiotic treatment [86,88]. Additionally, patients carrying this translocation do also present a poor response to alkylating agents such as cyclophosphamide or chlorambucil [89]. However, treatment with rituximab is active in monotherapy [90] or in combination with chlorambucil [91] or bendamustine [92]. For these reasons, testing for t(11;18)(q21;q21) at diagnosis is commonly recommended to guide treatment choice [93,94].

Patients with t(11;18) had more frequent monoclonal gammopathy, in particular of IgM subtype (31% v 8%), some of which developed class switch [86,95]. The link between high IgM and t(11;18) could have come via the CD40 pathway, which induces IgM secretion in B cells [96–98]. Finally, this translocation is rarely seen in transformed MALT lymphomas [99].

The t(14;18)(q32;q21) is the second most common among all balanced translocations in MALT lymphoma and brings the *MALT1* gene under the transcriptional control of the IgG enhancer, then MALT1 expression is deregulated fostering NF-kB activation [67,71,100–103]. MALT1 activation also produces its protease activities, causing specific cleavage and inactivation of NF-κB negative regulators including TNFAIP3 and CYLD, thus further enhancing NF-κB activation [104–107]. In addition, the lymphoma cells carrying *IGH/MALT1* show not only over-expression of MALT1, but also BCL10 accumulation in cytoplasm. This finding suggests that MALT1 may immobilize BCL10 in cytoplasm through their interaction [102]. Over-expression of MALT1, and also of BCL10, may promote the activation of non-canonical NF-κB pathway via up-regulation of BAFF expression [108]. This rearrangement is seen in 5–20% of MALT lymphomas, especially in the liver (17%), skin (10%), lung (6–9%) and ocular adnexa (7%) [50,67,100,102,109,110]. Other described sites are the salivary gland, dura and kidney among others [111–113]. This translocation is also described in rare cases of diffuse large B-cell lymphoma [114,115].

The t(1;14)(p22;q32) juxtaposes the *BCL10* gene under the regulatory control of the *IGH* gene, resulting in deregulated expression [116]. In normal conditions, BCL10 links BCR signalling to the canonical NF-kB pathway, being expressed in the cytoplasm of reactive B-cells [117]. However, BCL10 is aberrantly expressed in the nuclei of lymphoma cells with t(1;14)(p22;q32)/*BCL10-IGH*. Over-expression of BCL10 and formation of CBM signalosome via oligomers uniting the CARD domain results in NF-κB activation [81].

t(1;14)(p22;q32) is particularly associated with MALT lymphomas, albeit it is infrequent (1–2% of MALT lymphomas). This translocation may be seen in MALT lymphoma of the lung (9%) and stomach (4%), but it is rare in other sites: ocular adnexa, salivary gland, thyroid and skin [50,67]. The clinical utility of t(1;14)(p22;q32) is not yet fully characterized. However, retrospective studies suggest that gastric MALT lymphomas with strong BCL10 nuclear expression or t(1;14)(p22;q32) do not respond to *H. pylori* eradication [81,85].

t(3;14)(p14.1;q32), with rearrangement of *IGH* and *FOXP1*, is found in approximately 10% of MALT lymphomas, mainly from cases arising in the thyroid, ocular adnexa and skin. MALT lymphomas from the stomach and the lung, NMZL and SMZL are typically negative. Most MALT patients carrying t(3;14)(p14.1;q32) also harbor additional genetic abnormalities, such as trisomy 3 [118].

Several novel chromosome translocations in occasional cases of MALT lymphoma have been described: t(3;14)(p13;q32)/*FOXP1-IGH* [118–120], t(1;14)(p21;q32)/*CNN3-IGH*, t(5;14)(q34;q32)/*ODZ2-IGH*, t(9;14)(p24;q32)/*JMJD2C-IGH* [121], t(X;14)(p11.4;q32)/*GPR34-IGH* [122,123] and t(1;2)(p22;p12) [103,124]. These translocations typically juxtapose the oncogene involved to the *IGH* gene locus, (or with the kappa light chain gene) and cause their over-expression. For instance, FOXP1 over-expression though inhibition of apoptosis and plasma cell differentiation may contribute to the pathogenesis of MALT lymphomas [125,126]. The molecular mechanism causing the oncogenic activities of another aforementioned translocation remains to be investigated. Similar to that seen in the four leading translocations, these lesser common translocations are also restricted to specific sites. For instance, translocation t(3;14)/*FOXP1-IGH* is found in 7–56% of thyroid MALT lymphoma cases, [118,127,128], but is not evidenced in non-malignant thyroid disorders (Hashimoto's thyroiditis and benign tissue) [127]. Then, detection of t(3;14)/*FOXP1-IGH* may be useful for the differential diagnosis between primary MALT lymphoma of the thyroid and other thyroid disorders [127]. Furthermore, t(X;14)(p11.4;q32) which cause GPR34 over-expression is also restricted to MALT lymphoma of salivary gland, such as MALT lymphomas with *GPR34* mutation [122,123].

Beyond translocations, a spectrum of chromosomal numerical abnormalities has been described in MALT lymphomas. In the first cytogenetic study in MALT lymphomas from the Isaacson's group, numerical abnormalities of chromosomes 3 and 7 were found in a series of 23 MALT lymphomas [129]. Currently, multiple studies have investigated cytogenetic alterations in MALT lymphomas through several techniques, but in contrast with the aforementioned chromosomal translocations, the role of aneuploidies in lymphomagenesis is less clear and may represent secondary genetic events.

The most common numerical alterations found in MALT lymphomas are trisomy of chromosome 3 or 18, although the frequencies at which these trisomies occur vary markedly with the primary site of disease [130,131]. In cytogenetic studies, trisomy 3 is the most common aberration in MALT lymphomas with a frequency from 20–35% [132,133] to 55–60% [129,131,134], being mainly observed in gastrointestinal, parotid gland and thyroid. By FISH, the prevalence of trisomy 3 is also heterogeneous, from 5–20% [135,136] to 43–85% [131,137–139]. These differences could be the result of different primary sites of MALT lymphoma analyzed but also of different technical approaches. Trisomy 3 can co-occurs with trisomy 18 in up to 30% of cases [140] but is mutually exclusive with the translocation t(11;18)(q21;q21). In CGH analysis, partial gain of 3q affecting the regions 3q21-23 and 3q25-29 is reported, indicating that the latter regions are of particular importance and might point to genes involved in the pathogenesis of MZL [141,142].

The genetic mechanisms by which trisomy 3 contributes to lymphomagenesis are not fully clarified. However, the biological effects of chromosomal trisomies are likely to be explained by an enhanced gene dosage effect resulting from larger copy numbers of genes crucial to lymphoma development. Several candidate genes, such as the protooncogene *BCL6* [143], the transcription factor *FOXP1* [143] or the chemokine receptor *CCR4* [144], all found on chromosome 3, have been linked to lymphomagenesis. In addition, trisomy 3 has been recently associated to cause changes at transcriptome levels similar to that seen in the presence of the *BIRC3-MALT1* rearrangement [145]. Of note, patients harboring trisomy 3 were resistant to *H. pylori* eradication treatment in one study [132].

Trisomy 18 has an approximate frequency around 20% [146,147]. Its presence was associated with a tendency to predict recurrence in the stomach [82] and in the ocular adnexa [110]. By CGH analysis, gain of material of chromosome 18 is the second most frequent alteration, and the most common over-represented region can be delineated to bands 18q21-23 [142].

Other trisomies, such as trisomies 7, 12 and others, have been observed non-randomly but less frequently than trisomy 3 or 18. It is worth mentioning that different from other lymphoma types, copy-neutral LOH did not appear to be a common event in MZL [142].

Improvements in the cytogenetic tools have allowed the identification of lesions with relevant role in the lymphomagenesis of MALT lymphomas. Structural aberrations of chromosome 1 frequently involved the chromosomal regions 1p22, 1p34 and 1q21 [129,148] and gains of chromosomes 1q have been associated with progression or lymphoma relapse [141]. Isolated cases of 8q with a common region in 8q22-24 containing *C-MYC* are reported to have rapid disease progression [141]. C-MYC activation via amplification represents a well-known mechanism of disease progression in a wide spectrum of malignant disorders. Loss of material of chromosome 17, especially of 17p, is the most frequent chromosomal loss observed in MZL [141]. Alterations of *TP53* have also been described in a considerable proportion of gastric MALT lymphomas [149,150] and have been associated with high-grade transformation [149].

Other genomic imbalances have also been found using array-CGH [142,151,152]. For instance, deletion of *TNFAIP3* (*A20*) was detected in MALT lymphomas of the ocular adnexa (19%), thyroid (11%), salivary gland (8%), and liver (0.5%), but not in the lung, stomach, and skin [142,153–156]. In ocular adnexal MALT lymphoma, complete *TNFAIP3* inactivation is associated with reduced lymphoma-free survival [153,157]. TNFAIP3 can inactivate some NF-kB positive regulators including RIP1/2, TRAF6, Ubc13 and NEMO through removing the K63-linked ubiquitin chain, catalyzing the K48-linked polyubiquitination, or direct binding to the linear polyubiquitin chain of its targets [158]. However, *TNFAIP3* inactivation alone is not sufficient for malignant transformation but nonetheless may represent a promising future therapeutic target. In addition, deletion of *CD274* (*PD-L1*) are frequently found in MALT lymphomas of the thyroid, together with mutation in up to 68% of cases (see later) [128].

4. Mutations

Although mutational profiling of hematologic neoplasms currently predominates in the area of myeloid neoplasms, there is a growing wealth of literature describing common and highly characteristic genetic alterations in lymphomas. Certain mutations are enriched in specific lymphoma types, and new discoveries continue to emerge at a rapid pace.

The mutational landscape of MALT lymphomas is wide and, in the last decade, has been characterized using high-throughput technologies such as whole exome sequencing, whole genome sequencing and customized NGS panels. The data available to date show frequent lesions affecting chromatin remodeling and transcription regulation, BCR and NF-κB signalling, NOTCH pathways and immune surveillance. Not surprisingly, MALT lymphomas show considerable variations in the incidence and spectrum of genetic mutations among different sites, similar to what happens with translocations. Overall, the most frequent mutations are: *TNFAIP3* (29%; including deletions), *CREBBP* (22%), *KMT2C* (19%), *TET2* and *SPEN* (17%, each), *KMT2D*, *LRP1B*, and *PRDM1* (15%, each), *EP300* (13%; includes deletion), *TNFRSF14* (11%; includes deletion), *NOTCH1/NOTCH2* (11%, each) and *B2M* (10%; includes deletion) [145]. Other mutations detected in other studies have been *GPR34* (1–19%) and *CCR6* (1–8%) [159]. Similar to what occurs in follicular lymphoma and DLCBCL, mutations in *KMT2C*, *KMT2D*, *CREBBP* and *EP300* tended to coexist [145] (Figure 1 and Supplementary Table S1).

Some mutations deserve their separate discussion. A study prior the NGS era showed that *TP53* was mutated in 18.8% of gastric MALT lymphoma, and the frequency raised up to 33.3% in those transformed to DLBCL. Only 2% of gastric MALT patients showed the concomitance of *TP53* mutation and allele loss, but 22% of DLBCL displayed both *TP53* mutation and allele loss, suggesting that TP53 partial inactivation might play a role in the development of low-grade MALT lymphomas, whereas complete inactivation might be associated with high-grade transformation [149]. However, in recent studies using NGS technologies, *TP53* has not been usually found to be mutated at presentation in MALT lymphomas from several sites [145,159–161].

MYD88 mutation is infrequent in MALT lymphomas altogether [160,162,163], which is in contrast to primary ocular adnexa MALT lymphoma (OAMZL) where *MYD88* mutation, mainly L265P, occurs at frequencies about 6–7% [159,164,165]. The clinical characteristics are similar in patients with and without *MYD88* mutation, including lesion size, lymphoma stage, recurrence, and response to treatment [163]. This gain-of-function mutation enables MYD88 assembling an active complex containing IRAK1 and IRAK4, triggering signaling cascade to activate NF-κB, STAT3 and AP1 transcription factors [166].

As previously mentioned, *TNFAIP3* (*A20*) inactivation by mutation and/or deletion is frequent in MALT lymphomas, in particular in those arising in the ocular adnexa (29–54%) [145,153,167,168], although it has been described in other locations such as the dura (36%) [169], salivary gland (3%) [159] and thyroid (8%) [159], among others. The vast majority of *TNFAIP3* mutations are deleterious changes (frameshift indels and nonsense mutations), resulting in a truncated protein. Interestingly, *TNFAIP3* mutations rarely co-existed with mutations with other genes, supporting their important pathogenetic role in these lymphomas [170]. *TNFAIP3* truncation mutants show a substantial impairment in repression of NF-kB activation. *TNFAIP3* is a key regulator of inflammation signaling pathways as well as a negative regulator of the NF-κB pathway, which inhibits NF-κB activity triggered by signaling from a variety of surface receptors [171]. Thus, *TNFAIP3* inactivation can increase the activation of the canonical NF-κB pathway triggered by signalling from several receptors including BCR, TLR and TNFR1 due to loss of negative regulation on several signalling molecules (IKKγ, TRAF6 and RIP1/2) downstream of their receptors [172–174]. Similarly, *TRAF3* inactivation promotes the activation of the non-canonical NF-κB pathway due to impaired control on NIK degradation [175]. Thus, in gastric MALT lymphoma, alterations of *TRAF3* and *TNFAIP3* were mutually exclusive [176]. Beyond *TNFAIP3* and *MYD88* mutations, MALT lymphoma shows rare or no mutations in other members of NF-kB pathway such as *CD79A*, *CD79B*, *CARD11*, *BIRC3*, and *TNFRSF11A*, which are frequently seen in other B-cell lymphomas with constitutive NF-kB activation.

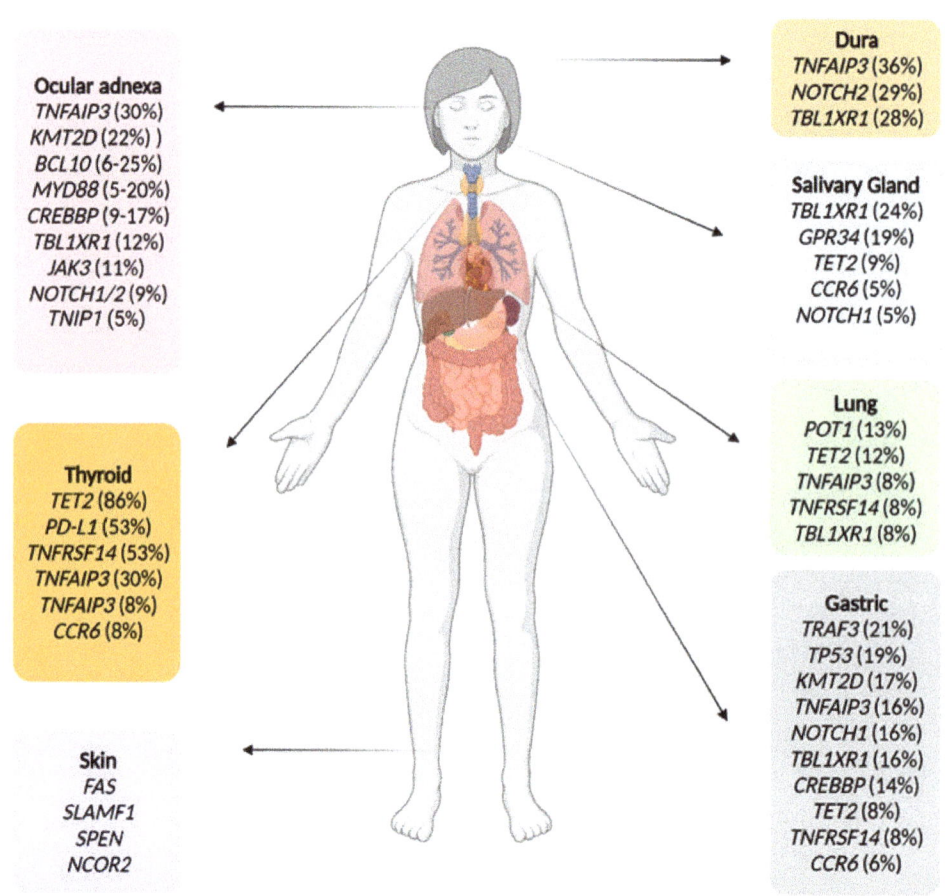

Figure 1. Recurrently mutated genes in MALT lymphoma according to site of origin. Created with BioRender.com.

NOTCH signalling regulates multiple aspects of lymphoid development and function. Although NOTCH inhibits the earliest stage of B lymphopoiesis, it is nevertheless necessary for the development and maintenance of marginal zone lymphocytes [177–179]. However, sustained constitutive NOTCH2 expression alone is insufficient for B-cell lymphomagenesis [180]. Recurrent mutations have been described in *NOTCH1* and *NOTCH2*, but mainly in MALT lymphomas of the ocular adnexa (8–10%) [160] and dura (29%) [169]. These mutations mainly resulted in a shortened *NOTCH1/2* product lacking TAD or PEST domains, which governs protein stability and degradation [181]. NOTCH1/2 mutations have been associated to aggressive course in some lymphoproliferative disorders [182–186], but the prognostic impact in MALT lymphomas remains to be determined. In a study of gastric

MALT lymphoma, *NOTCH1* mutations were enriched in patients who failed to *H. pylori* eradication [176]. In addition to *NOTCH1/2*, genetic lesions in additional NOTCH pathway modulators or members, including *SPEN* (17%) and *DELTEX1*, have been identified [145]. These mutations represent activation modifications that are likely to improve *NOTCH* stability and activity [187].

Several chromatin remodeling and transcriptional regulators are recurrently mutated in MALT lymphoma of different sites, including *TBL1XR1, TET2, MLL2/KMT2D* and *CREBBP* [37,145,159–161,176]. *TBL1XR1* mutations are found in MALT lymphoma of the salivary gland (24%) [159], ocular adnexa (6–18%) [159–161,168,188], and in *H. pylori*-resistant gastric MALT lymphoma (16%) [176]. In dural extranodal MZL, recurrent *TBL1XR1* mutations were only seen in association with *NOTCH2* mutations (4/11, 36%), which might indicate a co-operative role for these mutations in lymphomagenesis [169]. The majority of *TBL1XR1* mutations are missense changes affecting regions or residues critical for interaction with NCoR, and may increase TBL1XR1 binding to NCoR and facilitate its degradation, consequently promoting NF-κB and JUN target gene expression [37,159]. *TET2* mutations are frequently found in MALT lymphoma of the thyroid (62%) [128] and will be discussed later. Loss of function *MLL2/KMT2D* mutations have been described in several B-cell lymphomas, and the frequency in MALT lymphomas is variable among studies (5–25%) [145,160,161]. *CREBBP* mutations are also frequent observed (4–22%) [37,145,168,188,189].

Genetic abnormalities that regulate B and T cell interactions have also been described in MALT lymphomas. Mutations in *TNFRSF14* are frequently seen in those arising in the thyroid (46–52%) [128,159] but are also detected in lymphomas from other sites [37,145,159]. Most *TNFRSF14* mutations are deleterious changes such as nonsense, frameshift alterations, thus most likely inactivating or impairing the protein function. Thereby, *TNFRSF14* inactivation may enable malignant B-cells to gain more T-cell help.

As previously discussed, mutations in MALT lymphoma can vary widely depending on the site of origin and, therefore, characteristic locations have been the subject of specific genetic studies.

OAMZL have been the focus of mutation investigations by several groups. Initial studies found recurrent mutations in *TNFAIP3* (30%), *MYD88* (5–20%), and *BCL10* (6–25%), whereas other genes were rarely or not mutated in the cases analyzed [165,167,190] Later, other studies using whole exome sequencing (WES) or customized NGS panels have found mutations in many other genes, albeit with disparate frequencies. These differences could be attributed to regional variances or different sensibilities in the techniques used that could potentially identify subclonal mutations. Using a NGS panel, Johansson et al., besides validation of mutations previously described, found mutations in *KMT2D* (22%), *NOTCH1* (8%), *NOTCH2* (8%), *TNIP1* (5%), *NFKBIA* (4%), and in other genes at lower frequencies [160]. Using WES, Moody et al., also found a high proportion of patients with *TNFAIP3* mutations (36%), and also recurrent mutations in *MYD88* (7%), *TBL1XR1* (6%), *TNFRSF14* (5%) and *TET2* (4%), besides a few less frequently mutated genes [159]. A further mutation studies identified mutations in additional genes such as *CREBBP* (9–17%) [161,168] and *LRP1B* (6%) [161]. Interestingly, Vela et al., described that up to 65% MALT lymphomas harbored mutations of NF-κB compounds, raising the possibility of precision therapy with BCR inhibitors in refractory cases to conventional treatment. Other genome-wide mutation study identified mutations in *JAK3* (11%) that were located at sites known to alter the protein function and leading to activation of the JAK/STAT signaling pathway by causing a gain of function of *JAK3* [188]. Patients carrying *JAK3* mutation had shorter progression free survival, but not reduced overall survival [188]. Identification of activating *JAK3* mutations in OAML opens the option for potential precision therapeutics by targeting the JAK/STAT pathway with JAK inhibitors. Other newly identified genes recurrently mutated (5–10%) included members of the collagen family (*COL12A1* and *COL1A2*) and *DOCK8* which is involved in RhoGTPase signaling [188].

In SGMZL, G-protein coupled receptors have been found mutated at high frequency (*TBL1XR1* = 24%, *GPR34* = 19%) [159]. Interestingly, *GPR34* mutation is almost exclusive of this site and mutations in *GPR34* and *CCR6*, both members of the GPCR family, are mutually exclusive [159].

In MALT lymphomas of the thyroid, Wu et al., have found frequent deleterious mutations of *TET2* (86%), and also mutations in *CD274* (53%), *TNFRSF14* (53%), and *TNFAIP3* (30%) [128]. Both *TNFRSF14* and *TET2* had a significantly higher variant allele frequency than *TNFAIP3*, suggesting that *TNFAIP3* mutations may occur later than *TET2* and *TNFRSF14* changes. In patients carrying *TET2* mutations, 46% of them had two mutations and also had a significantly higher number of somatic variants compared with those without. Most *TET2* mutations are deleterious alterations, inactivating or impairing its dioxygenase activity, hence its role in DNA demethylation, consequently affecting a wide spectrum of gene expression [159,191]. In MALT lymphomas, *TET2* inactivation may deregulate the expression of transcriptional factors indispensable for B-cell function, and thus potentially cooperate with receptor signalling, including those by the enhanced T-helper cell signals, indirectly triggered by *PD-L1/TNFRSF14* inactivation in malignant B-cells [128].

Kiesewetter et al., have recently investigated the genetic characterization of *H. pylori*-negative gastric MALT lymphoma. In addition to reconfirming that the *MALT1* translocation is the most frequent genetic alteration (39%, most likely t(11;18)(q21;q21)/*BIRC3-MALT1*) and *IGH* translocation was further seen in 40% of MALT1-negative cases, mutations in NF-kB signaling pathways were detected in 40% of cases (*TNFAIP3* = 23%, *CARD11* = 9%, *MAP3K14* = 9%). The NF-kB pathway mutations were mutually exclusive from MALT1, albeit not IGH translocation, in total occurring in 86% of cases [189]. Then, *H. pylori*- negative gastric MALT lymphomas harbor activating mutations that affect both canonical and non-canonical NF-kB pathways [192].

Other studies analyzing the mutational landscape of MALT lymphomas at several sites have been conducted and the list of involved genes keeps growing [193].

5. MicroRNAs

MicroRNAs are small non-coding RNAs that modulate gene expression on a post-transcriptional level, playing critical roles in cellular proliferation, apoptosis and differentiation [194,195]. MicroRNAs have important roles as tumor suppressor genes and oncogenes in human malignancies, including in lymphomas [196,197]. Only a few studies have analyzed the role of microRNAs in MALT lymphomas, as diagnostic or prognostic tools.

In *H. pylori*-associated gastric MALT lymphoma, Craig et al., identified miR-203 as one of the most strongly downregulated miRNAs in comparison with normal lymphoid tissue, suggesting that might be a key player in the transformation from chronic gastritis to MALT lymphoma. In addition, since ABL1 is the target of miR-203, treatment with imatinib and dasatinib (BCR/ABL inhibitors) prevented tumor cell growth [198]. Zhang et al., have found 53 upregulated and 25 downregulated miRNAs in gastric MALT lymphoma. Subsequently, they found upregulated miR-320a, miR-940, and miR-622, and downregulated miR-331-3p and miR-429 miRNA, and after bioinformatic analysis, miR-320a, miR-622, and miR-429 were found likely to be functionally related to each other as they have the same targets, such as *C-MYC* [199].

miR-142-5p and miR-155 have also been found overexpressed in gastric MALT lymphoma [200]. miR-155, observed during *H. pylori* infection, may be a potential predictor of resistance to *H. pylori* eradication therapy, independently of *API2/MALT1* fusion gene [200]. Inhibition of miRNAs with chemically engineered oligonucleotides, known as "antagomirs", has been shown to work as specific inhibitors of endogenous miRNAs in mice, and they could be used to silence miR-142 and miR-155 for the treatment of gastric MALT lymphomas resistant to *H. pylori* eradication [201,202].

Our group found through analyses of expression of 384 miRNAs that gastric MALT lymphomas are characterized by specific miRNA expression profile, different to that seen in chronic gastritis and reactive lymphoid tissue. In addition, 17 differentially miRNAs were expressed between patients carrying or not t(11;18)(q21;q21). Overexpression of miR-142-3p and miR-155 and downregulation of miR-203 were detected in gastric MALT lymphomas in comparison with chronic gastritis. These finding suggest that expression levels of these miRNAs might be useful for the differential diagnosis between chronic gastritis and gastric MALT lymphoma [203].

In conjunctival MALT lymphoma, some upregulated miRNAs, such as miR-150/155, as well as downregulated miRNAs, such as miR-184, miR-200a/b/c, and miR-205, have also been identified. Dysregulation of the miR-200 family might be involved in the pathogenesis and progression of the lymphoma [204]. The miRNA-200 family inhibits the initiating step of metastasis, the epithelial-mesenchymal transition, by maintaining the epithelial phenotype through directly targeting the transcriptional repressors [205].

All of these miRNAs may be important in the pathomechanisms of MALT lymphoma. However, further studies are needed to clarify their role in the pathogenesis and also its utility in the clinical practice.

6. Transcriptomics

Understanding the transcriptome, the complete set of transcripts in a cell and their quantity, is crucial for interpreting the functional elements of the genome and revealing the molecular constituents of cells and tissues, and also for understanding development and disease [206]. Integration of transcriptome data allows for screening of molecular alterations in deregulated B cells, as well as identification of downstream target genes and pathways, shedding light on the understanding of the lymphomagenesis and in the development of novel therapeutics.

The gene expression profile of MALT lymphomas of the lung was analyzed by Chng et al., who described a prominent T-cell signature and a marginal zone/memory B-cell profile [207]. Gene expression profile also revealed one molecular subset characterized by *MALT1* translocations, having overexpression of NF-KB pathway genes and enrichment for chemokine signaling pathways (CXCR6 and the ligand of CCR5, CCL5). Another subset displayed increased plasma cells and a prominent plasma cell gene signature [207]. In addition, clusters with different biologic characteristics were identified through the analysis of several genes with very high expression in individual samples, such as cases with *MALT1* translocations with high expression of MALT1 and RARA, samples with plasmocytic differentiation having high FKBP11 expression, and cases with high RGS13 expression tending to have trisomy 3 and reactive follicles [207]. CCR4 (3p22.3) was found to be overexpressed in MALT lymphoma bearing trisomy 3 [144].

In 33 MZL cases (18 MALT lymphomas), gains affecting chromosomes 3q and 18 seemed to influence B-cell receptor signaling pathways, cell cycle, Wnt signaling, and apoptosis, whereas genes associated with 3p and 18p gains formed transcripts involved in chemokine and cytokine signaling pathway, ubiquitin proteasome pathway, Ras signaling, and in tight junction regulation [142]. *FOXP1* (3p14.1) is overexpressed in a few MALT lymphomas due to its juxtaposition to the immunoglobulin heavy chain gene promoter after chromosomal translocation [118].

Translocation-positive MALT lymphomas (from all sites) are characterized by an enhanced expression of NF-kB target genes, mainly *TLR6*, chemokine, *CD69*, *CCR2* and *BCL2*, while translocation-negative cases are characterized by active inflammatory and immune responses, such as interleukin-8, CD86, CD28 and ICOS [208]. The expression of these NF-kB target genes was higher in cases with *MYD88* mutation than in those without the mutation, with TLR6 showing a significant difference [165].

Recently, the transcriptome of MALT lymphomas of the lung harbouring *BIRC3-MALT1* fusion was analysed by Cascione et al. [145], identifying enrichment in MYC target genes, oxidative phosphorylation and DNA repair, genes related to cell cycle, among others. Members of the TNF-receptor superfamily, *TNFSF12-TNFSF13 (TWE-PRIL)*, *TNFRSF17*

(*BCMA*), *LTB* (*lymphotoxin β*), and *CXCR3* were among the most upregulated genes in this subset of patients.

In *H. pylori*-positive gastric MALT lymphoma cells, Zou et al., have found 15 pathways differentially enriched, including the Wnt, the mTOR, the NOD-like receptor and the Hippo signalling pathways. By deregulating these pathways, *H. pylori* might influence gastric lymphomagenesis through modulating the proliferation of cells, inducing autophagy and fostering inflammatory responses and epithelial mesenchymal transition. By proteomic analysis, they also identified 116 differentially expressed proteins, most of them previously associated with cancer that can be used as biomarkers for lymphoma diagnosis or as potential therapeutic targets [209].

Zhang et al., conducted a study to identify transcriptomic biomarkers in *H. pylori*-infected gastritis and gastric cancer or MALT lymphoma [210]. In gastric MALT lymphoma, lncRNA GHRLOS and another 44 mRNA were aberrantly expressed, in agreement with previous studies showing upregulation of lncRNA GHRLOS in different solid tumours [211]. In addition, several molecules such as CXCL13, CCL18, CCL19, CCL 20 and TLR 10 were found to be dysregulated in MALT lymphoma, suggesting that not only modulate *H. pylori* infection but also affect the risk of MALT lymphoma [210].

7. Epigenetics and Methylation

Epigenetic alterations such as disturbances of DNA methylation and histone modification are common in B-cell lymphomas, contributing to lymphomagenesis [212]. Alterations involving epigenetic regulators have been described in MALT lymphomas from different sites. Inactivation of chromatin remodeling genes are frequently observed in MALT lymphomas, with the most common mutated genes being *TET2, KMT2D, CREBBP, TBL1X1, KMT2C, MT2C, EP300*, among others [37,145,156,157,159,167,169,176] (Figure 1 and Supplemental Table S1).

In thyroid MALT lymphomas, as previously mentioned, *TET2* mutations were very common with frequencies up to 85.5% [128,159]. Mutations in TET2 has been associated with increased DNA methylation. Interestingly, genes with hypermethylated promoters in TET2 mutated cases were mostly enriched for the PRC2-complex (*EZH2, EED* and *SUZ12*) targets, genes bearing histone H3 dimethylation at K4 (H3K4me2) and trimethylation at K27 (H3K27me3). *TET2* mutations have been also described (in percentages below 10%) in the salivary gland, ocular adnexa, stomach, and lung (among others). Since *TET2* mutations are associated with higher response rate to demethylating agents in myeloid leukemias, it is reasonable to investigate the role of demethylating agents in patients with *TET2* mutated MALT lymphomas.

In OAMZL, the most commonly reported epigenetic mutated gene is *KMT2D* with frequencies varying from 14% to 22% [160,161,168], and in *Helicobacter pylori*-negative gastric MALT lymphoma, *KMT2D* (17%) and *CREBBP* (14%) are the two most epigenetic regulator gene mutations [189]. In fact, as previously discussed, mutations in *CREBBP* are found in 4–22% of MALT lymphomas [37,145,168,188,189]. The *CREBBP* gene encodes a lysine acetyltransferase (KAT) protein that activates gene expression through acetylation of histone H3 lysine 18 (H3K18Ac), histone H3 lysine 27 (H3K27Ac), and other residues. KAT domain mutation of *CREBBP* inhibit its catalytic activity and leads to a dominant-repressive effect by preventing the participation of redundant acetyltransferases in transactivation complexes, leading to loss of antagonism to BCL6-mediated gene repression and reduced expression of antigen presentation and interferon signaling genes in germinal-center lymphomas [213]. By using HDAC3-selective inhibitors, these genes can be restored in *CREBBP* mutant cells [214]. This suggests that epigenetic modulation of immune response with HDAC3 inhibitors (or EZH2 inhibitors) may be explored in *CREBBP*-mutant MALT lymphomas, alone or in combination with PD1/PD-L1 blockade (to prevent interferon-induced adaptive immune suppression).

While classical mutations in genes are region-limited, epimutations often occur early in cancer development and have a genome-wide impact. CpG island hypermethylation of

TP15 and *TP73* genes was detected more frequently in gastric MALT lymphomas than in gastric or nodal DLBCL [215]. Hypermethylation of *DAP-k* (72.2%), *GSTP1* (50%), *MGMT* (27.2%) and *TP73* (9%) have been found in MALT lymphomas [216]. Inactivation of the extrinsic pathway of apoptosis through DAP-k methylation, genetic instability favoring acquisition of DNA point mutation caused by MGMT hypermethylation and scavenging reactive oxygen species causing an inflammatory microenvironment by GSTP1 inactivation through promoter methylation may represent pathogenetic events in gastric MALT lymphomagenesis [216]. In MALT lymphomas of the lung, p16 gene methylation was detected at a frequently of 60%, similar to that found in DLBCL (55%), and was not correlated with API2-MALT1 fusion, serum LDH, clinical stage, and increased large cells [217]. The same group showed in MALT lymphoma of the skin that hypermethylation of the CpG islands of the tumor suppressor genes *DAPK* and *TP16^{INK4a}* was frequently observed at its initial presentation, but not at tumor progression [72]. These observations suggest that hypermethylation of various genes may be early molecular events that contribute in early MALT lymphomagenesis.

Furthermore, aberrant methylation has also been implicated in tumor progression. Dugge et al., investigated the DNA methylation changes associated with progression of gastric MALT lymphoma through genome-wide DNA methylation profiling and observed that 7698 CpG loci associated with 2419 genes were significantly differentially methylated during gastric MALT lymphoma progression [218]. Among these loci, enrichment of CpGs associated with the promoter was seen and the loci were also enriched in the CpG-rich regions, with most of loci being located within CpG islands [219]. As CpG islands are sites of transcription initiation whose methylation affects chromatin structure, the differentially methylated loci locate to regions involved in transcriptional regulation, which may influence the gene expression. However, no significant changes in the RNA expression levels in the majority of differentially methylated genes were identified. Nevertheless, morphological differences were reflected between gastric MALT lymphoma transformed to large cell lymphoma by characteristic DNA methylation profiles

Since epigenetic changes are potentially reversible, epigenetic therapy, both alone or in combination with established treatment regimens, has a promising future, leading to potentially less toxic and more effective approaches that standard chemotherapy.

8. Applicability in the Real-World

Davis et al., have explored the clinical and practical diagnostic utility of a targeted NGS within mature lymphoid neoplasms (MLN) [220]. They studied the integration of a 40 gene lymphoid panel in 534 MLN during 1-year into the routine comprehensive characterization of lymphomas and found that this practice is not of current diagnostic value in most cases. Improved diagnostic outcomes that led to changing, refining, and facilitating diagnoses were evident in only 5.5% of cases when such testing was applied empirically. Nevertheless, there remains the potential for better outcomes if the practice is standardized [220]. In MZL, from 52 cases, 25 disease-associated variants, 10 variants of uncertain significance, 14 no variant and 3 QLF (qualitative failure due to inadequate DNA quality) were observed. In this study, refinements of diagnoses were most frequently reported due to either the presence or absence of *MYD88* mutations in distinguishing LPL from MZL or the presence of *NOTCH2* and *TNFAIP3* mutations in favoring a diagnosis of MZL over LPL [220].

Pillonel et al., reported a 3-year experience with a 68-gene lymphoma NGS panel applied to 80 cases [221]. The analysis was useful in most cases, helping to confirm or support diagnoses in 35 of 50 histologically difficult cases. However, while it may appear that the diagnostic utility rate is much higher than reported by Davis (70% vs. 5.5%), it should be noted that cases included in the Swiss group were highly selected, based upon a predetermined perceived need for mutational analysis, resulting in only ~1% of all cases being analyzed. NGS analysis was useful to detect potentially therapy or matching drugs were still not available/accessible. However, no patients directly benefited from a matched targeted therapy, which might be mainly linked to the lack of approved agents in lymphoma management. Recently, tazemetostat, a methyltransferase inhibitor, has been approved by FDA for relapsed or refractory follicular lymphoma whose tumors are positive for an *EZH2* mutation and who have received at least 2 prior systemic therapies and also for relapsed or refractory follicular lymphoma who have no suitable alternative treatment options [222]. This precision therapy will change the usefulness of NGS panels for lymphomas in the near future.

Currently, NGS analysis is not generally applied to patients as first-line investigational approach, but rather applicable to further define diagnosis in highly selected otherwise equivocal instances and/or to identify mutations that will guide treatment decisions in cases in which standard treatment options are scarce or suboptimal [221].

9. Conclusions

MALT lymphomas are a diverse group of lymphoid neoplasms that exhibit a wide range of genetic features depending on the site of origin. Despite the fact that MALT lymphoma of different anatomic locations shares many common clinicopathological characteristics, there are substantial variances in the aetiology, Ig gene usage, and acquired genetic alterations. Then, it is crucial to better characterize the somatic mutation profile of MALT lymphomas and unravel their molecular oncogenic complexity applying the latest NGS platforms.

Excitingly, the majority of the genetic changes affects NF-KB signal pathway-related genes, resulting in constitutive NF-kB pathway activation. At the same time, since targeted gene sequencing panels have been recently applied to MALT lymphomas, we have learned that other genes are also frequently affected such as those involved in chromatin remodeling, BCR/TLR and NOTCH pathways. The growing knowledge of its genetic landscape, methylation, and transcriptome features raises the possibility of applying new agents to treat a subset of MALT lymphoma patients and also push forward the concept of precision medicine in this type of lymphoma.

Supplementary Materials: The following are available online at https://www.mdpi.com/article/10.3390/cancers14010176/s1, Table S1. Recurrently mutated genes in MALT lymphomas.

Author Contributions: Study concept and design: A.S.; methodology, literature review, data collection, analysis and interpretation: J.J.R.-S. and A.S.; writing-original draft manuscript: J.J.R.-S. and A.S.; figure editing: J.J.R.-S.; review-original final manuscript: J.J.R.-S. and A.S. All authors have read and agreed to the published version of the manuscript. We apologize to authors of several high-profile articles whose work was not included owing to space limitations.

Funding: This research received no external funding.

Acknowledgments: This study was supported in part by ISCIII, FIS-FEDER PI19/00034, GILEAD GLD18/00117, 2017SGR205, PT17/0015/0011 and Xarxa de Banc de Tumors de Catalunya.

Conflicts of Interest: The authors declare no conflict of interest.

References

1. Isaacson, P.; Wright, D.H. Malignant lymphoma of mucosa-associated lymphoid tissue. A distinctive type of B-cell lymphoma. *Cancer* **1983**, *52*, 1410–1416. [CrossRef]
2. Swerdlow, S.H.; World Health Organization, International Agency for Research on Cancer. *WHO Classification of Tumours of Haematopoietic and Lymphoid Tissues*; World Health Organization: Geneva, Switzerland; IARC: Lyon, France, 2017.
3. Teras, L.R.; DeSantis, C.E.; Cerhan, J.R.; Morton, L.M.; Jemal, A.; Flowers, C.R. 2016 US lymphoid malignancy statistics by World Health Organization subtypes. *CA Cancer J. Clin.* **2016**, *66*, 443–459. [CrossRef]
4. Cerhan, J.R.; Habermann, T.M. Epidemiology of Marginal Zone Lymphoma. *Ann. Lymphoma* **2021**, *5*, 1. [CrossRef] [PubMed]
5. Luminari, S.; Cesaretti, M.; Marcheselli, L.; Rashid, I.; Madrigali, S.; Maiorana, A.; Federico, M. Decreasing incidence of gastric MALT lymphomas in the era of anti-*Helicobacter pylori* interventions: Results from a population-based study on extranodal marginal zone lymphomas. *Ann. Oncol.* **2010**, *21*, 855–859. [CrossRef] [PubMed]
6. Zucca, E.; Bertoni, F. The spectrum of MALT lymphoma at different sites: Biological and therapeutic relevance. *Blood* **2016**, *127*, 2082–2092. [CrossRef]
7. Isaacson, P.G.; Du, M.-Q. MALT lymphoma: From morphology to molecules. *Nat. Rev. Cancer* **2004**, *4*, 644–653. [CrossRef]

8. Ferreri, A.J.M.; Govi, S.; Ponzoni, M. Marginal zone lymphomas and infectious agents. *Semin. Cancer Biol.* **2013**, *23*, 431–440. [CrossRef]
9. Zucca, E.; Conconi, A.; Pedrinis, E.; Cortelazzo, S.; Motta, T.; Gospodarowicz, M.K.; Patterson, B.J.; Ferreri, J.M.; Ponzoni, M.; Devizzi, L.; et al. Nongastric marginal zone B-cell lymphoma of mucosa-associated lymphoid tissue. *Arbor Cienc. Pensam. Cult.* **2003**, *101*, 2489–2495. [CrossRef]
10. Isaacson, P.G. Gastrointestinal lymphoma. *Hum. Pathol.* **1994**, *25*, 1020–1029. [CrossRef]
11. Morgner, A.; Lehn, N.; Andersen, L.P.; Thiede, C.; Bennedsen, M.; Trebesius, K.; Neubauer, B.; Neubauer, A.; Stolte, M.; Bayerdörffer, E. *Helicobacter heilmannii*-associated primary gastric low-grade MALT lymphoma: Complete remission after curing the infection. *Gastroenterology* **2000**, *118*, 821–828. [CrossRef]
12. Ponzoni, M.; Ferreri, A.J.M.; Guidoboni, M.; Lettini, A.A.; Cangi, M.G.; Pasini, E.; Sacchi, L.; Pecciarini, L.; Grassi, S.; Dal Cin, E.; et al. Chlamydia Infection and Lymphomas: Association Beyond Ocular Adnexal Lymphomas Highlighted by Multiple Detection Methods. *Clin. Cancer Res.* **2008**, *14*, 5794–5800. [CrossRef]
13. Ferreri, A.J.M.; Guidoboni, M.; Ponzoni, M.; De Conciliis, C.; Dell'Oro, S.; Fleischhauer, K.; Caggiari, L.; Lettini, A.A.; Dal Cin, E.; Ieri, R.; et al. Evidence for an association between *Chlamydia psittaci* and ocular adnexal lymphomas. *J. Natl. Cancer Inst.* **2004**, *96*, 586–594. [CrossRef]
14. Goodlad, J.R.; Davidson, M.M.; Hollowood, K.; Ling, C.; MacKenzie, C.; Christie, I.; Batstone, P.J.; Ho-Yen, D.O. Primary cutaneous B-cell lymphoma and *Borrelia burgdorferi* infection in patients from the highlands of Scotland. *Am. J. Surg. Pathol.* **2000**, *24*, 1279–1285. [CrossRef]
15. Cerroni, L.; Zöchling, N.; Pütz, B.; Kerl, H. Infection by *Borrelia burgdorferi* and cutaneous B-cell lymphoma. *J. Cutan. Pathol.* **1997**, *24*, 457–461. [CrossRef]
16. Lecuit, M.; Abachin, E.; Martin, A.; Poyart, C.; Pochart, P.; Suarez, F.; Bengoufa, D.; Feuillard, J.; Lavergne, A.; Gordon, J.I.; et al. Immunoproliferative Small Intestinal Disease Associated with *Campylobacter jejuni*. *N. Engl. J. Med.* **2004**, *350*, 239–248. [CrossRef] [PubMed]
17. Adam, P.; Czapiewski, P.; Colak, S.; Kosmidis, P.; Tousseyn, T.; Sagaert, X.; Boudova, L.; Okoń, K.; Morresi-Hauf, A.; Agostinelli, C.; et al. Prevalence of *Achromobacter xylosoxidans* in pulmonary mucosa-associated lymphoid tissue lymphoma in different regions of Europe. *Br. J. Haematol.* **2014**, *164*, 804–810. [CrossRef] [PubMed]
18. Wöhrer, S.; Troch, M.; Streubel, B.; Zwerina, J.; Skrabs, C.; Formanek, M.; Hauff, W.; Hoffmann, M.; Müllauer, L.; Chott, A.; et al. MALT lymphoma in patients with autoimmune diseases: A comparative analysis of characteristics and clinical course. *Leukemia* **2007**, *21*, 1812–1818. [CrossRef] [PubMed]
19. Galanina, N.; Bejar, R.; Choi, M.; Goodman, A.; Wieduwilt, M.; Mulroney, C.; Kim, L.; Yeerna, H.; Tamayo, P.; Vergilio, J.A.; et al. Comprehensive genomic profiling reveals diverse but actionable molecular portfolios across hematologic malignancies: Implications for next generation clinical trials. *Cancers* **2019**, *11*, 11. [CrossRef] [PubMed]
20. Hussell, T.; Isaacson, P.G.; Spencer, J. Proliferation and differentiation of tumour cells from B-cell lymphoma of mucosa-associated lymphoid tissue in vitro. *J. Pathol.* **1993**, *169*, 221–227. [CrossRef] [PubMed]
21. Noy, A.; de Vos, S.; Thieblemont, C.; Martin, P.; Flowers, C.R.; Morschhauser, F.; Collins, G.P.; Ma, S.; Coleman, M.; Peles, S.; et al. Targeting Bruton tyrosine kinase with ibrutinib in relapsed/refractory marginal zone lymphoma. *Blood* **2017**, *129*, 2224–2232. [CrossRef]
22. Aarts, W.M.; Bende, R.J.; Steenbergen, E.J.; Kluin, P.M.; Ooms, E.C.M.; Pals, S.T.; Van Noesel, C.J.M. Variable heavy chain gene analysis of follicular lymphomas: Correlation between heavy chain isotype expression and somatic mutation load. *Blood* **2000**, *95*, 2922–2929. [CrossRef]
23. Hallas, C.; Greiner, A.; Peters, K.; Müller-Hermelink, H.K. Immunoglobulin V(H) genes of high-grade mucosa-associated lymphoid tissue lymphomas show a high load of somatic mutations and evidence of antigen-dependent affinity maturation. *Lab. Investig.* **1998**, *78*, 277–287. [PubMed]
24. Qin, Y.; Greiner, A.; Trunk, M.J.F.; Schmausser, B.; Ott, M.M.; Müller-Hermelink, H.K. Somatic Hypermutation in Low-Grade Mucosa-Associated Lymphoid Tissue-Type B-Cell Lymphoma. *Blood* **1995**, *86*, 3528–3534. [CrossRef] [PubMed]
25. Bende, R.J.; Aarts, W.M.; Riedl, R.G.; De Jong, D.; Pals, S.T.; Van Noesel, C.J.M. Among B cell non-Hodgkin's lymphomas, MALT lymphomas express a unique antibody repertoire with frequent rheumatoid factor reactivity. *J. Exp. Med.* **2005**, *201*, 1229–1241. [CrossRef]
26. Du, M.; Diss, T.C.; Xu, C.; Peng, H.; Isaacson, P.G.; Pan, L. Ongoing mutation in MALT lymphoma immunoglobulin gene suggests that antigen stimulation plays a role in the clonal expansion. *Leukemia* **1996**, *10*, 1190–1197.
27. Bertoni, F.; Cazzaniga, G.; Bosshard, G.; Roggero, E.; Barbazza, R.; De Boni, M.; Capella, C.; Pedrinis, E.; Cavalli, F.; Biondi, A.; et al. Immunoglobulin heavy chain diversity genes rearrangement pattern indicates that MALT-type gastric lymphoma B cells have undergone an antigen selection process. *Br. J. Haematol.* **1997**, *97*, 830–836. [CrossRef]
28. Tierens, A.; Delabie, J.; Pittaluga, S.; Driessen, A.; De Wolf-Peeters, C.; DeWolf-Peeters, C. Mutation analysis of the rearranged immunoglobulin heavy chain genes of marginal zone cell lymphomas indicates an origin from different marginal zone B lymphocyte subsets. *Blood* **1998**, *91*, 2381–2386. [CrossRef] [PubMed]
29. Xochelli, A.; Bikos, V.; Polychronidou, E.; Galigalidou, C.; Agathangelidis, A.; Charlotte, F.; Moschonas, P.; Davis, Z.; Colombo, M.; Roumelioti, M.; et al. Disease-biased and shared characteristics of the immunoglobulin gene repertoires in marginal zone B cell lymphoproliferations. *J. Pathol.* **2019**, *247*, 416–421. [CrossRef]

30. Craig, V.J.; Arnold, I.; Gerke, C.; Huynh, M.Q.; Wündisch, T.; Neubauer, A.; Renner, C.; Falkow, S.; Müller, A. Gastric MALT lymphoma B cells express polyreactive, somatically mutated immunoglobulins. *Blood* 2010, *115*, 581–591. [CrossRef]
31. Du, M.-Q. Mucosa-associated lymphoid tissue lymphoma of various sites: Common molecular mechanisms but different players. *Ann. Lymphoma* 2020, *4*, 8. [CrossRef]
32. Bende, R.J.; Janssen, J.; Beentjes, A.; Wormhoudt, T.A.M.; Wagner, K.; Haacke, E.A.; Kroese, F.G.M.; Guikema, J.E.; van Noesel, C.J.M. Salivary gland MALT lymphomas of Sjögren's syndrome patients in majority express rheumatoid factors affinity-selected for IgG. *Arthritis Rheumatol.* 2020, in press. [CrossRef]
33. Hoogeboom, R.; Bende, R.J.; Van Noesel, C.J.M. MALT lymphoma-derived rheumatoid factors are nonpolyreactive high-affinity antibodies. *Blood* 2010, *116*, 1818–1819. [CrossRef]
34. Coupland, S.E.; Foss, H.D.; Anagnostopoulos, I.; Hummel, M.; Stein, H. Immunoglobulin V(H) gene expression among extranodal marginal zone B-cell lymphomas of the ocular adnexa. *Investig. Ophthalmol. Vis. Sci.* 1999, *40*, 555–562.
35. Mannami, T.; Yoshino, T.; Oshima, K.; Takase, S.; Kondo, E.; Ohara, N.; Nakagawa, H.; Ohtsuki, H.; Harada, M.; Akagi, T. Clinical, histopathological, and immunogenetic analysis of ocular adnexal lymphoproliferative disorders: Characterization of MALT lymphoma and reactive lymphoid hyperplasia. *Mod. Pathol.* 2001, *14*, 641–649. [CrossRef]
36. Bahler, D.W.; Szankasi, P.; Kulkarni, S.; Tubbs, R.R.; Cook, J.R.; Swerdlow, S.H. Use of similar immunoglobulin VH gene segments by MALT lymphomas of the ocular adnexa. *Mod. Pathol.* 2009, *22*, 833–838. [CrossRef]
37. Moody, S.; Escudero-Ibarz, L.; Wang, M.; Clipson, A.; Ruiz, E.O.; Dunn-Walters, D.; Xue, X.; Zeng, N.; Robson, A.; Chuang, S.-S.; et al. Significant association between TNFAIP3 inactivation and biased immunoglobulin heavy chain variable region 4-34 usage in mucosa-associated lymphoid tissue lymphoma. *J. Pathol.* 2017, *243*, 3–8. [CrossRef]
38. van Maldegem, F.; Wormhoudt, T.A.M.; Mulder, M.M.S.; Oud, M.E.C.M.; Schilder-Tol, E.; Musler, A.R.; Aten, J.; Saeed, P.; Kersten, M.J.; Pals, S.T.; et al. *Chlamydia psittaci*-negative ocular adnexal marginal zone B-cell lymphomas have biased VH4-34 immunoglobulin gene expression and proliferate in a distinct inflammatory environment. *Leukemia* 2012, *26*, 1647–1653. [CrossRef] [PubMed]
39. Dagklis, A.; Ponzoni, M.; Govi, S.; Cangi, M.G.; Pasini, E.; Charlotte, F.; Vino, A.; Doglioni, C.; Davi, F.; Lossos, I.S.; et al. Immunoglobulin gene repertoire in ocular adnexal lymphomas: Hints on the nature of the antigenic stimulation. *Leukemia* 2012, *26*, 814–821. [CrossRef] [PubMed]
40. Richardson, C.; Chida, A.S.; Adlowitz, D.; Silver, L.; Fox, E.; Jenks, S.A.; Palmer, E.; Wang, Y.; Heimburg-Molinaro, J.; Li, Q.-Z.; et al. Molecular Basis of 9G4 B Cell Autoreactivity in Human Systemic Lupus Erythematosus. *J. Immunol.* 2013, *191*, 4926–4939. [CrossRef] [PubMed]
41. Zhu, D.; Ikpatt, O.F.; Dubovy, S.R.; Lossos, C.; Natkunam, Y.; Chapman-Fredricks, J.R.; Fan, Y.-S.; Lossos, I.S. Molecular and genomic aberrations in *Chlamydophila psittaci* negative ocular adnexal marginal zone lymphomas. *Am. J. Hematol.* 2013, *88*, 730–735. [CrossRef]
42. Thiede, C.; Alpen, B.; Morgner, A.; Schmidt, M.; Ritter, M.; Ehninger, G.; Stolte, M.; Bayerdörffer, E.; Neubauer, A. Ongoing somatic mutations and clonal expansions after cure of *Helicobacter pylori* infection in gastric mucosa-assiociated lymphoid tissue B-cell lymphoma. *J. Clin. Oncol.* 1998, *16*, 3822–3831. [CrossRef] [PubMed]
43. Michaeli, M.; Tabibian-Keissar, H.; Schiby, G.; Shahaf, G.; Pickman, Y.; Hazanov, L.; Rosenblatt, K.; Dunn-Walters, D.K.; Barshack, I.; Mehr, R. Immunoglobulin gene repertoire diversification and selection in the stomach—From gastritis to gastric lymphomas. *Front. Immunol.* 2014, *5*, 264. [CrossRef]
44. Hashimoto, Y.; Nakamura, N.; Kuze, T.; Ono, N.; Abe, M. Multiple lymphomatous polyposis of the gastrointestinal tract is a heterogenous group that includes mantle cell lymphoma and follicular lymphoma: Analysis of somatic mutation of immunoglobulin heavy chain gene variable region. *Hum. Pathol.* 1999, *30*, 581–587. [CrossRef]
45. Matsubara, J.; Ono, M.; Negishi, A.; Ueno, H.; Okusaka, T.; Furuse, J.; Furuta, K.; Sugiyama, E.; Saito, Y.; Kaniwa, N.; et al. Identification of a predictive biomarker for hematologic toxicities of gemcitabine. *J. Clin. Oncol.* 2009, *27*, 2261–2268. [CrossRef] [PubMed]
46. Sakuma, H.; Nakamura, T.; Uemura, N.; Chiba, T.; Sugiyama, T.; Asaka, M.; Akamatsu, T.; Ueda, R.; Eimoto, T.; Goto, H.; et al. Immunoglobulin VH gene analysis in gastric MALT lymphomas. *Mod. Pathol.* 2007, *20*, 460–466. [CrossRef] [PubMed]
47. Thieblemont, C.; Bertoni, F.; Copie-Bergman, C.; Ferreri, A.J.M.; Ponzoni, M. Chronic inflammation and extra-nodal marginal-zone lymphomas of MALT-type. *Semin. Cancer Biol.* 2014, *24*, 33–42. [CrossRef] [PubMed]
48. Zhu, D.; Bhatt, S.; Lu, X.; Guo, F.; Veelken, H.; Hsu, D.K.; Liu, F.T.; Alvarez Cubela, S.; Kunkalla, K.; Vega, F.; et al. *Chlamydophila psittaci*-negative ocular adnexal marginal zone lymphomas express self polyreactive B-cell receptors. *Leukemia* 2015, *29*, 1587–1599. [CrossRef]
49. Du, M.Q. MALT lymphoma: Recent advances in aetiology and molecular genetics. *J. Clin. Exp. Hematop.* 2007, *47*, 31–42. [CrossRef]
50. Streubel, B.; Simonitsch-Klupp, I.; Müllauer, L.; Lamprecht, A.; Huber, D.; Siebert, R.; Stolte, M.; Trautinger, F.; Lukas, J.; Püspök, A.; et al. Variable frequencies of MALT lymphoma-associated genetic aberrations in MALT lymphomas of different sites. *Leukemia* 2004, *18*, 1722–1726. [CrossRef]
51. Farinha, P.; Gascoyne, R.D. Molecular Pathogenesis of Mucosa-Associated Lymphoid Tissue Lymphoma. *J. Clin. Oncol.* 2005, *23*, 6370–6378. [CrossRef]

52. Ruefli-Brasse, A.A.; French, D.M.; Dixit, V.M. Regulation of NF-κB-Dependent Lymphocyte Activation and Development by Paracaspase. *Science* **2003**, *302*, 1581–1584. [CrossRef] [PubMed]
53. Lucas, P.C.; Yonezumi, M.; Inohara, N.; McAllister-Lucas, L.M.; Abazeed, M.E.; Chen, F.F.; Yamaoka, S.; Seto, M.; Núñez, G. Bcl10 and MALT1, Independent Targets of Chromosomal Translocation in MALT Lymphoma, Cooperate in a Novel NF-κB Signaling Pathway. *J. Biol. Chem.* **2001**, *276*, 19012–19019. [CrossRef] [PubMed]
54. Akagi, T.; Motegi, M.; Tamura, A.; Suzuki, R.; Hosokawa, Y.; Suzuki, H.; Ota, H.; Nakamura, S.; Morishima, Y.; Taniwaki, M.; et al. A novel gene, MALT1 at 18q21, is involved in t(11;18) (q21;q21) found in low-grade B-cell lymphoma of mucosa-associated lymphoid tissue. *Oncogene* **1999**, *18*, 5785–5794. [CrossRef]
55. Morgan, J.; Yin, Y.; Borowsky, A.; Kuo, F.; Nourmand, N.; Koontz, J.; Reynolds, C.; Soreng, L.; Griffin, C.; Graeme-Cook, F.; et al. Breakpoints of the t(11;18)(q21;q21) in mucosa-associated lymphoid tissue (MALT) lymphoma lie within or near the previously undescribed gene MALT1 in chromosome 18. *Cancer Res.* **1999**, *59*, 6205–6213. [PubMed]
56. Baens, M.; Maes, B.; Steyls, A.; Geboes, K.; Marynen, P.; De Wolf-Peeters, C. The product of the t(11;18), an API2-MLT fusion, marks nearly half of gastric MALT type lymphomas without large cell proliferation. *Am. J. Pathol.* **2000**, *156*, 1433–1439. [CrossRef]
57. Sanchez-Izquierdo, D.; Buchonnet, G.; Siebert, R.; Gascoyne, R.D.; Climent, J.; Karran, L.; Marin, M.; Blesa, D.; Horsman, D.; Rosenwald, A.; et al. MALT1 is deregulated by both chromosomal translocation and amplification in B-cell non-Hodgkin lymphoma. *Blood* **2003**, *101*, 4539–4546. [CrossRef] [PubMed]
58. Ruland, J.; Duncan, G.S.; Wakeham, A.; Mak, T.W. Differential requirement for Malt1 in T and B cell antigen receptor signaling. *Immunity* **2003**, *19*, 749–758. [CrossRef]
59. Remstein, E.D.; James, C.D.; Kurtine, P.J. Incidence and subtype specificity of API2-MALT1 fusion translocations in extranodal, nodal, and splenic marginal zone lymphomas. *Am. J. Pathol.* **2000**, *156*, 1183–1188. [CrossRef]
60. Lucas, P.C.; Kuffa, P.; Gu, S.; Kohrt, D.; Kim, D.S.L.; Siu, K.; Jin, X.; Swenson, J.; McAllister-Lucas, L.M. A dual role for the API2 moiety in API2-MALT1-dependent NF-kappaB activation: Heterotypic oligomerization and TRAF2 recruitment. *Oncogene* **2007**, *26*, 5643–5654. [CrossRef]
61. Zhou, H.; Du, M.-Q.; Dixit, V.M. Constitutive NF-??B activation by the t(11;18)(q21;q21) product in MALT lymphoma is linked to deregulated ubiquitin ligase activity. *Cancer Cell* **2005**, *7*, 425–431. [CrossRef]
62. Baens, M.; Fevery, S.; Sagaert, X.; Noels, H.; Hagens, S.; Broeckx, V.; Billiau, A.D.; De Wolf-Peeters, C.; Marynen, P. Selective expansion of marginal zone B cells in Emicro-API2-MALT1 mice is linked to enhanced IkappaB kinase gamma polyubiquitination. *Cancer Res.* **2006**, *66*, 5270–5277. [CrossRef]
63. Dierlamm, J.; Baens, M.; Wlodarska, I.; Stefanova-Ouzounova, M.; Hernandez, J.M.; Hossfeld, D.K.; De Wolf-Peeters, C.; Hagemeijer, A.; Van den Berghe, H.; Marynen, P. The Apoptosis Inhibitor Gene API2 and a Novel 18q Gene, MLT, Are Recurrently Rearranged in the t(11;18)(q21;q21) Associated With Mucosa-Associated Lymphoid Tissue Lymphomas. *Blood* **1999**, *93*, 3601–3609. [CrossRef]
64. Rosebeck, S.; Madden, L.; Jin, X.; Gu, S.; Apel, I.J.; Appert, A.; Hamoudi, R.A.; Noels, H.; Sagaert, X.; Loo, P.V.; et al. Cleavage of NIK by the API2-MALT1 fusion oncoprotein leads to noncanonical NF-kappaB activation. *Science* **2011**, *331*, 468–472. [CrossRef]
65. Nie, Z.; Du, M.-Q.; McAllister-Lucas, L.M.; Lucas, P.C.; Bailey, N.G.; Hogaboam, C.M.; Lim, M.S.; Elenitoba-Johnson, K.S.J. Conversion of the LIMA1 tumour suppressor into an oncogenic LMO-like protein by API2–MALT1 in MALT lymphoma. *Nat. Commun.* **2015**, *6*, 5908. [CrossRef]
66. Streubel, B.; Seitz, G.; Stolte, M.; Birner, P.; Chott, A.; Raderer, M. MALT lymphoma associated genetic aberrations occur at different frequencies in primary and secondary intestinal MALT lymphomas. *Gut* **2006**, *55*, 1581–1585. [CrossRef]
67. Remstein, E.D.; Kurtin, P.J.; Einerson, R.R.; Paternoster, S.F.; Dewald, G.W. Primary pulmonary MALT lymphomas show frequent and heterogeneous cytogenetic abnormalities, including aneuploidy and translocations involving API2 and MALT1 and IGH and MALT1. *Leukemia* **2004**, *18*, 156–160. [CrossRef]
68. Gallardo, F.; Bellosillo, B.; Espinet, B.; Pujol, R.M.; Estrach, T.; Servitje, O.; Romagosa, V.; Barranco, C.; Boluda, S.; García, M.; et al. Aberrant nuclear BCL10 expression and lack of t(11;18)(q21;q21) in primary cutaneous marginal zone B-cell lymphoma. *Hum. Pathol.* **2006**, *37*, 867–873. [CrossRef]
69. Schreuder, M.I.; Hoefnagel, J.J.; Jansen, P.M.; van Krieken, J.H.J.M.; Willemze, R.; Hebeda, K.M. FISH analysis of MALT lymphoma-specific translocations and aneuploidy in primary cutaneous marginal zone lymphoma. *J. Pathol.* **2005**, *205*, 302–310. [CrossRef]
70. Dierlamm, J.; Baens, M.; Stefanova-Ouzounova, M.; Hinz, K.; Wlodarska, I.; Maes, B.; Steyls, A.; Driessen, A.; Verhoef, G.; Gaulard, P.; et al. Detection of t(11;18)(q21;q21) by interphase fluorescence in situ hybridization using API2 and MLTspecific probes. *Blood* **2000**, *96*, 2215–2218. [CrossRef]
71. Murga Penas, E.M.; Hinz, K.; Röser, K.; Copie-Bergman, C.; Wlodarska, I.; Marynen, P.; Hagemeijer, A.; Gaulard, P.; Löning, T.; Hossfeld, D.K.; et al. Translocations t(11;18)(q21;q21) and t(14;18)(q32;q21) are the main chromosomal abnormalities involving MLT/MALT1 in MALT lymphomas. *Leukemia* **2003**, *17*, 2225–2229. [CrossRef]
72. Takino, H.; Li, C.; Hu, S.; Kuo, T.-T.; Geissinger, E.; Muller-Hermelink, H.K.; Kim, B.; Swerdlow, S.H.; Inagaki, K. Primary cutaneous marginal zone B-cell lymphoma: A molecular and clinicopathological study of cases from Asia, Germany, and the United States. *Mod. Pathol.* **2008**, *21*, 1517–1526. [CrossRef]

73. Dierlamm, J.; Murga Penas, E.; Daibata, M.; Tagushi, H.; Hinz, K.; Baens, M.; Cools, J.; Schilling, G.; Michaux, L.; Marynen, P.; et al. The novel t(11;12;18)(q21;q13;q21) represents a variant translocation of the t(11;18)(q21;q21) associated with MALT-type lymphoma. *Leukemia* **2002**, *16*, 1863–1864. [CrossRef]
74. Kubonishi, I.; Sugito, S.; Kobayashi, M.; Asahi, Y.; Tsuchiya, T.; Yamashiro, T.; Miyoshi, I. A unique chromosome translocation, t(11;12;18)(q21;q13;q21) [correction of t(11;12;18)(q13;q13;q12)], in primary lung lymphoma. *Cancer Genet. Cytogenet.* **1995**, *82*, 54–56. [CrossRef]
75. Murga Penas, E.M.; Callet-Bauchu, E.; Ye, H.; Hinz, K.; Albert, N.; Copie-Bergman, C.; Gazzo, S.; Berger, F.; Salles, G.; Bokemeyer, C.; et al. The translocations t(6;18;11)(q24;q21;q21) and t(11;14;18)(q21;q32;q21) lead to a fusion of the API2 and MALT1 genes and occur in MALT lymphomas. *Haematologica* **2007**, *92*, 405–409. [CrossRef]
76. Alpen, B.; Neubauer, A.; Dierlamm, J.; Marynen, P.; Thiede, C.; Bayerdörffer, E.; Stolte, M. Translocation t(11;18) absent in early gastric marginal zone B-cell lymphoma of MALT type responding to eradication of *Helicobacter pylori* infection. *Blood* **2000**, *95*, 4014–4015. [CrossRef]
77. Liu, H.; Ye, H.; Ruskone-Fourmestraux, A.; De Jong, D.; Pileri, S.; Thiede, C.; Lavergne, A.; Boot, H.; Caletti, G.; Wündisch, T.; et al. T(11;18) is a marker for all stage gastric MALT lymphomas that will not respond to *H. pylori* eradication. *Gastroenterology* **2002**, *122*, 1286–1294. [CrossRef]
78. Montalban, C.; Santón, A.; Redondo, C.; García-Cosio, M.; Boixeda, D.; Vazquez-Sequeiros, E.; Norman, F.; de Argila, C.M.; Alvarez, I.; Abraira, V.; et al. Long-term persistence of molecular disease after histological remission in low-grade gastric MALT lymphoma treated with *H. pylori* eradication. Lack of association with translocation t(11;18): A 10-year updated follow-up of a prospective study. *Ann. Oncol.* **2005**, *16*, 1539–1544. [CrossRef]
79. Nakamura, S.; Matsumoto, T.; Nakamura, S.; Jo, Y.; Fujisawa, K.; Suekane, H.; Yao, T.; Tsuneyoshi, M.; Iida, M. Chromosomal translocation t(11;18)(q21;q21) in gastrointestinal mucosa associated lymphoid tissue lymphoma. *J. Clin. Pathol.* **2003**, *56*, 36–42. [CrossRef]
80. Iwano, M.; Okazaki, K.; Uchida, K.; Nakase, H.; Ohana, M.; Matsushima, Y.; Inagaki, H.; Chiba, T. Characteristics of gastric B-cell lymphoma of mucosa-associated lymphoid tissue type involving multiple organs. *J. Gastroenterol.* **2004**, *39*, 739–746. [CrossRef]
81. Yeh, K.H.; Kuo, S.H.; Chen, L.T.; Mao, T.L.; Doong, S.L.; Wu, M.S.; Hsu, H.C.; Tzeng, Y.S.; Chen, C.L.; Lin, J.T.; et al. Nuclear expression of BCL10 or nuclear factor kappa B helps predict *Helicobacter pylori*-independent status of low-grade gastric mucosa-associated lymphoid tissue lymphomas with or without t(11;18)(q21;q21). *Blood* **2005**, *106*, 1037–1041. [CrossRef]
82. Nakamura, S.; Ye, H.; Bacon, C.M.; Goatly, A.; Liu, H.; Banham, A.H.; Ventura, R.; Matsumoto, T.; Iida, M.; Ohji, Y.; et al. Clinical impact of genetic aberrations in gastric MALT lymphoma: A comprehensive analysis using interphase fluorescence in situ hybridisation. *Gut* **2007**, *56*, 1358–1363. [CrossRef] [PubMed]
83. Ye, H.; Liu, H.; Attygalle, A.; Wotherspoon, A.C.; Nicholson, A.G.; Charlotte, F.; Leblond, V.; Speight, P.; Goodlad, J.; Lavergne-Slove, A.; et al. Variable frequencies of t(11;18)(q21;q21) in MALT lymphomas of different sites: Significant association with CagA strains of *H. pylori* in gastric MALT lymphoma. *Blood* **2003**, *102*, 1012–1018. [CrossRef] [PubMed]
84. Kuo, S.H.; Chen, L.T.; Yeh, K.H.; Wu, M.S.; Hsu, H.C.; Yeh, P.Y.; Mao, T.L.; Chen, C.L.; Doong, S.L.; Lin, J.T.; et al. Nuclear expression of BCL10 or nuclear factor kappa B predicts *Helicobacter pylori*-independent status of early-stage, high-grade gastric mucosa-associated lymphoid tissue lymphomas. *J. Clin. Oncol.* **2004**, *22*, 3491–3497. [CrossRef] [PubMed]
85. Ye, H.; Gong, L.; Liu, H.; Ruskone-Fourmestraux, A.; De Jong, D.; Pileri, S.; Thiede, C.; Lavergne, A.; Boot, H.; Caletti, G.; et al. Strong BCL10 nuclear expression identifies gastric MALT lymphomas that do not respond to *H. pylori* eradication. *Gut* **2006**, *55*, 137–139. [CrossRef] [PubMed]
86. Toyoda, K.; Maeshima, A.M.; Nomoto, J.; Suzuki, T.; Yuda, S.; Yamauchi, N.; Taniguchi, H.; Makita, S.; Fukuhara, S.; Munakata, W.; et al. Mucosa-associated lymphoid tissue lymphoma with t(11;18)(q21;q21) translocation: Long-term follow-up results. *Ann. Hematol.* **2019**, *98*, 1675–1687. [CrossRef] [PubMed]
87. Dong, G.; Liu, C.; Ye, H.; Gong, L.; Zheng, J.; Li, M.; Huang, X.; Huang, X.; Huang, Y.; Shi, Y.; et al. BCL10 nuclear expression and t(11;18)(q21;q21) indicate nonresponsiveness to *Helicobacter pylori* eradication of Chinese primary gastric MALT lymphoma. *Int. J. Hematol.* **2009**, *88*, 516–523. [CrossRef] [PubMed]
88. Salar, A.; Bellosillo, B.B.; Serrano, S.; Besses, C. Persistent residual disease in t(11;18)(q21;q21) positive gastric mucosa-associated lymphoid tissue lymphoma treated with chemotherapy or rituximab. *J. Clin. Oncol.* **2005**, *23*, 7361–7362. [CrossRef]
89. Lévy, M.; Copie-Bergman, C.; Gameiro, C.; Chaumette, M.T.; Delfau-Larue, M.H.; Haioun, C.; Charachon, A.; Hemery, F.; Gaulard, P.; Leroy, K.; et al. Prognostic value of translocation t(11;18) in tumoral response of low-grade gastric lymphoma of mucosa-associated lymphoid tissue type to oral chemotherapy. *J. Clin. Oncol.* **2005**, *23*, 5061–5066. [CrossRef]
90. Martinelli, G.; Laszlo, D.; Ferreri, A.J.M.M.; Pruneri, G.; Ponzoni, M.; Conconi, A.; Crosta, C.; Pedrinis, E.; Bertoni, F.; Calabrese, L.; et al. Clinical activity of rituximab in gastric marginal zone non-Hodgkin's lymphoma resistant to or not eligible for anti-*Helicobacter pylori* therapy. *J. Clin. Oncol.* **2005**, *23*, 1979–1983. [CrossRef]
91. Lévy, M.; Copie-Bergman, C.; Molinier-Frenkel, V.; Riou, A.; Haioun, C.; Gaulard, P.; Delfau-Larue, M.-H.H.; Sobhani, I.; Leroy, K.; Delchier, J.-C.C. Treatment of t(11;18)-positive gastric mucosa-associated lymphoid tissue lymphoma with rituximab and chlorambucil: Clinical, histological, and molecular follow-up. *Leuk. Lymphoma* **2010**, *51*, 284–290. [CrossRef]

92. Salar, A.; Domingo-Domenech, E.; Panizo, C.; Nicolás, C.; Bargay, J.; Muntañola, A.; Canales, M.; Bello, J.L.; Sancho, J.M.; Tomás, J.F.; et al. First-line response-adapted treatment with the combination of bendamustine and rituximab in patients with mucosa-associated lymphoid tissue lymphoma (MALT2008-01): A multicentre, single-arm, phase 2 trial. *Lancet Haematol.* **2014**, *1*, e104–e111. [CrossRef]
93. Ruskone-Fourmestraux, A.; Fischbach, W.; Aleman, B.M.P.; Boot, H.; Du, M.Q.; Megraud, F.; Montalban, C.; Raderer, M.; Savio, A.; Wotherspoon, A.; et al. EGILS consensus report. Gastric extranodal marginal zone B-cell lymphoma of MALT. *Gut* **2011**, *60*, 747–758. [CrossRef]
94. Zucca, E.; Arcaini, L.; Buske, C.; Johnson, P.W.; Ponzoni, M.; Raderer, M.; Ricardi, U.; Salar, A.; Stamatopoulos, K.; Thieblemont, C.; et al. Marginal zone lymphomas: ESMO Clinical Practice Guidelines for diagnosis, treatment and follow-up. *Ann. Oncol.* **2020**, *31*, 17–29. [CrossRef]
95. Kobayashi, Y.; Nakata, M.; Maekawa, M.; Takahashi, M.; Fujii, H.; Matsuno, Y.; Mitsuhiro, F.; Hiroyuki, O.; Daizo, S.; Takeaki, T.; et al. Detection of t(11; 18) in MALT-type lymphoma with dual-color fluorescence in situ hybridization and reverse transcriptase-polymerase chain reaction analysis. *Diagn. Mol. Pathol.* **2001**, *10*, 207–213. [CrossRef]
96. Fecteau, J.F.; Néron, S. CD40 stimulation of human peripheral B lymphocytes: Distinct response from naive and memory cells. *J. Immunol.* **2003**, *171*, 4621–4629. [CrossRef]
97. Chen, J.; Chen, Z.J. Signaling to NF-kappaB: Regulation by ubiquitination. *Cold Spring Harb. Perspect. Biol.* **2010**, *2*, a003350.
98. Du, M.-Q. MALT lymphoma: Genetic abnormalities, immunological stimulation and molecular mechanism. *Best Pract. Res. Clin. Haematol.* **2017**, *30*, 13–23. [CrossRef]
99. Takada, S.; Yoshino, T.; Taniwaki, M.; Nakamura, N.; Nakamine, H.; Oshima, K.; Sadahira, Y.; Inagaki, H.; Oshima, K.; Tadaatsu, A. Involvement of the chromosomal translocation t(11;18) in some mucosa-associated lymphoid tissue lymphomas and diffuse large B-cell lymphomas of the ocular adnexa: Evidence from multiplex reverse transcriptase-polymerase chain reaction and fluorescence in situ hybridization on using formalin-fixed, paraffin-embedded specimens. *Mod. Pathol.* **2003**, *16*, 445–452. [PubMed]
100. Streubel, B.; Lamprecht, A.; Dierlamm, J.; Cerroni, L.; Stolte, M.; Ott, G.; Raderer, M.; Chott, A. T(14;18)(q32;q21) involving IGH and MALT1 is a frequent chromosomal aberration in MALT lymphoma. *Blood* **2003**, *101*, 2335–2339. [CrossRef]
101. Thome, M. CARMA1, BCL-10 and MALT1 in lymphocyte development and activation. *Nat. Rev. Immunol.* **2004**, *4*, 348–359. [CrossRef] [PubMed]
102. Ye, H.; Gong, L.; Liu, H.; Hamoudi, R.A.; Shirali, S.; Ho, L.; Chott, A.; Streubel, B.; Siebert, R.; Gesk, S.; et al. MALT lymphoma with t(14;18)(q32;q21)/IGH-MALT1 is characterized by strong cytoplasmic MALT1 and BCL10 expression. *J. Pathol.* **2005**, *205*, 293–301. [CrossRef]
103. Achuthan, R.; Bell, S.M.; Carr, I.M.; Leek, J.P.; Roberts, P.; Horgan, K.; Markham, A.F.; Selby, P.J.; MacLennan, K.A. BCL10 in malignant lymphomas—An evaluation using fluorescence in situ hybridization. *J. Pathol.* **2002**, *196*, 59–66. [CrossRef] [PubMed]
104. Coornaert, B.; Baens, M.; Heyninck, K.; Bekaert, T.; Haegman, M.; Staal, J.; Sun, L.; Chen, Z.J.; Marynen, P.; Beyaert, R. T cell antigen receptor stimulation induces MALT1 paracaspase—Mediated cleavage of the NF-κB inhibitor A20. *Nat. Immunol.* **2008**, *9*, 263–271. [CrossRef]
105. Düwel, M.; Welteke, V.; Oeckinghaus, A.; Baens, M.; Kloo, B.; Ferch, U.; Darnay, B.G.; Ruland, J.; Marynen, P.; Krappmann, D. A20 negatively regulates T cell receptor signaling to NF-kappaB by cleaving Malt1 ubiquitin chains. *J. Immunol.* **2009**, *182*, 7718–7728. [CrossRef] [PubMed]
106. Kirchhofer, D.; Vucic, D. Protease activity of MALT1: A mystery unravelled. *Biochem. J.* **2012**, *444*, e3–e5. [CrossRef]
107. Hailfinger, S.; Nogai, H.; Pelzer, C.; Jaworski, M.; Cabalzar, K.; Charton, J.E.; Guzzardi, M.; Décaillet, C.; Grau, M.; Dörken, B.; et al. Malt1-dependent RelB cleavage promotes canonical NF-kappaB activation in lymphocytes and lymphoma cell lines. *Proc. Natl. Acad. Sci. USA* **2011**, *108*, 14596–14601. [CrossRef] [PubMed]
108. Tusche, M.W.; Ward, L.A.; Vu, F.; McCarthy, D.; Quintela-Fandino, M.; Ruland, J.; Gommerman, J.L.; Mak, T.W. Differential requirement of MALT1 for BAFF-induced outcomes in B cell subsets. *J. Exp. Med.* **2009**, *206*, 2671. [CrossRef]
109. Zhang, S.; Wei, M.; Liang, Q.; Johnson, D.; Dow, N.; Nelson, A.; Aguilera, N.; Auerbach, A.; Wang, G. The t(14;18)(q32;q21)/IGH-MALT1 translocation in gastrointestinal extranodal marginal zone lymphoma of mucosa-associated lymphoid tissue (MALT lymphoma). *Histopathology* **2014**, *64*, 791–798. [CrossRef]
110. Tanimoto, K.; Sekiguchi, N.; Yokota, Y.; Kaneko, A.; Watanabe, T.; Maeshima, A.M.; Matsuno, Y.; Harada, M.; Tobinai, K.; Kobayashi, Y. Fluorescence in situhybridization (FISH) analysis of primary ocular adnexal MALT lymphoma. *BMC Cancer* **2006**, *6*, 249. [CrossRef]
111. Wongchaowart, N.T.; Kim, B.; Hsi, E.D.; Swerdlow, S.H.; Tubbs, R.R.; Cook, J.R. t(14;18)(q32;q21) involving IGH and MALT1 is uncommon in cutaneous MALT lymphomas and primary cutaneous diffuse large B-cell lymphomas. *J. Cutan. Pathol.* **2006**, *33*, 286–292. [CrossRef]
112. Garcia, M.; Konoplev, S.; Morosan, C.; Abruzzo, L.V.; Bueso-Ramos, C.E.; Medeiros, L.J. MALT lymphoma involving the kidney: A report of 10 cases and review of the literature. *Am. J. Clin. Pathol.* **2007**, *128*, 464–473. [CrossRef] [PubMed]
113. Bhagavathi, S.; Greiner, T.C.; Kazmi, S.A.; Fu, K.; Sanger, W.G.; Chan, W.C. Extranodal marginal zone lymphoma of the dura mater with IgH/MALT1 translocation and review of literature. *J. Hematop.* **2008**, *1*, 131–137. [CrossRef] [PubMed]

114. Kuper-Hommel, M.J.J.; Schreuder, M.I.; Gemmink, A.H.; van Krieken, J.H.J.M. T(14;18)(q32;q21) involving MALT1 and IGH genes occurs in extranodal diffuse large B-cell lymphomas of the breast and testis. *Mod. Pathol.* **2013**, *26*, 421–427. [CrossRef] [PubMed]
115. Cook, J.R.; Sherer, M.; Craig, F.E.; Shekhter-Levin, S.; Swerdlow, S.H. T(14;18)(q32;q21) involving MALT1 and IGH genes in an extranodal diffuse large B-cell lymphoma. *Hum. Pathol.* **2003**, *34*, 1212–1215. [CrossRef] [PubMed]
116. Maes, B.; Demunter, A.; Peeters, B.; De Wolf-Peeters, C. BCL10 mutation does not represent an important pathogenic mechanism in gastric MALT-type lymphoma, and the presence of the API2-MLT fusion is associated with aberrant nuclear BCL10 expression. *Blood* **2002**, *99*, 1398–1404. [CrossRef]
117. Ye, H.; Dogan, A.; Karran, L.; Willis, T.G.; Chen, L.; Wlodarska, I.; Dyer, M.J.; Isaacson, P.G.; Du, M.Q. BCL10 expression in normal and neoplastic lymphoid tissue. Nuclear localization in MALT lymphoma. *Am. J. Pathol.* **2000**, *157*, 1147–1154. [CrossRef]
118. Streubel, B.; Vinatzer, U.; Lamprecht, A.; Raderer, M.; Chott, A. T(3;14)(p14.1;q32) involving IGH and FOXP1 is a novel recurrent chromosomal aberration in MALT lymphoma. *Leukemia* **2005**, *19*, 652–658. [CrossRef]
119. Wlodarska, I.; Veyt, E.; De Paepe, P.; Vandenberghe, P.; Nooijen, P.; Theate, I.; Michaux, L.; Sagaert, X.; Marynen, P.; Hagemeijer, A.; et al. FOXP1, a gene highly expressed in a subset of diffuse large B-cell lymphoma, is recurrently targeted by genomic aberrations. *Leukemia* **2005**, *19*, 1299–1305. [CrossRef]
120. Fenton, J.A.L.; Schuuring, E.; Barrans, S.L.; Banham, A.H.; Rollinson, S.J.; Morgan, G.J.; Jack, A.S.; van Krieken, J.H.J.M.; Kluin, P.M. t(3;14)(p14;q32) Results in aberrant expression of FOXP1 in a case of diffuse large B-cell lymphoma. *Genes Chromosom. Cancer* **2006**, *45*, 164–168. [CrossRef]
121. Vinatzer, U.; Gollinger, M.; Müllauer, L.; Raderer, M.; Chott, A.; Streubel, B. Mucosa-associated lymphoid tissue lymphoma: Novel translocations including rearrangements of ODZ2, JMJD2C, and CNN3. *Clin. Cancer Res.* **2008**, *14*, 6426–6431. [CrossRef]
122. Ansell, S.M.; Akasaka, T.; McPhail, E.; Manske, M.; Braggio, E.; Price-Troska, T.; Ziesmer, S.; Secreto, F.; Fonseca, R.; Gupta, M.; et al. t(X;14)(p11;q32) in MALT lymphoma involving GPR34 reveals a role for GPR34 in tumor cell growth. *Blood* **2012**, *120*, 3949–3957. [CrossRef] [PubMed]
123. Baens, M.; Ferreiro, J.F.; Tousseyn, T.; Urbankova, H.; Michaux, L.; de Leval, L.; Dierickx, D.; Wolter, P.; Sagaert, X.; Vandenberghe, P.; et al. t(X;14)(p11.4;q32.33) is recurrent in marginal zone lymphoma and up-regulates GPR34. *Haematologica* **2012**, *97*, 184–188. [CrossRef] [PubMed]
124. Chuang, S.; Liu, H.; Ye, H.; Martín-Subero, J.I.; Siebert, R.; Huang, W. Pulmonary mucosa-associated lymphoid tissue lymphoma with strong nuclear B-cell CLL/lymphoma 10 (BCL10) expression and novel translocation t(1;2)(p22;p12)/immunoglobulin κ chain-BCL10. *J. Clin. Pathol.* **2007**, *60*, 727. [CrossRef] [PubMed]
125. Van Keimpema, M.; Grüneberg, L.J.; Mokry, M.; Van Boxtel, R.; Van Zelm, M.C.; Coffer, P.; Pals, S.T.; Spaargaren, M. The forkhead transcription factor FOXP1 represses human plasma cell differentiation. *Blood* **2015**, *126*, 2098–2109. [CrossRef] [PubMed]
126. van Keimpema, M.; Grüneberg, L.J.; Mokry, M.; van Boxtel, R.; Koster, J.; Coffer, P.J.; Pals, S.T.; Spaargaren, M. FOXP1 directly represses transcription of proapoptotic genes and cooperates with NF-κB to promote survival of human B cells. *Blood* **2014**, *124*, 3431. [CrossRef] [PubMed]
127. Sasaki, Y.; Shiozawa, E.; Watanabe, N.; Homma, M.; Noh, J.Y.; Ito, K.; Takimoto, M.; Yamochi-Onizuka, T. t(3;14)(p14.1;q32)/FOXP1-IGH translocation in thyroid extranodal marginal zone lymphoma of mucosa-associated lymphoid tissue (MALT lymphoma). *Leuk. Res.* **2020**, *95*, 106399. [CrossRef]
128. Wu, F.; Watanabe, N.; Tzioni, M.-M.; Akarca, A.; Zhang, C.; Li, Y.; Chen, Z.; Cucco, F.; Carmell, N.; Noh, J.Y.; et al. Thyroid MALT lymphoma: Self-harm to gain potential T-cell help. *Leukemia* **2021**, *35*, 3497–3508. [CrossRef]
129. Wotherspoon, A.C.; Pan, L.; Diss, T.C.; Isaacson, P.G. Cytogenetic study of B-cell lymphoma of mucosa-associated lymphoid tissue. *Cancer Genet. Cytogenet.* **1992**, *58*, 35–38. [CrossRef]
130. Whang-Peng, J.; Knutsen, T.; Jaffe, E.; Raffeld, M.; Zhao, W.P.; Duffey, P.; Longo, D.L. Cytogenetic study of two cases with lymphoma of mucosa-associated lymphoid tissue. *Cancer Genet. Cytogenet.* **1994**, *77*, 74–80. [CrossRef]
131. Dierlamm, J.; Michaux, L.; Wlodarska, I.; Pittaluga, S.; Zeller, W.; Stul, M.; Criel, A.; Thomas, J.; Boogaerts, M.; Delaere, P.; et al. Trisomy 3 in marginal zone B-cell lymphoma: A study based on cytogenetic analysis and fluorescence in situ hybridization. *Br. J. Haematol.* **1996**, *93*, 242–249. [CrossRef]
132. Taji, S.; Nomura, K.; Matsumoto, Y.; Sakabe, H.; Yoshida, N.; Mitsufiji, S.; Nishida, K.; Horiike, S.; Nakamura, S.; Morita, M.; et al. Trisomy 3 may predict a poor response of gastric MALT lymphoma to *Helicobacter pylori* eradication therapy. *World J. Gastroenterol.* **2005**, *11*, 89–93. [CrossRef] [PubMed]
133. Ott, G.; Katzenberger, T.; Greiner, A.; Kalla, J.; Rosenwald, A.; Heinrich, U.; Ott, M.M.; Müller-Hermelink, H.K. The t(11;18)(q21;q21) Chromosome Translocation Is a Frequent and Specific Aberration in Low-Grade but not High-Grade Malignant Non-Hodgkin's Lymphomas of the Mucosa-associated Lymphoid Tissue (MALT-) Type. *AACR* **1997**, *57*, 3944–3948.
134. Clark, H.M.; Jones, D.B.; Wright, D.H. Cytogenetic and molecular studies of t(14;18) and t(14;19) in nodal and extranodal B-cell lymphoma. *J. Pathol.* **1992**, *166*, 129–137. [CrossRef] [PubMed]
135. Wotherspoon, A.C.; Finn, T.M.; Isaacson, P.G. Trisomy 3 in Low-Grade B-Cell Lymphomas of Mucosa-Associated Lymphoid Tissue. *Blood* **1995**, *85*, 2000–2004. [CrossRef] [PubMed]
136. Ott, G.; Kalla, J.; Steinhoff, A.; Rosenwald, A.; Katzenberger, T.; Roblick, U.; Ott, M.M.; Müller-Hermelink, H.K. Trisomy 3 Is Not a Common Feature in Malignant Lymphomas of Mucosa-Associated Lymphoid Tissue Type. *Am. J. Pathol.* **1998**, *153*, 689. [CrossRef]

137. Blanco, R.; Lyda, M.; Davis, B.; Kraus, M.; Fenoglio-Preiser, C. Trisomy 3 in gastric lymphomas of extranodal marginal zone B-cell (mucosa-associated lymphoid tissue) origin demonstrated by FISH in intact paraffin tissue sections. *Hum. Pathol.* **1999**, *30*, 706–711. [CrossRef]
138. Zhang, Y.; Cheung, A.N.; Chan, A.C.; Shen, D.H.; Xu, W.S.; Chung, L.P.; Ho, F.C. Detection of trisomy 3 in primary gastric B-cell lymphoma by using chromosome in situ hybridization on paraffin sections. *Am. J. Clin. Pathol.* **1998**, *110*, 347–353. [CrossRef]
139. Brynes, R.K.; Almaguer, P.D.; Leathery, K.E.; McCourty, A.; Arber, D.A.; Medeiros, L.J.; Nathwani, B.N. Numerical cytogenetic abnormalities of chromosomes 3, 7, and 12 in marginal zone B-cell lymphomas. *Mod. Pathol.* **1996**, *9*, 995–1000. [PubMed]
140. Krugmann, J.; Tzankov, A.; Dirnhofer, S.; Fend, F.; Wolf, D.; Siebert, R.; Probst, P.; Erdel, M. Complete or partial trisomy 3 in gastro-intestinal MALT lymphomas co-occurs with aberrations at 18q21 and correlates with advanced disease stage: A study on 25 cases. *World J. Gastroenterol.* **2005**, *11*, 7384. [CrossRef] [PubMed]
141. Dierlamm, J.; Rosenberg, C.; Stul, M.; Pittaluga, S.; Wlodarska, I.; Michaux, L.; Dehaen, M.; Verhoef, G.; Thomas, J.; De Kelver, W.; et al. Characteristic pattern of chromosomal gains and losses in marginal zone B cell lymphoma detected by comparative genomic hybridization. *Leukemia* **1997**, *11*, 747–758. [CrossRef]
142. Rinaldi, A.; Mian, M.; Chigrinova, E.; Arcaini, L.; Bhagat, G.; Novak, U.; Rancoita, P.M.V.; de Campos, C.P.; Forconi, F.; Gascoyne, R.D.; et al. Genome-wide DNA profiling of marginal zone lymphomas identifies subtype-specific lesions with an impact on the clinical outcome. *Blood* **2011**, *117*, 1595–1604. [CrossRef]
143. Dierlamm, J.; Wlodarska, I.; Michaux, L.; Stefanova, M.; Hinz, K.; Van Den Berghe, H.; Hagemeijer, A.; Hossfeld, D.K. Genetic abnormalities in marginal zone b-cell lymphoma. *Hematol. Oncol.* **2000**, *18*, 1–13. [CrossRef]
144. Deutsch, A.J.A.; Aigelsreiter, A.; Steinbauer, E.; Fruhwirth, M.; Kerl, H.; Beham-Schmid, C.; Schaider, H.; Neumeister, P. Distinct signatures of B-cell homeostatic and activation-dependent chemokine receptors in the development and progression of extragastric MALT lymphomas. *J. Pathol.* **2008**, *215*, 431–444. [CrossRef] [PubMed]
145. Cascione, L.; Rinaldi, A.; Bruscaggin, A.; Tarantelli, C.; Arribas, A.J.; Kwee, I.; Pecciarini, L.; Mensah, A.A.; Spina, V.; Chung, E.Y.L.; et al. Novel insights into the genetics and epigenetics of MALT lymphoma unveiled by next generation sequencing analyses. *Haematologica* **2019**, *104*, E558–E561. [CrossRef]
146. Remstein, E.D.; Dogan, A.; Einerson, R.R.; Paternoster, S.F.; Fink, S.R.; Law, M.; Gordon, W.; Kurtin, P.J. The incidence and anatomic site specificity of chromosomal translocations in primary extranodal marginal zone B-cell lymphoma of mucosa-associated lymphoid tissue (MALT lymphoma) in North America. *Am. J. Surg. Pathol.* **2006**, *30*, 1546–1553. [CrossRef] [PubMed]
147. Joao, C.; Farinha, P.; Da Silva, M.G.; Martins, C.; Crespo, M.; Cabecadas, J. Cytogenetic abnormalities in MALT lymphomas and their precursor lesions from different organs. A fluorescence in situ hybridization (FISH) study. *Histopathology* **2007**, *50*, 217–224. [CrossRef]
148. Dierlamm, J.; Pittaluga, S.; Wlodarska, I.; Stul, M.; Thomas, J.; Boogaerts, M.; Michaux, L.; Driessen, A.; Mecucci, C.; Cassiman, J. Marginal Zone B-Cell Lymphomas of Different Sites Share Similar Cytogenetic and Morphologic Features. *Blood* **1996**, *87*, 299–307. [CrossRef]
149. Du, M.; Peng, H.; Singh, N.; Isaacson, P.G.; Pan, L. The Accumulation of p53 Abnormalities Is Associated With Progression of Mucosa-Associated Lymphoid Tissue Lymphoma. *Blood* **1995**, *86*, 4587–4593. [CrossRef] [PubMed]
150. Peng, H.; Chen, G.; Du, M.; Singh, N.; Isaacson, P.G.; Pan, L. Replication error phenotype and p53 gene mutation in lymphomas of mucosa-associated lymphoid tissue. *Am. J. Pathol.* **1996**, *148*, 643.
151. Rødahl, E.; Lybæk, H.; Arnes, J.; Ness, G.O. Chromosomal imbalances in some benign orbital tumours. *Acta Ophthalmol. Scand.* **2005**, *83*, 385–391. [CrossRef]
152. Matteucci, C.; Galieni, P.; Leoncini, L.; Lazzi, S.; Lauria, F.; Polito, E.; Martelli, M.; Mecucci, C. Typical genomic imbalances in primary MALT lymphoma of the orbit. *J. Pathol.* **2003**, *200*, 656–660. [CrossRef] [PubMed]
153. Chanudet, E.; Ye, H.; Ferry, J.; Bacon, C.; Adam, P.; Müller-Hermelink, H.; Radford, J.; Pileri, S.; Ichimura, K.; Collins, V.; et al. A20 deletion is associated with copy number gain at the TNFA/B/C locus and occurs preferentially in translocation-negative MALT lymphoma of the ocular adnexa and salivary glands. *J. Pathol.* **2009**, *217*, 420–430. [CrossRef] [PubMed]
154. Kim, W.S.; Honma, K.; Karnan, S.; Tagawa, H.; Kim, Y.D.; Oh, Y.L.; Seto, M.; Ko, Y.H. Genome-wide array-based comparative genomic hybridization of ocular marginal zone B cell lymphoma: Comparison with pulmonary and nodal marginal zone B cell lymphoma. *Genes Chromosomes Cancer* **2007**, *46*, 776–783. [CrossRef]
155. Honma, K.; Tsuzuki, S.; Nakagawa, M.; Karnan, S.; Aizawa, Y.; Kim, W.S.; Kim, Y.-D.; Ko, Y.-H.; Seto, M. TNFAIP3 is the target gene of chromosome band 6q23.3-q24.1 loss in ocular adnexal marginal zone B cell lymphoma. *Genes Chromosomes Cancer* **2008**, *47*, 1–7. [CrossRef]
156. Honma, K.; Tsuzuki, S.; Nakagawa, M.; Tagawa, H.; Nakamura, S.; Morishima, Y.; Seto, M. TNFAIP3/A20 functions as a novel tumor suppressor gene in several subtypes of non-Hodgkin lymphomas. *Blood* **2009**, *114*, 2467–2475. [CrossRef]
157. Chanudet, E.; Huang, Y.; Ichimura, K.; Dong, G.; Hamoudi, R.A.; Radford, J.; Wotherspoon, A.C.; Isaacson, P.G.; Ferry, J.; Du, M.-Q. A20 is targeted by promoter methylation, deletion and inactivating mutation in MALT lymphoma. *Leukemia* **2010**, *24*, 483–487. [CrossRef] [PubMed]
158. Catrysse, L.; Vereecke, L.; Beyaert, R.; van Loo, G. A20 in inflammation and autoimmunity. *Trends Immunol.* **2014**, *35*, 22–31. [CrossRef]

159. Moody, S.; Thompson, J.S.; Chuang, S.S.; Liu, H.; Raderer, M.; Vassiliou, G.; Wlodarska, I.; Wu, F.; Cogliatti, S.; Robson, A.; et al. Novel GPR34 and CCR6 mutation and distinct genetic profiles in MALT lymphomas of different sites. *Haematologica* **2018**, *103*, 1329–1336. [CrossRef]
160. Johansson, P.; Klein-Hitpass, L.; Grabellus, F.; Arnold, G.; Klapper, W.; Pförtner, R.; Dührsen, U.; Eckstein, A.; Dürig, J.; Küppers, R. Recurrent mutations in NF-κB pathway components, KMT2D, and NOTCH1/2 in ocular adnexal MALT-type marginal zone lymphomas. *Oncotarget* **2016**, *7*, 62627–62639. [CrossRef]
161. Jung, H.; Yoo, H.Y.; Lee, S.H.; Shin, S.; Kim, S.C.; Lee, S.; Joung, J.-G.; Nam, J.-Y.; Ryu, D.; Yun, J.W.; et al. The mutational landscape of ocular marginal zone lymphoma identifies frequent alterations in TNFAIP3 followed by mutations in TBL1XR1 and CREBBP. *Oncotarget* **2017**, *8*, 17038–17049. [CrossRef]
162. Cani, A.K.; Soliman, M.; Hovelson, D.H.; Liu, C.-J.; McDaniel, A.S.; Haller, M.J.; Bratley, J.; Rahrig, S.; Li, Q.; Briceño, C.A.; et al. Comprehensive Genomic Profiling of Orbital and Ocular Adnexal Lymphomas Identifies Frequent Alterations in MYD88 and Chromatin Modifiers: New Routes to Targeted Therapies. *Mod. Pathol.* **2016**, *29*, 685. [CrossRef]
163. Behdad, A.; Zhou, X.Y.; Gao, J.; Raparia, K.; Dittman, D.; Green, S.J.; Qi, C.; Betz, B.; Bryar, P.; Chen, Q.; et al. High Frequency of MYD88 L265P Mutation in Primary Ocular Adnexal Marginal Zone Lymphoma and Its Clinicopathologic Correlation: A Study From a Single Institution. *Arch. Pathol. Lab. Med.* **2019**, *143*, 483–493. [CrossRef] [PubMed]
164. Li, Z.M.; Rinaldi, A.; Cavalli, A.; Mensah, A.A.; Ponzoni, M.; Gascoyne, R.D.; Bhagat, G.; Zucca, E.; Bertoni, F. MYD88 somatic mutations in MALT lymphomas. *Br. J. Haematol.* **2012**, *158*, 662–664. [CrossRef] [PubMed]
165. Yan, Q.; Wang, M.; Moody, S.; Xue, X.; Huang, Y.; Bi, Y.; Du, M.Q. Distinct involvement of NF-κB regulators by somatic mutation in ocular adnexal malt lymphoma. *Br. J. Haematol.* **2013**, *160*, 851–854. [CrossRef] [PubMed]
166. Ngo, V.N.; Young, R.M.; Schmitz, R.; Jhavar, S.; Xiao, W.; Lim, K.H.; Kohlhammer, H.; Xu, W.; Yang, Y.; Zhao, H.; et al. Oncogenically active MYD88 mutations in human lymphoma. *Nature* **2011**, *470*, 115–121. [CrossRef]
167. Bi, Y.; Zeng, N.; Chanudet, E.; Huang, Y.; Hamoudi, R.A.; Liu, H.; Dong, G.; Watkins, A.J.; Ley, S.C.; Zou, L.; et al. A20 inactivation in ocular adnexal MALT lymphoma. *Haematologica* **2012**, *97*, 926–930. [CrossRef]
168. Vela, V.; Juskevicius, D.; Gerlach, M.M.; Meyer, P.; Graber, A.; Cathomas, G.; Dirnhofer, S.; Tzankov, A. High throughput sequencing reveals high specificity of TNFAIP3 mutations in ocular adnexal marginal zone B-cell lymphomas. *Hematol. Oncol.* **2020**, *38*, 284–292. [CrossRef] [PubMed]
169. Ganapathi, K.A.; Jobanputra, V.; Iwamoto, F.; Jain, P.; Chen, J.; Cascione, L.; Nahum, O.; Levy, B.; Xie, Y.; Khattar, P.; et al. The genetic landscape of dural marginal zone lymphomas. *Oncotarget* **2016**, *7*, 43052. [CrossRef]
170. Agathangelidis, A.; Xochelli, A.; Stamatopoulos, K. A gene is known by the company it keeps: Enrichment of TNFAIP3 gene aberrations in MALT lymphomas expressing IGHV4-34 antigen receptors. *J. Pathol.* **2017**, *243*, 403–406. [CrossRef]
171. Hayden, M.S.; Ghosh, S. Regulation of NF-κB by TNF family cytokines. *Semin. Immunol.* **2014**, *26*, 253–266. [CrossRef]
172. Vereecke, L.; Beyaert, R.; van Loo, G. The ubiquitin-editing enzyme A20 (TNFAIP3) is a central regulator of immunopathology. *Trends Immunol.* **2009**, *30*, 383–391. [CrossRef]
173. Boone, D.L.; Turer, E.E.; Lee, E.G.; Ahmad, R.C.; Wheeler, M.T.; Tsui, C.; Hurley, P.; Chien, M.; Chai, S.; Hitotsumatsu, O.; et al. The ubiquitin-modifying enzyme A20 is required for termination of Toll-like receptor responses. *Nat. Immunol.* **2004**, *5*, 1052–1060. [CrossRef]
174. Thome, M.; Tschopp, J. TCR-induced NF-kappaB activation: A crucial role for Carma1, Bcl10 and MALT1. *Trends Immunol.* **2003**, *24*, 419–424. [CrossRef]
175. Shi, J.H.; Sun, S.C. Tumor Necrosis Factor Receptor-Associated Factor Regulation of Nuclear Factor κB and Mitogen-Activated Protein Kinase Pathways. *Front. Immunol.* **2018**, *9*, 1849. [CrossRef] [PubMed]
176. Hyeon, J.; Lee, B.; Shin, S.H.; Yoo, H.Y.; Kim, S.J.; Kim, W.S.; Park, W.-Y.; Ko, Y.-H. Targeted deep sequencing of gastric marginal zone lymphoma identified alterations of TRAF3 and TNFAIP3 that were mutually exclusive for MALT1 rearrangement. *Mod. Pathol.* **2018**, *31*, 1418–1428. [CrossRef] [PubMed]
177. Pillai, S.; Cariappa, A.; Moran, S.T. Marginal Zone B Cells. *Annu. Rev. Immunol.* **2005**, *23*, 161–196. [CrossRef]
178. Pillai, S.; Cariappa, A. The follicular versus marginal zone B lymphocyte cell fate decision. *Nat. Rev. Immunol.* **2009**, *9*, 767–777. [CrossRef] [PubMed]
179. Saito, T.; Chiba, S.; Ichikawa, M.; Kunisato, A.; Asai, T.; Shimizu, K.; Yamaguchi, T.; Yamamoto, G.; Seo, S.; Kumano, K.; et al. Notch2 Is Preferentially Expressed in Mature B Cells and Indispensable for Marginal Zone B Lineage Development. *Immunity* **2003**, *18*, 675–685. [CrossRef]
180. Hampel, F.; Ehrenberg, S.; Hojer, C.; Draeseke, A.; Marschall-Schröter, G.; Kühn, R.; Mack, B.; Gires, O.; Vahl, C.J.; Schmidt-Supprian, M.; et al. CD19-independent instruction of murine marginal zone B-cell development by constitutive Notch2 signaling. *Blood* **2011**, *118*, 6321–6331. [CrossRef]
181. Zhang, X.; Shi, Y.; Weng, Y.; Lai, Q.; Luo, T.; Zhao, J.; Ren, G.; Li, W.; Pan, H.; Ke, Y.; et al. The Truncate Mutation of Notch2 Enhances Cell Proliferation through Activating the NF-κB Signal Pathway in the Diffuse Large B-Cell Lymphomas. *PLoS ONE* **2014**, *9*, e108747. [CrossRef]
182. Puente, X.S.; Pinyol, M.; Quesada, V.; Conde, L.; Ordonez, G.R.; Villamor, N.; Escaramis, G.; Jares, P.; Bea, S.; Gonzalez-Diaz, M.; et al. Whole-genome sequencing identifies recurrent mutations in chronic lymphocytic leukaemia. *Nature* **2011**, *475*, 101–105. [CrossRef]

183. Arcaini, L.; Rossi, D.; Lucioni, M.; Nicola, M.; Bruscaggin, A.; Fiaccadori, V.; Riboni, R.; Ramponi, A.; Ferretti, V.V.; Cresta, S.; et al. The NOTCH pathway is recurrently mutated in diffuse large B-cell lymphoma associated with hepatitis C virus infection. *Haematologica* **2015**, *100*, 246–252. [CrossRef]
184. Rossi, D.; Trifonov, V.; Fangazio, M.; Bruscaggin, A.; Rasi, S.; Spina, V.; Monti, S.; Vaisitti, T.; Arruga, F.; Famà, R.; et al. The coding genome of splenic marginal zone lymphoma: Activation of NOTCH2 and other pathways regulating marginal zone development. *J. Exp. Med.* **2012**, *209*, 1537–1551. [CrossRef]
185. Kiel, M.J.; Velusamy, T.; Betz, B.L.; Zhao, L.; Weigelin, H.G.; Chiang, M.Y.; Huebner-Chan, D.R.; Bailey, N.G.; Yang, D.T.; Bhagat, G.; et al. Whole-genome sequencing identifies recurrent somatic NOTCH2 mutations in splenic marginal zone lymphoma. *J. Exp. Med.* **2012**, *209*, 1553–1565. [CrossRef]
186. Karube, K.; Martínez, D.; Royo, C.; Navarro, A.; Pinyol, M.; Cazorla, M.; Castillo, P.; Valera, A.; Carrió, A.; Costa, D.; et al. Recurrent mutations of NOTCH genes in follicular lymphoma identify a distinctive subset of tumours. *J. Pathol.* **2014**, *234*, 423–430. [CrossRef]
187. Kuksin, C.A.; Minter, L.M. The Link between Autoimmunity and Lymphoma: Does NOTCH Signaling Play a Contributing Role? *Front. Oncol.* **2015**, *5*, 51. [CrossRef] [PubMed]
188. Johansson, P.; Klein-Hitpass, L.; Budeus, B.; Kuhn, M.; Lauber, C.; Seifert, M.; Roeder, I.; Pförtner, R.; Stuschke, M.; Dührsen, U.; et al. Identifying Genetic Lesions in Ocular Adnexal Extranodal Marginal Zone Lymphomas of the MALT Subtype by Whole Genome, Whole Exome and Targeted Sequencing. *Cancers* **2020**, *12*, 986. [CrossRef] [PubMed]
189. Kiesewetter, B.; Copie-Bergman, C.; Levy, M.; Wu, F.; Dupuis, J.; Barau, C.; Arcaini, L.; Paulli, M.; Lucioni, M.; Bonometti, A.; et al. Genetic Characterization and Clinical Features of *Helicobacter pylori* Negative Gastric Mucosa-Associated Lymphoid Tissue Lymphoma. *Cancers* **2021**, *13*, 2993. [CrossRef] [PubMed]
190. Zhu, J.; Wei, R.L.; Pi, Y.L.; Guo, Q. Significance of Bcl10 gene mutations in the clinical diagnosis of MALT-type ocular adnexal lymphoma in the Chinese population. *Genet. Mol. Res.* **2013**, *12*, 1194–1204. [CrossRef] [PubMed]
191. Shingleton, J.R.; Dave, S.S. TET2 Deficiency Sets the Stage for B-cell Lymphoma. *Cancer Discov.* **2018**, *8*, 1515–1517. [CrossRef] [PubMed]
192. Du, M.Q. MALT lymphoma: A paradigm of NF-κB dysregulation. *Semin. Cancer Biol.* **2016**, *39*, 49–60. [CrossRef] [PubMed]
193. Wen, S.; Liu, T.; Zhang, H.; Zhou, X.; Jin, H.; Sun, M.; Yun, Z.; Luo, H.; Ni, Z.; Zhao, R.; et al. Whole-Exome Sequencing Reveals New Potential Mutations Genes for Primary Mucosa-Associated Lymphoid Tissue Lymphoma Arising From the Kidney. *Front. Oncol.* **2021**, *10*, 609839. [CrossRef]
194. Bartel, D.P. MicroRNAs: Target recognition and regulatory functions. *Cell* **2009**, *136*, 215–233. [CrossRef] [PubMed]
195. Fernandez-Mercado, M.; Manterola, L.; Lawrie, C.H. MicroRNAs in Lymphoma: Regulatory Role and Biomarker Potential. *Curr. Genomics* **2015**, *16*, 349. [CrossRef] [PubMed]
196. Di Lisio, L.; Martinez, N.; Montes-Moreno, S.; Piris-Villaespesa, M.; Sanchez-Beato, M.; Piris, M.A. The role of miRNAs in the pathogenesis and diagnosis of B-cell lymphomas. *Blood* **2012**, *120*, 1782–1790. [CrossRef] [PubMed]
197. Lawrie, C.H. MicroRNAs and lymphomagenesis: A functional review. *Br. J. Haematol.* **2013**, *160*, 571–581. [CrossRef]
198. Craig, V.J.; Cogliatti, S.B.; Rehrauer, H.; Wündisch, T.; Müller, A. Epigenetic Silencing of MicroRNA-203 Dysregulates ABL1 Expression and Drives Helicobacter-Associated Gastric Lymphomagenesis. *Cancer Res.* **2011**, *71*, 3616–3624. [CrossRef]
199. Zhang, Y.; Liu, A.; Quan, L.; Qu, Y.; Gu, A. Three novel microRNAs based on microRNA signatures for gastric mucosa-associated lymphoid tissue lymphoma. *Neoplasma* **2018**, *65*, 339–348. [CrossRef]
200. Saito, Y.; Suzuki, H.; Tsugawa, H.; Imaeda, H.; Matsuzaki, J.; Hirata, K.; Hosoe, N.; Nakamura, M.; Mukai, M.; Saito, H.; et al. Overexpression of miR-142-5p and miR-155 in Gastric Mucosa-Associated Lymphoid Tissue (MALT) Lymphoma Resistant to *Helicobacter pylori* Eradication. *PLoS ONE* **2012**, *7*, e47396. [CrossRef]
201. Krützfeldt, J.; Rajewsky, N.; Braich, R.; Rajeev, K.G.; Tuschl, T.; Manoharan, M.; Stoffel, M. Silencing of microRNAs in vivo with "antagomirs". *Nature* **2005**, *438*, 685–689. [CrossRef]
202. Babar, I.A.; Cheng, C.J.; Booth, C.J.; Liang, X.; Weidhaas, J.B.; Saltzman, W.M.; Slack, F.J. Nanoparticle-based therapy in an in vivo microRNA-155 (miR-155)-dependent mouse model of lymphoma. *Proc. Natl. Acad. Sci. USA* **2012**, *109*, E1695–E1704. [CrossRef]
203. Fernández, C.; Bellosillo, B.; Ferraro, M.; Seoane, A.; Sánchez-González, B.; Pairet, S.; Pons, A.; Barranco, L.; Vela, M.C.; Gimeno, E.; et al. MicroRNAs 142-3p, miR-155 and miR-203 are deregulated in gastric MALT lymphomas compared to chronic gastritis. *Cancer Genom. Proteom.* **2017**, *14*, 75–82. [CrossRef]
204. Cai, J.; Liu, X.; Cheng, J.; Li, Y.; Huang, X.; Li, Y.; Ma, X.; Yu, H.; Liu, H.; Wei, R. MicroRNA-200 is commonly repressed in conjunctival MALT lymphoma, and targets cyclin E2. *Graefes Arch. Clin. Exp. Ophthalmol.* **2012**, *250*, 523–531. [CrossRef] [PubMed]
205. Park, S.M.; Gaur, A.B.; Lengyel, E.; Peter, M.E. The miR-200 family determines the epithelial phenotype of cancer cells by targeting the E-cadherin repressors ZEB1 and ZEB2. *Genes Dev.* **2008**, *22*, 894–907. [CrossRef] [PubMed]
206. Wang, Z.; Gerstein, M.; Snyder, M. RNA-Seq: A revolutionary tool for transcriptomics. *Nat. Rev. Genet.* **2009**, *10*, 57. [CrossRef] [PubMed]
207. Chng, W.J.; Remstein, E.D.; Fonseca, R.; Bergsagel, P.L.; Vrana, J.A.; Kurtin, P.J.; Dogan, A. Gene expression profiling of pulmonary mucosa-associated lymphoid tissue lymphoma identifies new biologic insights with potential diagnostic and therapeutic applications. *Blood* **2009**, *113*, 635–645. [CrossRef]

208. Hamoudi, R.A.; Appert, A.; Ye, H.; Ruskone-Fourmestraux, A.; Streubel, B.; Chott, A.; Raderer, M.; Gong, L.; Wlodarska, I.; De Wolf-Peeters, C. Differential expression of NF-kappaB target genes in MALT lymphoma with and without chromosome translocation: Insights into molecular mechanism. *Leukemia* **2010**, *24*, 1487–1497. [CrossRef]
209. Zou, Q.; Zhang, H.; Meng, F.; He, L.; Zhang, J.; Xiao, D. Proteomic and transcriptomic studies of BGC823 cells stimulated with *Helicobacter pylori* isolates from gastric MALT lymphoma. *PLoS ONE* **2020**, *15*, e0238379. [CrossRef]
210. Zhang, J.; Wei, J.; Wang, Z.; Feng, Y.; Wei, Z.; Hou, X.; Xu, J.; He, Y.; Yang, D. Transcriptome hallmarks in *Helicobacter pylori* infection influence gastric cancer and MALT lymphoma. *Epigenomics* **2020**, *12*, 661–671. [CrossRef] [PubMed]
211. Thomas, P.B.; Jeffery, P.; Gahete, M.D.; Whiteside, E.; Walpole, C.; Maugham, M.; Jovanovic, L.; Gunter, J.; Williams, E.; Nelson, C.; et al. The long non-coding RNA GHSROS reprograms prostate cancer cell lines toward a more aggressive phenotype. *PeerJ* **2021**, *9*, e10280. [CrossRef]
212. Lue, J.K.; Amengual, J.E.; O'Connor, O.A. Epigenetics and Lymphoma: Can We Use Epigenetics to Prime or Reset Chemoresistant Lymphoma Programs? *Curr. Oncol. Rep.* **2015**, *17*, 40. [CrossRef] [PubMed]
213. Yang, H.; Green, M.R. Harnessing lymphoma epigenetics to improve therapies. *Blood* **2020**, *136*, 2386–2391. [CrossRef] [PubMed]
214. Mondello, P.; Tadros, S.; Teater, M.; Fontan, L.; Chang, A.Y.; Jain, N.; Yang, H.; Singh, S.; Ying, H.-Y.; Chu, C.-S. Selective inhibition of HDAC3 targets synthetic vulnerabilities and activates immune surveillance in lymphoma. *AACR* **2020**, *10*, 440–459. [CrossRef] [PubMed]
215. Fung, M.K.L.; Au, W.Y.; Liang, R.; Srivastava, G.; Kwong, Y.L. Aberrant promoter methylation in gastric lymphomas. *Haematologica* **2003**, *88*, 231–232. [CrossRef]
216. Rossi, D.; Capello, D.; Gloghini, A.; Franceschetti, S.; Paulli, M.; Bhatia, K.; Saglio, G.; Vitolo, U.; Pileri, S.A.; Esteller, M.; et al. Aberrant promoter methylation of multiple genes throughout the clinico-pathologic spectrum of B-cell neoplasia. *Haematologica* **2004**, *89*, 154–164.
217. Takino, H.; Okabe, M.; Li, C.; Ohshima, K.; Yoshino, T.; Nakamura, S.; Ueda, R.; Eimoto, T.; Inagaki, H. p16/INK4a gene methylation is a frequent finding in pulmonary MALT lymphomas at diagnosis. *Mod. Pathol.* **2005**, *18*, 1187–1192. [CrossRef]
218. Dugge, R.; Wagener, R.; Möller, P.; Barth, T.F.E. Genome-wide DNA methylation analysis along the progression of gastric marginal zone B-cell lymphoma of mucosa-associated lymphoid tissue (MALT) type. *Br. J. Haematol.* **2021**, *193*, 369–374. [CrossRef]
219. Deaton, A.M.; Bird, A. CpG islands and the regulation of transcription. *Genes Dev.* **2011**, *25*, 1010–1022. [CrossRef]
220. Davis, A.R.; Stone, S.L.; Oran, A.R.; Sussman, R.T.; Bhattacharyya, S.; Morrissette, J.J.; Bagg, A. Targeted massively parallel sequencing of mature lymphoid neoplasms: Assessment of empirical application and diagnostic utility in routine clinical practice. *Mod. Pathol.* **2021**, *34*, 904–921. [CrossRef]
221. Pillonel, V.; Juskevicius, D.; Bihl, M.; Stenner, F.; Halter, J.P.; Dirnhofer, S.; Tzankov, A. Routine next generation sequencing of lymphoid malignancies: Clinical utility and challenges from a 3-Year practical experience. *Leuk. Lymphoma* **2020**, *61*, 2568–2583. [CrossRef]
222. Morschhauser, F.; Tilly, H.; Chaidos, A.; McKay, P.; Phillips, T.; Assouline, S.; Batlevi, C.L.; Campbell, P.; Ribrag, V.; Damaj, G.L.; et al. Tazemetostat for patients with relapsed or refractory follicular lymphoma: An open-label, single-arm, multicentre, phase 2 trial. *Lancet. Oncol.* **2020**, *21*, 1433–1442. [CrossRef]

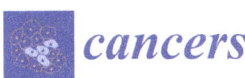

Review

Near-Haploidy and Low-Hypodiploidy in B-Cell Acute Lymphoblastic Leukemia: When Less Is Too Much

Oscar Molina [1,*], Alex Bataller [1,2], Namitha Thampi [1], Jordi Ribera [3], Isabel Granada [3,4], Pablo Velasco [5], José Luis Fuster [6,7] and Pablo Menéndez [1,7,8,9,*]

1. Josep Carreras Leukemia Research Institute, Campus Clinic, School of Medicine, University of Barcelona, 08036 Barcelona, Spain; ABATALLER@clinic.cat (A.B.); ntamphi@carrerasresearch.org (N.T.)
2. Hematology Department, Hospital Clínic de Barcelona, University of Barcelona, 08036 Barcelona, Spain
3. Acute Lymphoblastic Leukemia Group, Josep Carreras Leukemia Research Institute, Campus ICO-Germans Trias i Pujol, Autonomous University of Barcelona, 08916 Badalona, Spain; jribera@carrerasresearch.org (J.R.); igranada@iconcologia.net (I.G.)
4. Cytogenetics Laboratory, Hematology Department, Institut Català d'Oncologia (ICO), Hospital Germans Trias i Pujol, 08916 Badalona, Spain
5. Pediatric Oncology and Hematology Department, Hospital Vall d'Hebrón, 08035 Barcelona, Spain; pvelasco@vhebron.net
6. Pediatric Hematology and Oncology Department, Hospital Clínico Universitario Virgen de la Arrixaca, Instituto Murciano de Investigación Biosanitaria (IMIB), 30120 Murcia, Spain; josel.fuster@carm.es
7. Spanish Network for Advanced Therapies RICORS—TERAV, ISCIII, 28029 Madrid, Spain
8. Centro de Investigación Biomédica en Red de Cáncer (CIBER-ONC), ISCIII, 28029 Barcelona, Spain
9. Institució Catalana de Recerca i Estudis Avançats (ICREA), 08010 Barcelona, Spain
* Correspondence: omolina@carrerasresearch.org (O.M.); pmenendez@carrerasresearch.org (P.M.)

Simple Summary: B-cell acute lymphoblastic leukemia (B-ALL) is characterized by an uncontrolled proliferation of blood cells in the bone marrow. A small fraction of B-ALL patients shows abnormally low chromosome numbers, defined as hypodiploidy, in leukemic cells. Hypodiploidy with less than 40 chromosomes is a rare genetic abnormality in B-ALL and is associated to an extremely poor outcome, with low survival rates both in pediatric and adult cases. In this review, we describe the main clinical and genetic features of hypodiploid B-ALL subtypes with less than 40 chromosomes, the current treatment protocols and their clinical outcomes. Additionally, we discuss the potential cellular mechanisms involved on the origin of hypodiploidy, as well as its leukemogenic impact. Studies aiming to decipher the biological mechanisms involved in hypodiploid subtypes of B-ALL with less than 40 chromosomes are crucial to improve the poor survival rates in these patients.

Abstract: Hypodiploidy with less than 40 chromosomes is a rare genetic abnormality in B-cell acute lymphoblastic leukemia (B-ALL). This condition can be classified based on modal chromosome number as low-hypodiploidy (30–39 chromosomes) and near-haploidy (24–29 chromosomes), with unique cytogenetic and mutational landscapes. Hypodiploid B-ALL with <40 chromosomes has an extremely poor outcome, with 5-year overall survival rates below 50% and 20% in childhood and adult B-ALL, respectively. Accordingly, this genetic feature represents an adverse prognostic factor in B-ALL and is associated with early relapse and therapy refractoriness. Notably, half of all patients with hypodiploid B-ALL with <40 chromosomes cases ultimately exhibit chromosome doubling of the hypodiploid clone, resulting in clones with 50–78 chromosomes. Doubled clones are often the major clones at diagnosis, leading to "masked hypodiploidy", which is clinically challenging as patients can be erroneously classified as hyperdiploid B-ALL. Here, we summarize the main cytogenetic and molecular features of hypodiploid B-ALL subtypes, and provide a brief overview of the diagnostic methods, standard-of-care treatments and overall clinical outcome. Finally, we discuss molecular mechanisms that may underlie the origin and leukemogenic impact of hypodiploidy and may open new therapeutic avenues to improve survival rates in these patients.

Keywords: hypodiploidy; near-haploidy; B-cell acute lymphoblastic leukemia; clinical biomarkers; patient stratification

---

Citation: Molina, O.; Bataller, A.; Thampi, N.; Ribera, J.; Granada, I.; Velasco, P.; Fuster, J.L.; Menéndez, P. Near-Haploidy and Low-Hypodiploidy in B-Cell Acute Lymphoblastic Leukemia: When Less Is Too Much. *Cancers* **2022**, *14*, 32. https://doi.org/10.3390/cancers14010032

Academic Editor: François Guilhot

Received: 26 November 2021
Accepted: 18 December 2021
Published: 22 December 2021

Publisher's Note: MDPI stays neutral with regard to jurisdictional claims in published maps and institutional affiliations.

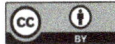

Copyright: © 2021 by the authors. Licensee MDPI, Basel, Switzerland. This article is an open access article distributed under the terms and conditions of the Creative Commons Attribution (CC BY) license (https://creativecommons.org/licenses/by/4.0/).

1. Introduction

Acute lymphoblastic leukemia (ALL) is a neoplasm arising from lymphoid precursor cells and can be classified as B-ALL or T-ALL based on the immunophenotype of the neoplastic cells [1]. The global incidence of ALL is ~3 cases per 100,000 people and shows a bimodal distribution, with a predominant peak early in life (1 to 15 years) and a second, much lower, peak in older groups (>55 years) [2] (Figure 1). ALL has a slightly higher incidence in males, with a male-to-female ratio of 1.2:1 [3]. The disease is characterized by the uncontrolled proliferation of leukemic cells, which invade the bone marrow (BM), peripheral blood (PB), and other hematopoietic tissues including spleen, liver, and lymph nodes, resulting in a hematopoietic displacement which is responsible for the cytopenias frequently observed at diagnosis. ALL cells also infiltrate commonly the central nervous system (CNS).

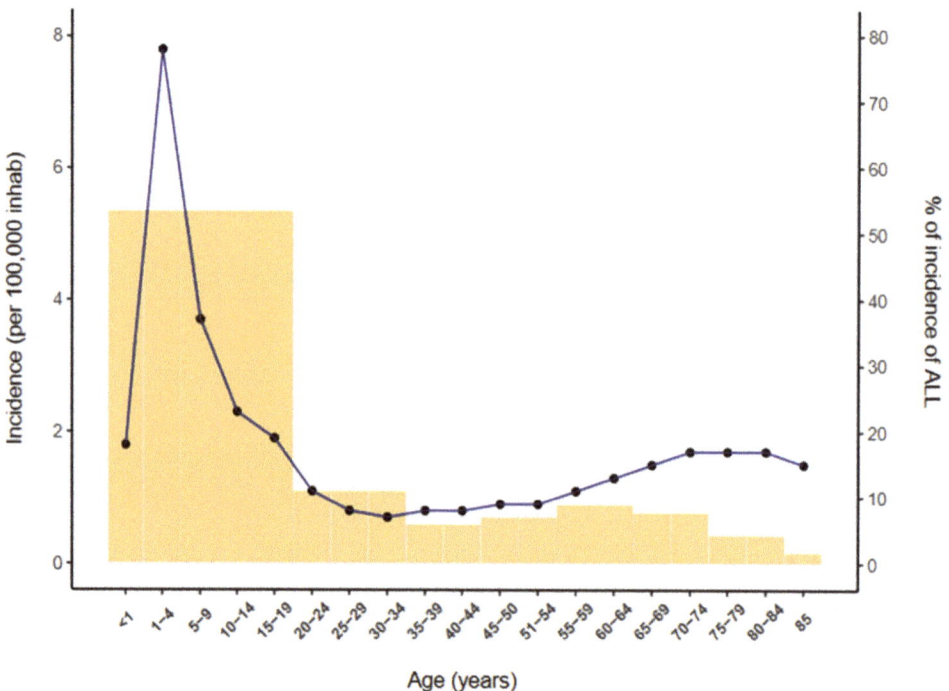

Figure 1. Incidence of ALL per 100,000 inhabitants by age (2014–2018) according to the SEER database [2].

B-cell precursor ALL (B-ALL) accounts for 80–85% of ALL cases and is characterized by small-medium sized leukemic blast cells staining almost always positive for the B-cell antigens CD19, cytoplasmic CD79a and CD22. Although BM and PB are involved in most cases, B-ALL occasionally presents with primary nodal or extranodal sites (B-lymphoblastic lymphoma), which predominantly affect skin, soft tissue, bone and lymph nodes [4]. Currently, B-ALL is classified by the World Health Organization as B-lymphoblastic leukemia/lymphoma with recurrent genetic abnormalities (Table 1) and B-lymphoblastic leukemia/lymphoma not otherwise specified. Among the B-ALL subtypes with recurrent genetic abnormalities, B-ALL with hypoploidy is classified as a well distinguished entity whose blasts contain <46 chromosomes (see below) [1].

Table 1. WHO classification of precursor lymphoid neoplasms.

Precursor Lymphoid Neoplasms
B-lymphoblastic leukemia/lymphoma not otherwise specified (NOS)
B-lymphoblastic leukemia/lymphoma with recurrent genetic abnormalities • B-lymphoblastic leukemia/lymphoma with t(9;22)(q34.1;q11.2); *BCR-ABL1* • B-lymphoblastic leukemia/lymphoma with t(v;11q23.3); *KMT2A*-rearranged • B-lymphoblastic leukemia/lymphoma with t(12;21)(p13.2;q22.1); *ETV6-RUNX1* • B-lymphoblastic leukemia/lymphoma with hyperdiploidy • B-lymphoblastic leukemia/lymphoma with hypodiploidy • B-lymphoblastic leukemia/lymphoma with t(5;14)(q31.1;q32.1); *IGH-IL3* • B-lymphoblastic leukemia/lymphoma with t(1;19)(q23;p13.3); *TCF3-PBX1* • B-lymphoblastic leukemia/lymphoma, BCR-ABL1-like • B-lymphoblastic leukemia/lymphoma with iAMP21
T-lymphoblastic leukemia/lymphoma • Early T-cell precursor lymphoblastic leukemia
NK-lymphoblastic leukemia/lymphoma

There has been an extraordinary improvement in outcomes for B-ALL during the last four decades, which have been more pronounced in children than in adults (5-year overall survival [OS] of ~90% compared with ~25% for patients >50 years) [5,6]. There are several known risk factors that can help to stratify patients with B-ALL, including adverse demographic factors such as age <1 or ≥10 years [7,8]; and also adverse clinical features at diagnosis, including CNS infiltration or high white blood cell (WBC) count (>50 × 10^9/L) [9]. Genetics and cytogenetics also have a direct impact on prognosis [10,11]. Among other genetic features, aneuploidy—defined as the gain or loss of one or more whole chromosomes—is an important prognostic factor [12], and will be examined in this review; specifically, the favorable risk of hyperdiploidy and the adverse risk of hypoploidy. Other genetic findings with prognostic impact used to stratify patients in treatment protocols have been recently discussed elsewhere [13,14]. Finally, one important risk factor with prognostic value is the response to treatment, evaluated as the detection of minimal residual disease (MRD) at specific timepoints of treatment [15].

2. Definition of Hypodiploid B-ALL Subgroups

Hypodiploidy -the loss of one or more whole chromosomes- is a rare cytogenetic finding (≤7%) in children and adults with B-ALL and is generally an adverse prognostic marker [12,16–26]. Most cases (~80%) of hypodiploid B-ALL present with 45 chromosomes and are classified as near-diploid B-ALL, a clinically distinct entity characterized by rearrangements that form dicentric chromosomes but that does not have outcomes as poor as those associated with hypodiploid B-ALL [21]. Hypodiploid B-ALL is strictly defined by most studies as ≤44 chromosomes and can be further subdivided based on chromosome number as: (i) high-hypodiploid B-ALL (40–44 chromosomes), (ii) low-hypodiploid (30–39 chromosomes), and (iii) near-haploid B-ALL (24–29 chromosomes) [17,20,24,26]. Additionally, a DNA index (determined by flow-cytometry) below 0.65 and between 0.65 to 0.82 may also be used to identify near-haploidy and low-hypodiploidy, respectively, in B-ALL samples [24]. The karyotypes and clinical outcomes of high-hypodiploid B-ALL cases differ from those of near-haploid and low-hypodiploid B-ALL, which display significantly poorer clinical outcomes across all age groups [21]. In the present review, we will focus on B-ALL with hypodiploidy of <40 chromosomes—near-haploidy and low-hypodiploidy subgroups—considered as separate cytogenetic entities associated with a very poor prognosis [27].

2.1. Demographic Features of B-ALL with Hypodiploidy <40 Chromosomes

Hypodiploidy is very rare in both childhood and adult B-ALL [27]. Near-haploidy is restricted to childhood B-ALL and represents ~0.5% of all B-ALL cases [21,28], while patients with low-hypodiploidy include both children and adults with frequencies of ~0.5% and ~4%, respectively [21,24,29]. Within the pediatric population, patients with near-haploidy present at a younger age (median age at diagnosis of 6.2 years), whereas low-hypodiploidy is more common in older children, with a median age at diagnosis of 12.9 years [17,21,23,24] (Table 2). Several studies have reported a higher proportion of males in the near-haploid and low-hypodiploid groups [22,24,26]. For example, in a retrospective analysis by the Ponte di Legno Childhood ALL Working Group (PDLWG), the male-to-female ratio was 1.46 in 101 cases with near-haploidy and 1.14 in 118 cases with low-hypodiploid B-ALL [24]. However, male predominance is not consistently reported in different studies [17,21] (Table 2).

Table 2. Clinical and biological features of patients with hypodiploid ALL.

Study	Near-Haploid							Low-Hypodiploid						
	M/F [1]	Age		WBC (×10^9/L) *			PreB/T Lineage	M/F [1]	Age		WBC (×10^9/L) *			PreB/T Lineage
		M [2]	<10 yo at dx *	M [2]	≤20	20–50	>50			M [2]	<10 yo at dx *	M [2]	≤20	20–50	>50	
SJCRH [16]	nr	4.5	3	nr				nr	nr	11	1	nr				nr
SJCRH-POG [17]	0.66	4.7	70	13	70	10	20	8/1 [3]	2	10.5	22.2	8.4	66.6	11.1	22.2	5/1 [3]
CCG [19]			63		50	13	38				nr		nr	nr	nr	nr
SJCRH [20]		7.3	100	2.5	100	0	0	4/0		nr	0	8.2	83.3	0	16.6	5/1
MRC [21]	0.75	7.4	64.3	67.3	38.5	30.8	30.8	13/0 [3]	1.1	21.6	7.1	11	85.7	7.1	7.1	12/0 [3,4]
Inc study [22]	1		69.6		39.1	41.3	19.6	nr	2.25		19.2		73	19.2	7.7	nr
SJTTS 15&16 [23]		3.6		8.1						13.9		5.6				
PDLWG [24]	1.46	6.2	73	21.8	49	20	31	99/1	1.14	12.9	26	7	85	10	4	99/1
Japanese study [25]	nr	nr	nr	nr	nr	nr	nr	3/0	nr	nr	nr	nr	nr	nr	nr	3/0

* Percentage of patients. [1] Male-to-female-ratio. [2] Median. [3] data not available from 4 patients in the SJCRH-PG study and in 1 patient in the MRC study. [4] one patient reported as "null" immunophenotype. Abbreviations: CCG, Children Cancer Group; CIBMTR, Centre for International Blood and Marrow Transplant Research; CNS, central nervous system; LH, low-hypodiploid; MRC, Medical Research Council; na, not applicable; NH, near-haploid; nr, not reported; PDLWG, Ponte di Legno childhood ALL Working group; POG, Pediatric Oncology Group; preB, B-cell precursor; SJCRH, Saint Jude Children's Research Hospital; SJTTS, Saint Jude Total Therapy Study; WBC, white blood cell count at presentation.

2.2. Clinical and Biological Features of B-ALL with Hypodiploidy <40 Chromosomes

Generally, patients with hypodiploid B-ALL present with a lower diagnostic WBC than patients with non-hypodiploid B-ALL [16]; however, some studies have reported a higher WBC in the near-haploid group [11,21,24]. The aforementioned PDLWG study [24] found a median WBC at presentation of 21.8×10^9/L in the near-haploid group against 7×10^9/L in the low-hypodiploid group. In addition, up to 49% of patients with a near-haploid karyotype presented with $\leq 20 \times 10^9$/L compared with 85% in the low-hypodiploid group, whereas 31% in the near-haploid group presented with $>50 \times 10^9$/L WBC compared with only 4% in the low-hypodiploid group. These findings are in line with previous reports [21,22,24] (Table 2).

Regarding cell morphology, French-American-British (FAB) L2/L1 or L2 subtypes were reported to be more frequent at presentation in patients with hypodiploid B-ALL. Indeed, up to 50% of near-haploid cases were non-L1 FAB subtype and 25% were L2 subtype in a series reported by the Children Cancer Group (CCG) [16,19]. Patients with B-ALL with hypodiploidy show a B-cell precursor immunophenotype, with positivity for CD19, CD34, CD22, cCD79a and TdT [22,27]. Near-haploid ALL is generally also positive for CD10, whereas low-hypodiploid ALL may exhibit a more immature B-cell precursor immunophenotype, lacking CD10 in a substantial proportion of cases, consistent with a pro-B ALL phenotype [30]. Additionally, a very small proportion of children with hypodiploid ALL present with a T-ALL immunophenotype, usually with positivity for TdT and expressing the T-cell specific markets CD1a, CD2, CD3, CD5, and CD7 [27,31,32]. In a larger series presented by the PDLWG, Nachman et al. and the UK Medical Research Council, only 1% of the total cases with hypodiploidy <40 chromosomes showed a T-cell immunophenotype (Table 2), whereas 11–15% of high-hypodiploid cases exhibited a T-ALL immunophenotype [21,22,24].

2.3. Extramedullary Involvement at Presentation

CNS involvement, which is defined as the presence of blasts in a sample of cerebrospinal fluid with ≥5 leukocytes/µL and <10 erythrocytes/µL or the presence of cranial nerve palsies (CNS3) [33], is rare at diagnosis and was recorded in only one out of 115 and 97 cases (1%) of near-haploid and low-hypodiploid ALL, respectively, in the PDLWG study [24,26]. Other frequent leukemic extramedullary involvements at diagnosis of near-haploid and low-hypodiploid B-ALL is at the spleen and liver, presenting as splenomegaly in 44% and 28% of cases, and hepatomegaly in 43% and 35%, respectively [24,26]. By contrast, mediastinal mass and lymphadenopathy is less frequent, with 7% and 13% and 30% and 14% of cases with near-haploid ALL and low-hypodiploid ALL, respectively [24]. Testicular disease at diagnosis is also rare in both types, with no reported cases in the AALL03B1 study and only 2 of 46 cases (4%) of near-haploid B-ALL in the PDLWG study [24]. Taking these findings together, it seems clear that most of the clinical and biological features in patients with near-haploid and low-hypodiploid B-ALL do not seem to be predictive of poor outcome.

3. Cytogenetic Characterization of B-ALL with Hypodiploidy <40 Chromosomes

Although traditionally defined as the loss of one or more chromosomes in a cell [34], hypodiploidy has been classified according to diverse criteria in different studies to define different hypodiploid B-ALL subtypes (Table 3), and a clear distinction between those cases with <40 chromosomes and those with 40–45 chromosomes has become generally accepted based on the evident differences in treatment response [21,35]. Hypodiploid cases with <40 chromosomes can be further subdivided into two groups based on the bimodal distribution of chromosome numbers: (i) near-haploidy, with 24–29 chromosomes (Figure 2A), and (ii) low-hypodiploidy, with 30–39 chromosomes (Figure 2B,C) [27] (Table 3). Although the modal number of chromosomes is variable, the most recurrent modal numbers are 25–28 for near-haploid and 33–39 for low-hypodiploid B-ALL [36]. Based on conventional chromosome banding analyses, hypodiploidy with <40 chromosomes shows a non-random loss of chromosomes: in near-haploid B-ALL, retained disomies generally comprise chromosomes 8, 10, 14, 18, 21, X and Y [21,22,30,37] whereas in low-hypodiploid cases, retained disomies are more variable and typically comprise chromosomes 1, 5, 6, 8, 10, 11, 14, 18, 19, 21, 22, X and Y, with retained disomies for chromosomes 1, 6, 11 and 18 being the most frequently observed. The most typically lost chromosomes are chromosome 3, 7, 9, 15, 16 and 17 [21,22,30,38,39] (Table 3). The non-random retention of chromosomes suggests that these chromosomes may harbor specific genes that enhance the oncogenic potential of leukemic cells.

Table 3. Cytogenetic characteristics of B-ALL patients with <40 chromosomes.

Age (Years)	Near-Haploid					Low-Hypodiploid					Reference
	MN	Retained chr	Lost chr	Doubled Clone	Frequency	MN	Retained chr	Lost chr	Doubled Clone	Frequency	
1–18	25–28	8, 10, 14, 18, 21 and sex chr.		yes	0.0046	30–40	1, 19, 21, 22 and sex chr.	3, 7, 13, 16, 17	yes	0.41	[17]

Table 3. Cont.

Age (Years)	Near-Haploid					Low-Hypodiploid					Reference
	MN	Retained chr	Lost chr	Doubled Clone	Frequency	MN	Retained chr	Lost chr	Doubled Clone	Frequency	
1–10	24–28	8, 10, 14, 18, 21 and sex chr.	7, 13, 14, 20, X	yes	0.0042	33–44		7, 13, 14, 20, X	nr	0.79	[19]
2–15	23–29	14, 18, 21 and sex chr.		yes	0.0039	33–39	1, 2, 5, 6, 8, 10, 11, 12, 14, 18, 19, 21, 22 and the sex chr.	7, 17	yes	0.39	[21]
15–84	-	-	-	-	-	30–39	1, 5, 6, 8, 10, 11, 15, 18, 19, 21, 22, X, Y	3, 7, 15, 16, 17	66 to 78 chr	0.05	[31]
15–55	-	-	-	-	-	33–39	nr	nr	nr	0.0008	[21]
15–55/>55	<30				0.0016	32–39	1	2, 3, 7, 9, 13, 15, 16, 17, 20, 4	64–74	3.85%	[40]
1–9/>10	24–29	14, 18, 21 and sex chr.	nr	nr	nr	33–39	nrec	3, 7, 16, 17	nr	nr	[10]
<31	24–31	14, 18, 21 and sex chr.	nr	yes	0.008	32–39	1, 8, 10, 11, 18, 19, 21 and 22	nr	nr	0.0064	[41]

Abbreviations: chr, chromosomes; MN, modal numbers; nr, non-reported; nrec, non-recurrent.

Structural chromosome aberrations (i.e., chromosomal translocations) in hypodiploidy of <40 chromosomes are extremely rare, especially in near-haploid B-ALL [21,22,38,42], suggesting that massive chromosomal loss alone may be sufficient for leukemogenesis. Patients with low-hypodiploid B-ALL show some additional alterations, albeit few, in the karyotype beyond monosomies (Figure 2B,C). It has been reported that pediatric patients with B-ALL with <36 chromosomes may show additional structural chromosome aberrations more frequently when compared with those with ≥36 [22]. It would be interesting to learn whether pediatric patients with additional structural alterations are also older than those without them, which would be consistent with different reports on adult B-ALL showing structural chromosome aberrations, especially unbalanced translocations and losses of chromosome arms, in 50% of low-hypodiploid cases [35,38].

"Masked Hypodiploidy": A Clinical Challenge

A feature common to patients with near-haploid and low-hypodiploid B-ALL is the presence of a clone with an exact or near-exact chromosome doubling of the hypodiploid clone, resulting in a clone with a modal chromosome number of 50–78, in the high-hyperdiploid or triploid range [17,21,22,41] (Table 3) (Figure 2A). Notably, some chromosomes are preferentially lost after chromosome doubling; typically, chromosomes 2, 5, 6, 10, 14 and 22 [38]. The presence of hypodiploid doubled clones has been observed in ~60–65% of patients with near-haploid and low-hypodiploid B-ALL in different studies, and is commonly observed as a mosaic with both hypodiploid and hyperdiploid (doubled) clones visible by standard cytogenetics, fluorescence in situ hybridization (FISH) or flow cytometry analysis of DNA content [21,41,43]. Furthermore, the doubled clone may be the only one detected at diagnosis, leading to the manifestation known as "masked hypodiploidy", which is clinically challenging since patients can be erroneously classified and treated for high-hyperdiploid B-ALL while being at higher risk of treatment failure. It has been reported that there is no difference in clinical outcome for patients with "masked hypodiploidy", those who are mosaic for a doubled clone and a hypodiploid clone, and those who have only a hypodiploid clone [22,35,41]. In addition, the hypodiploid clone tends to be quantitatively more frequent at relapse, suggesting that the actual hypodiploid clones may be more chemoresistant than their hyperdiploid (doubled) counterparts [20,44].

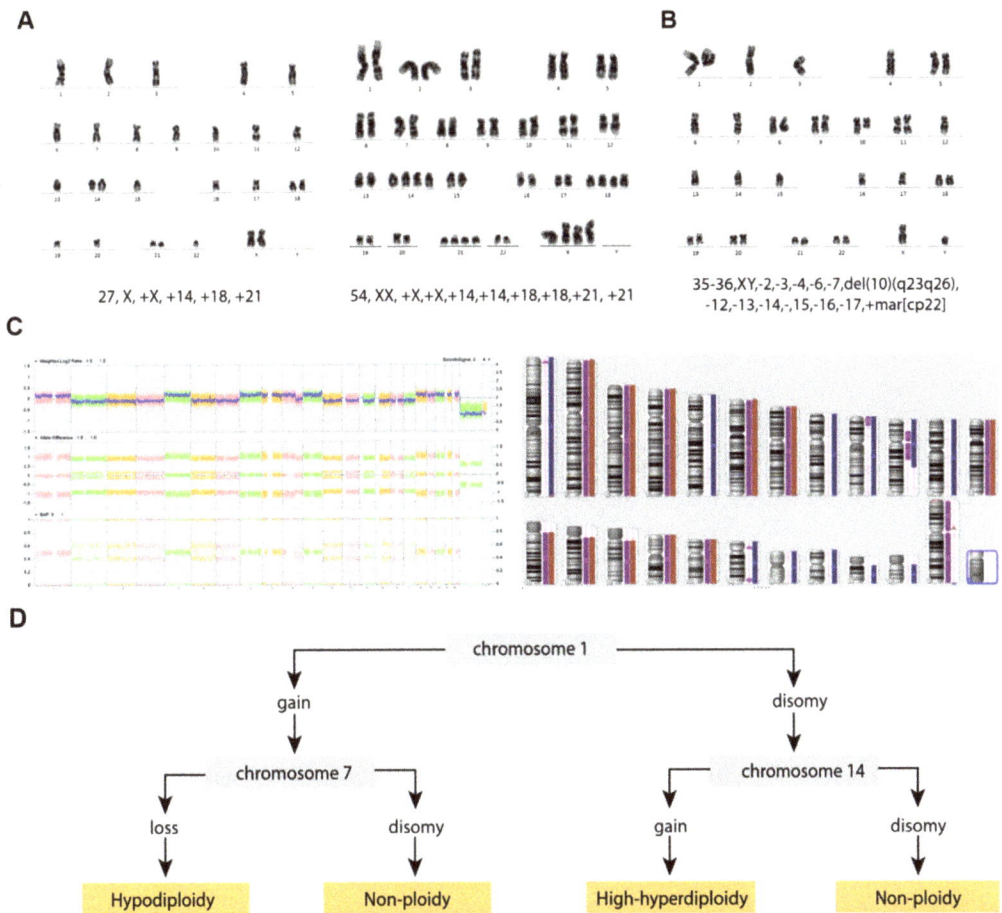

Figure 2. Cytogenetic characterization of B-ALL with <40 chromosomes. (**A**) G-banded karyotype of near-haploid B-ALL leukemic cells. *Left panel*, near-haploid clone. *Right panel*, chromosomally-doubled clone of the same patient. (**B**) G-banded karyotype of low-hypodiploid B-ALL leukemic cells. Karyotype formulas are indicated below. (**C**) SNP-array karyogram obtained for the low-hypodiploid B-ALL patient in B. *Right panel*, blue bars indicate chromosomal disomies of the duplicated/near-triploid clone, red bars indicate chromosomal losses, and purple bars indicate absence of heterozygosity. *Left panel*, Log2 ratio plot detailing whole chromosomal view for each chromosome, the figure demonstrates pattern of low-hypodiploidy where chromosomes with the lowest Log2 ratio represent the monosomies and a partial deletion of chromosome 10. Allele difference plot and B-allele frequency plot (BAF; BB, AB and AA alleles) indicates copy-neutral loss of heterozygosity. (**D**) Algorithm proposed by Creasey et al. [39] to distinguish hypodiploid with <40 chromosomes and high-hyperdiploid B-ALL cases based on specific chromosomal gains.

There is evidence to suggest that chromosomal doubling arises by endoreduplication [17]: for instance, (i) the hyperdiploid clone is an exact duplication of the near-haploid or low-hypodiploid clone; (ii) in rare cases, the structural chromosomal abnormalities are also shared in paired chromosomes; and (iii) hyperdiploid cell lines have been established in culture from near-haploid B-ALL patient samples [45,46]. However, studies aiming to elucidate the molecular mechanism(s) leading to the chromosomal doubling have not been performed to date.

Whole-genome doubling (WGD) is a common phenomenon in nature that generates cells referred to as "polyploid", containing multiple copies of the complete set of chromosomes [47]. Indeed, polyploidy has been reported to be indispensable for normal development and organ formation across various organisms, from fungi to humans [47,48], and has more recently been associated with wound healing and tissue homeostasis [48]. Additionally, polyploidization has been implicated in early carcinogenesis and neoplastic progression, as polyploid cells have been reported to be more permissive to aneuploidy through their ability to buffer deleterious mutations that affect cellular fitness [49,50]. In this line, it is tempting to speculate that WGD is even more relevant in near-haploid and low-hypodiploid cellular backgrounds, as it generates chromosomally-doubled clones with presumably lower cell-fitness costs and higher adaptation capacity than their hypodiploid counterparts. WGD arises as a consequence of alternative cell cycle programs referred to as endoreduplication or endocycles, through which cells successively duplicate genomic DNA without segregating their chromosomes during mitosis [47]. Only the most extreme abbreviations of the mitotic phase are correctly referred to as endoreduplication. The cell cycles that include some mitotic processes, such as chromosome condensation, nuclear envelope breakdown and spindle formation, are referred to as "endomitosis", which abort mitosis mostly during metaphase or anaphase and lack cytokinesis [47]. These cases are associated with mitotic defects leading to mitotic slippage. In both scenarios, the result is either a cell that maintains separate nuclei, generating multinucleate cells, or a cell with an enlarged single nucleus. Endoreduplication cycles use much of the same machinery that regulates the transition from G1 to S phase in normal "mitotic cell cycles". To convert the mitotic cell cycle into an endoreduplication cycle, the cell cycle must be altered in two essential ways. On the one hand, by bypassing the central processes of mitosis, chromosome segregation and cytokinesis, without blocking DNA replication. This is accomplished in plants and animal cells by downregulating the cyclin-dependent kinases (CDKs) that drive G2-to-M phase progression, while allowing continuous activity of the CDKs that drive G1-to-S progression. On the other hand, periodic inactivation of CDKs involved in G1-to-S phase transition to enable a G1-like gap with low S-phase-specific CDK activity during which pre-replication complexes can be reassembled [47,48]. The precise mechanism underlying WGD in near-haploid and low-hypodiploid B-ALL is currently not known, but as this phenomenon is very common and exclusive of these subtypes of B-ALL, it could be hypothesized that it has an important role on the development of these subtypes of ALL.

4. Molecular Characterization of Hypodiploid B-ALL with <40 Chromosomes

In addition to the massive genetic losses, both near-haploid and low-hypodiploid B-ALL show characteristic and differentiated gene expression profiles, in addition to specific mutational and focal copy-number alteration (CNA) landscapes, those excluding whole chromosome losses [30]. Notably, near-haploid and low-hypodiploid B-ALL presenting with or without doubled clones show similar transcriptional and mutational profiles [30], most likely explaining the similar clinical outcomes between patients with and without chromosomal doubling [17,22,41].

4.1. Near-Haploid B-ALL

The mutational landscape of near-haploid B-ALL is characterized mainly by the presence of alterations involving receptor tyrosine kinases and activating RAS signaling alterations, with >70% of patients showing mutations or focal CNA involving genes in these pathways (Table 4) [30,38,51]. The different RAS signaling alterations have been shown to be mutually exclusive, suggesting that, in contrast to the convergent evolution for RAS mutations observed in infants with MLL-rearranged B-ALL [52], a single alteration in the pathway is sufficient to maintain constitutive RAS-pathway activation. Focal deletions or point mutations in *NF1* gene are the most recurrent genetic alterations of near-haploid B-ALL (≥44% of patients) [23,30,53]. *NF1* encodes a RAS–GTPase-activating protein that negatively regulates Ras signaling. Deletions affecting this gene are intragenic and involve exons 15–35 in the majority of cases, most likely due to illegitimate recombinase activating gene (RAG) activity [30]. Other recurrently mutated RAS pathway genes in near-haploid B-ALL are *NRAS* (15% of patients), *FLT3* (9% of patients), *KRAS* (3% of patients) and *PTPN11* (1.5% of patients) [30,38,51]. Some of these mutations have been described in patients diagnosed with Noonan syndrome, such as the *PTPN11* Gly503Arg substitution, and have been also described in remission samples or in T-cell lymphocytes, such as *NRAS* Gly12Ser [30], suggesting that the single-nucleotide variants (SNVs) are germline SNVs and that near-haploidy may be a manifestation of this cancer-predisposing syndrome in some instances. Additionally, alterations in *PAG1* (mostly deletions) have been reported in 10% of patients with near-haploid B-ALL [23,30]. Most of the deletions were homozygous and affected the upstream region and first exon of the gene, leading to a complete loss of gene expression [30]. *PAG1* encodes for a transmembrane adaptor protein that binds to the tyrosine kinase CSK protein, which negatively regulates SRC-family kinases involved in both Ras and B-cell receptor signaling pathways. Importantly, *PAG1* deletions together with positive MRD status have been associated with poorer outcomes and increased incidence of relapse in hypodiploid ALL [30]. Other recurrent focal CNAs in near-haploid B-ALL include *CDKN2A/B* at 9p21.3 (22% of patients), a histone cluster at 6p22 (19% of patients), *IKZF3/Aiolos* at 17q12 (13% of patients), *RB1* at 13q14.2 (9% of patients) and *PAX5* at 9p13.2 (7% of patients) [30]. As with other B-ALL subtypes, patients with near-haploid B-ALL have recurrent disruption, by deletion, insertion-deletions or point mutations, of the lysine acetyltransferase gene *CREBBP* (32% of patients) [30]. CREBBP mediates the expression of glucocorticoid-responsive genes and may play an active role in response to glucocorticoids, suggesting that patients harboring *CREBBP* alterations may be more prone to therapy failure and relapse [54]. Point mutations in other histone-modifier genes, such as *EP300* and *EZH2*, are also observed in near-haploid B-ALL albeit at lower frequencies (<5% of patients). Of note, alterations involving epigenetic modifiers are more frequently observed in relapsed B-ALL than at diagnosis, highlighting their role in leukemia progression and clonal evolution.

4.2. Low-Hypodiploid B-ALL

The genetic hallmark of low-hypodiploid B-ALL is *TP53* mutations, which are observed in >90% of patients in both childhood and adult low-hypodiploid B-ALL (Table 4) [30,38,51,55]. Most are missense mutations in exons 5–8, affecting the DNA-binding domain and the nuclear localization sequence [30,38]. Other characteristic and recurrent genetic alterations in the low-hypodiploid B-ALL subtype are *RB1* mutations or deletions (41% of cases), deletions of *IKZF2/Helios* (53% of cases) and deletions of *CDKN2A/B* genes (22% of cases) [30,38]. Mutations of *TP53* are found in homozygosity in virtually all low-hypodiploid B-ALL cases due to the very recurrent loss of chromosome 17. *TP53* mutations are frequently found in non-tumor hematopoietic cells in 50% of the cases of childhood low-hypodiploid B-ALL [38,51], suggesting that these cases may be a manifestation of Li-Fraumeni syndrome or other germline *TP53* cancer-predisposing mutations [30,55,56]. Accordingly, genetic counseling is recommended for children with low-hypodiploid B-ALL carrying *TP53* mutations, and their relatives [57,58]. In contrast to childhood cases, *TP53* mutations in low-hypodiploid adult B-ALL are somatic, are not found in healthy hematopoietic cells, and not detectable in remission samples [30,38].

Table 4. Molecular characteristics of hypodiploid <40 chromosomes B-ALL (Adapted from Holmfelt et al., 2013 [30]).

Genes	Cellular Pathway	Near-Haploid B-ALL			Low-Hypodiploid B-ALL		
		Mutation	Focal Deletion	Focal DEL + Mut	Mutation	Focal Deletion	Focal DEL + Mut
NF1	RTK/RAS pathway	11/68 (16%)	16/68 (24%)	3/68 (4%)	0	2/34 (6%)	0
KRAS		2/68 (3%)	0	0	0	0	0
NRAS		10/68 (15%)	0	0	0	0	0
PTPN11		1/68 (1%)	0	0	0	0	0
FLT3		6/68 (9%)	0	0	0	0	0
CRLF2		0	2/68 (3%) *	0	0	0	0
MAPK1		1/68 (1%)	0	0	0	0	0
GAB2		0	2/68 (3%)	0	0	1/34 (3%)	0
EPHA7		0	2/68 (3%)	0	0	0	0
RASA2		0	2/68 (3%)	0	0	0	0
IKZF1	B-cell development	0	3/68 (4%)	0	0	1/34 (3%)	0
IKZF2		1/68 (1%)	0	0	0	18/34 (53%)	0
IKZF3		1/68 (1%)	8/68 (12%)	0	0	1/34 (3%)	0
PAX5		1/68 (1%)	4/68 (6%)	0	0	2/34 (6%)	0
EBF1		0	0	0	0	0	0
VPREB1		0	3/68 (4%)	0	0	2/34 (6%)	0
CDKN2A/B	Cell cycle and apoptosis	0	15/68 (22%)	0	0	8/34 (24%)	0
TP53		2/68 (3%)	0	0	31/34 (91%)	0	0
RB1		2/68 (3%)	3/68 (4%)	1/68 (1%)	5/34 (15%)	8/34 (24%)	0
ETV6	Hematopoiesis	1/68 (1%)	3/68 (4%)	1/68 (1%)	0	0	0
Histone cluster (6p22)	Histone-related	0	13/68 (19%)	0	0	1/34 (3%)	0
ARID1B		0	2/68 (3%)	0	0	0	0
PAG1	BCR signalling	1/68 (1%)	6/68 (9%)	0	0	1/34 (3%)	0
ARPP21	Calmodulin signalling	0	1/68 (1%)	0	0	0	0
SLX4IP (C20orf194)	Telomere length maintenance	0	2/68 (3%)	0	0	0	0
CUL5	Ubiquitin pathway	0	2/68 (3%)	0	0	0	0
FAM53B	Wnt signalling	0	2/68 (3%)	0	0	0	0
PDS5B (APRIN)	Cohesin complex	0	2/68 (3%)	0	0	0	0
ANKRD11	Cell adhesion	0	0	0	0	2/34 (6%)	0
DMD		0	0	0	0	1/34 (3%)	0

* one patient encoding P2RY8-CRLF2.

Focal deletions involving lymphocyte development genes, such as *IKZF1*, *EBF1* or *LEF1*, are not particularly frequent in low-hypodiploid B-ALL samples. Instead, *IKZF2/Helios* loss at 2q34 is the most recurrent alteration involving genes associated with B-cell differentiation (53% in children and 36% in adults), being much more frequently observed in low-hypodiploid B-ALL than in any other B-ALL subtype, including near-haploid ALL (Table 4). *IKZF2/Helios* is highly expressed in common lymphoid progenitors and in pre-pro-B progenitor cells, which is consistent with the immunophenotype observed in low-hypodiploid B-ALL of lower frequencies of antigen-receptor rearrangements, CD19 and CD10 [30,59]. These findings reinforce the hypothesis that low-hypodiploidy targets a more immature lymphoid progenitor (pro-B stage or earlier) than other B-ALL subtypes with a pre-B immunophenotype. Indeed, in one study patients with *IKZF2/Helios* deletions had a poorer outcome than patients with wild-type *IKZF2/Helios* in an univariate analysis [30]. Beyond lymphocyte development, alterations of cell cycle regulators are also frequently observed in both childhood and adult low-hypodiploid B-ALL. As discussed earlier, alterations in *RB1* are observed in 41% and 19% of childhood and adult patients, respectively. Additionally, *CDKN2A/B* mutations are observed in 22% of both childhood and adult low-hypodiploid B-ALL samples, and are often mutually exclusive with *RB1* mutations [58]. The finding that *TP53* is ubiquitously perturbed in low-hypodiploid B-ALL suggests that mutations in an additional member of the TP53/RB1 pathway (either *RB1* or *CDKN2A/B*) would be sufficient to deregulate cell proliferation in these cases. Furthermore, mutations in histone-modifier genes, such as *CREBBP*, are detected in 60% of patients with low-hypodiploid B-ALL [30]. Strikingly, while patients with low-hypodiploid B-ALL do not show recurrent mutations in genes associated with RAS pathway activation, as do patients with near-haploid B-ALL, transcriptomic analyses of pathway activation in low-hypodiploid B-ALL revealed constitutive signaling of *RAS* and *PI3K* pathways [30].

A recent study by the Japan Association Childhood Leukemia Study Group (JACLS) reported a high frequency of mutations in *CIC* in both low-hypodiploid and near-haploid B ALL, present in 5 of 9 patients [53]. *CIC* is a member of the high mobility group (HMG)-box superfamily of transcriptional repressors and is recurrently mutated in oligodendrogliomas and in round cell sarcomas. However, the germline status of *CIC* in B-ALL with hypodiploidy of <40 chromosomes is unknown and raises the question of whether it could be more prevalent in Asian ancestors than in non-Asian populations [53].

4.3. Proper Identification of Hypodiploid B-ALL with <40 Chromosomes

As previously mentioned, "masked hypodiploidy" represents an important diagnostic challenge, as it may be mis-diagnosed with high-hyperdiploidy of 51–65 chromosomes (Figure 2A). Conventional cytogenetic G-banding analysis provides the modal number of chromosomes, which is essential for the differentiation between these cytogenetic groups with <40 chromosomes, high-hyperdiploid B-ALL and, especially, for those B-ALL cases presenting with >65 chromosomes (near-triploidy), which should always be considered as doubled clones from a low-hypodiploid B-ALL. Cases between 51 and 65 chromosomes, in the range of the high-hyperdiploidy and masked near-haploidy, are especially difficult to define and a detailed analysis of the gained chromosomes is crucial to distinguish between the two B-ALL entities. The major cytogenetic characteristic of masked near-haploid B-ALL is the presence of mainly tetrasomies, which is in contrast to high-hyperdiploidy, which mainly shows trisomies (with the exception of chromosome 21). Accordingly, the presence of tetrasomies other than tetrasomy of chromosome 21 might suggest a masked hypodiploid clone. Moreover, the subsequent loss of some chromosomes is very frequently observed after chromosome doubling in cases of B-ALL with hypodiploidy of <40 chromosomes, suggesting certain levels of chromosome instability and, therefore, not all gained chromosomes are tetrasomic in the karyotypes of masked near-haploid samples [38].

Complementary techniques may be used when there is a suspicion of masked hypodiploidy, including interphase FISH or flow-cytometry analyses of DNA index. These techniques allow scoring a higher number of cells in the samples and may facilitate the detection of hypodiploid clones that were not detectable by conventional cytogenetics. Likewise, single nucleotide polymorphism (SNP)-arrays have emerged as a very reliable tool to identify masked hypodiploid clones, especially their capacity to detect loss of heterozygosity (LOH). Indeed, the presence of LOH in most chromosomes, especially those typically lost in the original hypodiploid clones (Table 3), is defining the near-haploid and low-hypodiploid entities. Some authors have recently provided simple and helpful algorithms for proper discrimination between masked hypodiploidy from high-hyperdiploid B-ALL using SNP-arrays and focusing on specific chromosome gains, such as chromosomes 1, 7 and 14 (Figure 2D) [39].

5. Etiology of Hypodiploidy in B-ALL

No preclinical models of near-haploid or low-hypodiploid B-ALL subtypes are currently available, preventing the direct study of the biological causes and the pathogenic consequences of hypodiploidy in B-ALL. Indeed, most studies describing hypodiploid subtypes in B-ALL are clinical reports, patient sample analyses and retrospective analyses of clinical outcomes. Accordingly, there is only circumstantial evidence for the cellular mechanisms leading to hypodiploidy and its pathogenic consequences. Genomic analyses of these subtypes have been difficult given the limited number of cases; however, a study on a small cohort of 8 near-haploid and 4 low-hypodiploid B-ALL samples suggested that the massive loss of chromosomes is the primary oncogenic event, with other oncogenic insults occurring after hypodiploidy [37]. This is consistent with similar analyses in high-hyperdiploid B-ALL cases, the most frequent aneuploid entity in B-ALL, indicating that chromosome gains were the primary oncogenic event [60,61]. Thus, similar pathogenic mechanisms involving gross aneuploidies may be shared in these B-ALL subtypes. Furthermore, the genomic landscape of near-haploid and low-hypodiploid B-ALL subtypes, as well as that of high-hyperdiploid subtypes, is characterized by aneuploidy and subtype-specific mutations (see above), with significant fewer microdeletions and structural chromosomal rearrangements in comparison with other cytogenetic subtypes containing structural chromosomal reorganizations [30,60]. Collectively, these data strongly suggest that hypodiploidy has a direct impact on cell transformation and leukemogenesis rather than being solely a passenger event. The fact that severe hypodiploidy is observed in a wide spectrum of neoplasms further indicates that it is indeed a major contributor of tumorigenesis [62].

Although the functional impact of extreme hypodiploidy on leukemia initiation is poorly understood, a common assumption is that the widespread LOH resulting from hypodiploidy leads to the unmasking of recessive alleles or to gene-dosage imbalances affecting oncogenes, tumor-suppressor genes, and also protein imbalances affecting different aspects of cell physiology, proliferation and/or survival [30,37,51]. Indeed, loss-of-function mutations of *TP53* are a hallmark of both childhood and adult low-hypodiploid B-ALL [30], suggesting that alterations in this gene are an important event in the pathogenesis of this B-ALL subtype. Alternative mechanisms for tumor suppressor pathway inactivation may be involved in the pathogenesis of near-haploid B-ALL; for instance, microdeletions of *CDKN2A/B* loci on chromosome 9, typically monosomic in near-haploid B-ALL, are common in this hypodiploid subtype [30]. These proteins are involved in the control of the tumor-suppressor *RB1* and their inactivation leads to a dysregulation of the G1-to-S checkpoint leading to uncontrolled proliferation [30,51].

Remarkably, the pattern of chromosomal retention in near-haploid B-ALL is similar to the pattern of commonly gained chromosomes in the high-hyperdiploid group [17,30]. Thus, retention of both homologs of specific chromosomes, especially 14, 18, 21 and X, may play an important role in leukemogenesis in these cases. Elucidating the role and cooperativity of the genes on these chromosomes, and their contribution to different cellular pathways, should shed new light on the pathogenic mechanisms resulting from hypodiploidy in B-ALL. In particular, the contribution of alterations in the RAS signaling pathway, Ikaros-family alterations and/or *TP53* alterations in leukemogenesis are a subject of active current investigation [58].

6. Origin of Near-Haploidy and Low-Hypodiploidy

While the near-haploid and low-hypodiploid chromosomal patterns have been recognized for many years [16], the factors driving the generation of these aneuploidies and their associated genomic alterations remain poorly understood. They may originate through successive loss of chromosomes or by a single erroneous mitosis event in an early hematopoietic stem/progenitor cell. The latter hypothesis is currently the most accepted owing to the bimodal distribution of chromosome numbers reported in the literature for these hypodiploid B-ALL subtypes [37]. Multipolar mitosis or an abnormal partial mitotic pairing of homologous chromosomes appear to be the most feasible mechanisms underlying hypodiploidy [17,62], but no experimental evidence has been provided to support this hypothesis. Remarkably, high-resolution microscopic analyses of dividing primary hypodiploid B-ALL cells stained with antibodies that recognize different cytoskeleton structures revealed an increase in the frequency of multipolar spindles when compared with non-hypodiploid B-ALL cells (data not previously published) [63], suggesting that multipolar spindles could indeed be a crucial cellular mechanism leading to hypodiploidy. However, whether these multipolar spindles are the cause or a consequence of the chromosome losses remains an open question.

Given that the immunophenotype of both near-haploid and low hypodiploid B-ALL is consistent with that of a common pre-B or pro-B leukemia, respectively [17,30], it is likely that hypodiploidy arises in a similar hematopoietic progenitor as most B-ALLs. Notably, pre-leukemic clones with different chromosome rearrangements and high-hyperdiploidy have been observed in cord blood samples and in neonatal heel prick tests from patients that later develop childhood B-ALL [64]. This finding suggests that the primary genetic abnormalities arise in utero during fetal hematopoiesis and act as pre-leukemic initiating events that remain clinically silent upon the acquisition of secondary cooperating genetic alterations, which are necessary to promote leukemia development [65]. Of note, although no direct evidence has been provided for near-haploid and low-hypodiploid B-ALL subtypes, it is tempting to speculate that hypodiploidy in childhood B-ALL also arises in utero as a consequence of an aberrant mitosis event in early hematopoietic progenitors. The pathogenic mechanisms of extreme hypodiploidy and their contribution to leukemogenesis are the subject of investigation, as the identification of novel therapeutic targets are crucial for developing new treatments to improve the dismal outcome of these rare subtypes of B-ALL.

7. Outcome and Treatment Strategies for B-ALL with Hypodiploidies <40 Chromosomes

7.1. Event-Free Survival and Overall Survival Rates

Patients with hypodiploid B-ALL have an overall very poor clinical outcome, particularly in those cases with <40 chromosomes [17]. While the survival rates are increasingly dismal with decreasing modal chromosome numbers, the outcome of patients with either near-haploidy and low-hypodiploidy do not significantly differ, being similarly poor in both groups with modal numbers below 40 chromosomes [20,21,24]. The poor prognostic impact conferred by hypodiploidy with <40 chromosomes is maintained in multivariate analyses after adjustment for important risk factors including age, WBC count, and Philadelphia/t(9;22) status [19]. Indeed, the MRC UK-ALL trials of childhood B-ALL cases reported 3-year event-free survival (EFS) rates of 29% versus 65% in hypodiploidy below and above 40 chromosomes, respectively [21]. Its prognosis in adults remains extremely poor, with 5-year EFS rates ~20%, despite stratification by high-risk treatment protocols [27]. Importantly, the poor outcome and low EFS rates of B-ALL with hypodiploidy with <40 chromosomes has been consistently reported by different studies (Table 5).

Table 5. Event-free survival reported for patients with hypodiploid B-ALL by several relevant studies. Colored cells indicate statistical comparisons (blue, between chromosome numbers; orange, between other variables).

Study group	Years	Outcome variable	MN	Other variables	n	Mean (%)	p-value	Reference
Total Therapy Studies IX–XI Pediatric Oncology Group (POG)	1979–1988 1986-1988	3-year-DFS	<30 chr 30–40 chr 41–44 chr		109 8	40 33 37		[17]
Children's Cancer Group (CCG)	1988–1995	6-year-EFS	33–34 chr 29–32 chr 24–28 chr 30–40 chr 41–44 chr		15 0 8	40 NA 25		[19]
Total Therapy protocols T11–T14	1984–1999	5-years EFS	36–44 chr 25–29 chr ≥45 chr <45 chr			17 26 75 20	<0.001	[20]
Medical Research Council, UK ALL trial protocols	1990–2002	3-year-EFS	42–45 chr 25–39 chr		121 20	65 29	0.0002	[21]
AIEOP-3; BFM-5; CCG-33; COALL-3; DANA FARBER-4; POG-44; SJCRH-6; UK-20; NOPHO-6; and EORTC-15	1986–1996	8-year EFS	44 chr 40–43 chr 33–39 chr 30–32 chr 24–29 chr		50 8 26 0 46	52 19 37 NA 28		[22]
COG AALL0031	2002–2006	4-year EFS	<30–44 chr	Chemotherapy alone Chemotherapy + BMT	26 13	50 62	0.65	[66]
St. Jude Total Therapy Study XV&XVI	2000–2014	5-year EFS	24–31 chr 32–39 chr	MRD EOI neg MRD EOI pos	8 12 14 6	73 75 85 44	0.8 0.03	[23]
CIBMTR-All BMT in CR1 or CR2	1990–2010	5-year-DFS	44–45 chr ≤43 chr		39 39	64 37	0.01	[67]
Children's Healthcare of Atlanta	2004–2016	2-year DFS	32–39 chr 24–31 chr	MRD EOI neg MRD EOI pos Age ≥ 10 years Age < 10 years	5 7 10 2 6 6	60 71 69 50 33 100	0.853 0.021	[57]
COG AALL03B1-COG AALL0331 and AALL0232 *	2003–2011	5-year EFS	>46 chr <44 chr	BMT en CR1 No BMT MRD pos MRD neg Standard NCI risk group High NCI risk group Chemotherapy [1] HSCT [1]	NR 131 61 52 30 74 48 83	85 52 56 49 26 64 60 47 4 7	<0.01 0.62 0.026 0.13	[26]

Table 5. Cont.

Study group	Years	Outcome variable	MN	Other variables	n	Mean (%)	p-value	Reference
Ponte di Legno Childhood ALL Working Group- ≤44 chromosomas	1997–2013	5-year EFS	44 chr		40	74		[24]
			40–43 chr		13	58		
			30–39 chr		118	50		
			24–29 chr		101	56		
				HCT in LH	21	64	0.89	
				No HCT in LH	93	62		
				HCT in NH	19	51	0.6	
				No HCT in NH	82	44		
TCCSG, JACLS, Japanese Children's Cancer and Leukemia Study Group, Kyushu-Yamaguchi Children's Cancer Study Group	1997–2012	5-year EFS	45 chr		101	73	<0.036	[25]
			44 chr		8	88		
			<44 chr		8	38		
				Relapse rate in patients < 44 chr	5	63		

* B-ALL patients 1–30-years-old. [1] The 5-year cumulative incidence of SMN. Abbreviations: chr, chromosomes; DFS, disease-free survival; EFS, event-free survival; HCT, hematopoietic stem cell transplant; LH, low-hypodiploidy; NH, near-haploidy.

The low EFS rates observed in near-haploid and low-hypodiploid groups are related to a high relapse rate mostly from isolated BM relapses, and succumbing to the disease after first remission [24,25] (Table 5). According to the review by Groeneveld-Krentz et al. on patients with relapsed BCP-ALL [68], those with pediatric B-ALL with hypodiploidy <40 chromosomes show specific characteristics compared with other B-ALL groups, including: (i) association with older age at initial diagnosis, (ii) shorter time to first relapse, (iii) more frequent allocation to the high-risk treatment arm of the relapse trial, and (iv) inferior second remission rates [68]. Remarkably, patients with hypodiploidy with <40 chromosomes presenting with a predominant doubled clone or masked hypodiploidy had late relapses and more often achieved a second remission, as compared with patients with a predominant or exclusive hypodiploid clone. Despite these differences, however, the outcome of these patients is similarly poor, highlighting that all hypodiploidies with <40 chromosomes should be classified as high-risk irrespective of time to relapse [68].

7.2. Relationship of Genetic and Clinical Features with Patient Outcome

The EFS is not significantly different between patients with near-haploid or low-hypodiploid B-ALL, including those cases with "masked hypodiploidy" [23,24,57]. In some cases, hypodiploidy may accompany other primary genetic abnormalities, such as *BCR-ABL1*, *TCF3-PBX1*, *ETV6-RUNX1* and *KMT2A* rearrangements, which modulate the prognosis of the disease. Accordingly, some authors have suggested that these patients should be treated based on the primary structural abnormalities rather than the hypodiploidy, and on their MRD values after induction [24]. The high presence of germline *TP53* mutations among patients with low-hypodiploidy confer an increased risk of relapse in this group and is associated with the development of secondary neoplasms [24]. Therefore, it is highly recommended that all patients with low-hypodiploid B-ALL are tested for germline *TP53* mutations [24,69]. Strikingly, the germline *TP53* mutations in these cases have been associated with increased mortality due to second neoplastic malignancies following hematopoietic stem cell transplantation (HSCT), highlighting the importance of the germline study in low-hypodiploid B-ALL to assess HSCT versus less toxic alternative therapies [26,67,70]. The presence of other recurrent mutations in near-haploid and low-hypodiploid B-ALL cases, such as alterations in the RAS-pathway, *IKZF* or *RB1*, has not shown a clear association with patient prognosis [23]. However, the small sample sizes, owing to the rarity of these B-ALL subtypes, may mask a significant association of these mutations with patient outcomes. Interestingly, a study by The Children's Healthcare of Atlanta found that patients with hypodiploid B-ALL with <40 chromosomes and age ≥10 years display significant worse 2-year EFS rates (33.3% vs. 100%) [57]. Noteworthy, the impact of age on prognosis has also been reflected in other studies of adult B-ALL [35], where low-hypodiploid B-ALL patients < 35 years had survival rates of 71% against 21% in those patients >35 years.

The most important prognostic factor for near-haploid and low-hypodiploid B-ALL groups is the MRD status at the end of induction (EOI) [23]. Univariateanalyses including different clinical factors, such as National Cancer Institute (NCI) risk groups, MRD EOI status or HSCT, showed that only MRD EOI <0.01% was a significant prognostic factor for EFS in these cases [26]. Despite the poor prognosis of hypodiploid B-ALL with <40 chromosomes, the outcome improves significantly if the MRD EOI is negative, with 5-year EFS of 68–85% vs. 44–50% for MRD negative and positive patients, respectively [22,23,26,57,67] (Table 5). In view of these data, several groups have intensified treatments based on MRD-based stratification protocols, which has proven to be the most appropriate strategy associated with more favorable outcomes [24].

7.3. Current Treatment Protocols

Different study groups, such as the UKALL, NOPHO, AALL0031 and COG studies, consistently stratify near-haploid and low-hypodiploid B-ALL subtypes as high-risk based on the poor prognosis of the patients, which does not depend on treatment era or on the NCI risk group in which they are classified [24,26,71]. In view of the poor prognosis of patients with hypodiploid B-ALL, they have been classically treated with high-dose chemotherapy followed by allogeneic transplantation. However, different studies assessing the impact of HSCT on B-ALL with near-haploidy and low-hypodiploidy failed to demonstrate a clear benefit of HSCT in MRD positive or negative patients [23,24,57,66] (Table 5). Notwithstanding these findings, the outcome of hypodiploid B-ALL with <40 chromosomes has been substantially improved by MRD-guided therapy, which intensifies treatments based on the MRD EOI status [23]. MRD-stratified treatment protocols are associated with a favorable outcome after adjusting for sex, age, and leukocyte count, with a 5-year EFS of 62% [24,72]. Interestingly, Jeha et al. described a 5-year EFS of 100% in a series of 6 patients with hypodiploidy of <44 chromosomes using MRD-guided therapy, and even in 1 patient with positive MRD EOI [72]. The favorable impact of treating patients according to protocols stratified by MRD EOI is likely related to the identification of chemosensitive patients, those that are MRD EOI negative, for whom HSCT does not represent any benefit, and to not undertreat MRD-positive patients. To evaluate the real impact of HSCT in this setting, trials comparing HSCT with chemotherapy alone in patients with positive MRD EOI would be necessary, but this would be difficult due to the low incidence and poor prognosis of these patients with only chemotherapy treatment [73]. Given the low survival in this group despite HSCT, it seems imperative to investigate novel treatments and therapeutic approaches. Interestingly, fit adult patients with hypodiploid B-ALL would likely benefit from pediatric-adapted more intensive chemotherapy schemes [74]; however, this is difficult to assess clinically due to the very low incidence and dismal prognosis of hypodiploid B-ALL adult patients.

7.4. Novel Therapeutic Targets and Approaches to Treat B-ALL with <40 Chromosomes

New treatments aiming to target recently identified biological drivers of hypodiploidies as well as immunotherapy strategies are currently being explored to achieve better responses before HSCT or to be used as alternative approaches. The recent discovery of near-universal *TP53* alterations in low-hypodiploid B-ALL has highlighted a key role for this gene in leukemogenesis. Investigation of this germinal mutation in this population is recommended when evaluating treatment with chemotherapy and HSCT. It remains to be demonstrated, however, whether therapies directed at this genetic lesion have an effect on low-hypodiploidy [58]. The anti-apoptotic protein BCL-2, has been identified as an effective therapeutic target for hypodiploid B-ALL with <40 chromosomes [75], and the efficacy of

BCL-2 inhibitors (mainly venetoclax) has been demonstrated in ex vivo models of B-ALL with near-haploidy and low-hypodiploidy, especially in cases with elevated levels of the apoptosis-related factors BIM or BAD. Other authors have investigated the sensitivity of hypodiploid B-ALL cell lines and xenografts to MEK, PI3K, and the dual PI3K/mTOR inhibitors [30]. The PI3K and dual PI3K/mTOR inhibitors substantially inhibited proliferation of all tumors examined, suggesting that inhibition of the PI3K pathway may serve as a novel alternative therapy to treat hypodiploid B-ALL with <40 chromosomes [30].

Immunotherapy has shown encouraging results in relapsed/refractory B-ALL with high-risk cytogenetics, such as near-haploidy and low-hypodiploidy. Chimeric antigen receptor (CAR) T-cell and monoclonal antibodies or bi-specific T-cell engagers (BiTE), such as inotuzumab and blinatumomab, are the main immunotherapy approaches currently in use. It has been described that the patient response to CAR T-cell therapy does not depend on the cytogenetic risk group, with hypodiploid B-ALL representing up to 3.5% of cases according to the series [73]. Some of these cases have shown a promising response to CAR T-cell therapy, including an adult patient with low-hypodiploidy B-ALL in first relapse who received CD19-specific CAR T-cell therapy consolidated with HSCT [76]. Trials with CAR T-cell therapies as frontline approaches remain scarce and in some of them patients with hypodiploidy <40 chromosomes were excluded, such as the AALL1721/Cassiopeia trial (NCT03876769), a phase II single-arm trial of tisagenlecleucel (CD19-specific CAR T) in children and young adults with high risk B-ALL and persistent MRD at end of consolidation [77]. Blinatumomab, a BiTE antibody that directs T-cells to CD19-positive cells, has proven to be effective in adult patients with low-hypodiploid B-ALL, with 2 of the 4 patients reaching a complete response in one study [78]. It has also been used as an additional therapeutic approach in high-risk group protocols, which may induce a more in-depth response in these groups of B-ALL [79]. On the other hand, studies treating patients with inotuzumab ozogamicin, a humanized anti-CD22 antibody-drug conjugate, have not shown any specific high efficacy in patients with hypodiploid B-ALL [80]. Among the 3 patients with <40 chromosomes included in the study, 1 patient did not reach complete remission and the remaining patients did not reach a negative MRD EOI. In conclusion, new targeted treatments and immunotherapy approaches are very promising strategies, with ongoing protocols and active trials being conducted in patients with a very poor prognosis such as hypodiploidy ALL.

8. Concluding Remarks

1. Both near-haploid and low-hypodiploid B-ALL represent very rare entities, associated with a dismal clinical outcome. Such a low disease incidence represents a challenge to develop pre-clinical models aimed to study the etiology and pathogenesis of the disease and also represents a barrier to design statistically robust clinical trials.
2. Cutting-edge cytogenetic and genetic assays must be implemented in routine diagnostic laboratories to distinguish between high-hyperdiploid and masked hypodiploid B-ALL patients since this has a major impact on patient treatment stratification and clinical outcome.
3. The pathogenic effect(s) of chromosome losses and its contribution to leukemogenesis is currently not known. Furthermore, the biological contribution of chromosome doublings occurring in most of hypodiploid B-ALL cases with <40 chromosomes is poorly understood. Future studies aiming to decipher the biological mechanisms involved in the progression of hypodiploid B-ALL will help in the identification of innovative targeted treatments and/or diagnostic biomarkers to improve survival in these patients.

Author Contributions: Conceptualization, O.M.; Conducted literature review: O.M., A.B., N.T., J.R., I.G., P.V. and J.L.F.; writing-original draft preparation, O.M. and P.M.; writing-review, all authors; supervision, O.M.; All authors have read and agreed to the published version of the manuscript.

Funding: This work was supported by Spanish Ministry of Economy and Competitiveness (PID2019-108160RB-I00/AEI/10.13039/501100011033), the European Research Council (CoG-2014-646903 and PoC-2018-811220), the Spanish Association of Cancer Research (AECC, INVES211226MOLI).

Acknowledgments: We thank Centres de Recerca de Catalunya (CERCA)/Generalitat de Catalunya, the Fundació Josep Carreras, and the Obra Social 'la Caixa' for their institutional support. Work in the laboratory of P.M. is supported by the Spanish Ministry of Economy and Competitiveness (PID2019-108160RB-I00/AEI/10.13039/501100011033), the European Research Council (CoG-2014-646903 and PoC-2018-811220), the Spanish Association of Cancer Research (AECC), the Fundación Uno entre Cienmil and la Caixa Foundation Health Research. O.M. is supported by an investigator fellowship from the AECC (INVES211226MOLI). A.B. is supported by Fundación Española de Hematología y Hemoterapia (FEHH).

Conflicts of Interest: The authors declare no conflict of interest.

References

1. Swerdlow, S.H.; Campo, E.; Pileri, S.A.; Harris, N.L.; Stein, H.; Siebert, R.; Advani, R.; Ghielmini, M.; Salles, G.A.; Zelenetz, A.D.; et al. The 2016 revision of the World Health Organization classification of lymphoid neoplasms. *Blood* **2016**, *127*, 2375–2390. [CrossRef]
2. Howlader, N.; Noone, A.; Krapcho, M.; Miller, D.; Brest, A.; Yu, M.; Ruhl, J.; Tatalovich, Z.; Mariotto, A.; Lewis, D.; et al. SEER Cancer Statistics Review (CSR), 1975–2018. Available online: https://seer.cancer.gov/csr/1975_2018/ (accessed on 5 November 2021).
3. Siegel, R.L.; Miller, K.D.; Jemal, A. Cancer statistics, 2020. *CA Cancer J. Clin.* **2020**, *70*, 7–30. [CrossRef]
4. Maitra, A.; McKenna, R.W.; Weinberg, A.G.; Schneider, N.R.; Kroft, S.H. Precursor B-cell lymphoblastic lymphoma. A study of nine cases lacking blood and bone marrow involvement and review of the literature. *Am. J. Clin. Pathol.* **2001**, *115*, 868–875. [CrossRef] [PubMed]
5. Pulte, D.; Gondos, A.; Brenner, H. Improvement in survival in younger patients with acute lymphoblastic leukemia from the 1980s to the early 21st century. *Blood* **2009**, *113*, 1408–1411. [CrossRef]
6. Pulte, D.; Jansen, L.; Gondos, A.; Katalinic, A.; Barnes, B.; Ressing, M.; Holleczek, B.; Eberle, A.; Brenner, H.; Group, G.C.S.W. Survival of adults with acute lymphoblastic leukemia in Germany and the United States. *PLoS ONE* **2014**, *9*, e85554. [CrossRef] [PubMed]
7. Kadan-Lottick, N.S.; Ness, K.K.; Bhatia, S.; Gurney, J.G. Survival variability by race and ethnicity in childhood acute lymphoblastic leukemia. *JAMA* **2003**, *290*, 2008–2014. [CrossRef]
8. Shuster, J.J.; Wacker, P.; Pullen, J.; Humbert, J.; Land, V.J.; Mahoney, D.H., Jr.; Lauer, S.; Look, A.T.; Borowitz, M.J.; Carroll, A.J.; et al. Prognostic significance of sex in childhood B-precursor acute lymphoblastic leukemia: A Pediatric Oncology Group Study. *J. Clin. Oncol.* **1998**, *16*, 2854–2863. [CrossRef] [PubMed]
9. Smith, M.; Arthur, D.; Camitta, B.; Carroll, A.J.; Crist, W.; Gaynon, P.; Gelber, R.; Heerema, N.; Korn, E.L.; Link, M.; et al. Uniform approach to risk classification and treatment assignment for children with acute lymphoblastic leukemia. *J. Clin. Oncol.* **1996**, *14*, 18–24. [CrossRef] [PubMed]
10. Pui, C.H.; Relling, M.V.; Downing, J.R. Acute lymphoblastic leukemia. *N. Engl. J. Med.* **2004**, *350*, 1535–1548. [CrossRef]
11. Moorman, A.V.; Ensor, H.M.; Richards, S.M.; Chilton, L.; Schwab, C.; Kinsey, S.E.; Vora, A.; Mitchell, C.D.; Harrison, C.J. Prognostic effect of chromosomal abnormalities in childhood B-cell precursor acute lymphoblastic leukaemia: Results from the UK Medical Research Council ALL97/99 randomised trial. *Lancet Oncol.* **2010**, *11*, 429–438. [CrossRef]
12. Molina, O.; Abad, M.A.; Sole, F.; Menendez, P. Aneuploidy in Cancer: Lessons from Acute Lymphoblastic Leukemia. *Trends Cancer* **2021**, *7*, 37–47. [CrossRef]
13. Inaba, H.; Mullighan, C.G. Pediatric acute lymphoblastic leukemia. *Haematologica* **2020**, *105*, 2524–2539. [CrossRef] [PubMed]
14. Malard, F.; Mohty, M. Acute lymphoblastic leukaemia. *Lancet* **2020**, *395*, 1146–1162. [CrossRef]
15. Bassan, R.; Spinelli, O.; Oldani, E.; Intermesoli, T.; Tosi, M.; Peruta, B.; Rossi, G.; Borlenghi, E.; Pogliani, E.M.; Terruzzi, E.; et al. Improved risk classification for risk-specific therapy based on the molecular study of minimal residual disease (MRD) in adult acute lymphoblastic leukemia (ALL). *Blood* **2009**, *113*, 4153–4162. [CrossRef]
16. Pui, C.H.; Williams, D.L.; Raimondi, S.C.; Rivera, G.K.; Look, A.T.; Dodge, R.K.; George, S.L.; Behm, F.G.; Crist, W.M.; Murphy, S.B. Hypodiploidy is associated with a poor prognosis in childhood acute lymphoblastic leukemia. *Blood* **1987**, *70*, 247–253. [CrossRef] [PubMed]
17. Pui, C.H.; Carroll, A.J.; Raimondi, S.C.; Land, V.J.; Crist, W.M.; Shuster, J.J.; Williams, D.L.; Pullen, D.J.; Borowitz, M.J.; Behm, F.G.; et al. Clinical presentation, karyotypic characterization, and treatment outcome of childhood acute lymphoblastic leukemia with a near-haploid or hypodiploid less than 45 line. *Blood* **1990**, *75*, 1170–1177. [CrossRef] [PubMed]

18. Chessels, J.M.; Swansbury, G.J.; Reeves, B.; Bailey, C.C.; Richards, S.M. Cytogenetics and prognosis in childhood lymphoblastic leukaemia: Results of MRC UKALL X. Medical Research Council Working Party in Childhood Leukaemia. *Br. J. Haematol.* **1997**, *99*, 93–100. [CrossRef]
19. Heerema, N.A.; Nachman, J.B.; Sather, H.N.; Sensel, M.G.; Lee, M.K.; Hutchinson, R.; Lange, B.J.; Steinherz, P.G.; Bostrom, B.; Gaynon, P.S.; et al. Hypodiploidy with less than 45 chromosomes confers adverse risk in childhood acute lymphoblastic leukemia: A report from the children's cancer group. *Blood* **1999**, *94*, 4036–4045.
20. Raimondi, S.C.; Zhou, Y.; Mathew, S.; Shurtleff, S.A.; Sandlund, J.T.; Rivera, G.K.; Behm, F.G.; Pui, C.H. Reassessment of the prognostic significance of hypodiploidy in pediatric patients with acute lymphoblastic leukemia. *Cancer* **2003**, *98*, 2715–2722. [CrossRef] [PubMed]
21. Harrison, C.J.; Moorman, A.V.; Broadfield, Z.J.; Cheung, K.L.; Harris, R.L.; Reza Jalali, G.; Robinson, H.M.; Barber, K.E.; Richards, S.M.; Mitchell, C.D.; et al. Three distinct subgroups of hypodiploidy in acute lymphoblastic leukaemia. *Br. J. Haematol.* **2004**, *125*, 552–559. [CrossRef]
22. Nachman, J.B.; Heerema, N.A.; Sather, H.; Camitta, B.; Forestier, E.; Harrison, C.J.; Dastugue, N.; Schrappe, M.; Pui, C.H.; Basso, G.; et al. Outcome of treatment in children with hypodiploid acute lymphoblastic leukemia. *Blood* **2007**, *110*, 1112–1115. [CrossRef] [PubMed]
23. Mullighan, C.G.; Jeha, S.; Pei, D.; Payne-Turner, D.; Coustan-Smith, E.; Roberts, K.G.; Waanders, E.; Choi, J.K.; Ma, X.; Raimondi, S.C.; et al. Outcome of children with hypodiploid ALL treated with risk-directed therapy based on MRD levels. *Blood* **2015**, *126*, 2896–2899. [CrossRef]
24. Pui, C.H.; Rebora, P.; Schrappe, M.; Attarbaschi, A.; Baruchel, A.; Basso, G.; Cave, H.; Elitzur, S.; Koh, K.; Liu, H.C.; et al. Outcome of Children With Hypodiploid Acute Lymphoblastic Leukemia: A Retrospective Multinational Study. *J. Clin. Oncol.* **2019**, *37*, 770–779. [CrossRef]
25. Ishimaru, S.; Okamoto, Y.; Imai, C.; Sakaguchi, H.; Taki, T.; Hasegawa, D.; Cho, Y.; Kakuda, H.; Sano, H.; Manabe, A.; et al. Nationwide survey of pediatric hypodiploid acute lymphoblastic leukemia in Japan. *Pediatr. Int.* **2019**, *61*, 1103–1108. [CrossRef] [PubMed]
26. McNeer, J.L.; Devidas, M.; Dai, Y.; Carroll, A.J.; Heerema, N.A.; Gastier-Foster, J.M.; Kahwash, S.B.; Borowitz, M.J.; Wood, B.L.; Larsen, E.; et al. Hematopoietic Stem-Cell Transplantation Does Not Improve the Poor Outcome of Children With Hypodiploid Acute Lymphoblastic Leukemia: A Report From Children's Oncology Group. *J. Clin. Oncol.* **2019**, *37*, 780–789. [CrossRef] [PubMed]
27. Safavi, S.; Paulsson, K. Near-haploid and low-hypodiploid acute lymphoblastic leukemia: Two distinct subtypes with consistently poor prognosis. *Blood* **2017**, *129*, 420–423. [CrossRef]
28. Gibbons, B.; MacCallum, P.; Watts, E.; Rohatiner, A.Z.; Webb, D.; Katz, F.E.; Secker-Walker, L.M.; Temperley, I.J.; Harrison, C.J.; Campbell, R.H.; et al. Near haploid acute lymphoblastic leukemia: Seven new cases and a review of the literature. *Leukemia* **1991**, *5*, 738–743. [PubMed]
29. Moorman, A.V. The clinical relevance of chromosomal and genomic abnormalities in B-cell precursor acute lymphoblastic leukaemia. *Blood Rev.* **2012**, *26*, 123–135. [CrossRef]
30. Holmfeldt, L.; Wei, L.; Diaz-Flores, E.; Walsh, M.; Zhang, J.; Ding, L.; Payne-Turner, D.; Churchman, M.; Andersson, A.; Chen, S.C.; et al. The genomic landscape of hypodiploid acute lymphoblastic leukemia. *Nat. Genet.* **2013**, *45*, 242–252. [CrossRef]
31. Groupe Francais de Cytogenetique Hematologique. Cytogenetic abnormalities in adult acute lymphoblastic leukemia: Correlations with hematologic findings outcome. A Collaborative Study of the Group Francais de Cytogenetique Hematologique. *Blood* **1996**, *87*, 3135–3142.
32. Moorman, A.V.; Harrison, C.J.; Buck, G.A.; Richards, S.M.; Secker-Walker, L.M.; Martineau, M.; Vance, G.H.; Cherry, A.M.; Higgins, R.R.; Fielding, A.K.; et al. Karyotype is an independent prognostic factor in adult acute lymphoblastic leukemia (ALL): Analysis of cytogenetic data from patients treated on the Medical Research Council (MRC) UKALLXII/Eastern Cooperative Oncology Group (ECOG) 2993 trial. *Blood* **2007**, *109*, 3189–3197. [CrossRef]
33. Pui, C.H.; Howard, S.C. Current management and challenges of malignant disease in the CNS in paediatric leukaemia. *Lancet. Oncol.* **2008**, *9*, 257–268. [CrossRef]
34. McGowan-Jordan, J.; Hastings, R.J.; Moore, S. *An International System for Human Cytogenomic Nomenclature (ISCN 2020)*; Karger: Basel, Switzerland, 2020; ISBN 978-3-318-06706-4.
35. Ribera, J.; Granada, I.; Morgades, M.; Vives, S.; Genesca, E.; Gonzalez, C.; Nomdedeu, J.; Escoda, L.; Montesinos, P.; Mercadal, S.; et al. The poor prognosis of low hypodiploidy in adults with B-cell precursor acute lymphoblastic leukaemia is restricted to older adults and elderly patients. *Br. J. Haematol.* **2019**, *186*, 263–268. [CrossRef]
36. Mitelman, F.; Johansson, B.; Mertens, F. Mitelman Database of Chromosome Aberrations and Gene Fusions in Cancer. 2021. Available online: https://www.clinicalgenetics.lu.se/division-clinical-genetics/database-chromosome-aberrations-and-gene-fusions-cancer (accessed on 5 November 2021).
37. Safavi, S.; Forestier, E.; Golovleva, I.; Barbany, G.; Nord, K.H.; Moorman, A.V.; Harrison, C.J.; Johansson, B.; Paulsson, K. Loss of chromosomes is the primary event in near-haploid and low-hypodiploid acute lymphoblastic leukemia. *Leukemia* **2013**, *27*, 248–250. [CrossRef]

38. Muhlbacher, V.; Zenger, M.; Schnittger, S.; Weissmann, S.; Kunze, F.; Kohlmann, A.; Bellos, F.; Kern, W.; Haferlach, T.; Haferlach, C. Acute lymphoblastic leukemia with low hypodiploid/near triploid karyotype is a specific clinical entity and exhibits a very high TP53 mutation frequency of 93%. *Genes Chromosomes Cancer* **2014**, *53*, 524–536. [CrossRef]
39. Creasey, T.; Enshaei, A.; Nebral, K.; Schwab, C.; Watts, K.; Cuthbert, G.; Vora, A.; Moppett, J.; Harrison, C.J.; Fielding, A.K.; et al. Single nucleotide polymorphism array-based signature of low hypodiploidy in acute lymphoblastic leukemia. *Genes Chromosomes Cancer* **2021**, *60*, 604–615. [CrossRef] [PubMed]
40. Charrin, C.; Thomas, X.; Ffrench, M.; Le, Q.H.; Andrieux, J.; Mozziconacci, M.J.; Lai, J.L.; Bilhou-Nabera, C.; Michaux, L.; Bernheim, A.; et al. A report from the LALA-94 and LALA-SA groups on hypodiploidy with 30 to 39 chromosomes and near-triploidy: 2 possible expressions of a sole entity conferring poor prognosis in adult acute lymphoblastic leukemia (ALL). *Blood* **2004**, *104*, 2444–2451. [CrossRef] [PubMed]
41. Carroll, A.J.; Shago, M.; Mikhail, F.M.; Raimondi, S.C.; Hirsch, B.A.; Loh, M.L.; Raetz, E.A.; Borowitz, M.J.; Wood, B.L.; Maloney, K.W.; et al. Masked hypodiploidy: Hypodiploid acute lymphoblastic leukemia (ALL) mimicking hyperdiploid ALL in children: A report from the Children's Oncology Group. *Cancer Genet.* **2019**, *238*, 62–68. [CrossRef]
42. Paietta, E.; Roberts, K.G.; Wang, V.; Gu, Z.; Buck, G.A.N.; Pei, D.; Cheng, C.; Levine, R.L.; Abdel-Wahab, O.; Cheng, Z.; et al. Molecular classification improves risk assessment in adult BCR-ABL1-negative B-ALL. *Blood* **2021**, *138*, 948–958. [CrossRef]
43. Harrison, C.J.; Moorman, A.V.; Barber, K.E.; Broadfield, Z.J.; Cheung, K.L.; Harris, R.L.; Jalali, G.R.; Robinson, H.M.; Strefford, J.C.; Stewart, A.; et al. Interphase molecular cytogenetic screening for chromosomal abnormalities of prognostic significance in childhood acute lymphoblastic leukaemia: A UK Cancer Cytogenetics Group Study. *Br. J. Haematol.* **2005**, *129*, 520–530. [CrossRef]
44. Stark, B.; Jeison, M.; Gobuzov, R.; Krug, H.; Glaser-Gabay, L.; Luria, D.; El-Hasid, R.; Harush, M.B.; Avrahami, G.; Fisher, S.; et al. Near haploid childhood acute lymphoblastic leukemia masked by hyperdiploid line: Detection by fluorescence in situ hybridization. *Cancer Genet. Cytogenet.* **2001**, *128*, 108–113. [CrossRef]
45. Kohno, S.; Minowada, J.; Sandberg, A.A. Chromosome evolution of near-haploid clones in an established human acute lymphoblastic leukemia cell line (NALM-16). *J. Natl. Cancer Inst.* **1980**, *64*, 485–493. [PubMed]
46. Aburawi, H.E.; Biloglav, A.; Johansson, B.; Paulsson, K. Cytogenetic and molecular genetic characterization of the 'high hyperdiploid' B-cell precursor acute lymphoblastic leukaemia cell line MHH-CALL-2 reveals a near-haploid origin. *Br. J. Haematol.* **2011**, *154*, 275–277. [CrossRef] [PubMed]
47. Edgar, B.A.; Zielke, N.; Gutierrez, C. Endocycles: A recurrent evolutionary innovation for post-mitotic cell growth. *Nat. Rev. Mol. Cell Biol.* **2014**, *15*, 197–210. [CrossRef]
48. Shu, Z.; Row, S.; Deng, W.M. Endoreplication: The Good, the Bad, and the Ugly. *Trends Cell Biol.* **2018**, *28*, 465–474. [CrossRef]
49. Bielski, C.M.; Zehir, A.; Penson, A.V.; Donoghue, M.T.A.; Chatila, W.; Armenia, J.; Chang, M.T.; Schram, A.M.; Jonsson, P.; Bandlamudi, C.; et al. Genome doubling shapes the evolution and prognosis of advanced cancers. *Nat. Genet.* **2018**, *50*, 1189–1195. [CrossRef]
50. Storchova, Z.; Kuffer, C. The consequences of tetraploidy and aneuploidy. *J. Cell Sci.* **2008**, *121*, 3859–3866. [CrossRef] [PubMed]
51. Safavi, S.; Olsson, L.; Biloglav, A.; Veerla, S.; Blendberg, M.; Tayebwa, J.; Behrendtz, M.; Castor, A.; Hansson, M.; Johansson, B.; et al. Genetic and epigenetic characterization of hypodiploid acute lymphoblastic leukemia. *Oncotarget* **2015**, *6*, 42793–42802. [CrossRef]
52. Agraz-Doblas, A.; Bueno, C.; Bashford-Rogers, R.; Roy, A.; Schneider, P.; Bardini, M.; Ballerini, P.; Cazzaniga, G.; Moreno, T.; Revilla, C.; et al. Unravelling the cellular origin and clinical prognostic markers of infant B-cell acute lymphoblastic leukemia using genome-wide analysis. *Haematologica* **2019**, *104*, 1176–1188. [CrossRef]
53. Ueno, H.; Yoshida, K.; Shiozawa, Y.; Nannya, Y.; Iijima-Yamashita, Y.; Kiyokawa, N.; Shiraishi, Y.; Chiba, K.; Tanaka, H.; Isobe, T.; et al. Landscape of driver mutations and their clinical impacts in pediatric B-cell precursor acute lymphoblastic leukemia. *Blood Adv.* **2020**, *4*, 5165–5173. [CrossRef]
54. Mullighan, C.G.; Zhang, J.; Kasper, L.H.; Lerach, S.; Payne-Turner, D.; Phillips, L.A.; Heatley, S.L.; Holmfeldt, L.; Collins-Underwood, J.R.; Ma, J.; et al. CREBBP mutations in relapsed acute lymphoblastic leukaemia. *Nature* **2011**, *471*, 235–239. [CrossRef] [PubMed]
55. Stengel, A.; Schnittger, S.; Weissmann, S.; Kuznia, S.; Kern, W.; Kohlmann, A.; Haferlach, T.; Haferlach, C. TP53 mutations occur in 15.7% of ALL and are associated with MYC-rearrangement, low hypodiploidy, and a poor prognosis. *Blood* **2014**, *124*, 251–258. [CrossRef]
56. Moorman, A.V. Does TP53 guard ALL genomes? *Blood* **2014**, *124*, 160–161. [CrossRef] [PubMed]
57. Miller, L.; Kobayashi, S.; Pauly, M.; Lew, G.; Saxe, D.; Keller, F.; Qayed, M.; Castellino, S. Evaluating approaches to enhance survival in children with hypodiploid acute lymphoblastic leukaemia (ALL). *Br. J. Haematol.* **2019**, *185*, 613–616. [CrossRef]
58. Comeaux, E.Q.; Mullighan, C.G. TP53 Mutations in Hypodiploid Acute Lymphoblastic Leukemia. *Cold Spring Harb. Perspect. Med.* **2017**, *7*, a026286. [CrossRef]
59. Lafage-Pochitaloff, M.; Baranger, L.; Hunault, M.; Cuccuini, W.; Lefebvre, C.; Bidet, A.; Tigaud, I.; Eclache, V.; Delabesse, E.; Bilhou-Nabera, C.; et al. Impact of cytogenetic abnormalities in adults with Ph-negative B-cell precursor acute lymphoblastic leukemia. *Blood* **2017**, *130*, 1832–1844. [CrossRef] [PubMed]
60. Paulsson, K.; Lilljebjorn, H.; Biloglav, A.; Olsson, L.; Rissler, M.; Castor, A.; Barbany, G.; Fogelstrand, L.; Nordgren, A.; Sjogren, H.; et al. The genomic landscape of high hyperdiploid childhood acute lymphoblastic leukemia. *Nat. Genet.* **2015**, *47*, 672–676. [CrossRef]

61. Paulsson, K. High hyperdiploid childhood acute lymphoblastic leukemia: Chromosomal gains as the main driver event. *Mol. Cell. Oncol.* **2016**, *3*, e1064555. [CrossRef]
62. Mandahl, N.; Johansson, B.; Mertens, F.; Mitelman, F. Disease-associated patterns of disomic chromosomes in hyperhaploid neoplasms. *Genes Chromosomes Cancer* **2012**, *51*, 536–544. [CrossRef] [PubMed]
63. Molina, O. (Josep Carreras Leukemia Research Institute, Barcelona, Spain). High-resolution confocal microscopy analyses of mitotic progression using PDX samples derived from near-haploid and low-hypodiploid B-ALL. 2021; material not intended for publication.
64. Gruhn, B.; Taub, J.W.; Ge, Y.; Beck, J.F.; Zell, R.; Hafer, R.; Hermann, F.H.; Debatin, K.M.; Steinbach, D. Prenatal origin of childhood acute lymphoblastic leukemia, association with birth weight and hyperdiploidy. *Leukemia* **2008**, *22*, 1692–1697. [CrossRef]
65. Greaves, M. A causal mechanism for childhood acute lymphoblastic leukaemia. *Nat. Rev. Cancer* **2018**, *18*, 471–484. [CrossRef]
66. Schultz, K.R.; Devidas, M.; Bowman, W.P.; Aledo, A.; Slayton, W.B.; Sather, H.; Zheng, H.W.; Davies, S.M.; Gaynon, P.S.; Trigg, M.; et al. Philadelphia chromosome-negative very high-risk acute lymphoblastic leukemia in children and adolescents: Results from Children's Oncology Group Study AALL0031. *Leukemia* **2014**, *28*, 964–967. [CrossRef] [PubMed]
67. Mehta, P.A.; Zhang, M.J.; Eapen, M.; He, W.; Seber, A.; Gibson, B.; Camitta, B.M.; Kitko, C.L.; Dvorak, C.C.; Nemecek, E.R.; et al. Transplantation Outcomes for Children with Hypodiploid Acute Lymphoblastic Leukemia. *Biol. Blood Marrow Transplant.* **2015**, *21*, 1273–1277. [CrossRef]
68. Groeneveld-Krentz, S.; Schroeder, M.P.; Reiter, M.; Pogodzinski, M.J.; Pimentel-Gutierrez, H.J.; Vagkopoulou, R.; Hof, J.; Chen-Santel, C.; Nebral, K.; Bradtke, J.; et al. Aneuploidy in children with relapsed B-cell precursor acute lymphoblastic leukaemia: Clinical importance of detecting a hypodiploid origin of relapse. *Br. J. Haematol.* **2019**, *185*, 266–283. [CrossRef] [PubMed]
69. Shetty, D.; Amare, P.K.; Mohanty, P.; Talker, E.; Chaubal, K.; Jain, H.; Tembhare, P.; Patkar, N.; Chaturvedi, A.; Subramanian, P.G.; et al. Investigating the clinical, hematological and cytogenetic profile of endoreduplicated hypodiploids in BCP-ALL. *Blood Cells Mol. Dis.* **2020**, *85*, 102465. [CrossRef]
70. Winter, G.; Kirschner-Schwabe, R.; Groeneveld-Krentz, S.; Escherich, G.; Moricke, A.; von Stackelberg, A.; Stanulla, M.; Bailey, S.; Richter, L.; Steinemann, D.; et al. Clinical and genetic characteristics of children with acute lymphoblastic leukemia and Li-Fraumeni syndrome. *Leukemia* **2021**, *35*, 1475–1479. [CrossRef]
71. Lee, S.H.R.; Li, Z.; Tai, S.T.; Oh, B.L.Z.; Yeoh, A.E.J. Genetic Alterations in Childhood Acute Lymphoblastic Leukemia: Interactions with Clinical Features and Treatment Response. *Cancers* **2021**, *13*, 4068. [CrossRef] [PubMed]
72. Jeha, S.; Choi, J.; Roberts, K.G.; Pei, D.; Coustan-Smith, E.; Inaba, H.; Rubnitz, J.E.; Ribeiro, R.C.; Gruber, T.A.; Raimondi, S.C.; et al. Clinical significance of novel subtypes of acute lymphoblastic leukemia in the context of minimal residual disease-directed therapy. *Blood Cancer Discov.* **2021**, *2*, 326–337. [CrossRef]
73. Talleur, A.C.; Maude, S.L. What is the role for HSCT or immunotherapy in pediatric hypodiploid B-cell acute lymphoblastic leukemia? *Hematol. Am. Soc. Hematol. Educ. Program* **2020**, *2020*, 508–511. [CrossRef]
74. Ribera, J.M.; Oriol, A.; Morgades, M.; Montesinos, P.; Sarra, J.; Gonzalez-Campos, J.; Brunet, S.; Tormo, M.; Fernandez-Abellan, P.; Guardia, R.; et al. Treatment of high-risk Philadelphia chromosome-negative acute lymphoblastic leukemia in adolescents and adults according to early cytologic response and minimal residual disease after consolidation assessed by flow cytometry: Final results of the PETHEMA ALL-AR-03 trial. *J. Clin. Oncol.* **2014**, *32*, 1595–1604. [CrossRef] [PubMed]
75. Diaz-Flores, E.; Comeaux, E.Q.; Kim, K.L.; Melnik, E.; Beckman, K.; Davis, K.L.; Wu, K.; Akutagawa, J.; Bridges, O.; Marino, R.; et al. Bcl-2 Is a Therapeutic Target for Hypodiploid B-Lineage Acute Lymphoblastic Leukemia. *Cancer Res.* **2019**, *79*, 2339–2351. [CrossRef] [PubMed]
76. Fang, M.; Becker, P.S.; Linenberger, M.; Eaton, K.D.; Appelbaum, F.R.; Dreyer, Z.; Airewele, G.; Redell, M.; Lopez-Terrada, D.; Patel, A.; et al. Adult Low-Hypodiploid Acute B-Lymphoblastic Leukemia With IKZF3 Deletion and TP53 Mutation: Comparison With Pediatric Patients. *Am. J. Clin. Pathol.* **2015**, *144*, 263–270. [CrossRef]
77. Diorio, C.; Maude, S.L. CAR T cells vs allogeneic HSCT for poor-risk ALL. *Hematol. Am. Soc. Hematol. Educ. Program* **2020**, *2020*, 501–507. [CrossRef]
78. Zhao, Y.; Aldoss, I.; Qu, C.; Crawford, J.C.; Gu, Z.; Allen, E.K.; Zamora, A.E.; Alexander, T.B.; Wang, J.; Goto, H.; et al. Tumor-intrinsic and -extrinsic determinants of response to blinatumomab in adults with B-ALL. *Blood* **2021**, *137*, 471–484. [CrossRef]
79. Wang, L.; Ashraf, D.C.; Kinde, B.; Ohgami, R.S.; Kumar, J.; Kersten, R.C. Hypodiploid B-Lymphoblastic Leukemia Presenting as an Isolated Orbital Mass Prior to Systemic Involvement: A Case Report and Review of the Literature. *Diagnostics* **2020**, *11*, 25. [CrossRef] [PubMed]
80. Bhojwani, D.; Sposto, R.; Shah, N.N.; Rodriguez, V.; Yuan, C.; Stetler-Stevenson, M.; O'Brien, M.M.; McNeer, J.L.; Quereshi, A.; Cabannes, A.; et al. Inotuzumab ozogamicin in pediatric patients with relapsed/refractory acute lymphoblastic leukemia. *Leukemia* **2019**, *33*, 884–892. [CrossRef]

MDPI
St. Alban-Anlage 66
4052 Basel
Switzerland
www.mdpi.com

Cancers Editorial Office
E-mail: cancers@mdpi.com
www.mdpi.com/journal/cancers

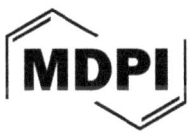

Disclaimer/Publisher's Note: The statements, opinions and data contained in all publications are solely those of the individual author(s) and contributor(s) and not of MDPI and/or the editor(s). MDPI and/or the editor(s) disclaim responsibility for any injury to people or property resulting from any ideas, methods, instructions or products referred to in the content.

www.ingramcontent.com/pod-product-compliance
Lightning Source LLC
LaVergne TN
LVHW070136100526
838202LV00015B/1836